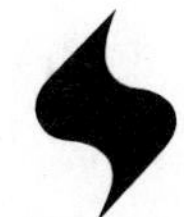

Stedman's

SURGERY WORDS

INCLUDES
ANATOMY,
ANESTHESIA,
& PAIN MANAGEMENT

SECOND EDITION

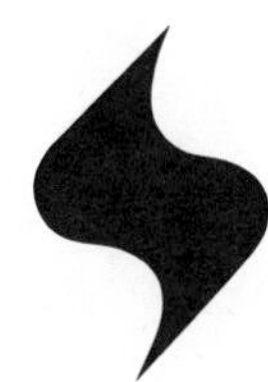

Stedman's

SURGERY WORDS

INCLUDES
ANATOMY,
ANESTHISIA,
& PAIN MANAGEMENT

SECOND EDITION

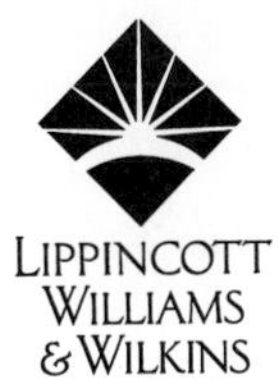

LIPPINCOTT
WILLIAMS
& WILKINS

Publisher: Rhonda M. Kumm, RN, MSN
Senior Manager: Julie K. Stegman
Senior Managing Editor: Nancy S. Wachter
Associate Managing Editor: Trista A. DiPaula
Associate Managing Editor: William A. Howard
Art Program Coordinator: Jennifer Clements
Assistant Production Manager: Kevin Iarossi
Typesetter: Peirce Graphic Services, Inc.
Printer & Binder: Malloy Litho, Inc.

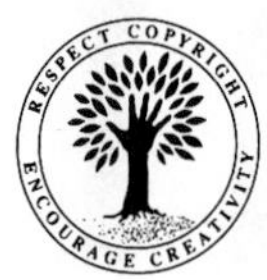

Printed in the United States of America

Second Edition, 2002

Library of Congress Cataloging-in-Publication Data

Stedmans surgery words : includes anatomy, anesthesia & pain management.—2nd ed.
p. cm.
ISBN 0-7817-3831-8 (alk. paper)
1. Surgery—Terminology. I. Title: Surgery words. II. Stedman, Thomas Lathrop, 1853–1938. III. Lippincott Williams & Wilkins.

RD16 .S74 2002
617'.001'4—dc21

2002066124
01
1 2 3 4 5 6 7 8 9 10

Contents

Contents

Acknowledgments

An important part of our editorial process is the involvement of medical transcriptionists—as advisors, reviewers, and/or editors.

We extend special thanks to Jeanne Bock, CSR, MT, and Marty Cantu, CMT, for editing the manuscript, helping resolve many difficult questions, and contributing material for the appendix sections. We are grateful to our MT Editorial Advisory Board members, including Marty Cantu, CMT; Lin Harvell; Nancy Hill, MT; Helen Littrell; Robin Koza; and Wendy Ryan, RHIT, who were instrumental in the development of this reference. They recommended sources and shared their valuable judgment, insight, and perspective.

We also extend thanks to Jeanne Bock, CSR, MT, for working on the appendix. Additional thanks to Helen Littrell for performing the final prepublication review. Other important contributors to this edition include Shemah Fletcher; Nancy Hill, MT; Sandy Kovacs, CMT; Robin Koza; Lin Harvell; Wendy Ryan, RHIT; and Tina Whitecotton, MT.

And, as always, Barb Ferretti played an integral role in the process by reviewing the content files for format, updating the database, and providing a final quality check.

As with all our *Stedman's* word references, this resource incorporates the suggestions and expertise of our many contacts in the medical transcriptionist community. Thanks to all of our advisory board participants, reviewers, and editors; AAMT meeting attendees; and others who have written us with requests and comments—keep talking, and we'll keep listening.

Editor's Preface

At the start of my career as a medical transcriptionist, I had the good fortune to work for a wonderful woman, the supervisor for a local office of a major transcription service. During my training, she told me of her passion for operative reports. I still remember her words . . . When I'm transcribing an operative report, Jeanne, I feel as though I am in the operating room, standing alongside the surgeon, with my gloved hands inside the patient. What a perfect description for the experience we have, as medical transcriptionists transcribing operative reports! We are present in the operating room with the surgeon, and the steps of the operation come alive for us as we transcribe the words dictated, forming them into an integral part of the patient's permanent medical record.

That being said, let's consider the medical field of surgery. There have been dramatic changes in surgery through the years. Once was the time when the answer to any ailment was bleeding a patient, and many succumbed in the process of receiving this "cure." During the Revolutionary War, soldiers most often died of infection, the all-too-common complication resulting from the surgery undertaken in an effort to save their lives. Thankfully, we have moved far beyond those scenarios, and many an illness once deemed a death sentence is now curable through surgery, making the need for a complete surgical word book all the more essential.

The most challenging aspects of surgery dictation involve anatomical references, surgical procedures, and equipment terminology. This new edition contains the names of numerous surgical procedures and the terminology used in describing those procedures. For a complete listing of equipment, you will find *Stedman's Equipment Words, Third Edition,* an invaluable tool and companion book to *Stedman's Surgery Words, Second Edition.*

I am very excited that we have enhanced this book by including a compilation of pain management terminology, anatomical illustrations depicting surgical positions and surgical block applications, as well as a variety of sample pain treatment procedures, including trigger point injections, epidural steroid injections, and an intrathecal pump implantation.

Next time you prepare to enter the operating room for a day of surgical procedure transcription, don't enter without *Stedman's Surgery Words, Second Edition,* and *Stedman's Equipment Words, Third Edition,* within easy reach. These reference tools are as essential to an MT as sterile preparation, draping, and a scalpel are to a surgeon.

My thanks go to Marty Cantu, CMT, for working with me on this project. As always, I extend my heartfelt thanks and appreciation to Barb Ferretti, our superb database editor.

Jeanne Bock, CSR, MT

Publisher's Preface

Stedman's Surgery Words, Second Edition, offers an authoritative assurance of quality and exactness to the wordsmiths of the healthcare professions—medical transcriptionists, medical editors and copyeditors, health information management personnel, court reporters, and the many other users and producers of medical documentation.

We have received many requests for updates to *Stedman's Surgery Words.* As a result, we have published this new edition that includes surgical, anatomical, anesthesia, and pain management terminology. In this new edition, we have opted to omit equipment terminology. You will find *Stedman's Equipment Words, Third Edition* to be an excellent companion source for verifying equipment terminology.

In *Stedman's Surgery Words, Second Edition,* users will find thousands of words as they relate to the specialties of surgery, gross anatomy, anesthesia, and pain management. Users will also find terms for protocols, diagnostic and therapeutic procedures, new techniques, lab tests, clinical research terms, as well as abbreviations with their expansions. The appendix sections provide anatomical illustrations with useful captions and labels, sample reports, common terms by procedure, a pain glossary, pain management techniques, an explanation of dermatomes, American Academy of Pain Management (AAPM)-accredited pain programs, drugs commonly used in pain practice, drugs used for anesthesia, and drugs by indication.

This compilation of more than 100,000 entries, fully cross-indexed for quick access, was built from a base vocabulary of approximately 66,000 medical words, phrases, abbreviations, and acronyms. The extensive A-Z list was developed from the database of *Stedman's Medical Dictionary, 27th Edition,* and supplemented by terminology found in current medical literature (see References on page xvi).

We at Lippincott Williams & Wilkins strive to provide you with the most up-to-date and accurate word references available. Your use of this word book will prompt new editions, which we will publish as often as updates and revisions justify. We welcome your suggestions for improvements, changes, corrections, and additions—whatever will make this *Stedman's* product more useful to you. Please complete the postpaid card at the back of this book, and send your recommendations care of "Stedman's" at Lippincott Williams & Wilkins.

Explanatory Notes

Medical transcription is an art as well as a science. Both approaches are needed to correctly interpret the dictation of a physician, whose language is a product of education, training, and experience. This variety in medical language means that there are several acceptable ways to express certain terms, including jargon. *Stedman's Surgery Words, Second Edition,* provides variant spellings and phrasings for many terms. These elements, in addition to complete cross-indexing, make *Stedman's Surgery Words, Second Edition,* a valuable resource for determining the validity of terms as they are encountered.

Alphabetical Organization

Alphabetization of main entries is letter by letter as spelled, ignoring punctuation, spaces, prefixed numbers, or other characters. For example:

Coats white ring
cobalt-60 moving strip technique
cobalt therapy

Terms beginning or ending with Greek letters show the Greek letters spelled out and listed alphabetically. For example:

alpha, α
a. adrenoreceptor

In subentry alphabetization, the abbreviated singular form or the spelled-out plural form of the noun main entry word is ignored.

Format and Style

All main entries are in **boldface** to expedite locating a sought-after term, to enhance distinction between main entries and subentries, and to relieve the textual density of the pages.

Irregular plurals and variant spellings are shown on the same line as the singular or preferred form of the word. For example:

dorsum, pl. **dorsa**
hypophysial, hypophyseal

Hyphenation

As a rule of style, multiple eponyms (e.g., Mears-Rubash approach) are hyphenated. Also, hyphens have been added between a manufacturer and one or more eponyms (e.g., Vital-Metzenbaum dissecting scissors). Please note that in many cases, hyphenation is a question of style, not of accuracy, and thus is a matter of choice.

Possessives

Possessive forms have been dropped in this reference for the sake of consistency and conformance with the guidelines of the American Association for Medical Transcription (AAMT) and other groups. Please note, however, that in many cases, retaining the possessive, like hyphenating, is a question of style, not of accuracy, and thus is a matter of choice. To form the possessive of a word, simply add the apostrophe or apostrophe "s" to the end of the word.

Cross-indexing

The word list is in an index-like main entry-subentry format that contains two combined alphabetical listings:

(1) A *noun* main entry-subentry organization, which is typical of the A-Z section of medical dictionaries like *Stedman's:*

lymphocyte
B phenotypic l.
l. cell
l. migration

osteotomy
Simmons o.
o. site
sliding oblique o.

(2) An *adjective* main entry-subentry organization, which lists words and phrases as you hear them. The main entries are the adjectives or modifiers in a multiword term. The subentries are the nouns around which the terms are constructed and to which the adjectives or modifiers pertain:

alveolar
a. adenoma
a. artery
a. body

interrupted
i. aortic arch
i. respiration
i. suture technique

This format provides the user with more than one way to locate and identify a multiword term. For example:

syndrome
vibration s.

vibration
v. syndrome

tricuspid
t. valve annuloplasty

annuloplasty
tricuspid valve a.

It also allows the user to see together all terms that contain a particular descriptor, as well as all types, kinds, or variations of a noun entity. For example:

trigeminal
t. cave
t. cavity
t. decompression.

wall
orbital w.
posterior oropharyngeal w.
w. push maneuver

Wherever possible, abbreviations are separately defined and cross-referenced. For example:

LNP
laparoscopic Nissen fundoplication

laparoscopic
l. Nissen fundoplication (LNP)

fundoplication
laparoscopic Nissen f. (LNP)

References

In addition to the manufacturers' literature we gather at various medical meetings, scientific reports from hospitals, and the lists of our MT Editorial Advisory Board members (from their daily transcription work), we used the following sources for new terms in *Stedman's Surgery Words, Second Edition.*

Books

Abram SE, Haddox JD. The Pain Clinic Manual, 2nd Edition. Philadelphia: Lippincott Williams & Wilkins, 2000.

Ballantyne J. The Massachusetts General Handbook of Pain Management, 2nd Edition. Philadelphia: Lippincott Williams & Wilkins, 2002.

Barash PG, Cullen BF, Stoelting RK. Clinical Anesthesia, 4th Edition. Philadelphia: Lippincott Williams & Wilkins, 2000.

Drake E. Sloane's Medical Word Book, 4th Edition. Philadelphia: Saunders, 2001.

General Surgery/GI Words and Phrases. Modesto, CA: Health Professions Institute, 2001.

Greenfield LJ, Mulholland MW, Oldham KT, Zelenock GB, Lilemoe KD. Surgery: Scientific Principles and Practice, 3rd Edition. Philadelphia: Lippincott Williams & Wilkins, 2001.

Hiatt JL, Gartner LP. Textbook of Head and Neck Anatomy, 3rd Edition. Philadelphia: Lippincott Williams & Wilkins, 2000.

Hollinshead WH. Anatomy for Surgeons, The Head and Neck, 3rd Edition. Philadelphia: Lippincott Williams & Wilkins, 1982.

Lance LL. Quick Look Drug Book 2002. Baltimore: Lippincott Williams & Wilkins, 2002.

Lawrence PF. Essentials of General Surgery, 3rd Edition. Philadelphia: Lippincott Williams & Wilkins, 1999.

Loeser JD, Butler SH, Chapman CR, Turk DC. Bonica's Management of Pain, 3rd Edition. Philadelphia: Lippincott Williams & Wilkins, 2000.

McCaffery M, Pasero C. Pain Clinic Manual, 2nd Edition. Philadelphia: Saunders, 1999.

Olson T. A.D.A.M. Student Atlas of Anatomy. Philadelphia: Lippincott Williams & Wilkins, 1996.

Schwartz SI, Shires GT, Spencer FC, Galloway AC. Principles of Surgery, 7th Edition. Columbus: McGraw-Hill, 1998.

Stedman's Medical Dictionary, 27th Edition. Baltimore: Lippincott Williams & Wilkins, 2000.

Stedman's Surgery Words. Baltimore: Lippincott Williams & Wilkins, 1998.

Tessier C. The AAMT Book of Style. Modesto, CA: AAMT, 1995.

Tessier C. The Surgical Word Book, 2nd Edition. Philadelphia: Saunders, 1991.

Vera Pyle's Current Medical Terminology, 8th Edition. Modesto, CA: Health Professions Institute, 2000.

Journals

Anesthesia & Analgesia. Baltimore: Lippincott Williams & Wilkins, 2001.

Anesthesiology. Baltimore: Lippincott Williams & Wilkins, 2001.

Annals of Surgery. Baltimore: Lippincott Williams & Wilkins, 1999–2001.

Clinical Journal of Pain. Baltimore: Lippincott Williams & Wilkins, 1999–2001.

Computer Aided Surgery. New York: John Wiley & Sons, Inc., 1997–2000.

Journal of the American College of Surgeons. New York: Elsevier Science, 1997–2001.

Laparoscopic Update. Baltimore: Lippincott Williams & Wilkins, 1998–2001.

Latest Word. Philadelphia: Saunders, 1999–2001.

Surgical Laparoscopy Endoscopy & Percutaneous Techniques. Baltimore: Lippincott Williams & Wilkins, 1999–2001.

Topics in Pain Management. Baltimore: Lippincott Williams & Wilkins, 2001.

CD

Lippincott's Interactive Anesthesia Library v3.0. Philadelphia: Lippincott Williams & Wilkins, 2001.

Websites

http://carecure.rutgers.edu/spinewire/Articles/SpinalLevels.html

http://my.webmd.com/index

http://surgery.medscape.com/Home/Topics/surgery/surgery.html

http://www.aapainmange.org

http://www.anesthesiology.org

http://www.asahq.org

http://www.aspmn.org

http://www.centerwatch.com

http://www.facs.org

http://www.gasnet.com

http://www.hpisum.com

http://www.jnjgateway.com

http://www.laparoscopy.com

http://www.lapsurgery.com

http://www.mtdaily.com

http://www.mtdesk.com

http://www.mtmonthly.com

http://www.pain.com

http://www.sls.org

http://www.theasgs.org

http://www.ussurg.com

A

AA
anterior apical
AA segment
AAA
abdominal aortic aneurysm
AAC
acute acalculous cholecystitis
AACLR
arthroscopic anterior cruciate ligament reconstruction
AANA
American Association of Nurse Anesthetists
AAST
American Association for the Surgery of Trauma
AB
anterior basal
AB segment
ab
ab externo filtering operation
ab externo incision
ab interno incision
ABA
American Board of Anesthesiology
Abbe
A. flap
A. operation
A. vaginal construction
Abbe-Estlander operation
Abbe-McIndoe
A.-M. procedure
A.-M. vaginal reconstruction
Abbe-McIndoe-Williams procedure
Abbe-Wharton-McIndoe procedure
Abbott
A. esophagogastroscopy
A. esophagogastrostomy
A. knee approach
A. method
Abbott-Carpenter posterior approach
Abbott-Gill
A.-G. epiphysial plate exposure
A.-G. osteotomy
Abbott-Lucas shoulder operation
Abbreviated Injury Scale (AIS)
ABC
airway, breathing, and circulation
abdomen
accordion a.
acute surgical a.
apertures of a.
boatlike a.
boat-shaped a.
carinate a.
concave a.
diffusely tender a.
distended a.
doughy a.
dull to percussion a.
exquisitely tender a.
fascia of a.
flabby a.
flat a.
hostile a.
hyperdistended a.
hyperresonant a.
navicular a.
nondistended a.
pendulous a.
postlymphangiography a.
postsurgical a.
protuberant a.
prune-belly a.
resonant a.
scaphoid a.
soft a.
splinting of a.
stiff a.
surgical a.
tympanitic a.
abdominal
a. abscess
a. adhesiolysis
a. adipose tissue
a. agitation
a. air collection
a. angina
a. angiography
a. aorta
a. aortic aneurysm (AAA)
a. aortic artery
a. aortic plexus
a. aponeurosis
a. approach
a. apron
a. brace position
a. canal
a. cardiac reflex
a. cavity
a. colectomy
a. colic
a. compartment syndrome
a. complication
a. content
a. cramp
a. distention
a. domain
a. drainage
a. evisceration

abdominal *(continued)*
a. examination
a. exploration
a. external oblique muscle
a. fasciocutaneous flap
a. fat
a. fat pad
a. film
a. fissure
a. fluid collection
a. fluid wave
a. girth
a. guarding
a. gunshot wound
a. gutter
a. hemorrhage
a. hydatid disease
a. hysterectomy
a. hysteropexy
a. hysterotomy
a. imaging
a. impalement
a. incisional hernia
a. incision dehiscence
a. internal oblique muscle
a. iron deposition
a. irradiation
a. kidney
a. lavage
a. lipectomy
a. lymph node biopsy
a. malignancy
a. midline incisional hernioplasty
a. migraine
a. muscle deficiency syndrome
a. myomectomy
a. nephrectomy
a. ostium
a. panniculus
a. paracentesis
a. peritoneum
a. pool
a. pregnancy
a. pressure
a. pressure technique
a. procedure
a. proctocolectomy
a. pull-through
a. pulse
a. rectopexy
a. reflux
a. region
a. respiration
a. respiratory motion
a. rigidity
a. ring
a. sac
a. sacropexy
a. salpingo-oophorectomy
a. salpingotomy
a. section
a. space
a. splenectomy
a. stoma
a. stool
a. structure
a. tap
a. tenderness
A. Trauma Index (ATI)
a. tumor
a. vascular accident
a. view
a. viscus
a. volume
a. wall closure
a. wall fistula
a. wall hernia
a. wall incision
a. wall lifting
a. wall mass
a. wall mobility
a. wall rhabdomyosarcoma
a. wall venous pattern
a. wound closure
a. x-ray (AXR)
a. zone

abdominalis
abdominal-perineal resection
abdominal-sacral colpoperineopexy
abdominis
abdominocentesis
abdominocystic
abdominogenital
abdominohysterectomy
abdominohysterotomy
abdominoinguinal incision
abdominojugular reflux
abdominopelvic
a. abscess
a. cavity
a. irradiation
a. mass
a. splanchnic nerve
a. viscus

abdominoperineal
a. excision
a. proctectomy
a. resection (APR)

abdominoplasty
abdominosacral resection
abdominoscopy
abdominoscrotal
abdominothoracic
a. arch
a. incision

abdominovaginal hysterectomy

abdominovesical
abducens nerve
abducent
abduction
a. deformity
a. external rotation test
a. osteotomy
a. traction technique
abduction-external
a.-e. rotation
a.-e. rotation fracture
abductor
a. digiti minimi muscle
a. digiti minimi opponensplasty
a. digiti quinti opponensplasty
a. hallucis muscle
a. longus muscle
a. magnus muscle
a. osteotomy
a. pollicis brevis muscle
a. pollicis longus muscle
a. pollicis longus tendon
abductorplasty
flexor pollicis longus a.
Smith flexor pollicis longus a.
abductory wedge osteotomy
Abell-Kendall method
Abell method
Aberdeen knot
Abernethy
A. fascia
A. operation
A. sarcoma
aberrancy
acceleration-dependent a.
aberrant
a. bile duct
a. bronchial origin
a. ductule
a. ganglion
a. goiter
a. obturator artery
a. obturator vein
a. pancreas
a. regeneration
a. third nerve degeneration
a. tissue
a. umbilical stomach
a. vessel
aberrantes
aberration
angle of a.
chromatic lens a.
color a.
coma a.
curvature a.
dioptric a.
distantial a.
distortion a.
intraventricular a.
lateral a.
lens a.
longitudinal a.
meridional a.
monochromatic a.
newtonian a.
oblique a.
optical a.
regeneration a.
sexual a.
spherical lens a.
ventricular a.
ability
tumor-targeting a.
ablate
ablation
accessory conduction a.
adrenal a.
androgen a.
atrioventricular junctional a.
carbon dioxide laser plaque a.
catheter a.
celiac alcohol a.
cold forceps a.
cold snare a.
Concept a.
continuous-wave laser a.
coronary rotational a.
cryogenic a.
cryosurgical a.
dioiodine a.
direct-current shock a.
electrical catheter a.
endometrial a.
endoscopic mucosal a.
ethanol a.
fast-pathway radiofrequency a.
His bundle a.
homogeneous a.
Kent bundle a.
laparoscopic uterine nerve a.
laser uterosacral nerve a.
liver wire TC a.
marrow a.

NOTES

ablation *(continued)*
mucosal a.
Nd:YAG laser a.
needle a.
neoadjuvant total androgen a.
nerve rootlet a.
organ a.
ovarian a.
panretinal a.
parathyroid tumor a.
percutaneous ethanol a.
percutaneous radical cryosurgical a.
percutaneous radiofrequency catheter a.
percutaneous tumor a.
peripheral panretinal a.
photothermal laser a.
pituitary a.
pulsed laser a.
radiofrequency catheter a. (RFCA)
radiofrequency thermal a. (RFTA)
radioiodine a.
rectoscopic endometrial a.
renal cyst a.
rollerball endometrial a.
rotational a.
slow-pathway a.
stereotactic surgical a.
surgical a.
surgical estrogen a.
a. therapy
thermal a.
thyroid nodule a.
tissue a.
toric a.
transcatheter a.
transurethral needle a.
tumor a.
valve a.
visual laser a.

ablative
a. cardiac surgery
a. laser angioplasty
a. laser therapy
a. procedure
a. technique

ABMT
autologous bone marrow transplantation

ABMTR
Autologous Bone Marrow Transplant Registry

abnormal
a. bleeding
a. clotting
a. cytology
a. fetal urogenital tract
a. mammogram
a. parathyroid gland
a. preoperative localization signal

abnormality, pl. **abnormalities**
anatomic a.
bleeding a.
caliceal a.
clotting a.
cytologic a.
dislocation contour a.
diverticulation a.
DNA ploidy a.
electrical activation a.
electrolyte a.
extremity a.
genetic a.
ictal a.
limb reduction a.
mammographic a.
migration a.
mucosal a.
nondermatomal sensory a. (NDSA)
nonpalpable mammographic a.
oral cavity a.
persistent breast a.
pulmonary vascular a.
regional wall motion a. (RWMA)
renal a.
reproductive tract a.
rostrocaudal extent signal a.
segmental wall motion a. (SWMA)
skeletal a.
small bowel congenital a.
soft-tissue a.
structural a.
suspicious a.
tissue texture a.
urinary tract a.
vascular a.
ventilation/perfusion a.
ventricular depolarization a.

abnormally
a. feeding blood vessel
a. hyperplastic gland

ABO barrier

aborad

abortion
menstrual extraction a.

abortive infection

above-elbow (AE)
a.-e. amputation (AEA)

above-knee (AK)
a.-k. amputation (AKA)
a.-k. amputation conversion

ABPI
ankle-brachial pressure index

abraded wound

Abraham iridotomy

Abraham-Pankovich tendo calcaneus repair
Abrami disease
abrasion
- a. arthroplasty
- bobby-pin a.
- a. chondroplasty
- corneal a.
- perioperative corneal a.
- traumatic corneal a.

abrasive
- a. brush biopsy
- a. point

Abrikosov tumor
abrupt hemodynamic collapse
ABS
American Board of Surgery
abscess
- abdominal a.
- abdominopelvic a.
- actinomycotic brain a.
- acute a.
- amebic hepatic a.
- anal a.
- anastomotic a.
- anorectal a.
- aponeurotic a.
- appendiceal a.
- arthrifluent a.
- axillary a.
- Bezold a.
- bicameral a.
- blind a.
- bone a.
- bowel a.
- brain a.
- breast a.
- Brodi metaphysial a.
- buccal space a.
- button a.
- caseous a.
- cerebral a.
- chronic subareolar a.
- cold a.
- collar-button a.
- colonic a.
- corneal a.
- crypt a.
- cuff a.
- deep interloop a.
- diffuse a.
- Douglas a.
- draining a.
- dry a.
- echinococcal liver a.
- encapsulated brain a.
- enteroperitoneal a.
- epidural a.
- extradural a.
- fecal a.
- fluctuant a.
- a. formation
- frontal a.
- gallbladder wall a.
- gas a.
- gas-forming liver a.
- gravitation a.
- growth plate a.
- hepatic a.
- Highmore a.
- horseshoe a.
- hot a.
- hypostatic a.
- infraorbital space a.
- intermesenteric a.
- intersphincteric a.
- intraabdominal a.
- intradural a.
- intrahepatic a.
- intramural a.
- intramusculature a.
- intraosseous a.
- intraperitoneal a.
- ischiorectal a.
- kidney a.
- lacunar a.
- liver a.
- local a.
- localized a.
- lumbar epidural a.
- mesentery a.
- metaphysial a.
- metastatic a.
- midpalmar a.
- migrating a.
- miliary a.
- missile track a.
- necrotic a.
- pancreatic a.
- paranephric a.
- parapharyngeal space a.
- pelvic a.
- perforating a.
- perianal fistula a.

NOTES

abscess *(continued)*
periappendiceal a.
periesophageal a.
perihepatic a.
perineal a.
perinephric a.
perirectal a.
peritoneal cavity a.
periumbilical a.
periureteral a.
periurethral a.
phlegmonous a.
pilonidal a.
point of a.
postoperative a.
premasseteric space a.
prevertebral space a.
pterygomandibular space a.
pyogenic hepatic a.
residual a.
retrocecal a.
retroperitoneal-iliopsoas a.
retrorectal a.
ring a.
a. ring
satellite a.
soft-tissue a.
space of Retzius a.
spinal epidural a. (SEA)
stercoral a.
sterile a.
stitch a.
subdiaphragmatic a.
subdural a.
subgaleal a.
subhepatic a.
sublingual space a.
submandibular space a.
submasseteric space a.
submental space a.
subperiosteal a.
subphrenic a.
supralevator perirectal a.
tuberculous a.
tuboovarian a.
wandering a.
wound a.
abscise
abscission
corneal a.
absence
microscopic a.
absent
a. bowel sounds
a. gag reflex
a. peristalsis
a. respiration
***Absidia* infection**
absolute
a. construction
a. curative resection
a. humidity
a. noncurative resection
absorbable
absorbent
a. point
a. vessel
absorption
external a.
nutrient a.
reservoir mucosal a.
systemic a.
absorptive cell
abut
abutment
implant a.
screw-type a.
subperiosteal implant a.
AC
acromioclavicular
acalculous cholecystitis
acantha
acanthion
acanthocytosis
acanthoid
acantholysis
ACAS
Asymptomatic Carotid Atherosclerosis Study
accelerans
accelerated
a. respiration
a. transplant rejection
acceleration
angular a.
fetal growth a.
fetal heart rate a.
growth a.
a. injury
tibial a.
a. time
acceleration/deceleration injury
acceleration-dependent aberrancy
accelerator
a. fiber
linear a. (LINAC)
a. nerve
access
a. cavity
cavity a.
central venous a.
cutdown a.
a. emergency
exit a.
extrahepatic a.
a. flap

minimally invasive surgical a.
percutaneous a.
peritoneal a.
a. preparation
root canal a.
side-entry a.
surgical a.
transcervical tubal a.
transcutaneous a.
transjugular liver a.
vascular a.
venous a.
ventricular a.

accessible lesion
accessoria
accessoriae
accessorii
accessoril
accessorium
accessorius
accessory
a. adrenal
a. breast
a. cephalic vein
a. conduction ablation
a. duct stenting
a. flexor muscle
a. muscle activity
a. nerve
a. nerve root
a. nerve trunk
a. nipple
a. obturator artery
a. palatine canal
a. pancreas
a. pancreatic duct
a. papillotomy
a. parotid gland
a. plantar ligament
a. process
a. root canal
a. spleen
a. suprarenal gland
a. thyroid gland
a. tubercle
a. venous sinus of Verga
a. volar ligament

accident
abdominal vascular a.
cerebrovascular a.
intraoperative vascular a.
vascular a.

accidental
a. hemorrhage
a. hypothermia
a. pulp exposure

accommodation
a. curve
a. disorder
a. reflex

accordion
a. abdomen
a. graft
a. sign

Accreditation Council for Graduate Medical Education (ACGME)
accretion line
accumulation
collagen a.
third space fluid a.

accuracy
diagnostic a.

ACE
angiotensin-converting enzyme inhibitor
antegrade continence enema

Ace-Colles frame technique
acellular pannus tissue
acentric relation
acestoma
acetabula (*pl. of* acetabulum)
acetabular
a. artery
a. augmentation graft
a. branch
a. cavity
a. cup arthroplasty
a. extensile approach
a. lip
a. notch
a. protrusio deformity
a. rim fracture

acetabuloplasty
Pemberton a.
shelf a.

acetabulum, pl. **acetabula**
notch of a.

acetohydroxamic acid irrigation
acetowhite lesion
acetylcholine (Ach)
a. receptor

ACGME
Accreditation Council for Graduate Medical Education

NOTES

Ach
acetylcholine
achalasia
a. balloon dilation
a. cardiae
esophageal a.
Achilles
A. bursa
A. tendon
A. tendon rupture
achillis
bursa a.
tendo a.
achondrogenesis
achondroplasia
homozygous a.
achondroplastic
achondroplasty
achromic patch
acid
amino a.
a. anhydride method
a. aspiration
a. etch bonding technique
gastric chloric a.
a. gland
a. guanidine thiocyanate-phenol-chloroform method
a. hemolysis
mefenamic a.
phenylethylbarbituric a.
a. reflux
retinoic a.
stomach a.
acid-base
a.-b. balance
a.-b. disturbance
a.-b. equilibrium
a.-b. status
a.-b. value
acid-etched restoration
acidic fibroblast growth factor
acidification treatment
acidosis
concomitant a.
hepatocellular a.
lactic a.
metabolic a.
renal tubular a.
acinar tissue
acini (*pl. of* acinus)
acinic
a. cell tumor
acinous
a. cell carcinoma
a. gland
acinus, pl. **acini**
lobular a.
Ackerman-Proffitt classification of malocclusion
ACL
anterior cruciate ligament
ACL reconstruction
ACL repair
acneform lesion
acneiform rash
acorn treatment
Acosta classification
acoupedic method
acoustic
a. canal
a. method
a. nerve
a. neuroma
A. Neuroma Registry
a. pressure
a. quantification
a. reflection measurement
a. reflectometry
a. shadowing
a. stimulation study
a. stimulation test
AC-PC line
acquired
a. centric relation
a. cornification disorder
a. deformity
a. diverticulum
a. eccentric jaw relation
a. hernia
acquisition
image a.
multiple gated a. (MUGA)
acral lentiginous melanoma (ALM)
Acrel ganglion
acridine orange method
acrobrachycephaly
acrocephalia
acrocephalic
acrocephalopolysyndactyly
acrocephalosyndactyly type I-IV
acrocephalous
acrocephaly
acrocyanosis
acrodysplasia
acrofacial syndrome
acromegaly
acromial
a. arterial network
a. artery
a. articular facies
a. articular surface
a. branch
a. extremity
a. process
acromialis

acromii
acromioclavicular (AC)
a. articulation
a. disk
a. injury classification
a. joint dislocation
a. joint repair
a. ligament
a. space
acromioclaviculare
acromioclavicularis
acromiocoracoid
acromiohumeral
acromion
acromionectomy
Armstrong a.
acromioplasty
anterior a.
McLaughlin a.
McShane-Leinberry-Fenlin a.
Neer a.
acromioscapular
acromiothoracic
a. approach
a. artery
acroosteolysis
acroosteolytica
ACS
American College of Surgeons
ACT
activated clotting time
actinomycetoma
actinomycoma
actinomycotic brain abscess
actinomyoma
action
anesthesia a.
a. of anesthetic
ball valve a.
a. line
nonstereospecific a.
stereospecific a.
activated
a. clotting time (ACT)
a. coagulation time
a. protein-C resistance
activating solution
activation
baroreflex a.
cortical a.
egg a.
hypothalamic a.
a. map-guided surgical resection
a. moment
very late a.
activation-sequence mapping
activator
a. modification
recombinant tissue-type plasminogen a. (RTPA, rtPA)
active
a. appliance therapy
a. assistive motion therapy
a. chronic inflammation
a. core cooling
a. hemorrhage
a. reciprocation
a. source of bleeding
a. specific immunotherapy (ASI)
a. systemic bacterial infection
actively bleeding varix
activity
accessory muscle a.
antithrombotic a.
duodenal migrating a.
efferent nerve a.
inspiratory intercostal a.
jejunal fasting motor a.
mitotic a.
motor a.
a. pattern analysis
postprandial motor a.
sympathetic nerve a. (SNA)
actuation
direct mechanical ventricular a.
acuminatum
condyloma a.
acuology
acupuncture anesthesia
acusection
acute
a. abscess
a. acalculous cholecystitis (AAC)
a. allergic extrinsic alveolitis
a. allograft rejection
a. aortic dissection
a. blood transfusion
a. calculous cholecystitis
a. cardiac event
a. cellular rejection
a. and chronic inflammation
a. compression triad
a. coronary syndrome
a. digestive bleeding

NOTES

acute *(continued)*
a. disconnection syndrome
a. fracture
a. gastric mucosal lesion
a. graft-versus-host disease
a. hemorrhagic inflammation
a. hemorrhagic ulceration
a. hepatic coma
a. hepatic rupture
a. inflammatory exudate
a. inflammatory membrane
a. intermittent porphyria
a. intestinal obstruction
a. ischemic stroke
A. Low Back Pain Screening Questionnaire (ALBPSQ)
a. lung rejection
a. mesenteric venous thrombosis
a. normovolemic hemodilution (ANH)
a. pancreatitis (AP)
a. physiologic assessment and chronic health evaluation
a. physiology and chronic health evaluation (APACHE)
a. physiology prognostic scoring index
a. presentation
a. pyogenic membrane
a. radiation pneumonitis
a. recurrent rhabdomyolysis
a. rejection of liver transplant
a. respiratory distress syndrome (ARDS)
a. respiratory failure
a. subdural hematoma
a. surgical abdomen
a. symptom
a. traumatic lesion
a. tubular necrosis (ATN)
a. vascular rejection
a. wound
acyltransferase
lecithin-cholesterol a. (LCAT)
acystia
adactylous
adactyly
adamantine membrane
adamantinoblastoma
adamantinocarcinoma
adamantinoma
adamantinum
Adams
A. hip operation
A. position
A. procedure
Adam's apple
adaptable
adaptation
arterial a.
a. disease
a. syndrome of Selye
adaptational approach
adaptive
a. correction
a. relaxation
adaxial
Adden herniorrhaphy
addiction
a. acknowledgment scale
a. potential scale
A. Severity Index
Addison
A. maneuver
A. point
additional canal
additive interaction
additivity
adduction
a. deformity
a. osteotomy
a. traction technique
adduction-internal rotation deformity
adductor
a. canal
a. hiatus
a. longus muscle rupture
a. magnus tendon
a. tenotomy
adductorius
adductovarus deformity
addustorius
adenectomy
adenoacanthoma
adenoameloblastoma
adenocanthoma
adenocarcinoma
alveolar a.
ampullary a.
anaplastic a.
annular a.
appendiceal a.
bile duct a.
bronchial a.
bronchiolar a.
bronchioloalveolar a.
bronchogenic a.
cervical a.
colonic a.
colorectal a.
cystic a.
duct cell a.
duodenal a.
endometrial a.
esophageal a.
gastric a.

infiltrating duct a.
invasive a.
kidney a.
medullary a.
mesonephric a.
metastatic a.
mucinous a.
ovarian clear cell a.
pancreatic a.
peritoneal a.
primary a.
prostatic a.
renal a.
sebaceous a.
secretory a.
serous a.
signet-ring a.
spontaneous a.
stomach a.
sweat-gland a.
undifferentiated a.
uterine a.
vaginal a.
vulvar adenoid cystic a.

adenochondroma
adenocystic carcinoma
adenocystoma
adenodiastasis
adenoepithelioma
adenofibroma
adenofibromyoma
adenohypophysial
adenohypophysis
adenoid
a. cystic carcinoma
a. pad
a. squamous cell carcinoma
a. tumor

adenoidal pad
adenoidal-pharyngeal-conjunctival (A-P-C)
a.-p.-c. virus

adenoidea
adenoidectomy
lateral a.
tonsillectomy and a.

adenoleiomyofibroma
adenolipoma
adenolymphocele
adenolymphoma
adenolysis
adenoma
adnexal a.
adrenal a.
bile duct a.
a. of breast
bronchial a.
colonic a.
colorectal a.
double a.'s
ductal a.
duodenal a.
ectopic parathyroid a.
fibroid a.
hepatic a.
kidney a.
malignant a.
monoclonal a.
papillary a.
parathyroid a.
pituitary a.
prostatic a.
renal a.
a. sebaceum
sessile a.
single a.
sporadic pituitary a.
sweat-gland a.
thyroid a.
tracheal a.
tubulovillous a.
upper a.
well-localized a.

adenoma-hyperplastic polyp ratio
adenoma-nonadenoma ratio
adenomatosis
endocrine a.

adenomatous
a. hyperplasia
a. polyp
a. polyposis coli (APC)

adenomectomy
adenomyosarcoma
adenopathy
axillary a.
cervical a.
metastatic a.
retroperitoneal a.

adenosarcoma
adenose
adenosine-regulating agent
adenosis
sclerosing a.

NOTES

adenosquamous carcinoma
adenotomy
adenotonsillectomy
adenoviral
a. infection
a. transfer
adenovirus infection
adequate hydration
adherence obstruction
adherens
adherent
a. leukoma
a. zone
adhesed
adhesiectomy
adhesio
adhesiolysis
abdominal a.
adhesion
anomalous mesenteric a.
attic a.
banjo-string a.
a. barrier
cell-cell a.
cell-extracellular matrix a.
dense a.
fibrinous a.
fibrous a.
filmy a.
a. formation
hard a.
intraabdominal a.
intraperitoneal a.
laparoscopic lysis of a.
lysis of a.
a. lysis
membranous a.
peritoneal a.
piano-wire a.
primary a.
secondary a.
serologic a.
tenacious a.
adhesiotomy
adhesive
a. arachnoiditis
a. band
a. bonding
a. capsulitis
a. disease
a. ileus
a. inflammation
a. otitis media
a. peritonitis
a. resin-bonded bridge
a. resin-bonded cast restoration
a. syndrome
adipectomy
adipocele
adipodermal graft
adipolysis
adiposa
adipose
a. body
a. capsule
a. connective tissue
a. fold
a. graft
a. infiltration
a. tissue extract
adiposus
aditus
adjunct
surgical a.
a. therapy
adjunctive
a. balloon angioplasty
a. chemotherapy
a. screw fixation
a. suppressive medical therapy
adjustable ring gastroplasty
adjustable-suture strabismus surgery
adjuvant
anesthesia a.
a. chemoradiation therapy
a. chemotherapy
a. diagnostic modality
a. drug therapy
a. irradiation
a. nephrectomy
a. radiotherapy
a. regimen
Adkins
A. spinal fusion
A. technique spinal arthrodesis
Adler operation
admaxillary gland
admedial
administered
spinally a.
administration
altering route of a.
buccal drug a.
concomitant a.
drug a.
epidural a.
interpleural a.
intraocular a.
intraperitoneal drug a.
intraspinal a.
intrathecal a.
intravenous a.
oral a.
oxygen a.
parenteral a.
postischemic a.

preischemic a.
route of a.
sequential a.
transdermal a.
transnasal a.
vasodilator a.

admixture
a. lesion
venous a.

adnexa
ocular a.

adnexal
a. adenoma
a. carcinoma
a. infection
a. mass
a. metastasis

adnexectomy

adnexopexy

adrenal
a. ablation
accessory a.
a. adenoma
a. androgen
a. body
a. branch
a. capsule
a. carcinoma
a. cortex
a. cystic mass
a. feminization syndrome
a. gland
a. gland biopsy
a. hemorrhage
a. incidentaloma
Marchand a.
a. medulla graft
a. medulla transplantation
a. metastasis
a. pathology
a. pheochromocytoma
a. primary aldosteronism
a. vein

adrenalectomy
bilateral total a.
complete a.
ipsilateral a.
laparoscopic a.
open a.
transperitoneal laparoscopic a.

adrenergic

adrenic

adrenocortical
a. carcinoma
a. extract

adrenoprival

adrenoreceptor
alpha a.
beta a.

Adson
A. maneuver
A. test

Adson-Coffey scalenotomy

adsorption theory of narcosis

adsternal

adterminal

adult
a. cardiovascular surgery
a. familial hyaline membrane disease
a. intussusception
a. patient
a. population
a. recipient
a. respiratory distress syndrome (ARDS)
a. scoliosis surgery
a. wandering spleen

adulthood astrocytoma

adult-to-adult living related donor living transplant

advanced
a. disease
a. local invasion
a. retroperitoneal rhabdomyosarcoma
a. therapeutic endoscopy
a. trauma life support (ATLS)
a. tumor perforation

advancement
a. flap graft
Johnson pronator a.
LeFort III facial a.
mandibular osteotomy a.
mucosal a.
a. procedure
a. of rectal flap
transanal pouch a.
V-Y a.

advance to regular diet

adventitia

adverse event

AE
above-elbow
aryepiglottic

NOTES

AEA
above-elbow amputation
Aeby
A. muscle
A. plane
aeration of lung
aerobe
gram-negative a.
aerobic
a. flora
a. gram-negative organism
a. infection
a. respiration
aerobilia
aerocele
aerocystoscopy
aerodigestive tract
aerodynamic size
aerosol
inhalation a.
respirable a.
a. therapy
aerosolized
a. medication
a. pollutant exposure
aesthetic procedure
A-exotropia
AFBG
aortofemoral bypass graft
affect
congruent a.
afferens
afferent
a. clot
a. glomerular arteriole
a. jejunostomy
a. limb
a. loop syndrome
a. lymphatic vessel
PGA a.
PJA a.
a. projection
a. spinal
a. vagal
affrication
AFH
anterior facial height
afterload
decreased a.
a. reduction
afterloading technique
afterpain, after-pain
afterroot amputation restoration
aganglionic rectum
aganglionosis
total colonic a.
agar diffusion method
age
a., distant metastases, extent of local size (AMES)
fertilization a.
Agee force-couple splint reduction
agenesis
tracheal a.
agenetic fracture
agent
adenosine-regulating a.
alpha-adrenergic a.
alpha-sympatholytic a.
anesthetic induction a.
antiadhesion a.
antibacterial a.
antifibrinolytic a.
antifungal a.
antimotility a.
antineoplastic a.
beta-sympathomimetic a.
cavity lining a.
chemoprevention a.
chemopreventive a.
endogenous algogenic a.
hemostatic a.
inhalation a.
neuroleptic a.
neuromuscular blocking a.
oral antimotility a.
prothrombogenic a.
sympatholytic a.
sympathomimetic a.
thrombolytic a.
topical antibacterial a.
topical hemostatic a.
vasodilator a.
ventilation a.
volatile anesthetic a.
age-related macular degeneration
agglutinant
agglutinate
agglutination technique
aggregate gland
aggregation
platelet a.
aggressive
a. lesion
a. renal angiomyolipoma
a. surgical approach
aging degenerative change
agitation
abdominal a.
emergence a.
Agliette supracondylar osteotomy
aglossia-adactylia syndrome
aglossostomia
agminate gland
agnathia

agnathous
Agnew
A. canthoplasty
A. operation
Agnew-Verhoeff incision
agonadal
agonal
a. clot
a. respiration
agonist
alpha-1-adrenergic a.
alpha-2-adrenergic a.
alpha-adrenergic receptor a.
alpha-2-adrenoreceptor a.
beta-adrenergic a.
beta-receptor a.
muscarinic a.
opioid a.
Agrikola operation
AH
atypical hyperplasia
ahaustral
Ahern knot
AHI
Arthritis Helplessness Index
air
bowel loop a.
a. collection
colonic a.
a. critical-care transport
a. cyst
a. embolism
a. embolus
a. enema
a. entrainment
a. entry
a. exchange
expired a.
extrapleural a.
free a.
a. injection
inspired a.
a. insufflation
intramural colonic a.
intramyocardial a.
intraperitoneal a.
minimal a.
oxygen in a.
a. sac
a. sinus
a. space
a. space disease
a. test
a. vesicle
air-bone-tissue boundary
airborne infection
airbrasive technique
air-contrast barium enema
air-filled loop
air-fluid
a.-f. exchange
a.-f. line
air-gap technique
airplane position
airway
anatomic a.
anatomical a.
a., breathing, and circulation (ABC)
a. compromise
a. elastance
a. gas monitoring
large mask a.
laryngeal mask a. (LMA)
a. management
nasal a.
nasopharyngeal a.
a. obstruction
a. occlusion technique
oral pharyngeal a.
oropharyngeal a.
a. pattern
pediatric a.
pharyngeal a.
a. pressure
a. pressure release ventilation (APRV)
a. protection
a. reactivity
a. responsiveness
a. score
a. shunting
a. smooth muscle (ASM)
a. suction
AIS
Abbreviated Injury Scale
Aitken epiphysial fracture classification
AJCC
American Joint Committee on Cancer
AJCC TNM tumor classification
Ajmalin liver injury
AJPBD
anomalous junction of the pancreatobiliary duct

NOTES

AK
above-knee
AKA
above-knee amputation
Akerlund deformity
Akin
A. bunionectomy
A. procedure
A. proximal phalangeal osteotomy
Akiyama procedure
ala, pl. **alae**
sacral a.
alanine amino transaminase (ALT)
Alanson amputation
alar
a. base reduction
a. cartilage
a. fascia
a. fold
a. groove
a. incision
a. lamina
a. ligament
a. reconstruction
a. spine
a. wedge excision
alares
alaria
alarm
alba
linea a.
albae
Albarran
A. gland
A. y Dominguez tubule
Albee-Delbert procedure
Albee spinal fusion
Albert-Lembert gastroplasty
Albert suture technique
Albinus muscle
ALBPSQ
Acute Low Back Pain Screening Questionnaire
Albrecht bone
Albright-Chase arthroplasty
Albright synovectomy
albugineotomy
albumin
radiolabeled serum a.
Alcock canal
alcohol
a. dependence scale
a. fixation
a. used disorders identification test
alcohol-fixed gastric biopsy
alcoholic
a. coma
a. liver
Alcon aspiration
Alden loop gastric bypass
Alder-Reilly anomaly
aldosterone-producing carcinoma
aldosteronism
adrenal primary a.
Aldrete score
Aldridge sling procedure
Aldridge-Studdefort urethral suspension
Alexander
A. incision
A. operation
A. technique
Alexander-Adams
A.-A. hysteropexy
A.-A. uterine suspension
algesimeter
Al-Ghorab
A.-G. modification
A.-G. procedure
alginate
algology
algoscopy
alignment
extramedullary a.
normal anatomic a.
alimentarium
alimentary
a. apparatus
a. canal
a. tract
a. tract duplication
alimentation
central venous a.
enteral a.
forced a.
intravenous a.
peripheral intravenous a.
rectal a.
total parenteral a.
alinasal
aliquorrhea
spontaneous a.
aliquot
alkaline
a. phosphatase-antiphosphatase
a. reflux
Alken approach
alkylation resistance
Allain method
allantoic
a. circulation
a. sac
allele
Allen
A. correction
A. maneuver
A. operation

A. reduction
A. test
allergen exposure
allergic
a. fungal sinusitis
a. inflammation
a. manifestation
a. shock
Allgöwer stitch
alligator skin
all-inside repair
Allis-Abramson breast biopsy
Allis maneuver
Allison
A. gastroesophageal reflux repair
A. hiatal hernia repair
A. suture technique
Alliston
A. GE reflux correction
A. procedure
Allman acromioclavicular injury classification
allocation
dynamic storage a.
fresh tissue a.
static storage a.
storage a.
a. of treatment
allodynia
compression-evoked a.
allogenic, allogeneic
a. blood
a. blood component
a. blood transfusion
a. bone graft
a. bone marrow
a. fetal graft
a. transplantation
allogenous bone graft
allograft
a. corneal rejection
cryopreserved heart-valve a.
a. extraction
femoral cortical ring a.
functioning a.
hepatic a.
intestinal a.
liver a.
organ a.
osteoarticular a.
osteochondral a.
pancreaticoduodenal a.
renal a.
a. transplantation
allografting
nerve a.
peripheral nerve a.
allokeratoplasty
allongement
allopathic keratoplasty
alloplastic chin augmentation
alloplasty
all-or-nothing phenomenon
allotransplantation
inlet a.
liver a.
alloy restoration
Allport operation
ALM
acral lentiginous melanoma
ALND
axillary lymph node dissection
alone
pancreatic transplantation a. (PTA)
Alonso-Lej classification
alopecia
pressure a.
traction a.
alpha
a. adrenoreceptor
alpha-2-adrenoreceptor agonist
alpha-adrenergic
a.-a. agent
a.-a. antagonist
a.-a. receptor
a.-a. receptor agonist
alpha-1-adrenergic
a.-a. agonist
a.-a. antagonist
alpha-2-adrenergic
a.-a. agonist
a.-a. receptor
a.-a. receptor antagonist
alpha-loop maneuver
alpha-sympatholytic agent
Alport syndrome
Alsus-Knapp operation
ALT
alanine amino transaminase
serum ALT
Altemeier repair of rectal prolapse
alteration
dentin crystal a.
alterative inflammation

NOTES

altercursive intubation
altered gene product
altering route of administration
alternate-day therapy
alternating suture technique
alternation
alternative
cost-effective a.
a. introduction site
a. medicine
a. practitioner
a. surgical approach
therapeutic a.
a. therapy
a. treatment
altitude simulation study
aluminum
a. cranioplasty
implant alloy a.
alveodental suppuration
alveolar
a. adenocarcinoma
a. artery
a. body
a. canal
a. carbon dioxide pressure
a. cavity
a. cell carcinoma
a. dead space
a. dead-space fraction
a. diffusion measurement
a. ectasia
a. end-capillary difference
a. fistula
a. foramina
a. gas equation
a. hemorrhage
a. hyperventilation
a. hypoventilation
a. index
a. oxygen partial pressure (PAO_2)
a. partial pressure
a. plateau
a. plate fenestration
a. point
a. point-meatus plane
a. point-nasal point line
a. point-nasion line
a. process
a. process fracture
a. rhabdomyosarcoma
a. sac
a. socket wall fracture
a. tumor
a. ventilation
a. ventilation per minute (V_A)
a. yoke
alveolar-arterial
a.-a. oxygen gradient
a.-a. pressure difference
alveolar-capillary membrane
alveolaris
alveolarization
alveolectomy
partial a.
alveoli (*pl. of* alveolus)
alveolitis
acute allergic extrinsic a.
chronic extrinsic a.
extrinsic allergic a.
alveolobasilar line
alveolocapillary
a. membrane
a. partial pressure gradient
alveolodental membrane
alveololabial groove
alveolomerotomy
alveolonasal line
alveoloplasty
interradicular a.
intraseptal a.
alveolotomy
alveolus, pl. **alveoli**
alveoplasty
alvine calculus
alvinolith
Alvis operation
AM
anterior midpapillary
AM segment
amalgam
a. condensation
a. restoration
Amato body
amaurosis
intoxication a.
pressure a.
Amberg lateral sinus line
ambiens
ambient
a. cisterna
a. oxygen concentration
a. temperature
ambiguous external genitalia
amblyopia
deprivation a.
eclipse a.
ex a.
exertional a.
ambulatory
a. anesthesia
a. gynecologic laparoscopy
a. hemorrhoidectomy
a. pneumoperitoneum
a. setup

a. surgery
a. surgery center
amebic, amoebic
a. colitis
a. cyst
a. hepatic abscess
a. infection
a. perforation
a. peritonitis
ameboma
ameliorating myocardial stunning liposomal coenzyme
amelioration
ameloblastic
a. carcinoma
a. fibroma
ameloblastoma
American
A. Association of Nurse Anesthetists (AANA)
A. Association for the Surgery of Trauma (AAST)
A. Association for Surgery of Trauma Organ Injury Scale classification
A. Board of Anesthesiology (ABA)
A. Board of Surgery (ABS)
A. College of Surgeons (ACS)
A. Heart Association classification
A. Joint Committee on Cancer (AJCC)
A. laryngectomy technique
A. Pediatric Surgical Association (APSA)
A. Rheumatism Association index
A. Society of Anesthesiologists (ASA)
A. Society of Anesthesiologists classification
A. Society of Anesthesiology score
A. Society for Colon and Rectal Surgeons (ASCRS)
A. Society for Gastrointestinal Endoscopy (ASGE)
A. Urological Association symptom index
AMES
age, distant metastases, extent of local size
AMES criteria
ametropia
position a.
amidation
amino acid
aminoglycoside
a. toxicity
a. tubular necrosis
AML
angiomyolipoma
AMLR
auditory middle-latency response
Ammon
A. canthoplasty
A. operation
amnesia
patch a.
amnestic effect
amnioma
amnion
a. ring
a. rupture
amnioscopy
amniotic
a. band amputation
a. cavity
a. fluid embolism
a. fold
a. hernia
a. infection syndrome
a. membrane
a. sac
amniotomy
amobarbital
amoebic (*var. of* amebic)
amphibolic fistula
amphibolous fistula
amphoric respiration
Amplatz technique
amplitude
a. of fusion
a. modulation
amplitude-summation
a.-s. interferential current
a.-s. interferential current therapy
ampulla, pl. **ampullae**
duodenal a.
hepatopancreatic a.
rectal a.
Thoma a.
Vater a.
ampullaris
ampullary
a. adenocarcinoma
a. aneurysm

NOTES

ampullary *(continued)*
a. cancer
a. carcinoma
a. crura
a. granulation tissue
a. sulcus
a. tumor
ampullectomy
ampulloma
amputation
above-elbow a. (AEA)
above-knee a. (AKA)
Alanson a.
amniotic band a.
Béclard a.
below-elbow a. (BEA)
below-knee a. (BKA)
Berger interscapular a.
Bier a.
bilateral a.
birth a.
bloodless a.
border ray a.
Boyd ankle a.
Bunge a.
Burgess below-knee a.
Callander a.
central ray a.
cervical a.
chop a.
Chopart a.
circular open a.
closed flap a.
congenital above-elbow a.
congenital below-elbow a.
consecutive a.
corporectomy a.
disarticular a.
dry a.
extremity a.
Farabeuf a.
fingertip a.
fishmouth a.
forearm a.
forequarter a.
Gordon-Taylor hindquarter a.
Gritti-Stokes a.
guillotine a.
hand a.
hindfoot a.
hindquarter a.
immediate a.
incomplete a.
index ray a.
interilioabdominal a.
interinnominoabdominal a.
intermediate a.
interpelviabdominal a.
interphalangeal a.
intrapyretic a.
intrauterine a.
Jaboulay a.
Kendrick method below-knee a.
King-Steelquist hindquarter a.
Lisfranc a.
major a.
minor a.
multiple ray a.
one-stage a.
open a.
pathologic a.
penile a.
Pirogoff a.
primary a.
pulp a.
quadruple a.
ray a.
rectangular a.
root a.
secondary a.
shoulder a.
Sorondo-Ferré hindquarter a.
spontaneous a.
supracondylar a.
Syme ankle disarticulation a.
tarsal a.
tarsometatarsal a.
tendinomyoplastic a.
tertiary a.
through-knee a.
transcarpal a.
transiliac a.
transmetatarsal a.
transpelvic a.
traumatic a.
two-stage Syme a.
Wagner modification of Syme a.
Wagner two-stage Syme a.
Wilms a.
amputee
unilateral a.
Amreich vaginal extirpation
Amsler operation
Amspacher-Messenbaugh
A.-M. closing wedge osteotomy
A.-M. technique
Amstutz-Wilson osteotomy
Amussat
A. incision
A. operation
A. valvula
amygdaline
amygdalohippocampectomy
amygdalotomy
amyloid
a. angiopathy

a. kidney
a. oral cavity disease
anabolic response
anaclitic therapy
anacrotic notch
anadidymus
anaerobe
anaerobic
a. ocular infection
a. respiration
anaeroplasty
anagenesis
Anagnostakis operation
anal
a. abscess
a. anastomosis
a. canal
a. canal artery
a. canal rhythmic contraction
a. canal staining
a. cleft
a. column
a. condyloma
a. continence
a. crypt
a. dilation
a. electrical stimulation
a. endoscopy
a. fascia
a. fissure
a. fistula
a. foreign body
a. HPZ
a. incontinence
a. manometry
a. orifice
a. pecten
a. pouch
a. region
a. resting pressure
a. sinus
a. sphincter injury
a. sphincter reconstruction
a. sphincter repair
a. sphincter squeeze pressure
a. squamous intraepithelial lesion
a. stretch
a. transitional zone (ATZ)
a. triangle
a. ulceration
a. verge
analgesia
ceiling a.
conduction a.
dermatomal level of a.
fixed-dose patient-controlled a. (FDPCA)
inhalation a.
interpleural a.
intrathecal opioid labor a.
multimodal a.
opioid a.
parenteral a.
patient-controlled a. (PCA)
patient-controlled epidural a. (PCEA, PEA)
patient-controlled intranasal a. (PCINA)
perineal a.
perioperative a.
a. permeation
postoperative a.
preemptive a.
preoperative a.
rescue a.
spinal a.
supplementary a.
thoracic epidural a.
tracheal topical a.
analgesic
a. abuse headache
a. effect
a. index
a. infusion
intranasal a.
intrathecal a.
intravenous a.
narcotic a.
NSAID a.
opioid a.
oral a.
parenteral a.
pediatric a.
postoperative a.
spinal a.
transdermal a.
analgetic
analogous
analogue
somatostatin a.
analysis, pl. **analyses**
activity pattern a.
blood-gas a.

NOTES

analysis *(continued)*
body composition a.
body-fluid a.
combined a.
deformity a.
displacement a.
failure a. (FA)
fixed-dose a.
frozen section a.
histopathologic a.
image a.
immunohistochemical a.
isobologram a.
isobolographic a.
Kruskal-Wallis nonparametric a.
mutation a.
neutron activation a.
peak pressure a.
power spectral a.
pressure-volume a.
p53 tumor suppressor gene a.
restriction endonuclease a.
retrospective a.
saturation a.
single strand conformation polymorphism a.
slot-blot hybridization a.
sound a.
total space a.
Vindelov method flow cytometry a.
visual a.
volumetric a.

analytic
a. method
a. reconstruction

anaphylactoid-type reaction

anaphylaxis
eosinophilic chemotactic factor of a. (ECF-A)

anaplastic
a. adenocarcinoma
a. astrocytoma
a. carcinoma
a. ependymoma

anapophysis

anastole

anastomose

anastomosed graft

anastomosis, pl. **anastomoses**
anal a.
aneurysm by a.
antecolic a.
antiperistaltic a.
aortic a.
arterial a.
arteriolovenular a.
arteriovenous a.
Baffe a.
Béclard a.
beveled a.
bidirectional superior cavopulmonary a.
biliary-enteric a.
biliary intestinal a.
biliodigestive a.
Billroth I, II gastrointestinal a.
bladder neck-to-urethra a.
bowel a.
Brackin ureterointestinal a.
Braun a.
carotid-basilar a.
carotid-vertebral a.
cavopulmonary a.
cervical a.
choledochocholedochostomy side-to-side a.
circular a.
Clado a.
cobra-head a.
Coffey ureterointestinal a.
coloanal a.
colocolic a.
colocolonic a.
coloendoanal a.
colonic pouch anal a.
colorectal a.
conjoined a.
cornual a.
Couvelaire ileourethral a.
cross-facial nerve graft a.
crucial a.
cruciate a.
crunch-stick a.
crushing a.
curved end-to-end a.
Daines-Hodgson a.
D-D a.
delayed direct coloanal a.
dismembered a.
distal a.
duct-to-duct a.
duct-to-mucosa a.
elliptical a.
endoanal a.
end-to-back bowel a.
end-to-end splenoadrenal a.
end-to-side a.
end-weave a.
esophageal-jejunal a.
esophagocolic a.
esophagogastric a.
extended end-to-end a.
extraabdominal a.
extracorporeal a.
extrapleural a.
extravesical a.

fishmouth a.
flexor tendon a.
Fontan atriopulmonary a.
Furniss a.
Galen a.
gastroduodenal a.
gastrointestinal a. (GIA)
gastrojejunal a.
genicular a.
Glenn a.
graft a.
Haight a.
handmade a.
handsewn a.
hand-sutured ileoanal a.
heel-toe a.
hepatojejunal a.
Hofmeister a.
Hofmeister-Pólya a.
Horsley a.
Hoyer a.
H-shaped ileal pouch-anal a.
hypoglossal facial nerve a.
Hyrtl a.
ileal pouch-anal a. (IPAA)
ileal pouch-distal rectal a.
ileal-sigmoid a.
ileoanal a.
ileorectal a. (IRA)
ileosigmoid a.
ileotransverse colon a.
ileovesical a.
intercoronary a.
intermesenteric arterial a.
intestinal a.
intracorporeal a.
intragastric a.
intrathoracic a.
intravesical a.
invaginating a.
isoperistaltic a.
jejunoileal a.
jejunojejunal a.
J-shaped ileal pouch-anal a.
Kocher a.
Kugel a.
laparoscopic bilioenteric a.
LeDuc a.
leptomeningeal a.
Lich-Gregoir a.
longitudinal side-to-side a.
lymphaticovenous a.
Martin-Gruber a.
mechanical a.
mesocaval a.
microneurovascular a.
microsurgical tubocornual a.
microvascular surgical a.
mucosa-to-mucosa a.
Nakayama a.
nerve a.
nondismembered a.
onlay patch a.
pancreatic a.
pancreaticogastric a.
pancreaticogastrointestinal a.
pancreaticogastrostomy a. (PGA)
pancreaticojejunal a.
pancreaticojejunostomy a. (PJA)
Parks ileoanal a.
percutaneous portocaval a.
Politano-Leadbetter a.
Pólya a.
portacaval a.
portal-systemic a.
portoportal a.
portopulmonary venous a.
portosystemic a.
Potts a.
Potts-Smith a.
precapillary a.
primary end-to-end a.
rectosigmoid a.
Riche-Cannieu a.
right-angled end-to-side a.
Riolan a.
Roux-en-Y hepaticojejunal a.
Schmidel a.
Schoemaker a.
side-to-side a.
spinal accessory nerve-facial nerve a.
splenoadrenal a.
splenorenal venous a.
S-shaped ileal pouch-anal a.
STA-MCA a.
stapled coloanal a.
stapled ileoanal a.
State end-to-end a.
stenotic esophagogastric a.
subcutaneous a.
Sucquet a.
Sucquet-Hoyer a.
supraoptic a.

NOTES

anastomosis *(continued)*
suture a.
sutureless bowel a.
temporal-cerebral arterial a.
tension-free a.
terminoterminal a.
transanal mucosectomy with handsewn a.
transureteroureteral a.
triple a.
two-layer a.
ureterocolonic a.
ureteroileal a.
ureterosigmoid a.
ureterotubal a.
ureteroureteral a.
urethrocecal a.
valved conduit a.
vascular a.
venous a.
venous-to-venous a.
vesicourethral a.
Von Haberer-Finney a.
Waterston extrapericardial a.
wide elliptical a.
wide-open a.
W-shaped ileal pouch-anal a.
Z-shaped a.

anastomotic
a. abscess
a. area
a. branch
a. breakdown
a. complication
a. complication rate
a. dehiscence
a. edge
a. failure
a. fiber
a. fistula
a. flow
a. healing
a. leakage
a. operation
a. stoma
a. stricture
a. stricture formation
a. stricture rate
a. stump
a. stump leak
a. ulceration
a. vein

anastomoticum

anastomoticus

anatomic
a. abnormality
a. airway
a. barrier
a. dead space
a. diagnosis
a. equator
a. event
a. fracture
a. fracture reduction principle
a. imaging
a. imaging information
a. insertion
a. integrity
a. landmark
a. localization
a. pathology
a. plane
a. position
a. repair
a. site
a. structure
a. variation

anatomical
a. airway
a. landmark
a. position
a. radical retropubic prostatectomy
a. root
a. site
a. situation
a. snuffbox
a. sphincter
a. tooth
a. tubercle
a. variation

anatomicosurgical

anatomique

anatomist

anatomy
anomalous a.
biliary a.
Billroth II a.
cervicothoracic pedicle a.
congenitally altered a.
coronary vessel a.
dental a.
designed after natural a. (DANA)
fetal intracranial a.
gingival a.
immune system a.
intracranial a.
intrahepatic a.
knee a.
Lowsley lobar a.
native coronary a.
neurovascular a.
normal planar MR a.
pathological a.
pedicle a.
peritoneal a.
plantar compartmental a.

surgical a.
vascular a.
zonal a.

anatrophic
a. nephrolithotomy
a. nephroscopy
a. nephrotomy

anchor
a. mastopexy
a. molar

anchorage
extramaxillary a.
extraoral a.
gastrophrenic a.

anchoring
a. point

anchovy procedure

ancipital

anconeal

anconeus
a. muscle
a. muscle flap

Andersch
A. ganglion
A. nerve

Anderson
A. ankle fusion
A. modification of Berndt-Harty classification
A. procedure

Anderson-D'Alonzo odontoid fracture classification

Anderson-Fowler
A.-F. calcaneal displacement osteotomy
A.-F. procedure

Anderson-Hutchins
A.-H. technique
A.-H. unstable tibial shaft fracture

Anderson-Hynes pyeloplasty

Anderson-Keys method

Andrews
A. iliotibial band reconstruction
A. technique

Andrews-type nonorthodontic normal crown angulation

androblastoma

androgen
a. ablation
adrenal a.
excess a.

androgenic

androgenization

android pelvis

Andy Gump deformity

anecdotal procedure

anechoic tissue

Anel
A. method
A. operation

anemia
Fanconi a.
a. of hemodialysis

anesthesia
a. action
acupuncture a.
a. adjuvant
ambulatory a.
ankle block a.
axillary block a.
balanced a.
barbiturate burst-suppression a.
basal a.
Bier block a.
block a.
bolus intravenous a.
brachial a.
a. breathing circuit
bypass a.
cardiac a.
cardiovascular a.
caudal a.
centroneuroaxis a.
cervical a.
circle absorption a.
closed a.
closed-circuit a.
cocaine a.
coinduction of a.
combined epidural-general a.
combined spinal-epidural a. (CSEA)
come-and-go a.
compression a.
computer-assisted a.
conduction a.
continuous epidural a.
continuous lumbar peridural a.
continuous spinal a.
corneal a.
crossed a.
dental a.
depth of a.
diagnostic a.
differential spinal a.

NOTES

anesthesia *(continued)*
digital block a.
dissociated a.
dissociative a.
a. dolorosa
ear a.
electric a.
endotracheal a.
epidural a. (EA)
exam under a.
extradural a.
failed a.
fast-track cardiac a.
field block a.
fitness for general a.
fractional epidural a.
fractional spinal a.
general a. (GA)
general endotracheal a.
geriatric a.
girdle a.
glove a.
graded spinal a.
gustatory a.
gynecologic a.
high spinal a.
hydrate microcrystal theory of a.
hyperbaric spinal a.
hypnosis a.
hypobaric spinal a.
hypotensive a.
hypothermic a.
hysterical a.
induction of a.
infiltration a.
infraorbital a.
inhalant a.
inhalational a.
inhalation mask a.
insufflation a.
intercostal a.
interpleural a.
intracavitary a.
intraligamentary a.
intramedullary a.
intranasal a.
intraoral a.
intraorbital a.
intraosseous a.
intraperitoneal a.
intrapulpal a.
intraspinal a.
intrathecal a.
intratracheal a.
intravenous block a.
intravenous regional a. (IVRA)
intravenous sedation a.
isobaric spinal a.
laryngeal a.
ligamental a.
local a.
low central venous pressure a.
low spinal a.
low thoracic level epidural a.
lumbar epidural a.
MAC a.
management of a.
maternal a.
modified Van Lint a.
monitored anesthesia care a.
muscular a.
neonatal a.
nerve block a.
nerve compression a.
neuroleptanalgesia a.
neurosurgical a.
newborn a.
nonrebreathing a.
nose a.
O'Brien a.
obstetric a.
olfactory a.
one-lung a.
open drop a.
ophthalmic a.
ophthalmologic a.
opioid a.
orbital a.
oropharyngeal a.
orthopedic a.
outpatient a.
painful a.
paracervical block a.
paravertebral a.
parenteral a.
patient-controlled epidural a.
patient-controlled intravenous a.
pediatric radiotherapy a.
peribulbar a.
peridural a.
perineal a.
perineural a.
periodontal ligament a.
peripheral nerve block a.
pharyngeal a.
Ponka technique for local a.
postcesarean a.
postoperative a.
preemptive a.
pregnancy-induced a.
preperitoneal a.
presacral a.
pressure a.
pudendal a.
rapid-sequence induction of a.
Raplon a.

rebreathing a.
a. record
rectal a.
refrigeration a.
regional a. (RA)
retrobulbar a.
risk of a.
risk management of a.
sacral a.
saddle block a.
segmental epidural a.
selective a.
semiclosed a.
semiopen a.
single-breath induction of a.
spinal a. (SA)
splanchnic a.
stellate ganglion block a.
stocking a.
stocking-glove a.
subarachnoid a.
supraclavicular brachial block a.
surgical a.
tactile a.
therapeutic a.
thermal a.
thermic a.
thoracic a.
throat a.
a. time
to-and-fro a.
toe-block a.
topical oropharyngeal a.
total intravenous a. (TIVA)
total spinal a.
transdermal a.
traumatic a.
unilateral a.
unmonitored local a.
urologic a.
Van Lint a.
variable-dose patient-controlled a. (VDPCA)
visceral a.
volatile a.

anesthesiologist
American Society of A.'s (ASA)

anesthesiology
American Board of A. (ABA)
critical care a.
a. critical care medicine

anesthetic
action of a.
a. approach
a. block
a. blockade
cardiac a.
a. circuit
a. consideration
a. cutoff
a. depth
a. emergence
EMLA a.
epidural a.
eutectic mixture of local a.'s (EMLA)
flammable a.
a. and fluid management
a. gas
gas a.
a. gas exposure
a. gas mixture
general a.
halogenated volatile a.
a. hepatitis
a. hepatotoxicity
hyperbaric local a.
a. immediate recovery
a. index
a. induction
a. induction agent
inhaled a.
injection of local a.
instillation of a.
intradermal a.
intramuscular a.
intraperitoneal a.
intrathecal a.
intravenous a.
a. leprosy
local a.
low-dose a.
a. management
a. monitoring
multiple mechanism inhaled a.
multiple site inhaled a.
opioid a.
oral a.
pediatric a.
polymer a.
a. potency
preoperative a.
primary a.

NOTES

anesthetic *(continued)*
a. record
rectal a.
regional a.
ring block digital a.
a. risk
secondary a.
a. shock
single mechanism inhaled a.
single site inhaled a.
spinal a.
a. system
a. technique
a. time
a. tolerance
topical a.
trace a.
a. vapor
volatile a.
walking epidural a.
anesthetic/hypnotic
anesthetist
American Association of Nurse A.'s (AANA)
certified registered nurse a. (CRNA)
nurse a.
anesthetization
anesthetize
aneuploid cell line
aneurysm
abdominal aortic a. (AAA)
ampullary a.
a. by anastomosis
anterior circulation a.
aortic a.
aortoiliac a.
arterial a.
arteriosclerotic a.
arteriovenous a.
atherosclerotic a.
axial a.
axillary artery a.
basilar artery a.
basilar bifurcation a.
basilar tip a.
Bérard a.
berry a.
bifurcation a.
celiac artery a.
circulation a.
clavicular fracture a.
a. clip ligation
coiled intracranial a.
complex intracranial a.
compound a.
congenital cerebral a.
consecutive a.
cylindroid a.
descending aortic a.
diffuse a.
dissecting a.
ectatic a.
endogenous a.
endovascular a.
exogenous a.
false a.
femoral artery a.
fusiform a.
hernial a.
iliac artery a.
infraclinoid a.
intracranial a.
isolated iliac artery a.
a. management
miliary a.
mitral valve a.
mycotic a.
peripheral a.
phantom a.
posterior circulation a.
Pott a.
a. repair
ruptured abdominal aortic a.
saccular a.
serpentine a.
subclavian artery a.
supraclinoid a.
thoracic a.
thoracoabdominal a.
a. tissue
traction a.
traumatic false a.
true a.
tubular a.
varicose a.
aneurysmal
a. dilatation
a. dilation
a. disease
a. hematoma
a. hemorrhage
a. rupture
a. sac
a. tissue
a. varix
aneurysmectomy
aortic a.
conventional aortic a.
elective a.
laparoscopic-assisted a.
Matas a.
aneurysmoplasty
aneurysmorrhaphy
aneurysmotomy

ANF
atrial natriuretic factor
Angelucci operation
angel-wing deformity
angiectasia
angiectatic
angiectopia
angiitis
hypersensitivity a.
necrotizing a.
angina
abdominal a.
unstable a.
angina-guided therapy
angioblastoma
angiocentric
a. immunoproliferative lesion
a. lymphoproliferative lesion
angiodysplastic lesion
angioembolization
angioendothelioma
angiofibrolipoma
angiofibroma, pl. **angiofibromata**
facial a.
angiogenesis
therapeutic a.
tumor a.
angiogram
mesenteric a.
multigated a.
angiographic
a. demonstration
a. embolization
a. evaluation
a. intervention
a. result
a. road-mapping technique
a. study
angiographically occult intracranial vascular malformation (AOIVM)
angiography
abdominal a.
fluorescein a.
magnetic resonance a. (MRA)
mesenteric a.
selective a.
angioinvasive lesion
angiokeratoma
angioleiomyoma
angiolipofibroma
angiolipoma
angiolith
angiolithic
angiolysis
angioma
arterial a.
bleeding a.
capillary a.
cavernous a.
cerebral a.
cherry a.
conjunctival a.
gastric a.
orbital a.
pulmonary a.
spider a.
spinal a.
strawberry a.
superficial a.
telangiectatic a.
venous a.
angiomatosis
skeletal-extraskeletal a.
angiomatous neoplastic tissue
angiomyofibroma
angiomyolipoma (AML)
aggressive renal a.
asymptomatic a.
hemorrhagic a.
malignant a.
renal a.
uncomplicated a.
visceral a.
angiomyoma
angiomyoneuroma
angiomyxoma
angioneurectomy
angioneuromyoma
angioneurotomy
angio-osteohypertrophy syndrome
angiopathy
amyloid a.
radiation a.
angioplany
angioplasty
ablative laser a.
adjunctive balloon a.
aortoiliac a.
balloon catheter a.
balloon coarctation a.
balloon coronary a.
balloon dilation a.
balloon laser a.
bootstrap two-vessel a.

NOTES

angioplasty *(continued)*
brachiocephalic vessel a.
carotid a.
complementary balloon a.
coronary artery a.
coronary balloon a.
culprit lesion a.
excimer laser coronary a.
facilitated a.
high-risk a.
Ho:YAG laser a.
iliac artery a.
infrapopliteal transluminal a.
Kinsey rotation atherectomy extrusion a.
kissing balloon a.
laser-assisted balloon a.
low-speed rotational a.
Osypka rotational a.
patch-graft a.
percutaneous balloon a.
percutaneous low-stress a.
percutaneous transluminal coronary a. (PTCA)
percutaneous transluminal renal a.
peripheral balloon a.
peripheral laser a.
postcoronary a.
renal a.
rescue a.
salvage balloon a.
subclavian vein patch a.
Tactilaze a.
thermal/perfusion balloon a.
thulium:YAG laser a.
tibioperoneal trunk a.
tibioperoneal vessel a.
transluminal coronary a.
vein patch a.
vibrational a.
angioplasty-related vessel occlusion
angioproliferative lesion
angioreticuloma
angiorrhaphy
angiorrhexis
angiosarcoma
angioscopy
fluorescein fundus a.
percutaneous transluminal a.
angioscotoma
angiostomy
angiotelectasis
angiotensin-converting enzyme inhibitor (ACE)
angiotensinogen
angiotomy
angle
a. of aberration
anomaly a.
anorectal a.
anterior angulation a.
axial line a.
biorbital a.
a. bisection technique
Böhler calcaneal a.
Broca basilar a.
Broca facial a.
buccoocclusal line a.
calcaneal inclination a.
calcaneal-second metatarsal angle inclination a.
cardiohepatic a.
cavity line a.
costal a.
Daubenton a.
declination a.
deformity a.
distobuccal line a.
distobuccoocclusal point a.
distolabial line a.
distolabioincisal point a.
distolingual line a.
distolinguoincisal point a.
distoocclusal point a.
duodenojejunal a.
elevation a.
epigastric a.
facial a.
a. of femoral torsion
filtration a.
Frankfort mandibular incisor a.
Frankfort mandibular plane a.
hepatic-renal a.
hepatorenal a.
a. of His
hypsiloid a.
incisal mandibular plane a.
infrasternal a.
iridocorneal a.
Jacquart facial a.
labioincisal line a.
line a.
linguoincisal line a.
linguoocclusal line a.
Louis a.
Ludwig a.
lumbosacral a.
magnetization precession a.
A. malocclusion classification
mesiobuccal line a.
mesiobuccoocclusal point a.
mesiolabial line a.
mesiolabioincisal point a.
mesiolingual line a.
mesiolinguoincisal point a.
mesiolinguo-occlusal point line a.

mesioocclusal line a.
metafacial a.
nail-to-nail bed a.
occipital a.
occlusal plane a.
ophryospinal a.
a. of orientation
parietal a.
pelvivertebral a.
Pirogoff a.
point a.
pubic a.
Quatrefages a.
a. of reflection
Serres a.
sharp a.
sphenoid a.
sphenoidal a.
splenorenal a.
sternal a.
sternoclavicular a.
subpubic a.
substernal a.
superior a.
a. suture technique
talocalcaneal a.
tip a.
Topinard facial a.
tracheal bifurcation a.
venous a.
y a.

angled blade plate fixation

Anglo-Saxon nomenclature

angular

a. acceleration
a. artery
a. deformity
a. incision
a. line
a. notch
a. osteotomy
a. phenolization
a. position
a. spine
a. vein

angularis

angulated

a. fracture
a. lesion

angulation

Andrews-type nonorthodontic normal crown a.
anterior a.
apex dorsal a.
bracket slot a.
built-in a.
caudal a.
coronal a.
a. deformity
a. fracture
horizontal a.
kyphotic a.
limb length a.
lower incisor a.
a. motion
a. osteotomy
palmar a.
plantar a.
radius of a.
RAO a.
rectoanal a.
right anterior oblique a.
screw a.
upper incisor a.
valgus a.
vertical a.
volar a.

ANH

acute normovolemic hemodilution

anhepatic stage of liver transplantation

anhydration

anhydrous facial foundation

ani (*pl. of* anus)

animal

animation

suspended a.

anisocoria

postoperative a.

anisotropic

a. rotation
a. tissue

ankle

a. block
a. block anesthesia
dorsiflexion of a.
a. fusion
lateral joint of a.
a. mortise diastasis
a. mortise fracture
a. region

ankle-brachial

ankle-brachial index
ankle-brachial pressure index (ABPI)

NOTES

ankle-brachial *(continued)*
a.-b. blood pressure ratio
a.-b. pressure measurement
ankyloglossia superior syndrome
ankylosing spondylitis
ankylosis
extraarticular a.
extracapsular a.
Ann
A. Arbor classification
A. Arbor classification of Hodgkin disease staging
A. Arbor Hodgkin
A. Arbor Hodgkin lymphoma stage I, IE, II, IIE, IIIE, IIIS, IIISE, IV
A. Arbor stage IE, IIE
annexectomy
annexopexy
annular
a. adenocarcinoma
a. cartilage
a. constricting lesion
a. corneal graft operation
a. pancreas
a. sphincter
annularis
annuloplasty
Carpentier a.
DeVega tricuspid valve a.
Gerbode a.
isolated a.
prosthetic ring a.
tricuspid valve a.
Wooler-type a.
annulorrhaphy
annulotomy
annulus (*See* anulus)
ano
fistula in a.
anociassociation
anococcygea
anococcygeal
a. body
a. ligament
anococcygei
anococcygeum
anocutanea
anocutaneous
a. line
a. stimulation
anoderm
anoderm-preserving hemorrhoidectomy
anodyne
anogenital raphe
anomalad
Pierre Robin a.
anomalous
a. anatomy
a. fixation
a. innominate artery compression syndrome
a. insertion
a. junction of the pancreatobiliary duct (AJPBD)
a. mesenteric adhesion
a. position
a. rectification
a. vertebral artery
anomaly
Alder-Reilly a.
a. angle
anorectal a.
arterial a.
atrioventricular connection a.
atrioventricular junction a.
Axenfeld a.
branchial a.
cardiac a.
cervical a.
Chiari a.
coloboma a.
congenital conotruncal a.
conjoined nerve-root a.
conotruncal a.
coronary artery a.
craniofacial a.
Cruveilhier-Baumgarten a.
dental a.
dentofacial a.
double-inlet ventricle a.
Duane a.
duplication a.
dysgnathic a.
Ebstein cardiac a.
eugnathic a.
facet a.
fetal cardiac a.
fetal chest a.
fetal gastrointestinal a.
fetal vascular a.
fixation a.
Freund a.
genetic a.
genitourinary a.
gestant a.
hand a.
heart a.
intracranial dural vascular a.
jugular bulb a.
kidney a.
Kimerle a.
Klippel-Feil a.
lacrimal angle duct a.
laryngeal a.

limb reduction a.
maxillofacial a.
megadolichovertebrobasilar a.
Michel a.
Moebius a.
Mondini a.
morning glory optic disk a.
müllerian duct a.
nevoid a.
numerary renal a.
occipitoatlantoaxial a.
oculocephalic vascular a.
oral a.
orthopedic a.
osseous a.
Peters a.
Poland a.
postsurgical motor a.
presacral a.
pulmonary valve a.
pulmonary venous connection a.
pulmonary venous return a.
renal a.
reticulate pigmented a.
root a.
segmentation a.
Shone a.
Sprengel a.
structural a.
Taussig-Bing a.
tracheobronchial a.
Uhl a.
umbilical cord a.
Undritz a.
urinary tract a.
urogenital a.
uterine a.
VACTERL a.
vaginal a.
vascular a.
ventricular inflow a.
vertebral, anus, tracheoesophageal, radial, and renal a.
viscerobronchial cardiovascular a.
vitelline duct a.
a. of Zahn

anopia

anoplasty
cutback a.
House advancement a.
House flap a.
Martin a.
a. treatment
Y-V a.

anopsia

anorchia

anorchism

anorectal
a. abscess
a. angle
a. anomaly
a. carcinoma
a. disorder
a. fistula
a. flexure
a. foreign body
a. function test
a. impalement
a. junction
a. line
a. malformation
a. manometry
a. melanoma
a. mucosal prolapse
a. myectomy
a. outlet obstruction
a. ring
a. septum
a. space
a. sphincter
a. surgery
a. variceal bleeding

anorectales

anorectoplasty
Laird-McMahon a.

anorectovaginoplasty

anorectum

anoscopy

anosigmoidoscopy

anosmia

anosmic

anospinal

anotia

anovesical

anovulation
persistent a.

anoxemia

anoxia
anoxic a.
diffusion a.
histotoxic a.
stagnant a.

anoxic anoxia

NOTES

ANP
autonomic nerve preservation
ansa, pl. **ansae**
a. cervicalis nerve
a. cervicalis root
Haller a.
Vieussens a.
anserina
anserine bursa
anserinus
anserinus
Anson-McVay
A.-M. hernia repair
A.-M. operation
ansotomy
antagonist
alpha-adrenergic a.
alpha-1-adrenergic a.
alpha-2-adrenergic receptor a.
antimuscarinic a.
beta-receptor a.
antagonistic muscle
antagonize
antalgesia
antalgic medication
antebrachial
a. fascia
a. flexor retinaculum
antebrachii
antecolic
a. anastomosis
a. long-loop isoperistaltic gastrojejunostomy
a. position
antecubital
a. approach
a. arteriovenous fistula
a. space
antegrade
a. approach
a. catheterization
a. continence enema (ACE)
a. continence enema procedure
a. double balloon-double wire technique
a. method
a. nailing
a. puncture
antegrade/retrograde cardioplegia technique
antemortem clot
antenatal dislocation
antenna procedure
antepartum hemorrhage
anteposition
anteprostate
anterior
a. abdominal injury
a. abdominal wall
a. acromioplasty
a. acromioplasty approach
a. angulation
a. angulation angle
a. antebrachial region
a. aortic wall
a. apical (AA)
a. aspiration
a. auricular artery
a. auricular groove
a. auricular muscle
a. auricular nerve
a. axillary approach
a. axillary fold
a. axillary line
a. basal (AB)
a. basal branch
a. basal segment
a. brachial region
a. calcaneal osteotomy
a. capsulolabral reconstruction
a. capsulotomy
a. carotid artery
a. cavernous sinus syndrome
a. cecal artery
a. cerebral artery
a. cervical diskectomy and fusion
a. cervical intertransverse muscle
a. cervical spine surgery
a. cervical surgery vocal cord damage
a. cervicothoracic junction surgery
a. chest wall syndrome
a. choroidal artery
a. ciliary artery
a. circulation aneurysm
a. circumflex humeral artery
a. clear space
a. clinoid process
a. column
a. column fracture
a. column osteosynthesis
a. commissure-posterior commissure line
a. communicating artery
a. complete dislocation
a. condylar canal
a. condyloid foramen
a. cord
a. cord compression
a. cornea
a. corneal curvature
a. corpectomy
a. correction
a. cortex
a. costotransverse ligament
a. cranial base

a. cranial fossa
a. cruciate ligament (ACL)
a. cruciate ligament reconstruction
a. crus
a. cutaneous branch
a. cutaneous nerve
a. cyst
a. descending artery
a. diskectomy
a. displacement
a. epineurotomy
a. esophagus
a. ethmoidal nerve
a. ethmoidectomy
a. extensile approach
a. extradural clinoidectomy
a. extremity
a. facial height (AFH)
a. focal point
a. fontanelle
a. forearm
a. fundoplasty
a. gastropexy
a. gastrotomy
a. great vessel
a. ground bundle
a. helical rim free flap
a. hip dislocation
a. humeral circumflex artery
a. incision
a. inferior cerebellar artery
a. inferior iliac spine
a. inferior segment
a. inguinal herniorrhaphy
a. innominate osteotomy
a. innominate rotation
a. intercostal artery
a. intermuscular septum
a. internal fixation
a. internal stabilization
a. intraoccipital joint
a. knee region
a. labial artery
a. labial commissure
a. labial nerve
a. labrum periosteum shoulder arthroscopic lesion
a. limiting ring
a. lingual gland
a. lip
a. lower cervical spine surgery
a. lumbar vertebral interbody fusion
a. mediastinal artery
a. mediastinal mass
a. mediastinum
a. meningeal artery
a. metallic fixation
a. midpapillary (AM)
a. midpapillary level
a. nasal meatus
a. nephrectomy
a. oblique position
a. oblique projection
a. parietal artery
a. partial laryngectomy
a. pelvic exenteration
a. plate fixation
a. Pólya procedure
a. and posterior (A&P)
a. and posterior repair
a. primary division
a. puncture
a. quadriceps musculocutaneous flap technique
a. radicular artery
a. rectopexy
a. rectus fascia
a. rectus muscle
a. rectus sheath
a. rectus sheath wall
a. resection
a. retroperitoneal decompression
a. retroperitoneal flank approach
a. rhizotomy
a. root
a. sandwich patch technique
a. scalene muscle
a. sclerotomy
a. screw fixation
a. scrotal nerve
a. semicircular canal
a. seromyotomy
a. serratus muscle
a. sheath
a. short-segment stabilization
a. shoulder dislocation
a. spinal artery
a. spinal artery syndrome
a. spinal fixation
a. spinal fusion
a. stabilization procedure
a. sternoclavicular ligament

NOTES

anterior *(continued)*
a. sternomastoid approach
a. superior alveolar artery
a. superior iliac spine
a. superior segment
a. supraclavicular nerve
a. surgical exposure
a. synechia formation
a. talofibular ligament rupture
a. temporal artery
a. thoracic wall
a. thoracotomy
a. tibial bursa
a. tibialis tendon
a. tibial muscle
a. tibial recurrent artery
a. tibiotalar ligament
a. transabdominal approach
a. transhepatic approach
a. translation
a. transthoracic approach
a. triangle
a. tubercle
a. ulnar recurrent artery
a. urethra
a. uveitis
a. vaginal fornix
a. vaginal trunk
a. vertical canal
a. view
a. vitrectomy
a. wound
anteriora
anteriores
anterior-inferior dislocation
anterior-posterior
a.-p. compression
a.-p. fusion with SSI
anterius
anterocrural celiac plexus block
anterograde
a. direction
a. transseptal technique
anterolateral
a. approach
a. compression fracture
a. cordotomy
a. dislocation
a. fontanelle
a. neck
a. thalamostriate artery
a. thoracotomy
a. thoracotomy incision
a. tractotomy
anterolaterales
anterolateralis
anterolateralium
anterolisthesis
anteromedial
a. arm
a. bundle
a. incision
a. retropharyngeal approach
a. thalamostriate artery
anteromediales
anteromesial temporal lobectomy
anteroposterior (AP)
a. chest x-ray
a. compression
a. correction
a. nail
a. projection
a. translation
anterosuperior external ilium movement
antevesical hernia
anthelix (*var. of* antihelix)
anthracosis
anthrone method
anthropoid pelvis
anthropometric evaluation
antiadhesion agent
antianalgesia
antiangiogenic effect
antiantibody formation
antiarrhythmic therapy
antibacterial agent
antibasement membrane
antibiotic
a. bead pouch
broad-spectrum a.
perioperative a.
postoperative a.
prophylactic a. (PA)
prophylactic intravenous a.
a. prophylaxis
systemic a.
a. therapy
topical a.
antibody
Bipolaris specific IgE, IgG a.
fungal a.
HCV a.
human monoclonal a.
a. linkage method
monoclonal a. (MAb)
unfractionated heparin a.
anticalculous
anticholinergic medication
anticipated blood loss
anticipatory coarticulation
anticoagulant
a. effect
lupus a.
a. monitoring
oral a.
a. therapy

anticoagulation
a. monitoring
a. monitoring requirement
oral a.
prophylactic a.
systemic a.
a. therapy
anticus
antidote
antidromic stimulation
antiembolic position
antiemetic
rescue a.
a. therapy
antiepileptic medication
antifibrinolytic agent
antifungal
a. agent
a. esophageal infection
a. prophylaxis
a. regimen
a. therapy
a. treatment
antifungal-resistant opportunistic infection
antigen
carbohydrate a. 19-9 (CA 19-9)
carcinoembryonic a. (CEA)
CTL-inducing peptide a.
hepatitis B surface a. (HB_s)
human leukocyte class II DR a.
proliferating cell nuclear a. (PCNA)
serum carcinoembryonic a.
tumor a.
antigen-extracted allogeneic bone
antigenic modulation
antiglaucoma surgery
antiglomerular
a. basement membrane
a. basement membrane antibody disease
antigravity muscle
antihelix, anthelix
antihemophilic
antihemorrhagic
antihormonal therapy
antiincontinence procedure
antiinflammatory medication
antilymphoid therapy
antimesenteric
a. enterotomy
a. fat pad
a. side
antimetabolite
antimotility agent
antimuscarinic antagonist
antimycotic
antineoplastic agent
antinephritic
antiniad
antinial
antinion
antinociception
intrathecal a.
antinociceptive
antioxidant
antiperistaltic
a. anastomosis
a. operation
antiphospholipid antibody assay
antiplatelet regimen
antipyogenic
antireflux
a. flap-valve mechanism
a. operation
a. procedure
a. surgery
a. therapy
a. ureteral implantation technique
antirefluxing colonic conduit
antisaccade
antisense
antisialagogue
antitension line
antithrombin
a. III (ATIII)
a. III plasma level
antithromboembolic prophylaxis
antithrombotic
a. activity
a. therapy
antitragicus muscle
antitragus
antitubular basement membrane
antra (*pl. of* antrum)
antral
a. biopsy
a. edema
a. exclusion
a. irrigation
a. membrane
a. sphincter
a. stenting

NOTES

antral *(continued)*
a. tumor
a. web
antrectomy
Roux-en-Y biliary bypass with a.
antroduodenectomy
antropyloric canal
antroscopy
antrostomy
inferior meatal a.
intraoral a.
nasal a.
antrotomy
antrum, pl. **antra**
gastric a.
a. of Highmore
mastoid a.
maxillary a.
pyloric a.
Willis a.
Antyllus method
anulus, pl. **anuli**
Haller a.
mitral valve a.
tricuspid valve a.
anum
per a.
anuria
anuric
anus, pl. **ani**
artificial a.
ectopic a.
imperforate a.
vaginal ectopic a.
anusitis
AO
AO classification
AO external fixation
AO procedure
AO rigid fixation
AO spinal internal fixation
AO technique
AOD
aortic occlusive disease
AOIVM
angiographically occult intracranial vascular malformation
aorta, pl. **aortae**
abdominal a.
appendicular a.
arcuate a.
coarctation of a.
deep articular a.
dissection of a.
infrarenal a.
posterior articular a.
proximal a.
pseudocoarctation of a.
recoarctation of a.
thoracic a.
aortectomy
aortic
a. anastomosis
a. aneurysm
a. aneurysmal disease
a. aneurysmectomy
a. aneurysm tissue
a. arch
a. arch disease
a. atheromatous disease
a. bifurcation
a. blood pressure
a. body
a. body tumor
a. clamping
a. conduit
a. cross-clamping
a. cuff
a. dicrotic notch pressure
a. dissection
a. foramen
a. graft placement
a. hiatus
a. hypoplasia
a. intramural hematoma
a. knob
a. laceration
a. neck
a. nipple
a. node metastasis
a. occlusion
a. occlusive disease (AOD)
a. patch
a. perfusion
a. pressure gradient
a. pullback pressure
a. reconstructive surgery
a. regurgitation murmur
a. ring
a. root reconstruction
a. root velocity waveform
a. rupture
a. sac
a. stump blow-out
a. transection
a. valve area
a. valve atresia
a. valve disease
a. valve gradient
a. valve insufficiency
a. valve leaflet
a. valve repair
a. valve replacement
a. valve resistance
a. valve restenosis
a. valve velocity profile

a. valvotomy
a. valvuloplasty
a. wall
a. wall deterioration
aortica
aorticorenal ganglion
aortic-pulmonic window
aorticum
aorticus
aortoannular ectasia
aortocaval
a. fistula
aortocoronary
aortoduodenal fistula
aortoenteric fistula
aortoesophageal fistula
aortofemoral
a. bypass
a. bypass graft (AFBG)
aortogastric fistula
aortograft duodenal fistula
aortoiliac
a. aneurysm
a. angioplasty
a. bypass
a. occlusive disease
aortoplasty
patch a.
aortopulmonary
a. fenestration
a. window
aortorenal
a. bypass
a. reconstruction
a. reimplantation
aortorrhaphy
aortosigmoid fistula
aortotomy
AP
acute pancreatitis
anteroposterior
A&P
anterior and posterior
A&P projection
A&P repair
APACHE
acute physiology and chronic health evaluation
APACHE-II
APACHE-II point
APACHE-II score
APACHE-II system
apatite calculus
APC
adenomatous polyposis coli
A-P-C
adenoidal-pharyngeal-conjunctival
apellous
aperta
Apert syndrome
apertura
aperture
inferior pelvic a.
inferior thoracic a.
laryngeal a.
lateral cerebral a.
superior pelvic a.
superior thoracic a.
upper thorax a.
apertures of abdomen
apex, pl. **apices**
corneal a.
a. dorsal angulation
a. fracture
lateral a.
Apgar score
aphakia
extracapsular a.
aphakic correction
aphthous
a. ulcer
a. ulceration
aphthous-type lesion
apical
anterior a. (AA)
a. fenestration
a. gland
a. infection
inferior a. (IA)
lateral a. (LA)
a. left ventricular puncture
a. lordotic projection
a. lordotic view
a. polar nephrectomy
a. ramification
a. segment
septal a. (SA)
a. space
a. suture
a. transverse (AP-T)
apicale
apicales
apically repositioned flap in mucogingival surgery

NOTES

apiceotomy
apices (*pl. of* apex)
apicoectomy
apicolysis
extrapleural a.
Semb a.
apicoposterior segment
apicoposterius
apicostomy
apicotomy
Apley
A. compression test
A. maneuver
apnea
induced a.
obstructive a.
posthyperventilation a.
postoperative a.
apneic
a. oxygenation
a. threshold
apneustic
a. breathing
a. respiration
apocrine
a. carcinoma
a. gland
a. metaplasia
APOLT
auxiliary partial orthotopic liver transplantation
APOLT technique
aponeurectomy
aponeurorrhaphy
aponeurosis, pl. **aponeuroses**
abdominal a.
Denonvilliers a.
epicranial a.
external oblique a.
internal oblique a.
Petit a.
temporal a.
thoracolumbar a.
transversus abdominis a.
triangular a.
aponeurotic
a. abscess
a. closure
a. defect
a. flap
a. layer
aponeurotica
aponeurotomy
apophysary point
apophysial, apophyseal
a. fracture
a. point
apophysis, pl. **apophyses**
iliac a.
ring a.
slipped vertebral a.
temporal a.
vertebral ring a.
apophysitis
calcaneal a.
apoplectic coma
apoplexy
apoptosis
resuscitation-induced pulmonary a.
selective lectin-triggered a.
apostaxis
apotreptic therapy
apparatus
alimentary a.
digestive a.
genitourinary a.
hyoid a.
lacrimal a.
urinary a.
urogenital a.
appearance
bat-wing a.
beads-on-a-string a.
beefy a.
cobblestone a.
coiled spring a.
collar-bone a.
corkscrew a.
dewy a.
gland a.
granular a.
ground-glass a.
hobnailed a.
honeycombed a.
lead-pipe a.
macroscopic a.
mammographic a.
meaty a.
moth-eaten a.
mottled a.
nutmeg a.
onion peel a.
sausage-shaped a.
signet-ring a.
speckled a.
steamy a.
string-of-beads a.
tigroid a.
whorled a.
appendage
epiploic a.
omental a.
testicular a.
vermiform a.
vesicular a.

appendectomy, appendicectomy
auricular a.
colonoscopic a.
emergency a.
emergent a.
incidental a.
a. incision
interval a.
inversion a.
inversion-ligation a.
laparoscopic a. (LA)
laser-assisted a.
McBurney a.
negative a.
open a. (OA)
percutaneous a.
appendiceal
a. abscess
a. adenocarcinoma
a. cancer
a. colic
a. CT
a. fecalith
a. gangrene
a. intussusception
a. mass
a. opening
a. orifice
a. perforation
appendices (*pl. of* appendix)
appendicitis
chronic a.
epiploic a.
gangrenous a.
appendicocele
appendicocystostomy
continent cutaneous a.
dismembered reimplanted a.
nonplicated a.
orthotopic a.
plicated a.
reversed reimplanted a.
appendicoenterostomy
appendicolithiasis
appendicolysis
appendicostomy
appendicovesicostomy
Mitrofanoff a.
appendicular
a. aorta
a. artery
a. colic
a. muscle
a. skeleton
a. vein
appendiculare
appendiculares
appendicularis
appendix, pl. **appendices**
cecal a.
ensiform a.
epiploic a.
a. mucocele
pelvic a.
vermiform a.
apperceptive mass
applanation
a. pressure
tension by a.
a. tonometry
apple
Adam's a.
apple-core lesion
appliance modification
application
arch bar a.
cast a.
clip a.
cold a.
force a.
frame a.
heat a.
ice a.
interpleural a.
Kumar a.
laparoscopic clip a.
paraspinal rod a.
pilot a.
topical iodine a.
traction a.
transverse fixator a.
Appolito
A. operation
A. suture technique
apponensplasty
ring sublimis a.
appose
apposition
a. of skull suture
stent a.
a. suture technique
approach
Abbott-Carpenter posterior a.
Abbott knee a.

NOTES

approach *(continued)*
abdominal a.
acetabular extensile a.
acromiothoracic a.
adaptational a.
aggressive surgical a.
Alken a.
alternative surgical a.
anesthetic a.
antecubital a.
antegrade a.
anterior acromioplasty a.
anterior axillary a.
anterior extensile a.
anterior retroperitoneal flank a.
anterior sternomastoid a.
anterior transabdominal a.
anterior transhepatic a.
anterior transthoracic a.
anterolateral a.
anteromedial retropharyngeal a.
axillary a.
Bailey-Badgley anterior cervical a.
Banks-Laufman a.
basal subfrontal a.
Bennett posterior shoulder a.
Berger-Bookwalter posterior a.
Berke a.
bilateral ilioinguinal a.
bilateral sacroiliac a.
Bosworth a.
Boyd a.
Boyd-Sisk a.
brachial artery a.
Brackett-Osgood posterior a.
Brodsky-Tullos-Gartsman a.
Broomhead medial a.
Brown knee a.
Brown lateral a.
Bruner a.
Bruser knee a.
Bruser lateral a.
Bryan-Morrey elbow a.
Bryan-Morrey extensive posterior a.
buccopharyngeal a.
buttonhole a.
Caldwell-Luc a.
Callahan a.
Campbell posterior shoulder a.
Campbell posterolateral a.
Carnesale acetabular extensile a.
Carnesale hip a.
case-by-case a.
Cave hip a.
Cave knee a.
central a.
cerebellopontine angle a.
cervical a.
cervicothoracic a.
choledochal fiberoscopic a.
Cloward cervical disk a.
cochleovestibular a.
Codman saber-cut shoulder a.
Colonna-Ralston ankle a.
Colonna-Ralston medial a.
combined anterior and posterior a.
combined laparoscopic and thoracoscopic a.
combined low cervical and transthoracic a.
combined presigmoid-transtransversarium intradural a.
combined transsylvian and middle fossa a.
consortial a.
Coonse-Adams knee a.
Cubbins shoulder a.
curved a.
deltoid-splitting shoulder a.
deltopectoral a.
Dickinson a.
distal interphalangeal joint a.
dorsal finger a.
dorsal midline a.
dorsalward a.
dorsolateral a.
dorsomedial a.
dorsoplantar a.
dorsoradial a.
dorsorostral a.
dorsoulnar a.
double-doughnut a.
double-seton modified surgical a.
Duran a.
DuVries a.
Endius a.
endovascular a.
extended iliofemoral a.
extended subfrontal a.
extensile a.
extrabursal a.
extralaryngeal a.
extraperitoneal a.
extrapharyngeal a.
extravesical Lich a.
extreme lateral transcondylar a.
Fahey a.
far lateral inferior suboccipital a.
fascial sling a.
femoral artery a.
Fernandez extensile anterior a.
flank a.
foraminal a.
fornix a.
Fowler-Philip a.
frontal cortical a.

frontotemporal a.
gasless laparoscopic a.
Gatellier-Chastang ankle a.
Gatellier-Chastang posterolateral a.
genetic a.
Gibson a.
Gordon a.
Guleke-Stookey a.
Hardinge lateral a.
Harmon cervical a.
Harmon modified posterolateral a.
Harmon shoulder a.
Harris anterolateral a.
Harris lateral a.
Hay lateral a.
Henderson posterolateral a.
Henderson posteromedial a.
Henry anterior strap a.
Henry anterolateral a.
Henry extensile a.
Henry posterior interosseous nerve a.
Henry radial a.
Hoffmann a.
Hoppenfeld-Deboer a.
Howorth a.
humeral a.
idiographic a.
Iliff a.
iliofemoral a.
ilioinguinal acetabular a.
immunocytochemical a.
inferior extradural a.
inferior-lateral endonasal transsphenoidal a.
inferior transvermian a.
infralabyrinthine a.
inframammary a.
infratemporal fossa a.
infratentorial supracerebellar a.
inguinal a.
interfascial a.
interforniceal a.
interhemispheric a.
interscalene a.
intradural a.
intranasal a.
intratentorial supracerebellar a.
Japanese a.
keyhole a.
Kikuchi-MacNap-Moreau a.
Kocher curved L a.
Kocher-Gibson posterolateral a.
Kocher-Langenbeck a.
Kocher lateral J a.
Koenig-Schaefer medial a.
Kraske parasacral a.
Kugel a.
labioglossomandibular a.
labiomandibular a.
laparoscopic a.
lateral deltoid splitting a.
lateral extracavitary a.
lateral Gatellier-Chastung a.
lateral J a.
lateral Kocher a.
Lazepen-Gamidov anteromedial a.
Leslie-Ryan anterior axillary a.
lesser sac a.
Letournel-Judet a.
limbal a.
lingual a.
Lortat-Jacob a.
Ludloff medial a.
lumbar a.
Mayo a.
McAfee a.
McConnell extensile a.
McConnell median and ulnar nerve a.
McFarland-Osborne lateral a.
McLaughlin a.
McWhorter posterior shoulder a.
Mears-Rubash a.
medial extradural a.
medial parapatellar capsular a.
midlateral a.
midline medial a.
midline spinal a.
minimally invasive a.
Minkoff-Jaffe-Menendez posterior a.
Mize-Bucholz-Grogen a.
Molesworth-Campbell elbow a.
Moore posterior a.
multidisciplinary a.
multiple-stage a.
neurosurgical a.
nonoperative a.
Ollier arthrodesis a.
Ollier lateral a.
open laparoscopic a.
operative a.
orbitozygomatic temporopolar a.
oropharyngeal a.

NOTES

approach *(continued)*
Osborne posterior a.
otomicrosurgical transtemporal a.
palmar a.
paramedian a.
pararectus a.
paraspinal a.
parietooccipital a.
patella turndown a.
percutaneous transhepatic a.
peroral a.
Perry extensile anterior a.
petrosal a.
Pfannenstiel transverse a.
Phemister medial a.
plantar a.
Pogrund lateral a.
posterior costotransversectomy a.
posterior inverted-U a.
posterior laparoscopic a.
posterior lumbar a.
posterior midline a.
posterior occipitocervical a.
posterior transolecranon a.
posterolateral a.
posteromedial a.
preperitoneal a.
presigmoid-transtransversarium intradural a.
proprioceptive neuromuscular facilitation a.
proximal interphalangeal joint a.
pterional a.
pulp a.
Putti posterior a.
rapid-volume a.
Redman a.
regressive-reconstructive a.
Reinert acetabular extensile a.
retrograde endoscopic a.
retrograde femoral a.
retrolabyrinthine presigmoid a.
retroperitoneal a.
retropharyngeal a.
retrosigmoid a.
rhinoseptal a.
Risdon a.
Roberts a.
Roos a.
Rowe posterior shoulder a.
saber-cut a.
sacral-foraminal a.
sacroperineal a.
screw-plate a.
sensorimotor stimulation a.
skull base a.
Smith-Petersen a.
Smith-Petersen-Cave-Van Gorder anterolateral a.
Smith-Robinson cervical disk a.
somatic gene-transfer a.
Somerville anterior a.
Southwick-Robinson anterior cervical a.
Spetzler anterior transoral a.
split-heel a.
split-patellar a.
stabilization a.
standard open a.
sternum-splitting a.
subchoroidal a.
subclavicular a.
subfrontal a.
subfrontal-transbasal a.
sublabial midline rhinoseptal a.
suboccipital-subtemporal a.
suboccipital-transmeatal a.
subtemporal-intradural a.
superior-intradural a.
supine-oblique a.
supracerebellar a.
supraclavicular a.
supraduodenal a.
supraorbital-pterional a.
supratentorial a.
surgical a.
suspended-pedicle a.
Swedish a.
sylvian a.
takedown abdominal a.
Taylor a.
therapeutic a.
Thompson anterolateral a.
Thompson anteromedial a.
Thompson posterior radial a.
thoracic a.
thoracoabdominal extrapleural a.
thoracoabdominal intrapleural a.
thoracolumbar retroperitoneal a.
thoracoscopic a.
thoracotomy a.
thumb metacarpophalangeal joint a.
transabdominal a.
transacromial a.
transanal a.
transantral a.
transantral ethmoidal a.
transaxillary a.
transbrachioradialis a.
transcallosal transventricular a.
transcanine a.
transcavernous transpetrous apex a.
transcerebellar hemispheric a.
transcervical a.
transclavicular a.

transcoccygeal a.
transcochlear a.
transcortical transventricular a.
transcranial frontal-temporal-orbital a.
transcranial-supraorbital a.
transcubital a.
transcystic a.
transduodenal a.
transfibular a.
transfrontal a.
transgluteal a.
transhepatic a.
transhiatal a.
translabyrinthine and suboccipital a.
transmandibular-glossopharyngeal a.
transmastoid a.
transmeatal a.
transmural a.
transolecranon a.
transoral a.
transpalatal a.
transpapillary a.
transpedicular a.
transperitoneal a.
transradial a.
transrectal a.
transseptal a.
transsinus a.
transsphenoidal a.
transsternal a.
transsylvian a.
transtentorial a.
transthoracic a.
transtorcular a.
transtrochanteric a.
transvaginal a.
transvenous a.
transverse a.
transxiphoid a.
trapdoor a.
triradiate acetabular extensile a.
triradiate transtrochanteric a.
unilateral a.
unilateral sacroiliac a.
vaginal wall a.
volar finger a.
volar midline a.
volar radial a.
volar ulnar a.
volarward a.
Wadsworth elbow a.
Wadsworth posterolateral a.
Wagoner posterior a.
Watson-Jones anterior a.
Watson-Jones lateral a.
Wiltberger anterior cervical a.
Wiltse-Spencer paraspinal a.
Yee posterior shoulder a.
zig-zag a.
Z-plasty a.

approximate
a. entropy
a. lethal concentration

approximation
Friedewald a.
skin a.
successive a.
a. suture technique
tissue a.
vocal fold a.
wound a.

APR
abdominoperineal resection
APR cement fixation

aproctia

apron
abdominal a.
fatty a.
a. flap
a. skin incision

APRV
airway pressure release ventilation

APSA
American Pediatric Surgical Association

AP-T
apical transverse
AP-T image

aquapuncture

aquatic stabilization program

aqueduct
Cotunnius a.
sylvian a.
a. veil

aqueductal intubation

aqueductus

aqueous
a. extract
a. humor
a. solution
a. vein

arachnoid
a. cyst
a. granulation

NOTES

arachnoid *(continued)*
a. hemorrhage
a. mater
a. membrane
a. retrocerebellar pouch
a. space
a. villus
arachnoiditis
adhesive a.
Araki-Sako technique
araldehyde-tanned bovine carotid artery graft
Arantius
A. body
canal of A.
A. duct
A. ligament
plate of A.
Arbor
Ann A. stage IE, IIE
arborization
a. block
pattern a.
pulmonary a.
Arbuthnot Lane disease
arc
bregmatolambdoid a.
flexion-extension a.
mobile a.
nasobregmatic a.
nasooccipital a.
Riolan a.
arcade
gastroepiploic a.
intestinal arterial a.
pancreaticoduodenal arterial a.
Riolan a.
arch
abdominothoracic a.
aortic a.
arterial a.
axillary a.
a. bar application
crural a.
deep crural a.
deep palmar a.
double aortic a.
expansion of the a.
extramedullary alignment a.
femoral a.
a. fracture
hemal a.
iliopectineal a.
interrupted aortic a.
jugular venous a.
Langer a.
neural a.
posterior a.
prepancreatic a.
pubic a.
Simon expansion a.
superciliary a.
superficial palmar a.
supraorbital a.
tendinous a.
transverse aponeurotic a.
Treitz a.
vertebral a.
wire a.
zygomatic a.
arch-and-slouch position
archenteronoma
archicerebellum
architectural pattern
architecture
lesion a.
tissue a.
arch-loop-whorl
arciform vein of kidney
arctation
arcuata
arcuate
a. aorta
a. artery
a. eminence
a. incision
a. line
a. nerve fiber bundle
a. pubic ligament
a. suture technique
a. transverse keratotomy
a. vein
a. zone
arcuation
arcuatum
arcus
corneal a.
arcutata
ARDS
acute respiratory distress syndrome
adult respiratory distress syndrome
area
anastomotic a.
aortic valve a.
articulation a.
bare a.
body surface a. (BSA)
cortical a.
cribriform a.
crural a.
denture foundation a.
end-diastolic cross-sectional a. (EDA)
end-systolic cross-sectional a.
fusion a.
gastric a.

jejunal puncture a.
Kiesselbach a.
Killian-Jamieson a.
Laimer a.
left ventricular end-diastolic a. (LVEDa)
left ventricular end-systolic a. (LVESa)
Little a.
mitral valve a.
Panum fusion a.
paraglottic a.
pericolostomy a.
pressure a.
pressure-sensitive a.
proliferation a.
pulmonary valve a.
right crural a.
skip a.
Stroud pectinated a.
tissue-bearing a.
total body surface a. (TBSA)
tricuspid valve a.
a. under curve (AUC)
valve orifice a.
visual association a.
voluntary a.

area-length method

areflexia
detrusor a.

areola, pl. **areolae**

areolar
a. complex
a. connective tissue
a. gland
a. incision
a. mastopexy

areolares

areolaris

argon
a. beam coagulation
a. laser endophotocoagulation
a. laser iridectomy
a. laser photocoagulation
a. laser therapy
a. laser trabeculopexy
a. laser trabeculoplasty

Argyll-Robertson
A.-R. operation
A.-R. suture technique

argyrophilic
a. nucleolar organizer region
a. nucleolar organizer region staining

arhinia

Aria coronary bypass

Aries-Pitanguy
A.-P. breast reduction
A.-P. mammaplasty
A.-P. operation

Arion operation

aristotelian method

Arlt
A. epicanthus repair
A. eyelid repair
A. line
A. operation
A. suture technique

Arlt-Jaesche
A.-J. excision
A.-J. operation

arm
anteromedial a.
brawny a.
dissected tissue a.
endosteal implant a.
a. flap
a. position
posterior a.

Armaly-Drance technique

armamentarium
endodontic a.

arm-extension position

Armistead
A. technique
A. ulnar lengthening operation

Armstrong acromionectomy

Arneth classification

Arnold
A. body
A. bundle
A. canal
foramen of A.
A. ganglion
A. nerve
A. tract

Arnold-Chiari
A.-C. deformity
A.-C. malformation
A.-C. syndrome

Aronson-Prager technique

around the clock (ATC)

around-the-clock
a.-t.-c. dosing

NOTES

around-the-clock *(continued)*
a.-t.-c. oral maintenance bronchodilator therapy
arrangement
lesion a.
array
epidural electrode a.
subdural electrode a.
arrector, pl. **arrectores**
arrectores pilorum
a. pilus
arrest
cardiac a.
circulatory a.
deep hypothermic circulatory a. (DHCA)
hypothermic circulatory a.
hypothermic hypokalemic cardioplegic a. (HHCA)
imminent cardiac a.
profoundly hypothermic circulatory a. (PHCA)
secondary a.
traumatic cardiac a.
vagal a.
arrested-heart
a.-h. revascularization
a.-h. revascularization technique
arrhenoblastoma
Arrhigi
point of A.
arrhythmia
atrial a.
exercise-induced a.
supraventricular a.
arrhythmogenic
Arrowhead operation
Arroyo
A. cataract extraction
A. dacryostomy
A. keratoplasty
A. operation
A. tenotomy
Arruga
A. cataract extraction
A. dacryostomy
A. keratoplasty
A. operation
A. tenotomy
Arruga-Berens operation
arsenal
therapeutic a.
arteria, pl. **arteriae**
arterial
a. adaptation
a. anastomosis
a. aneurysm
a. angioma
a. anomaly
a. arch
a. bleeding
a. bleeding site
a. blood collection
a. blood gas
a. blood pressure
a. branch
a. cannulation anesthetic technique
a. carbon dioxide
a. carbon dioxide pressure
a. catheterization
a. cerebral circle
a. chemoembolization
a. circulation
a. decortication
a. dicrotic notch pressure
a. disorder
a. embolectomy
a. embolization
a. entry site
a. flap
a. groove
a. hemorrhage
a. hypertension
a. inflow
a. injury
a. lactate level
a. mean line
a. occlusion
a. occlusive disease
a. oxygen desaturation
a. oxygen partial pressure (PaO_2)
a. oxygen saturation (SaO_2)
a. oxyhemoglobin saturation (SpO_2)
a. partial pressure
a. partial pressure of CO_2
a. reconstructive procedure
a. reconstructive surgery
a. revascularization
a. ring
a. stenosis
a. supply
a. switch operation
a. switch procedure
a. system
a. thrombosis
a. transfusion
umbilical a. (UA)
a. vein
a. wall dissection
a. wedge
arterial-arterial fistula
arterial-enteric fistula
arterialization
arterialized flap
arterial-portal fistula
arterial-selective intravenous vasodilator

arteriectomy
arteriobiliary fistula
arteriocapillary
arteriococcygeal gland
arteriogram
arteriographic presence
arteriography
arteriola, pl. **arteriolae**
arteriolar attenuation
arteriole
afferent glomerular a.
capillary a.
copper-wire a.
efferent glomerular a.
silver-wire a.
arteriolith
arteriolovenular anastomosis
arterionephrosclerosis
arterioplasty
arterioportal fistula
arterioportobiliary fistula
arteriorrhaphy
arteriorrhexis
arteriosa
arteriosclerosis obliterans (ASO)
arteriosclerotic
a. aneurysm
a. gangrene
a. kidney
arteriosinusoidal penile fistula
arteriostenosis
arteriosum
arteriosus
patent ductus a. (PDA)
arteriotomy
brachial a.
end-to-side a.
arteriovenosa
arteriovenous (A-V, AV)
a. anastomosis
a. aneurysm
a. dialysis
a. fistula (AVF)
a. hemofiltration
a. malformation (AVM)
a. subclavian fistula
arteritis
giant cell a.
inflammatory a.
Takayasu a.
temporal a.

artery
abdominal aortic a.
aberrant obturator a.
accessory obturator a.
acetabular a.
acromial a.
acromiothoracic a.
alveolar a.
anal canal a.
angular a.
anomalous vertebral a.
anterior auricular a.
anterior carotid a.
anterior cecal a.
anterior cerebral a.
anterior choroidal a.
anterior ciliary a.
anterior circumflex humeral a.
anterior communicating a.
anterior descending a.
anterior humeral circumflex a.
anterior inferior cerebellar a.
anterior intercostal a.
anterior labial a.
anterior mediastinal a.
anterior meningeal a.
anterior parietal a.
anterior radicular a.
anterior spinal a.
anterior superior alveolar a.
anterior temporal a.
anterior tibial recurrent a.
anterior ulnar recurrent a.
anterolateral thalamostriate a.
anteromedial thalamostriate a.
appendicular a.
arcuate a.
ascending cervical a.
ascending pharyngeal a.
atherosclerotic carotid a.
axillary a.
basilar a.
blood supply a.
brachial a.
brachiocephalic trunk a.
bronchial a.
buccal a.
buccinator a.
calcaneal a.
calcareous a.
calcarine a.
callosomarginal a.

NOTES

artery *(continued)*
caroticotympanic a.
carpal a.
caudal pancreatic a.
cecal a.
celiac a.
celiacomesenteric a.
central retinal a.
central sulcal a.
cerebellar a.
cerebral a.
cervicovaginal a.
choroidal a.
ciliary a.
cilioretinal a.
circumflex femoral a.
circumflex humeral a.
circumflex iliac a.
circumflex scapular a.
coarctation of pulmonary a.
coeliac a.
colic a.
collateral digital a.
colli a.
common femoral a. (CFA)
common femoral artery-superficial femoral a. (CFA-SFA)
common hepatic a.
common iliac a.
common interosseous a.
common palmar digital a.
common peroneal a.
common plantar digital a.
communicating a.
companion a.
copper-wire a.
cortical a.
costocervical a.
cricothyroid a.
cystic a.
deep auricular a.
deep brachial a.
deep cervical a.
deep circumflex inguinal a.
deep epigastric a.
deep femoral a.
deep profunda brachial a.
deep temporal a.
deferential a.
descending genicular a.
descending palatine a.
descending scapular a.
digital collateral a.
diploic a.
D-loop transposition of the great a.
dolichoectatic a.
dorsal digital a.
dorsal interosseous a.
dorsal pancreatic a.
dorsal scapular a.
dorsal thoracic a.
a. ectasia
ectatic carotid a.
endometrial spiral a.
epigastric a.
esophageal a.
ethmoidal a.
external acoustic meatus a.
external carotid a. (ECA)
external iliac a.
external mammary a.
external maxillary a.
external pudendal a.
external spermatic a.
extradural vertebral a.
facial a.
femoral a.
first metacarpal a.
frontal a.
gastric a.
gastroduodenal a.
gastroepiploic a.
gastroomental a.
genicular a.
gingival a.
gonadal a.
great anastomotic a.
greater palatine a.
great pancreatic a.
great radicular a.
great superior pancreatic a.
hepatic a.
Huebner recurrent a.
humeral a.
hyaloid a.
hypogastric a.
hypoglossal a.
hypophyseal a.
ileal a.
ileocolic a.
iliac a.
iliofemoral flap a.
iliolumbar a.
inferior alveolar a.
inferior carotid a.
inferior cerebral a.
inferior epigastric a.
inferior gluteal a.
inferior hemorrhoidal a.
inferior hypophysial a.
inferior internal parietal a.
inferior labial a.
inferior laryngeal a.
inferior lateral genicular a.
inferior medial genicular a.

inferior mesenteric a. (IMA)
inferior pancreatic a.
inferior pancreaticoduodenal a.
inferior phrenic a.
inferior rectal a.
inferior suprarenal a.
inferior thoracic a.
inferior thyroid a.
inferior ulnar collateral a.
inferior vesical a.
infragenicular popliteal a. (IGPA)
infraorbital a.
infrascapular a.
innominate a.
insular a.
intercostal a.
interlobular a.
intermediate temporal a.
internal auditory a.
internal carotid a. (ICA)
internal iliac a.
internal mammary a. (IMA)
internal maxillary a.
internal pudendal a.
internal rectal a.
internal spermatic a.
internal thoracic a.
intestinal a.
intramural a.
a. island flap
jejunal a.
labyrinthine a.
lacrimal a.
left coronary a.
left vertebral a.
lenticulostriate a.
lesser palatine a.
lienal a.
a. ligation
lingual a.
long thoracic a.
lower thyroid a.
lowest lumbar a.
lowest thyroid a.
lumbar a.
major a.
marginal a.
masseteric a.
mediastinal a.
medium-sized a.
medullary spinal a.
mental a.
mesenteric a.
metatarsal a.
middle cerebral a. (MCA)
muscular a.
musculophrenic a.
mylohyoid a.
Neubauer a.
nutrient a.
obturator a.
occipital a.
a. occlusion
ophthalmic a.
orbitofrontal a.
ovarian a.
palmar interosseous a.
palpebral a.
pancreatic a.
pancreaticoduodenal a.
a. of the pancreatic tail
parathyroid a.
parietal a.
parietooccipital a.
pericallosal a.
pericardiacophrenic a.
perineal a.
peroneal a.
petrosal a.
pontine a.
popliteal a.
postcentral sulcal a.
posterior alveolar a.
posterior auricular a.
posterior cecal a.
posterior cerebral a.
posterior choroidal a.
posterior circumflex humeral a.
posterior communicating a.
posterior humeral circumflex a.
posterior inferior cerebellar a.
posterior intercostal a. 1–11
posterior interosseous a.
posterior labial a.
posterior mediastinal a.
posterior meningeal a.
posterior pancreaticoduodenal a.
posterior parietal a.
posterior radicular a.
posterior spinal a.
posterior superior alveolar a.
posterior temporal a.
posterior tibial recurrent a.
posterior ulnar recurrent a.

NOTES

artery *(continued)*
posterolateral central a.
posteromedial central a.
precentral sulcal a.
precuneal a.
pre-rolandic a.
princeps cervicis a.
princeps pollicis a.
profunda brachii a.
profunda cervicalis a.
proper hepatic a.
proper palmar digital a.
proper plantar digital a.
pterygoid a.
pubic a.
pulmonary a. (PA)
pyloric a.
radial collateral a.
radial index a.
radial recurrent a.
radicular a.
a. reconstruction
recurrent interosseous a.
recurrent radial a.
recurrent ulnar a.
renal a.
retroduodenal a.
retroesophageal a.
retrograde vascularization of superior mesenteric a.
right colic a.
right femoral a.
right middle suprarenal a.
right obturator a.
right replaced hepatic a.
right subclavian a.
right testicular a.
rolandic a.
scrotal a.
second lumbar a.
sheathed a.
short central a.
short gastric a.
sigmoid a.
sphenopalatine a.
spinal a.
splenic a. (SA)
a. stenosis
sternal a.
sternocleidomastoid a.
sternomastoid a.
striate a.
stylomastoid a.
subclavian a.
subcostal a.
sublingual a.
submental a.
subscapular a.
sulcal a.
superficial brachial a.
superficial cervical a.
superficial circumflex iliac a.
superficial epigastric a.
superficial external pudendal a.
superficial palmar a.
superficial perineal a.
superficial temporal a.
superficial temporal artery to middle cerebral a. (STA-MCA)
superficial temporalis a.
superficial volar a.
superior alveolar a.
superior cerebellar a.
superior epigastric a.
superior gluteal a.
superior hemorrhoidal a.
superior hypophysial a.
superior intercostal a.
superior internal parietal a.
superior labial a.
superior lateral genicular a.
superior medial genicular a.
superior mesenteric a. (SMA)
superior pancreaticoduodenal a.
superior phrenic a.
superior rectal a.
superior suprarenal a.
superior thoracic a.
superior thyroid a.
superior ulnar collateral a.
superior vesical a.
supraduodenal a.
supragenicular popliteal a. (SGPA)
supraorbital a.
suprascapular a.
supratrochlear a.
supreme intercostal a.
sural a.
temporal a.
testicular a.
thoracoacromial a.
thoracodorsal a.
thymic a.
thyrocervical a.
thyroid ima a.
tortuous intercostal a.
transverse cervical a.
transverse facial a.
transverse pancreatic a.
transverse scapular a.
ulnar a.
umbilical a.
urethral a.
uterine a.
vaginal a.
vertebral a.

volar interosseous a.
Wilkie a.
a. of Willis
zygomaticofacial a.
zygomaticoorbital a.

arthralgia
asymmetrical a.
recurrent a.

arthrifluent abscess

arthritis, pl. **arthritides**
gonococcal a.
A. Helplessness Index (AHI)
hemophilic a.
juvenile rheumatoid a.
Lyme a.
pisotriquetral a.
psoriatic a.
pyogenic a.
reactive a.
rheumatoid a.
scaphotrapezial trapezoid a.
septic a.
tuberculous a.

arthrocele

arthrodesis
Adkins technique spinal a.
atlantoaxial a.
Batchelor-Brown extraarticular subtalar a.
beak modification with triple a.
Brockman-Nissen wrist a.
Charnley compression a.
compression a.
excisional a.
extension injury posterior atlantoaxial a.
extraarticular a.
resection a.
tarsometatarsal truncated-wedge a.
tibiocalcaneal a.
tibiotalocalcaneal a.
truncated tarsometatarsal wedge a.
truncated-wedge a.

arthrodial
a. articulation
a. cartilage
a. joint

arthrographic capsular distention and rupture technique

arthrology

arthropathy
cuff tear a.
hemophilic a.
hydroxyapatite a.
osteopulmonary a.
rotator cuff a.

arthrophyte

arthroplasty
abrasion a.
acetabular cup a.
Albright-Chase a.
Ashworth hand a.
Ashworth implant a.
Aufranc cup a.
Austin-Moore a.
autogenous interpositional shoulder a.
Bechtol a.
bipolar hip a.
Bryan a.
Campbell interpositional a.
Campbell resection a.
capitellocondylar total elbow a.
capsular interposition a.
carpometacarpal a.
Carroll a.
cemented total hip a.
cementless total hip a.
Charnley total hip a.
Clayton forefoot a.
Colonna trochanteric a.
condylar implant a.
constrained ankle a.
constrained shoulder a.
convex condylar implant a.
Coonrad-Morrey total elbow a.
Coonrad total elbow a.
Cracchiolo forefoot a.
Crawford-Adams cup a.
Cubbins a.
cuff tear a.
cup a.
Dewar-Barrington a.
distraction a.
duToit-Roux a.
Eaton implant a.
Eaton volar plate a.
Eden-Hybbinette a.
elbow a.
Ewald capitellocondylar total elbow a.
Ewald-Walker kinematic knee a.
excision a.
fascial a.

NOTES

arthroplasty *(continued)*
finger joint a.
forefoot a.
Girdlestone resection a.
Gristina-Webb total shoulder a.
Gunston a.
Harrington total hip a.
Head hip a.
Helal flap a.
hemiresection interposition a.
hip a.
Hungerford-Krackow-Kenna knee a.
ICLH double-cup a.
implant a.
Inglis triaxial total elbow a.
Insall-Burstein-Freeman knee a.
interpositional elbow a.
interpositional shoulder a.
intracapsular temporomandibular joint a.
Jones resection a.
Keller resection a.
knee a.
Kocher-McFarland hip a.
Kutes a.
Larmon forefoot a.
Mann-DuVries a.
Matchett-Brown hip a.
Mayo modified total elbow a.
Mayo resection a.
Memford-Gurd a.
metacarpophalangeal joint a.
Meuli a.
Millender a.
Miller-Galante knee a.
modified mold and surface replacement a.
mold acetabular a.
monospherical total shoulder a.
Morrey-Bryan total elbow a.
Mould a.
Mueller hip a.
Mumford-Gurd a.
NEB hip a.
Neer unconstrained shoulder a.
Niebauer trapeziometacarpal a.
noncemented total hip a.
Post total shoulder a.
prosthetic a.
Putti-Platt a.
resection a.
revision hip a.
rotator cuff tear a.
Schlein elbow a.
semiconstrained total elbow a.
shoulder a.
Silastic lunate a.
silicone implant a.
silicone rubber a.
silicone wrist a.
Smith-Petersen cup a.
Speed a.
Stanmore shoulder a.
Steffee thumb a.
Suave-Kapandji a.
surface replacement hip a.
Swanson Convex condylar a.
Swanson radial head implant a.
Swanson silicone wrist a.
tendon interposition a.
total ankle a.
total articular replacement a.
total articular resurfacing a.
total elbow a.
total hip a.
total joint a.
total knee a.
total patellofemoral joint a.
total shoulder a.
total wrist a.
triaxial total elbow a.
Tupper a.
ulnar hemiresection interposition a.
unconstrained shoulder a.
unicompartmental knee a.
Vaino MP a.
volar plate a.
Volz a.
Wilson-McKeever a.

arthroscopic
a. abrasion chondroplasty
a. anterior cruciate ligament reconstruction (AACLR)
a. augmentation
a. entry portal
a. examination
a. laser surgery
a. meniscectomy
a. microdiskectomy
a. synovectomy

arthroscopy
diagnostic and operative a.
Gillquist a.
laser a.
midcarpal a.
needle a.
operative a.
radiocarpal a.
Ringer a.
total knee a. (TKA)

arthrosia

arthrotomy
diagnostic arthroscopy, operative arthroscopy, and possible operative a.
Magnuson-Stack shoulder a.

operative a.
parapatellar a.

articular

a. bone loss
a. branch
a. capsule
a. cartilage
a. cartilage lesion
a. cavity
a. crescent
a. crest
a. disk
a. facet
a. fragment
a. manifestation
a. mass separation fracture
a. pillar fracture
a. process
a. recurrent nerve
a. vascular circle
a. vascular network

articulate

articulated

articulatio

articulation

acromioclavicular a.
a. area
arthrodial a.
articulator a.
atlantoaxial a.
atlantooccipital a.
balanced a.
bicondylar a.
calcaneocuboid a.
carpometacarpal a.
Chopart a.
condylar a.
coracoclavicular a.
coxofemoral a.
cricothyroid a.
a. curve
dental a.
deviant a.
a. disorder
glenohumeral a.
humeral a.
humeroradial a.
humeroulnar a.
incudomalleolar a.
a. index
infantile a.
intercarpal a.
interchondral a.
intermetacarpal a.
interphalangeal a.
Lisfranc a.
mandibular a.
metacarpophalangeal a.
metatarsocuneiform a.
metatarsophalangeal a.
patellofemoral a.
peg-and-socket a.
a. of pisiform bone
place of a.
proximal radioulnar a.
radiocapitellar a.
radiocarpal a.
radioulnar a.
sacroiliac a.
scapuloclavicular a.
secondary a.
spheroid a.
sternocostal a.
subtalar a.
superior tibial a.
talocalcaneal a.
talocalcaneonavicular a.
tarsometatarsal a.
temporomandibular joint a.
a. test
tibiofemoral a.
tibiofibular a.
triquetropisiform a.
trochoid a.
Vermont spinal fixator a.

articulationes

articulator articulation

articulatory procedure

artifact

pacemaker a.

artificial

a. anus
a. classification cavity
a. endocrine pancreas
a. erection test
a. fat pad
a. fistulation
a. intravaginal insemination
a. kidney
a. method
a. nose
a. respiration
a. sphincter

NOTES

artificial *(continued)*
a. ventilation
a. vertebral body
Arvidsson dimension-length method
arycorniculata
aryepiglottic (AE)
a. fold
a. muscle
aryepiglottica
aryepiglotticus
arytenoid
a. cartilage
a. gland
a. muscle
arytenoidal
arytenoideae
arytenoidectomy
arytenoidei
arytenoideus
arytenoidopexy
aryvocalis
ASA
American Society of Anesthesiologists
ASA physical status
A.S.A.-induced gastric ulceration
ascendens
ascending
a. anterior branch
a. aortic pressure
a. cervical artery
a. colon
a. lumbar vein
a. mesocolon
a. pathway of pain projection
a. pharyngeal artery
a. pharyngeal plexus
a. posterior branch
a. technique
Ascher
A. glass-rod phenomenon
A. syndrome
Aschoff body
ascites
bile a.
blood-tinged a.
chyliform a.
chylous a.
cloudy a.
exudative a.
fatty a.
gelatinous a.
hemorrhagic a.
marked a.
massive a.
milky a.
mucinous a.
mucoid a.
myxedema a.
progressive a.
pseudochylous a.
recurrent a.
straw-colored a.
transudative a.
tumor a.
ascitic fluid
ascitogenous
ASCRS
American Society for Colon and Rectal Surgeons
Aselli pancreas
asepsis
aseptic
a. peritonitis
a. surgery
a. technique
asepticism
ASGE
American Society for Gastrointestinal Endoscopy
Ashby differential agglutination method
Ashford retracted nipple operation
Ashhurst-Bromer ankle fracture classification
ash-leaf
a. patch
a. spot
Ashworth
A. hand arthroplasty
A. implant arthroplasty
ASI
active specific immunotherapy
ASIF screw fixation technique
Ask-Upmark kidney
ASM
airway smooth muscle
Asnis technique
ASO
arteriosclerosis obliterans
aspect
buccal a.
dorsal a.
inferomedial a.
laminar cortex posterior a.
medial a.
medicolegal a.
paraspinous a.
physiologic a.
plantar a.
posterior a.
posterolateral a.
puriform a.
spinous a.
volar a.
aspergilloma formation
aspergillosis infection
***Aspergillus* infection**

aspermatogenic
aspermia
asphyxia
asphyxial
asphyxiant
asphyxiate
asphyxiating thoracic dysplasia
asphyxiation
intrapartum a.
aspirate
endotracheal a.
percutaneous a.
transtracheal a.
aspirated foreign body
aspiration
acid a.
Alcon a.
anterior a.
a. biopsy cytology
bone marrow a.
breast cyst a.
cataract a.
cervical a.
cold knife cone a.
corporeal a.
a. of cortex
CT-directed needle a.
CT-guided fine-needle a.
CT scan-guided needle a.
cyst a.
endoscopic transesophageal fine-needle a.
epididymal sperm a.
EUS-guided fine-needle a.
fine-needle a. (FNA)
fluid a.
foreign body a.
full-thickness rectal a.
gastric fluid a.
guided fine-needle a.
hematoma a.
iliac crest bone a.
image-guided pancreatic core a.
irrigation and a.
joint a.
lateral a.
Mammotest Plus breast a.
meconium a.
medial a.
menstrual a.
Michele vertebral a.
microscopic epididymal sperm a.
microsurgical epididymal sperm a.
mineral oil a.
mucosal needle a.
myringotomy with a.
needle a.
a. needle biopsy
negative a.
percutaneous balloon a.
percutaneous CT-guided a.
percutaneous epididymal sperm a.
percutaneous fine-needle a.
peritoneal a.
pleural fluid a.
a. pneumonia
a. pneumonitis
a. portal
preoperative percutaneous a.
a. prophylaxis
pulmonary a.
real-time endoscopic ultrasound-guided fine-needle a.
recurrent a.
seminal vesicle a.
silent a.
sonography-guided a.
sperm a.
stereotactic a.
suction a.
suprapubic needle a.
tracheal a.
transbronchial needle a.
transthoracic needle a.
transtracheal a.
ultrasonic a.
ultrasound-guided fine-needle a.
uterine a.
vacuum a.
vitreous a.
asplenia
assay
antiphospholipid antibody a.
coagulation factor a.
immunoreactive parathyroid hormone a.
intact parathyroid hormone a.
intraoperative iPTH a.
iPTH a.
a. normalization
parathyroid hormone chemiluminescent a.
PTH chemiluminescent a.

NOTES

assay *(continued)*
- rapid intraoperative parathormone immunoradiometric a.
- a. technique

assessment
- awake neurological a.
- cytological a.
- echocardiographic a.
- endoscopic color Doppler a.
- extrapyramidal function a.
- histologic a.
- histological a.
- intraoperative a.
- jugular bulb catheter placement a.
- noninvasive a.
- nutritional a.
- peritoneal cytological a.
- weight estimation and a.

Assézat triangle

assimilation
- a. pelvis
- a. sacrum

assist
- hand a.

assistance
- laparoscopic a.

assist-control mode ventilation

assisted
- a. circulation
- a. medical procreation
- a. reproductive technique
- a. respiration
- a. ventilation

assisted-reproduction technology

associated
- a. injury
- a. myofascial trigger point

association
- American Pediatric Surgical A. (APSA)
- auditory-vocal a.
- a. cortex
- a. fiber
- law of a.
- a. mechanism
- megacystis-megaureter a.
- noncausal a.
- a. time
- a. tract
- VATER a.

asterion

asternal

asteroid body

asthma
- exercise-induced a.
- extrinsic a.

asthmatic
- steroid-dependent a.

asthmoid respiration

astigmatic keratotomy

astigmatism
- corneal a.
- a. correction

Astler-Coller
- A.-C. A, B1, B2, C1, C2 classification
- A.-C. modification of Dukes classification

astragalar

astragalocalcanean

astragaloscaphoid

astragalotibial

Astrand
- A. 30-beat stopwatch method
- A. 6-minute submaximal cycle ergometer test

astriction

astringent

astroblastoma

astrocyte
- fibrillary a.

astrocytoma
- adulthood a.
- anaplastic a.
- giant cell a.
- high-grade a.
- subependymal giant cell a.

Astwood-Coller staging system for carcinoma

asymmetric
- a. hyperplasia
- a. parathyroid enlargement
- a. surgery
- a. unit membrane

asymmetrical arthralgia

asymmetry

asymptomatic
- a. angiomyolipoma
- A. Carotid Atherosclerosis Study (ACAS)
- a. cholecystitis
- a. infection
- a. mass
- a. neoplasm
- a. patient

asynchronism

asynclitic
- a. position

ataractic

Atasoy
- A. palmar flap
- A. triangular advancement flap
- A. volar V-Y flap
- A. V-Y technique

Atasoy-Kleinert flap

Atasoy-type flap

atavistic epiphysis
ataxia
respiratory a.
ATC
around the clock
ATC dosing
atelectasis
ateral ligament
atherectomy
Auth a.
coronary angioplasty versus excisional a.
coronary rotational a.
directional coronary a.
high-speed rotational a.
a. index
Kinsey a.
percutaneous coronary rotational a.
rotational coronary a.
Simpson a.
transluminal extraction a.
atheroma embolism
atheromatous plaque
atherosclerosis
carotid a.
atherosclerotic
a. aneurysm
a. carotid artery
a. carotid artery lesion
a. heart disease
a. plaque
a. renal artery stenosis
ATI
Abdominal Trauma Index
ATIII
antithrombin III
Atkin epiphysial fracture
Atkinson
A. lid block
A. technique
atlantad
atlantal fracture
atlantica
atlantis
atlantoaxial
a. arthrodesis
a. articulation
a. dislocation
a. fracture-dislocation
a. fusion
a. instability
a. joint
a. lesion
a. rotatory fixation
a. stabilization
atlantoepistrophic
atlantooccipital
a. articulation
a. extension
a. fusion
a. joint
a. joint dislocation
a. ligament
a. membrane
a. stabilization
atlantooccipitalis
atlantooccipital transection
atlantoodontoid
atlas
atlas-axis combination fracture
atloaxoid
atloid
ATLS
advanced trauma life support
atmosphere
oxygen-enriched a.
a.s of pressure
ATN
acute tubular necrosis
atomic mass
atomizer
atonic bladder
atony
gastric a.
atopic line
ATP hydrolysis
atrabiliaris
atrabiliary capsule
atraumatic suture technique
atresia
aortic valve a.
biliary a.
extrahepatic biliary a.
pulmonary a.
urethral a.
atretocystia
atretogastria
atria (*pl. of* atrium)
atrial
a. activation mapping
a. arrhythmia
a. baffle operation
a. balloon septostomy
a. defibrillation threshold

NOTES

atrial *(continued)*
a. dissociation
a. ectopic tachycardia
a. extrastimulus method
a. fibrillation
a. fibrillation-flutter
a. filling pressure
a. natriuretic factor (ANF)
a. natriuretic peptide
a. ring
a. septal defect
a. septal resection
a. septectomy
a. stasis index
atrial-well technique
atriocaval shunt
atriocommissuropexy
atriodextrofascicular tract
atriofascicular tract
atrio hisian bypass tract
atrionodal bypass tract
atriopulmonary connection
atriotomy
pursestring a.
atrioventricular
a. bundle
a. canal
a. canal defect
a. conduction tissue
a. connection anomaly
a. dissociation
a. junctional ablation
a. junction anomaly
a. malformation
a. nodal function
a. node
a. reentry tachycardia
a. ring
a. septal defect
a. sulcus
a. valve insufficiency
atrium, pl. **atria**
atrophic
a. excavation
a. fenestration
a. fracture
a. inflammation
a. kidney
a. skin
atrophy
brown a.
cortical a.
crypt a.
endometrial a.
exhaustion a.
gastric a.
graft a.
healed yellow a.
intestinal villous a.
mammary a.
mucosal a.
multiple system a.
muscular a.
optic nerve a.
peroneal muscle a.
pressure a.
scapular peroneal a.
skeletal muscle a.
traction a.
villous a.
vocal cord a.
attached
a. cranial section
a. craniotomy
a. gingiva extension
attack
recurrent a.
transient ischemic a. (TIA)
attenuating tissue
attenuation
arteriolar a.
beam a.
broadband a.
a. correction
digital beam a.
heterogeneous a.
high a.
interaural a.
a. level
signal a.
a. of tendon
ultrasonic a.
attic adhesion
attollens
Attwood staining method
atypia
nuclear a.
atypical
a. dislocation
a. hyperplasia (AH)
a. junction
a. mycobacterial infection
a. regeneration
ATZ
anal transitional zone
AUC
area under curve
postprandial AUC
Auchincloss
A. modified radical mastectomy
A. operation
audioanalgesia
audiological evaluation
auditory
a. canal
a. closure

a. method
a. middle-latency response (AMLR)
a. tract
a. tube
a. tube nerve

auditory-vocal association

auditus

Auerbach
A. ganglion
A. plexus

Aufranc cup arthroplasty

augmentation
alloplastic chin a.
arthroscopic a.
bladder a.
breast a.
chin a.
connective tissue a.
a. cystoplasty
donor-specific bone marrow a.
endoscopic breast a.
extraarticular a.
gastroileac a.
a. genioplasty
gingival a.
a. graft
hamstring ligament a.
ileocecocystoplasty bladder a.
iliotibial band graft a.
Leach-Schepsis-Paul a.
Mainz pouch a.
a. mammaplasty
a. plaque
reverse a.
simultaneous areolar mastopexy and breast a. (SAMBA)
slotted acetabular a.
submucosal urethral a.
synthetic a.
a. therapy
thiol a.
transumbilical breast a. (TUBA)
ureteral bladder a.

augmentor nerve

aural fistula

auren

auricle

auricular
a. appendectomy
a. branch
a. canaliculus
a. cartilage
a. fibrillation
a. fissure
a. ganglion
a. index
a. ligament
a. muscle
a. notch
a. point
a. surface
a. triangle
a. tubercle
a. vein

auricularia

auriculocranial

auriculoinfraorbital plane

auriculomastoid

auriculotemporalis

auriculotemporal nerve

auriculoventricular groove

auscultation

Austin
A. bunionectomy
A. Flint murmur
A. Flint respiration
A. osteotomy

Austin-Moore arthroplasty

Autenrieth and Funk method

Auth atherectomy

autoamputation

autoaugmentation
bladder a.

autocastration

autocatheterization

autocaval fistula

autocystoplasty

autocytolysis

autodilation
Frank nonsurgical perineal a.

autodrainage

autogeneic graft

autogenous
a. bone graft
a. bone grafting
a. fascial heterograft
a. interpositional shoulder arthroplasty
a. keratoplasty
a. strip
a. tooth transplantation
a. vein

autograft
cultured epithelial a.

NOTES

autograft *(continued)*
a. fusion
a. harvesting
parathyroid a.
pulmonary a. (PA)
Russell fibular head a.
autografting
autoimmune
a. connective tissue disorder
a. demyelination
a. hepatitis
autoimmunization
surgical a.
autoinflation
autoinfusion
autokeratoplasty
autolesion
autologous
a. blood
a. blood donation
a. blood stem cell transplantation
a. blood unit
a. bone marrow transplant
a. bone marrow transplantation (ABMT)
A. Bone Marrow Transplant Registry (ABMTR)
a. clot
a. internal jugular vein
a. melanoma system
a. pericardial patch
a. RBC unit
autolytic débridement
automated
a. anesthesia record
a. boundary protection
a. large-core breast biopsy
a. percutaneous diskectomy
automatic ectopic tachycardia
autonephrectomy
silent a.
autonomic
a. blockade
a. dysreflexia
a. dysregulation
a. ganglion block
a. modulation
a. nerve
a. nerve block
a. nerve preservation (ANP)
a. neurogenic bladder
a. plexus
autonomici
autonomicorum
autonomous function
auto-PEEP
autoplasty
autopod
autopodium
autopsy
laparoscopic a.
autoreinfection
autorrhaphy
autoscopy
autosomal
a. dominant polycystic kidney disease
a. recessive
autosuture technique
autotransfusion
massive a.
autotransplant
autotransplantation
colostomy pyloric a.
pancreatic a.
posttraumatic a.
pyloric a.
renal a.
autotrophic fixation
autovaccination
Auvray incision
auxiliary
a. canal
a. partial orthotopic liver transplantation (APOLT)
a. transplant
A-V, AV
arteriovenous
A-V bundle
A-V dissociation
A-V fistula
A-V malformation
A-V nodal modification
avascular
a. fragment
a. necrosis
avascularization
average
a. extubation time
a. flow rate
a. mean pressure
AVF
arteriovenous fistula
avidin-biotin-peroxidase complex method
Avila technique
avium-intracellulare
Mycobacterium avium-intracellulare (MAI)
AVM
arteriovenous malformation
avoidance maneuver
avulse
avulsed
a. fragment
a. wound

avulsion
a. stress fracture
a. technique
a. trauma
awake
a. craniotomy
a. neurological assessment
awaken
failure to a.
awakening
planned a.
awareness
body a.
AXBF
axillobifemoral
Axenfeld
A. anomaly
A. suture technique
Axer
A. lateral opening wedge osteotomy
A. varus derotational osteotomy
Axer-Clark procedure
axes (*pl. of* axis)
axial
a. aneurysm
a. calcaneal projection
a. compression
a. compression injury
a. compression principle
a. compression test
a. fixation
a. flag flap
a. hiatal hernia
a. illumination
a. inclination
a. lesion
a. line angle
a. loading fracture
a. melanoma
a. muscle
a. pattern scalp flap
a. plane
a. point
a. rotation
a. rotation joint
a. section
a. sesamoid projection
a. skeleton
a. spin-echo image
a. surface cavity
axiale
axifugal
axil
axile
axilla, pl. **axillae**
hot a.
a. temperature
axillares
axillaris
axillary
a. abscess
a. adenopathy
a. approach
a. arch
a. artery
a. artery aneurysm
a. bed
a. block
a. block anesthesia
a. block anesthetic technique
a. endoscopic reduction
a. envelope
a. fascia
a. fat pad
a. flap
a. fold
a. fossa
a. hematoma
a. incision
a. insertion
a. line
a. lymphadenectomy
a. lymphadenopathy
a. lymph node dissection (ALND)
a. nerve
a. node dissection
a. node dissection mastectomy
a. node metastasis
a. node negative
a. perivascular technique
a. plexus
a. region
a. sheath
a. skin lesion
a. space
a. sweat gland
a. thoracotomy
a. triangle
a. vascular injury
a. vein
axilloaxillary bypass
axillobifemoral (AXBF)

NOTES

axillobifemoral *(continued)*
a. bypass
a. bypass graft
axillofemoral bypass
axillounifemoral (AXUF)
a. bypass
axiobuccolingual plane
axiolabiolingual plane
axiomesiodistal plane
axis, pl. **axes**
basibregmatic a.
basicranial a.
basifacial a.
celiac a.
cephalocaudal a.
coeliac a.
conjugate a.
craniofacial a.
facial a.
a. fixation
flexion-extension a.
a. fracture
hypothalamic-hypophysial-ovarian-endometrial a.
long a.
mesentericoportal a.
pelvic a.
a. pelvis
a. of rotation
thoracic a.
thyroid a.
axis-atlas combination fracture
axofugal
axon
corticospinal a.
axonal
a. demyelination
a. injury
a. regeneration
axotomy
AXR
abdominal x-ray
AXUF
axillounifemoral
Aylett operation
Ayoub-Shklar method
Ayre spatula-Zelsmyr cytobrush technique
azeotrope
azeotropic solution
azotemia
transient a.
azure lunula
azygoesophageal
a. line
a. recess
azygos
a. artery of vagina
a. fissure
a. vein
azygous

B
B cell line
B phenotypic lymphocyte
B point
B ring
Babcock
B. operation
B. suture technique
Bachmann
B. bundle
internodal tract of B.
back
b. gunshot wound
b. pain
b. projection
back-and-forth suture technique
backbone
backcut incision
backfire fracture
backflow
b. bleeding
pyelovenous b.
background illumination
back-knee deformity
back-propagation neural network program
back-up position
backward
b. coarticulation
b. position
Bacon-Babcock operation
bacteremia
perioperative b.
bacteremic donor
bacteria (*pl. of* bacterium)
bacterial
b. agar method
b. complication
b. contamination
b. endotoxin
b. flora
b. infection
b. mucosal infiltration
b. overgrowth
b. translocation
bactericidal concentration
bacteriologic data
bacteriolysis
bacteriopexy
bacteriospermia
bacteriostasis
bacteriostatic barrier
bacterium, pl. **bacteria**
probiotic bacteria
bacteriuria
BAD
bipolar affective disorder
Badal operation
Badenoch urethroplasty
Badgley
B. combination procedure
B. iliac wing resection
B. technique
Bado classification
Baehr-Lohlein lesion
Baffe anastomosis
baffle fenestration
bag-and-mask ventilation
bag extraction
bagged mask ventilation
bag-of-bones technique
bag-valve-mask
bag-valve-mask-assisted ventilation
Bailey-Badgley
B.-B. anterior cervical approach
B.-B. cervical spine fusion
B.-B. technique
Bailey-Dubow
B.-D. osteotomy
B.-D. technique
bailout valvuloplasty
Bailyn classification
Bain circle
Baker
B. cyst
B. patellar advancement operation
B. pyridine extraction
B. Sudan black method
B. technique
B. translocation operation
Baker-Hill osteotomy
Balacescu closing wedge osteotomy
Balacescu-Golden technique
balance
acid-base b.
heat b.
thermal b.
balanced
b. anesthesia
b. anesthetic technique
b. articulation
b. salt solution volume diuresis
balanic
balanitis
balanocele
balanoplasty
balanoposthitis
balanus
Balbiani body
Baldy operation

Baldy-Webster
B.-W. operation
B.-W. procedure
B.-W. uterine suspension
Balfour gastroenterostomy
Balkan nephrectomy
ball
B. operation
b. valve action
b. wedge
ball-and-socket
b.-a.-s. epiphysis
b.-a.-s. joint
b.-a.-s. trochanteric osteotomy
Ballard examination
Ball-Hoffman operation
ballistics
balloon
b. aortic valvotomy
b. aortic valvuloplasty
b. atrial septostomy
b. bronchoplasty
b. catheter angioplasty
b. catheter technique
b. cell formation
b. coarctation angioplasty
b. coronary angioplasty
b. counterpulsation
b. dilatation
b. dilation
b. dilation angioplasty
b. dilation valvuloplasty
b. dissection
b. embolectomy
b. epiphysis
b. esophagoplasty
b. expulsion test
b. fenestration procedure
b. inflation
b. laser angioplasty
b. mitral commissurotomy
b. mitral valvotomy
b. mitral valvuloplasty
b. occlusive intravascular lysis enhanced recanalization
b. photodynamic therapy
b. pulmonary valvotomy
b. pulmonary valvuloplasty
b. rupture
b. septectomy
b. tamponade technique
b. tricuspid valvotomy
b. tube tamponade
b. tuboplasty
B. Valvuloplasty Registry
b. valvulotomy
balloon-catheter and basket-retrieval technique
balloon-occluded retrograde transvenous obliteration (B-RTO)
ball-valve obstruction
banana fracture
band
adhesive b.
ciliary body b.
Clado b.
fracture b.
gastric b.
iliotibial b.
b. keratopathy
Ladd b.
Lane b.
b. ligation
Maissiat b.
Meckel b.
moderator b.
pecten b.
peritoneal b.
b. placement
b. sigmoidopexy
Simonart b.
zonular b.
bandage
compression b.
b. method
Band-Aid operation
bandeau defect
Bandi
B. procedure
B. technique
banding
Kuzmak gastric b.
laparoscopic adjustable silicone gastric b.
laparoscopic gastric b.
open adjustable silicone gastric b.
Banff classification
Bangerter
B. method of pleoptics
B. pterygium operation
banjo-string adhesion
bank
blood b.
shoulder dislocation bone b.
staple capsulorraphy bone b.
tissue b.
Traumatic Coma Data B.
Bankart
B. fracture
B. operation
B. procedure
B. reconstruction
B. shoulder dislocation
B. shoulder lesion
B. shoulder repair
Bankart-Putti-Platt operation

banking
cryopreserved tissue b.
Banks-Laufman
B.-L. approach
B.-L. incision
B.-L. technique
Bannayan-Riley-Ruvalcaba syndrome
Baptist
New England B. (NEB)
bar
b. bolt fixation
Mercier b.
Passavant b.
b. resection
b. section
barber
b. chair position
b. pole stripe transfer
barbiturate
b. burst-suppression anesthesia
b. coma
barbiturate-related hyperalgesia
barbotage
Barcat technique
Bard endoscopic suturing
bare
b. area
b. area diaphragm
b. scleral technique
bariatric
b. operation
b. surgery
barium
b. contrast x-ray
b. enema
b. enema finding
b. esophagogram
b. examination
b. peritonitis
b. swallow
b. swallow study
Barkan
B. double cyclodialysis operation
B. goniotomy operation
B. membrane
B. technique
Barkan-Cordes linear cataract operation
Barlow maneuver
Barnard operation
Barnett-Bourne acetic alcohol-silver nitrate method
Barnhart repair
barometric pressure
baroreceptor
b. nerve
b. test
baroreflex
b. activation
b. response
b. responsiveness
barostat method
barotrauma
Barr
B. body
B. open reduction and internal fixation
B. tendon transfer operation
B. tibial fracture fixation
barrage cryopexy
Barraquer
B. enzymatic zonulolysis operation
B. keratomileusis operation
B. method
B. suture technique
B. zonulolysis
barrel-hooping compression
barrel-shaped lesion
Barrett
B. epithelium
B. esophagus
B. metaplasia
Barrie-Jones canaliculodacryorhinostomy operation
barrier
ABO b.
adhesion b.
anatomic b.
bacteriostatic b.
blood-air b.
blood-brain b. (BBB)
blood-cerebral b.
blood-cerebrospinal fluid b.
blood-liquor b.
blood-ocular b.
blood-optic nerve b.
blood-retinal b.
blood-thymus b.
blood-urine b.
cerebrospinal fluid-brain b.
elastic b.
endothelial b.
epithelial b.
gastric mucosal b.
integumentary b.

NOTES

barrier *(continued)*
b. layer
b. method
motion b.
mucosal b.
ocular b.
pathologic b.
physical b.
physiologic b.
placental b.
posterior capsular zonular b.
b. protection
side-bending b.
sterile field b.
b. technique
b. zone
Barriers Pain Questionnaire
Barrio operation
Barrnett-Seligman
B.-S. dihydroxydinaphthyl disulfide method
B.-S. indoxyl esterase method
Barron
B. hemorrhoidal banding technique
B. ligation
Barroso-Moguel and Costero silver method
Barsky
B. cleft closure
B. macrodactyly reduction
B. procedure
B. technique
Barth hernia
Bartholin
B. cystectomy
B. duct
B. gland
Bartlett
B. nail fold
B. nail-fold excision
B. procedure
Barton-Smith fracture
basad
basal
b. anal canal pressure
b. anal sphincter pressure
b. anesthesia
anterior b. (AB)
b. body temperature
b. cell carcinoma
b. cell hyperplasia
b. cell membrane
b. cistern
b. ganglia hematoma
b. ganglion
b. ganglionic lesion
inferior b. (IB)
b. iridectomy
b. lamina
b. line
b. neck fracture
septal b. (SB)
b. skull fracture
b. sphincter
b. subfrontal approach
b. tentorial branch
b. vein
b. vein of Rosenthal
basalis
basaloid
bascule
cecal b.
base
anterior cranial b.
b. of bladder
cavity preparation b.
cement b.
cranial b.
b. deficit (BD)
extension b.
fixation b.
b. line
b. medication
National Cancer Data B. (NCDB)
b. plane
b. projection
saddle connector b.
tissue-supported b.
tissue-tissue-supported b.
b. wedge osteotomy
baseball
b. finger fracture
b. stitch
b. suture technique
baseline capacity evaluation
basement
b. membrane
b. membrane zone
base-of-the-neck osteotomy
base-ring tilt
bas-fond
basialis
basialveolar
basibregmatic axis
basicranial axis
basic technique
basifacial axis
basihyal
basihyoid
basilar
b. artery
b. artery aneurysm
b. artery migraine
b. bifurcation
b. bifurcation aneurysm
b. bone

b. cartilage
b. femoral neck fracture
b. fibrocartilage
b. index
b. invagination
b. lamina
b. membrane
b. osteotomy
b. process
b. skull fracture
b. suture
b. suture technique
b. tip aneurysm
b. venous plexus
b. venous sinus
b. vertebra
basilare
basilaris
basilateral
basilica
basilic vein
basin
lymph node b.
nonclassic nodal b.
portal lymph node b.
regional lymph node b.
retropancreatic lymph node b.
basinasal line
basioccipital bone
basiocciput
basioglossus
basion
basipetal
basipharyngeal canal
basis
basisphenoid bone
basitemporal
basivertebrales
basivertebralis
basivertebral vein
basket
b. extraction technique
b. fragmentation technique
b. impaction
basketing technique
basket-weave vacuolization
basolateral membrane
basosquamous cell carcinoma
Bass
B. method
B. technique
Basset radical vulvectomy
Bassini
B. inguinal hernia repair
B. inguinal herniorrhaphy
B. method
B. operation
B. procedure
B. technique
Bassini-Stetten hernia repair
bastard suture technique
Batchelor-Brown extraarticular subtalar arthrodesis
Batch least-squares method
Batch-Spittler-McFaddin
B.-S.-M. knee disarticulation
B.-S.-M. technique
bat ear surgery
Bateman
B. hemiarthroplasty
B. modification of Mayer transfer operation
bath
contrast b.
bathing trunk nevus
Batista procedure
batrachian position
Batson plexus
Battle
B. incision
B. operation
B. sign
battledore incision
Battle-Jalaguier-Kammerer incision
bat-wing appearance
Baudelocque operation
Bauer-Jackson classification
Bauer-Tondra-Trusler
B.-T.-T. operation
B.-T.-T. technique
Bauhin
B. gland
valve of B.
Baume classification
Baumgard-Schwartz tennis elbow technique
Baumgartner method
Baxter
B. VAMP
B. venous/arterial management protection
Baxter-D'Astous procedure
Bayne-Klug centralization
Baynton operation

NOTES

bayonet
b. canal
b. dislocation
b. fracture position
bayonet-curved canal
bayonet-type incision
BBB
blood-brain barrier
BCSS
breast cancer-specific survival
BCT
breast conservation therapy
BD
base deficit
BEA
below-elbow amputation
beach chair position
bead
b. bed
b. chain study
b. pouch
b. technique filling
beads-on-a-string appearance
beak
b. fracture
b. modification with triple arthrodesis
b. nail
Beall-Webel-Bailey technique
beam
b. attenuation
fluoroscopy b.
Beard-Cutler operation
Beard operation
beating-heart bypass surgery
Beatson ovariotomy
beat-to-beat variation of fetal heart rate
Beau line
Beaver direct smear method
Bechterew
line of B.
Bechtol arthroplasty
Beck
B. cardiopericardiopexy
B. gastrostomy
B. method
B. I, II operation
B. triad
Beckenbaugh
B. correction
B. technique
Becker
B. muscular dystrophy
B. technique
Béclard
B. amputation
B. anastomosis
B. hernia
B. suture technique
B. triangle
BeCoMo
Bernse Coping Modes
Becton
B. open reduction
B. technique
bed
axillary b.
bead b.
bone graft b.
fracture b.
gastric b.
graft b.
hot axillary b.
liver b.
mud b.
nail b.
parotid b.
tumor b.
vascular b.
bedroom fracture
bedside laparoscopy
beefy appearance
Beer operation
Begg light wire differential force technique
behavior
pain b.
behavioral
b. inhibition system (BIS)
b. technique
Behçet
B. disease
B. skin puncture test
B. syndrome
behind-sternum column esophagoplasty
Bell
B. muscle
B. palsy
B. respiratory nerve
bell-clapper deformity
Bell-Dally cervical dislocation
Bellemore-Barrett closing wedge osteotomy
Bell-Tawse
B.-T. open reduction technique
B.-T. procedure
belly
b. bath therapy
b. button
b. button augmentation mammaplasty
occipital b.
posterior b.
below-elbow amputation (BEA)
below-knee amputation (BKA)

Belsey
B. esophagoplasty
B. fundoplication method
B. fundoplication procedure
B. fundoplication technique
B. IV fundoplasty
B. Mark II, IV fundoplication
B. Mark IV antireflux operation
B. Mark IV cardioplasty
B. Mark IV 240-degree fundoplication
B. Mark IV gastropexy
B. Mark IV repair
B. partial fundoplication
B. two-thirds wrap fundoplication
belt
b. loop gastropexy
b. muscle
B. Technique
Belt-Fuqua hypospadias repair
Bence Jones body
bench
b. examination
b. surgery
b. surgical technique
Benchekroun stoma
Benedict orbit operation
Benedict-Talbot body surface area method
Benelli lollipop mastopexy
Bengston method
benign
b. bone lesion
b. bone tumor
b. duodenocolic fistula
b. dysphagia
b. esophageal disorder
b. fasciculation
b. giant cell synovioma
b. inflammatory disease
b. liver cyst
b. lymphoepithelial lesion
b. lymphoproliferative lesion
b. mass
b. mesothelioma
b. nature
b. papillomavirus infection
b. paroxysmal positional vertigo (BPPV)
b. pneumatic colonoscopy complication
b. process
b. prostatic hyperplasia (BPH)
b. prostatic hypertrophy
b. reading
b. stricture
b. subcutaneous cyst
b. vascular lesion
benign-acting renal cell carcinoma
Bennett
B. classification
B. comminuted fracture
B. dislocation
B. fracture-dislocation
B. lesion
B. nail biopsy
B. posterior shoulder approach
B. sulfhydryl method
Bennhold Congo red method
Bensley aniline-acid fuchsin-methyl green method
Bentall
B. composite graft technique
B. inclusion technique
B. procedure
bent-nail syndrome
benzodiazepine-induced hypoventilation
benzo sky blue method
Bérard aneurysm
Berci-Shore choledochoscopy
Berens
B. graft
B. pterygium transplant operation
B. sclerectomy operation
Berens-Smith
B.-S. cul-de-sac restoration
B.-S. operation
Berg chelate removal method
Berger
B. disease
B. interscapular amputation
B. operation
B. space
Berger-Bookwalter posterior approach
Bergey classification
Bergmann incision
Bergmann-Israel incision
Berke
B. approach
B. operation
Berke-Krönlein orbitotomy
Berke-Motais operation

NOTES

Berman-Gartland
B.-G. metatarsal osteotomy
B.-G. procedure
Bernard
B. canal
B. duct
B. lip reconstruction procedure
B. operation
B. puncture
Berndt-Harty classification
Bernoulli effect
Bernse Coping Modes (BeCoMo)
berry
b. aneurysm
B. ligament
Bertel position
Bertin column
Bertrandi suture technique
beta
b. adrenoreceptor
b. hemolytic streptococci infection
beta-2-adrenergic receptor
beta-adrenergic
b.-a. agonist
b.-a. blockade
b.-a. receptor
beta-blocker medication
beta-oxidation pathway
beta-receptor
b.-r. agonist
b.-r. antagonist
beta-sympathomimetic agent
betel carcinoma
Bethesda System for Pap smear classification
Bethke
B. iridectomy
B. operation
Bevan
B. abdominal incision
B. orchiopexy
bevel
beveled anastomosis
Beverly-Douglas lip-tongue adhesion technique
BeWo choriocarcinoma cell line
bezoar
medication b.
Bezold abscess
Bezold-Jarisch reflex
B.H. Moore procedure
biarticular
biasterionic
biaxial joint
BIB
biliointestinal bypass
bicameral abscess
bicanalicular sphincter
biceps
b. interval lesion
b. tendon
Bichat
B. canal
B. fat pad
B. fossa
B. membrane
bicipital
b. groove
b. rib
b. ridge
bicipitoradial bursa
bicipitoradialis
bursa b.
Bickel-Moe procedure
bicondylar
b. articulation
b. joint
b. T-shaped fracture
b. Y-shaped fracture
bicondylaris
bicoronal
b. incision
b. scalp flap
bicortical screw fixation
bicycle spoke fracture
bidirectional
b. ligation
b. superior cavopulmonary anastomosis
Biebl loop
Bielschowsky
B. maneuver
B. method
B. operation
B. three-step, head-tilt test
Bielschowsky-Parks head-tilt, three-step test
Bier
B. amputation
B. block
B. block anesthesia
B. method
Biesenberger technique of mastopexy
Biesiadecki fossa
bifemoral
bifid
b. penis
b. rib
b. thumb deformity
bifida
spina b.
bifocal fixation
bifoveal fixation
bifrontal
b. craniotomy
b. incision

bifurcated vascular graft
bifurcation
b. aneurysm
aortic b.
basilar b.
carotid artery b.
coronary b.
b. graft
b. involvement
b. lesion
b. osteotomy
portal b.
b. of root
Bigelow
B. litholapaxy
B. maneuver
B. septum
BIH
bilateral inguinal hernia
bikini skin incision
bilabe
bilaminar membrane
bilateral
b. adrenal hemorrhage
b. amputation
b. anterior thoracotomy
b. bundle branch block
b. ilioinguinal approach
b. inguinal hernia (BIH)
b. inguinal hernia repair
b. inguinal hernia repair method
b. inguinal hernia repair procedure
b. inguinal hernia repair technique
b. interfacetal dislocation
b. intrafacetal dislocation
b. lithotomy
b. lymphadenectomy
b. myocutaneous graft
b. neck dissection
b. neck exploration
b. nephroureterectomy
b. resection
b. sacroiliac approach
b. salpingo-oophorectomy
b. subcostal incision
b. subcutaneous mastectomy
b. temporary tarsorrhaphy
b. total adrenalectomy
b. transabdominal incision
b. ureterostomy takedown
b. vagotomy
b. ventral rhizotomy
b. V-Y Kutler flap
bilayer patch hernia repair
bile
b. acid circulation
b. ascites
b. content
b. duct
b. duct adenocarcinoma
b. duct adenoma
b. duct calculus
b. duct cannulation
b. duct carcinoma
b. duct catheterization
b. duct colic
b. duct cystadenocarcinoma
b. duct dilatation
b. duct epithelium
b. duct exploration
b. duct injury
b. duct ligation
b. duct lumen
b. duct manipulation
b. duct pressure
b. duct wall
b. encrustation
b. fluid examination
b. leak
b. leakage
b. papilla
b. sample
b. tract
b. tract drainage
bile-plug syndrome
bile-stained cyst content
bilevel positive airway pressure
bilharzial carcinoma
Bilhaut-Cloquet procedure
biliaris
biliary
b. anatomic variation
b. anatomy
b. atresia
b. calculus
b. canaliculus
b. cannulation
b. carcinoma
b. colic
b. conduit
b. dilation
b. drainage
b. duct

NOTES

biliary *(continued)*
- b. ductule
- b. endoprosthesis insertion
- b. endoscopy
- b. enteric bypass
- b. fistula
- b. intestinal anastomosis
- b. leakage
- b. lithiasis
- b. lithotripsy
- b. pancreatitis
- b. problem
- b. reconstruction
- b. saturation index
- b. secretion
- b. sphincterotomy
- b. sphincterotomy and stent placement
- b. stenting
- b. stent patency
- b. stricture
- b. system
- b. tract
- b. tract cancer
- b. tract disease
- b. tract infection
- b. tract obstruction
- b. tract pressure
- b. tract stone
- b. tract torsion
- b. tract tumor
- b. tree

biliary-bronchial fistula
biliary-cutaneous fistula
biliary-duodenal
- b.-d. fistula
- b.-d. pressure gradient

biliary-enteric
- b.-e. anastomosis
- b.-e. anastomosis operation
- b.-e. fistula

biliferi
biliocystic fistula
biliodigestive
- b. anastomosis
- b. origin

biliointestinal bypass (BIB)
biliopancreatic bypass (BPB)
biliopleural fistula
bilious
- b. colic
- b. empyema
- b. vomit

bilirubin
- b. concentration
- b. level
- serum b.

Billings method
Bill maneuver
billowing mitral valve syndrome
Billroth
- B. II anatomy
- B. I, II gastrectomy
- B. I gastroduodenostomy
- B. I, II gastroenterostomy
- B. I, II gastrointestinal anastomosis
- B. II gastrojejunostomy
- B. I method
- B. I, II operation
- B. II pancreatoduodenectomy
- B. I partial gastrectomy
- B. I, II procedure
- B. I, II reconstruction
- splenic cord of B.
- B. I, II technique

bilobar
- b. disease
- b. liver metastasis
- b. resection

bilobate
bilobectomy
bilobed
- b. polypoid lesion
- b. skin flap
- b. transposition flap

bilobular
bilocular
- b. femoral hernia
- b. joint
- b. stomach

biloma
bimalleolar ankle fracture
bimanual
- b. palpation
- b. pelvic examination

bimastoid line
bimodal method
bimucosa
- fistula b.

binaural
- b. fusion
- b. integration

Binet system of classification
Bing-Siebenmann malformation
Bing-Taussig heart procedure
binocular
- b. fixation
- b. fusion
- b. indirect ophthalmoscopy
- b. microscopy

bioavailability
- nitric oxide b.

biobehavioral response
biochemical
- b. evidence

b. metastasis
b. modulation
biocompatibility
implant b.
biofeedback
biofilm production
biologic
b. fixation
b. marker
biological
b. effect
biology
cellular b.
molecular b.
biomagnetic therapy
biomechanical preparation
bioprogressive technique
bioprosthesis
biopsy
abdominal lymph node b.
abrasive brush b.
adrenal gland b.
alcohol-fixed gastric b.
Allis-Abramson breast b.
antral b.
aspiration needle b.
automated large-core breast b.
Bennett nail b.
bite b.
blind percutaneous liver b.
bone marrow b.
bone marrow aspiration and b.
brain b.
breast b.
bronchial brush b.
bronchoscopic needle b.
brush b.
Campylobacter-like organism b.
catheter-guided b.
b. cavity
cervical cone b.
channel and core b.
chorionic villus b.
CLO b.
coin b.
cold cone b.
cold cup b.
colonoscopic b.
colorectal b.
computed tomography-guided b.
cone b.
core needle b.
corporal b.
cortical b.
Crosby-Kugler capsule for b.
CT-guided liver b.
CT-guided needle-aspiration b.
cutting needle b.
cytobrush b.
cytologic b.
diagnostic b.
diathermic loop b.
digitally-guided b.
direct-vision liver b.
Dunn b.
elliptical b.
embryo b.
endometrial b.
endomyocardial b.
endoscopic small bowel b.
endoscopic sphenoidal b.
ERCP-guided b.
esophageal b.
excision b.
excisional b.
fetal liver b.
fetal skin b.
fine-needle aspiration b.
FNA b.
forage core b.
Fosnaugh nail b.
four-point b.
guided transcutaneous b.
guillotine needle b.
hilar b.
hot b.
ileal b.
iliac crest b.
image-guided breast b. (IGBB)
image-guided fine-needle aspiration b.
image-guided stereotactic brain b.
incisional b.
internal mammary node b.
intestinal b.
intramedullary tumor b.
intraoperative b.
jejunal b.
jumbo b.
Kevorkian punch b.
Keyes punch b.
kidney b.
laparoscopic liver b.
large-core needle aspiration b.

NOTES

biopsy *(continued)*
large-particle b.
lift-and-cut b.
liver b.
lumbar spine b.
lung b.
lymph node b.
mammary node b.
mediastinal lymph node b.
Menghini technique for percutaneous liver b.
minimally invasive b.
mirror-image breast b.
mucosal b.
multiple core b.
muscle b.
nasopharyngeal b.
native renal b.
needle core b.
needle-localized open b. (NLOB)
negative breast b.
nerve b.
node b.
onion-bulb changes on b.
open brain b.
open liver b.
open lung b.
open surgical b.
optical b.
out-of-phase endometrial b.
outpatient b.
pancreatic b.
paracollicular b.
parathyroid b.
pelvic aspiration b.
percutaneous excisional breast b. (PEBB)
percutaneous fine-needle aspiration b.
percutaneous fine-needle pancreatic b.
percutaneous liver b.
percutaneous native renal b.
percutaneous needle liver b.
percutaneous pancreas b.
pericardial b.
peritoneal b.
peroral intestinal b.
PET-guided b.
pinch b.
Pipelle b.
pleural b.
point-in-space stereotactic b.
positron emission tomography-guided b.
pouch b.
preoperative b.
pseudotumor cerebrimeningeal b.
punch b.
random bladder b.
rectal suction b.
renal b.
b. sample
saucerized b.
scalene fat pad b.
scalene lymph node b.
scalene node b. (SNB)
scan-directed b.
Scher nail b.
secondary diagnostic b.
sentinel lymph node b.
sentinel node b. (SNB)
serial percutaneous liver b.
shave b.
single b.
b. site
skeletal b.
skin b.
skinny-needle b.
SLN b.
small bowel b.
snap-frozen b.
snare excision b.
snare loop b.
sonoguided b.
b. specimen
spinal infection b.
sponge b.
StereoGuide stereotactic needle core b.
stereotactic aspiration b.
stereotactic brain b.
stereotactic core breast b.
stereotactic-guided b.
stereotactic needle core b.
stereotactic percutaneous needle b.
strip b.
suction b.
supraclavicular lymph node b.
sural nerve b.
surface b.
surgical excision b.
synovial b.
systematic sextant b.
tangential b.
targeted brain b.
b. technique
temporal artery b.
testicular b.
thin-needle b.
thoracic spine b.
thyroid needle b.
total b.
transbronchial lung b.
transcutaneous b.
transfemoral liver b.

transgastric fine-needle aspiration b.
transitional zone b.
transjugular hepatic b.
transjugular liver b.
transnasal b.
transpapillary b.
transrectal ultrasound-guided sextant b.
transthoracic needle aspiration b.
transthoracic percutaneous fine-needle aspiration b.
transvenous liver b.
trephine needle b.
trophectoderm b.
Tru-Cut needle b. (TCNB)
ultrasonography-guided fine-needle aspiration b.
ultrasound-guided anterior subcostal liver b.
ultrasound-guided automated large-core breast b.
ultrasound-guided core breast b.
ultrasound-guided core-needle b. (US-CNB)
ultrasound-guided echo b.
ultrasound-guided fine-needle aspiration b. (US-FNAB)
ultrasound-guided needle b.
ultrasound-guided stereotactic b.
vaginal cone b.
Valls-Ottolenghim-Schajowicz needle b.
ventricular endomyocardial b.
Verman needle b.
Vertical lip b.
video-assisted excisional b.
Vim-Silverman technique for liver b.
b. volume
vulvar b.
Watson capsule b.
wedge hepatic b.
wedge liver b.
wire-guided breast b.
wound b.
Zaias nail b.

biopsy-proven metastasis
biorbital angle
biospectroscopy
biosurfactant
Biot
B. breathing
B. respiration
biotransformation
BiPAP nasal continuous positive airway pressure
biparietal
b. diameter (BPD)
b. suture technique
bipedicle dorsal flap
bipennate muscle
bipennatus
biperforate
biphase pin fixation
biplanar fluoroscopy
biplane
b. fluoroscopy
b. scan
b. trochanteric osteotomy
bipolar
b. affective disorder (BAD)
b. cauterization
b. coagulation
b. electrocautery
b. electrocoagulation
b. hip arthroplasty
Bipolaris specific IgE, IgG antibody
BIRADS
Breast Imaging Reporting and Data System
BIRADS classification
BIRADS score
biramous
Bircher operation
Bircher-Weber technique
Birch-Hirschfeld entropion operation
bird-beak deformity
bird's nest lesion
Birkett hernia
birth
b. amputation
b. canal
b. canal laceration
b. fracture
birthing position
BIS
behavioral inhibition system
bis
central b.
bisacromial
bisaxillary
Bischof myelotomy

NOTES

bisecting
b. angle cone position
b. angle technique
bisecting-the-angle technique
bisection
bisector line
bisegmentectomy
bisensory method
bisexual
Bishop classification
Bishop-Koop ileostomy
bisiliac
bismuth
b. benign bile duct stricture classification
b. bile duct stricture type I-V classification
b. line
b. type IV stricture
bispectral index
bissac
hernia en b.
bisubcostal incision
bite
b. biopsy
b. plane
b. plane therapy
bitemporal
biterminal
bitewing technique
biting pressure
bitrochanteric
biventer cervicis
biventral
bizygomatic
Björk method of Fontan procedure
Björk-Shiley graft
BKA
below-knee amputation
BL
blood lactate
buccolingual
black
b. blood clot
b. classification
b. epidermoidoma
b. line
b. patch syndrome
b. periodic acid method
b. repair
b. technique
Black-Broström staple technique
Blackburn technique
bladder
atonic b.
b. augmentation
b. autoaugmentation
autonomic neurogenic b.
base of b.
b. calculus
b. carcinoma
b. carcinoma classification
b. catheterization
b. chimney procedure
b. distention
b. diverticulectomy
b. drainage
b. fistula
b. flap
b. flap hematoma
b. hemorrhage
b. hernia
hyperreflexic b.
hypertonic b.
ileal b.
b. laceration
b. neck elevation test
b. neck preserving technique
b. neck suspension
b. neck-to-urethra anastomosis
neurogenic b.
neuropathic b.
orthotopic b.
b. outlet reconstruction
b. perforation
poorly compliant b.
b. pressure
pseudoneurogenic b.
reflex neurogenic b.
b. replacement urinary pouch
stammering of the b.
b. stone
b. temperature
trabeculated b.
uninhibited neurogenic b.
unstable b.
urinary b.
valve b.
blade
b. atrial septostomy
b. bone
b. plate fixation
shoulder b.
Blair
B. epicanthus repair
B. fusion
B. incision
B. operation
B. technique
Blair-Brown
B.-B. procedure
B.-B. skin graft
Blair-Byars hypospadias technique
Blaivas classification of urinary incontinence

Blalock-Hanlon
B.-H. atrial septectomy
B.-H. operation
B.-H. procedure
Blalock-Taussig
B.-T. operation
B.-T. procedure
B.-T. shunt ligation
blanchable red lesion
blanched cutaneous elevation
Bland-Altman method
Blandin gland
Blandin-Nuhn gland
blanket suture technique
Blaschko line
Blasius
B. duct
B. lid flap operation
Blaskovics
B. canthoplasty operation
B. dacryostomy operation
B. flap
B. lid operation
B. tarsectomy
blastic
b. lesion
b. metastasis
blast injury
blastocele
blastocytoma
blastolysis
blastoma
pulmonary b.
blastotomy
Blatt
B. operation
B. procedure
Blatt-Ashworth procedure
bleb
endothelial b.
b. resection
Bleck
B. method
B. recession technique
bleed
postgastrectomy b.
postpolypectomy b.
trocar wound b.
bleeding
abnormal b.
b. abnormality
active source of b.
acute digestive b.
b. angioma
anorectal variceal b.
arterial b.
backflow b.
chronic digestive b.
colorectal b.
b. complication
concomitant b.
b. controlled with direct pressure
b. controlled with electrocautery
digestive b.
distal b.
b. episode
esophageal variceal b.
esophagogastric variceal b.
excessive b.
external b.
gastric variceal b.
gastrointestinal b.
implantation b.
intraabdominal b.
intracranial b.
intraoperative b.
intrathoracic b.
b. lesion
massive lower GI b.
occult b.
painless rectal b.
pinpoint gastric mucosal defect b.
placentation b.
b. point
portal hypertensive b.
postcoital b.
postmenopausal b.
postoperative b.
retroperitoneal b.
b. risk
b. site
b. site ligation
b. site localization
b. time
b. time coagulation panel
b. tumor
upper gastrointestinal b.
variceal b.
b. vessel
Blenderm patch technique
blenorrhagic inflammation
blepharal
blepharectomy
blepharochalasis repair

NOTES

blepharon
blepharoplasty
Davis-Geck b.
reoperative b.
blepharoptosis repair
blepharorrhaphy
Elschnig b.
blepharospasm
blepharosphincterectomy
blepharotomy
blind
b. abscess
b. clamping
b. dilatation
b. end
b. fistula
b. foramen
b. gut
b. insertion
b. lithotripsy
b. loop syndrome
b. nasal intubation anesthetic technique
b. nasotracheal intubation
b. nasotracheal intubation anesthetic technique
b. osteotomy
b. percutaneous liver biopsy
b. pouch syndrome
b. rectal pouch
b. upper esophageal pouch
blind-spot projection technique
blister
fracture b.
pressure b.
subcorneal b.
bloc
en b.
Bloch-Paul-Mikulicz operation
block
b. anesthesia
anesthetic b.
ankle b.
anterocrural celiac plexus b.
arborization b.
Atkinson lid b.
autonomic ganglion b.
autonomic nerve b.
axillary b.
Bier b.
bilateral bundle branch b.
brachial plexus b. (BPB)
bundle-branch b.
caudal b.
celiac plexus b.
central b.
cervical plexus b.
ciliovitrectomy b.
complete left bundle-branch b.
complete right bundle-branch b.
depolarization b.
depolarizing b.
differential nerve b.
differential spinal b.
direct obturator nerve b.
epidural b.
exit b.
extradural b.
femoral nerve b.
field b.
ganglion impar b.
gasserian ganglion b.
glossopharyngeal nerve b.
greater occipital nerve b.
Hara infiltration b.
hepatic outflow b.
His bundle heart b.
iliohypogastric nerve b.
ilioinguinal-iliohypogastric nerve b. (IINB)
ilioinguinal nerve b.
incomplete right bundle-branch b.
indirect obturator nerve b.
infiltration b.
infraorbital nerve b.
inguinal field b.
inguinal perivascular b.
b. injection
intercostal fossa b.
intercostal nerve b.
interpleural b.
interscalene brachial plexus b.
intrapleural b.
laparoscopic celiac plexus pain b.
left bundle-branch b.
lower extremity nerve b.
lumbar plexus b.
lumbar sympathetic b.
mandibular nerve b.
maxillary nerve b.
mental nerve b.
motor point b.
nerve b.
neuraxial neurolytic b.
neurolytic celiac plexus b. (NCPB)
neuromuscular b.
nondepolarizing b.
obturator nerve b.
b. osteotomy
paracervical b.
paravertebral lumbar sympathetic b.
penile b.
peripheral nerve b.
phase I, II b.
phrenic nerve b.
preganglionic sympathetic b.

prognostic b.
psoas sheath b.
regional b.
retrobulbar nerve b.
retrocrural celiac plexus b.
right bundle-branch b.
sciatic nerve b.
sensory b.
sinoatrial exit b.
sinus exit b.
skull b.
spinal b.
Steinberg infiltration b.
stellate ganglion b.
subarachnoid b.
subclavian perivascular b.
subdural b.
supraclavicular b.
sympathetic nerve b.
therapeutic nerve b.
three-in-one b.
tibial augmentation b.
tracheal b.
two-point nerve b.
upper extremity nerve b.
uterosacral b.
Van Lint lid b.
wrist b.
yoke b.

blockade
anesthetic b.
autonomic b.
beta-adrenergic b.
cholinergic b.
epidural b.
epidural neural b.
flickering b.
ganglionic b.
gasserian ganglion b.
interscalene b.
lytic b.
myoneural b.
neuromuscular b. (NMB)
nondepolarizing b.
onset of b.
preganglionic cardiac sympathetic b.
pulmonary sympathetic b.
sensory b.
stellate ganglion b.
sympathetic b.
temporary nerve b.

blockage
complete b.
ganglion b.
shunt b.

blocker
calcium entry b.
dihydropyridine calcium channel b.
ganglion b.
H_2 b.
use-dependent sodium channel b.

blocking
b. procedure
tissue b.
vecuronium neuromuscular b.

Blom-Singer tracheoesophageal fistula

blood
b. alcohol concentration
allogenic b.
autologous b.
b. bank
b. calculus
b. cell count
cerebral b.
circulating b.
b. clot
b. coagulation
b. coagulation disorder
b. donation
b. flow
b. flow rate
intraoperatively donated autologous b.
intravenous b.
b. lactate (BL)
b. loss
b. marker
mediastinal shed b. (MSB)
MV b.
occult b.
b. oxygenation level-dependent
b. oxygenation level-dependent contrast
oxygen concentration in pulmonary capillary b.
oxygen saturation of the hemoglobin of arterial b.
b. patch
b. patch injection
b. perfusion
preoperatively donated autologous b.
b. pressure

NOTES

B

blood *(continued)*
b. pressure monitoring
b. pressure support
b. product
b. product transfusion
b. stream infection
b. substitute
b. supply
b. supply artery
b. transfusion volume
b. tumor
UA b.
umbilical artery b.
umbilical vein b.
UV b.
b. vessel
b. vessel formation
b. vessel invasion (BVI)
b. vessel tumor
blood-air barrier
blood-borne infection
blood-brain
b.-b. barrier (BBB)
b.-b. equilibration time
blood-cerebral barrier
blood-cerebrospinal fluid barrier
blood-gas
b.-g. analysis
b.-g. exchange
Bloodgood syndrome
bloodless
b. amputation
b. decerebration
b. field
b. operation
b. phlebotomy
b. zone of necrosis
bloodletting
general b.
local b.
blood-liquor barrier
blood-ocular barrier
blood-optic nerve barrier
blood-retinal barrier
bloodstream infection
blood-substitute resuscitation
blood-thymus barrier
blood-tinged
b.-t. ascites
b.-t. CSF
blood-urine barrier
bloody peritoneal fluid
Bloom-Raney
B.-R. modification
B.-R. modification of Smith-Robinson technique
blot hemorrhage
Blount
B. displacement osteotomy
B. technique for osteoclasis
B. tracing technique
blowhole
b. decompressing colostomy
b. ileostomy
blow-in fracture
blow-out
aortic stump b.-o.
b.-o. fracture
blue
b. dome breast cyst
b. line
b. staining
b. toe syndrome
blue-black monofilament suture
blue-gray lesion
Blumenbach clivus
Blumensaat line
Blumenthal lesion
Blumer shelf
Blundell-Jones technique
blunderbuss apical canal
blunt
b. carotid injury
b. eversion carotid endarterectomy
b. hepatic trauma
b. liver injury
b. and sharp dissection
b. torso injury
blur point
blush
tumor b.
BMI
body mass index
B-mode imaging
BNP
brain natriuretic peptide
Boari
B. bladder flap
B. bladder flap procedure
B. ureteral flap repair
Boari-Ockerblad flap
Boas point
boatlike abdomen
boat nail
boat-shaped abdomen
Bobath method
bobby-pin abrasion
Bochdalek
B. gap
B. hernia
Bock
B. ganglion
B. nerve
Boden-Gibb tumor staging
Bodian method

body
adipose b.
adrenal b.
alveolar b.
Amato b.
anal foreign b.
anococcygeal b.
anorectal foreign b.
aortic b.
Arantius b.
Arnold b.
artificial vertebral b.
Aschoff b.
aspirated foreign b.
asteroid b.
b. awareness
Balbiani b.
Barr b.
Bence Jones b.
Bracht-Wachter b.
brassy b.
cancer b.
carotid b.
cartilaginous loose b.
b. cast syndrome
caudate b.
cavernous b.
b. cavity
b. cell mass
central fibrous b.
chromaffin b.
chromatinic b.
ciliary b.
coccidian b.
coccygeal b.
colloid b.
colonic foreign b.
b. composition analysis
compressed b.
compressible cavernous b.
corneal foreign b.
Creola b.
crescent b.
cystoid b.
cytoid b.
dense b.
duodenal foreign b.
Dutcher b.
Ehrlich inner b.
Elschnig b.
esophageal foreign b.
esophageal Lewy b.
external geniculate b.
fat b.
b. fat
fibrous loose b.
b. fluid
foreign b.
b. of gallbladder
Gamna-Gandy b.
gastric foreign b.
gelatin compression b.
geniculate b.
glomus b.
Goldmann-Larson foreign b.
Gordon elementary b.
b. habitus
Hamazaki-Wesenberg b.
Harting b.
Hassall b.
Heinz b.
Heinz-Ehrlich b.
b. hematocrit-venous hematocrit ratio
hematoxylin b.
Henle b.
Hensen b.
Highmore b.
Hirano b.
Howell-Jolly b.
hyaline b.
hyaloid b.
b. image
infrapatellar fat b.
ingested foreign b.
intraarticular loose b.
intraluminal foreign b.
intraocular foreign b.
intraorbital foreign b.
intrauterine foreign b.
intravascular foreign b.
Jaworski b.
juxtaglomerular b.
juxtarestiform b.
Kelvin b.
Lallemand b.
Lallemand-Trousseau b.
Landolt b.
lateral geniculate b.
Lieutaud b.
loose intraarticular b.
lower GI tract foreign b.
Luys b.
lyssa b.

NOTES

body *(continued)*
malpighian b.
mamillary b.
Maragiliano b.
b. mass index (BMI)
Maxwell b.
May-Hegglin b.
melon seed b.
metallic foreign b.
mineral oil foreign b.
Mott b.
Müller duct b.
multilamellar b.
Neill-Mooser b.
newtonian b.
nigroid b.
olivary b.
osteocartilaginous loose b.
osteochondral loose b.
owl eye inclusion b.
pampiniform b.
pancreatic b.
paranephric b.
paraterminal b.
pectinate b.
pedunculated loose b.
perineal b.
pineal b.
pituitary b.
b. position
Prowazek-Greeff b.
psammoma b.
pubic b.
pyknotic b.
radiopaque foreign b.
rectal foreign b.
refractile b.
Reilly b.
removal of foreign b.
residual b.
restiform b.
retained foreign b.
rice b.
b. righting reflex
rigid b.
Rosenmüller b.
Ross b.
round b.
Rucker b.
sand b.
Sandström b.
Savage perineal b.
b. scanning
Schaumann b.
b. schema
Schiller-Duvall b.
Seidelin b.
selenoid b.
b. side integration
spongy b.
S-shaped b.
b. stalk
striate b.
suprarenal b.
b. surface area (BSA)
b. surface burned
b. surface Laplacian mapping
Symington anococcygeal b.
b. temperature
thoracic vertebral b.
thrombogenic foreign b.
thyroid b.
tracheobronchial foreign b.
trapezoid b.
b. tumor
upper GI tract foreign b.
vagal b.
vaginal foreign b.
vermiform b.
vertebral b.
vitreous foreign b.
wall of b.
b. weight
Wesenberg-Hamazaki b.
Winkler b.
wolffian b.
X b.
Y b.
yellow b.

body-fluid
b.-f. analysis
b.-f. exchange

Boehler
B. calcaneal view
B. lumbosacral view

Boerema
B. anterior gastropexy
B. hernia repair

Boerhaave
B. gland
B. syndrome

Bogros space

Böhler calcaneal angle

Bohlman
B. anterior cervical vertebrectomy
B. cervical fusion technique
B. triple-wire technique

Böhm operation

Bohr
B. effect
B. equation
B. isopleth method

Boitzy open reduction

bolster suture technique

bolt fixation

Bolton-nasion line

Bolton point
bolus
fluid b.
b. injection
b. intravenous anesthesia
b. intravenous anesthetic technique
b. thermodilution (BTD)
Bonaccolto-Flieringa vitreous operation
bonded cast restoration
bonding
adhesive b.
bone
b. abscess
Albrecht b.
antigen-extracted allogeneic b.
articulation of pisiform b.
b. autogenous graft
basilar b.
basioccipital b.
basisphenoid b.
blade b.
b. block procedure
breast b.
Breschet b.
bundle b.
calcaneal b.
calf b.
capitate b.
central b.
cheek b.
b. chip
b. chip graft
collar b.
compact b.
cornua of hyoid b.
cortical b.
coxal b.
cranial b.
cuboid b.
cuneiform b.
b. cyst excision
b. cyst fracture probability
b. destruction
b. disease
b. dissection
dorsal talonavicular b.
ear b.
ectopic b.
enchondroma of b.
endochondral b.
epactal b.
epipteric b.
episternal b.
ethmoid b.
exoccipital b.
b. exposure
facial b.
first cuneiform b.
flank b.
b. flap
b. flap osteitis
flower b.
b. formation
b. fragment
frontal b.
Goethe b.
b. graft bed
b. graft collapse
b. graft decompression
b. graft extrusion
b. graft incorporation
b. graft placement
b. graft repair
b. graft substitute graft
greater multangular b.
hamate b.
heel b.
hip b.
hollow b.
hooked b.
b. hunger
hyoid b.
iliac b.
incarial b.
innominate b.
intermediate cuneiform b.
interparietal b.
irregular b.
ischial b.
jaw b.
jugal b.
Krause b.
lacrimal b.
lentiform b.
lingual b.
long b.
b. loss
lunate b.
lyophilization of b.
b. marrow aspiration
b. marrow aspiration and biopsy
b. marrow biopsy
b. marrow dysfunction
b. marrow examination

NOTES

bone *(continued)*
b. marrow failure
b. marrow graft
b. marrow infiltration
b. marrow lesion
b. marrow pressure
b. marrow puncture
b. marrow transplantation
b. mass
b. matrix
mesethmoid b.
metacarpal b.
b. metastasis
metatarsal b.
multangular b.
navicular b.
occipital b.
osteonal lamellar b.
osteoporotic b.
b. pain
palatine b.
parietal b.
b. peg graft
periotic b.
petrosal b.
pipe b.
Pirie b.
pisiform b.
pneumatic b.
postsphenoid b.
preinterparietal b.
presphenoid b.
pubic b.
pyramidal b.
b. resection
Riolan b.
sacred b.
scaphoid b.
second cuneiform b.
semilunar b.
sesamoid b.
shank b.
shin b.
short b.
sieve b.
sphenoid b.
sphenoidal turbinated b.
suprainterparietal b.
suprasternal b.
sutural b.
tail b.
b. technique
temporal b.
thigh b.
three-cornered b.
tongue b.
triangular b.
triquetral b.
b. tumor
tympanic b.
tympanohyal b.
unciform b.
upper jaw b.
Vesalius b.
wedge b.
b. wedge
wormian b.
yoke b.
zygomatic b.

bone-cement interface
bone-implant interface
bone-ingrowth fixation
bone-ligament dissection
bone-patellar tendon-bone preparation
bone-retinaculum-bone autograft graft
bone-screw interface strength
bone-tendon-bone graft
bone-to-bone graft
Bonferroni correction
Bonfiglio
B. bone graft
B. modification
B. modification of Phemister technique

Bonfiglio-Bardenstein technique
Bonnaire method
Bonner position
Bonnet
B. capsule
B. enucleation operation

Bonney
B. abdominal hysterectomy
B. test

Bonola technique
bony
b. bridge resection
b. deformity
b. demineralization
b. dissection
b. element destruction
b. excrescence
b. exposure
b. fragment
b. labyrinth
b. landmark
b. lesion
b. mass
b. metastasis
b. necrosis and destruction
b. procedure
b. projection
b. semicircular canal
b. structure

Bonzel operation
book thoracotomy
boomerang-shaped lesion

boost technique
bootstrap
- b. dilation
- b. two-vessel angioplasty
- b. two-vessel technique

boot-top fracture
Boplant graft
Bora
- B. centralization
- B. operation
- B. technique

Borchgrevink method
border
- frontal b.
- interosseous b.
- b. involvement
- mesenteric b.
- nasal b.
- occipital b.
- parietal b.
- b. ray amputation
- squamous b.
- b. tissue
- b. tissue of Jacoby
- b. tissue movement
- vermilion b.

Borggreve
- B. limb rotation
- B. method

Borggreve-Hall technique
Borg treadmill exertion scale
boron neutron-capture therapy
Borrmann
- B. gastric cancer classification
- B. gastric cancer typing systems (types I–IV) classification
- B. type I-IV carcinoma

Bose
- B. nail-fold excision
- B. operation
- B. procedure

Bosniak classification
boss
- carpal b.

Bossalino blepharoplasty operation
bosselation
Bosworth
- B. approach
- B. femoroischial transplantation
- B. fracture
- B. spinal fusion
- B. tendo calcaneus repair

both-bone fracture
both-column fracture
Böttcher
- B. canal
- B. space

botulinum A toxin
Bouchut respiration
bougienage technique
bounce point
boundary
- air-bone-tissue b.
- inferior b.
- superior b.

boutonnière
- b. deformity
- b. hand dislocation
- b. incision

Bovero muscle
Bovie
- B. cauterization
- B. coagulation

bovied
bovina
bowel
- b. abscess
- b. anastomosis
- b. bypass
- b. bypass syndrome
- b. cleansing
- compliant b.
- b. continuity
- denuded b.
- dilated loop of b.
- b. dilation
- edematous b.
- b. function
- b. habits
- b. injury
- b. lavage
- b. length
- b. loop
- b. loop air
- b. movement
- Noble surgical plication of b.
- obstructed b.
- b. obstruction
- b. perforation
- b. preparation
- prepared large b.
- b. refashioning procedure
- b. resection
- b. sounds

NOTES

bowel *(continued)*
b. stoma
supple b.
b. wall
b. wall hematoma
weakened b.
Bowen cavity primer
Bowers technique
bowing
b. deformity
b. fracture
bowleg deformity
Bowles technique
bowl fistula
Bowman
B. gland
B. membrane
B. operation
B. space
bow-tie
b.-t. knot
b.-t. stitch
boxer fracture
Box technique
Boyce
longitudinal nephrotomy of B.
B. position
Boyce-Vest procedure
Boyd
B. ankle amputation
B. approach
B. classification
B. hip disarticulation
B. operation
B. point
Boyd-Anderson
B.-A. biceps tendon repair
B.-A. technique
Boyd-Bosworth procedure
Boyden
B. chamber technique
B. sphincter
Boyd-Griffin trochanteric fracture classification
Boyd-Ingram-Bourkhard treatment
Boyd-McLeod
B.-M. procedure
B.-M. tennis elbow technique
Boyd-Sisk
B.-S. approach
B.-S. posterior capsulorrhaphy
Boyer bursa
Boyes brachioradialis transfer technique
Boytchev procedure
Bozeman
B. operation
B. position
B. suture technique
BPB
biliopancreatic bypass
brachial plexus block
BPCF
bronchopleurocutaneous fistula
BPD
biparietal diameter
bronchopulmonary dysplasia
BP fistula
BPH
benign prostatic hyperplasia
BPI
Brief Pain Inventory
BPPV
benign paroxysmal positional vertigo
Braasch bulb technique
brachia (*pl. of* brachium)
brachial
b. anesthesia
b. arteriotomy
b. artery
b. artery approach
b. cleft cyst
b. fascia
b. gland
b. muscle
b. plexus
b. plexus block (BPB)
b. plexus block anesthetic technique
b. plexus infiltration
b. plexus nerve
b. plexus repair
b. plexus traction injury
brachiales
brachialis
brachii
brachioaxillary bridge graft fistula
brachiocephalic
b. trunk
b. trunk artery
b. vein
b. vessel angioplasty
brachiocephalicus
brachioplasty
brachioradialis
b. flap
brachioradial muscle
brachiosubclavian
b. bridge graft
b. bridge graft fistula
brachium, pl. **brachia**
Bracht maneuver
Bracht-Wachter
B.-W. body
B.-W. lesion
brachybasocamptodactyly
brachybasophalangia

brachycheilia
brachydactyly
brachyfacial
brachygnathia
brachymorphic
brachypellic pelvis
brachyprosopic
brachyrhinia
brachyrhynchus
brachystaphyline
brachysyndactyly
brachytherapy
endobronchial b.
interstitial b.
bracing
external b.
fracture b.
bracket
b. modification
b. slot angulation
Brackett-Osgood posterior approach
Brackett-Osgood-Putti-Abbott technique
Brackett osteotomy
Brackin
B. incision
B. technique
B. ureterointestinal anastomosis
Bradford fusion
Bradley method of prepared childbirth
Brady-Jewett technique
bradykinesia
Bragg peak proton-beam therapy
Brahms procedure
braid-like lesion
Brailey operation
brain
b. abscess
b. biopsy
b. concussion
b. congestion
b. contusion
b. death
b. edema
b. herniation
b. infection
b. injury
b. laceration
b. mass
b. metastasis
b. natriuretic peptide (BNP)
b. neoplasm
b. puncture
b. region
respirator b.
b. revascularization
b. stimulation
b. temperature
b. transplantation
b. tumor
b. tumor headache
B. Tumor Registry
brain-dead patient
brainstem
b. compression
b. evoked response
b. hemorrhage
b. lesion
braking radiation
branch
acetabular b.
acromial b.
adrenal b.
anastomotic b.
anterior basal b.
anterior cutaneous b.
arterial b.
articular b.
ascending anterior b.
ascending posterior b.
auricular b.
basal tentorial b.
buccal b.
capsular b.
carotid sinus b.
caudate b.
celiac b.
cervical b.
clavicular b.
coeliac b.
communicating b.
deep palmar b.
deep plantar b.
deltoid b.
descending anterior b.
descending posterior b.
digastric b.
dorsal b.
epiploic b.
esophageal b.
external b.
faucial b.
frontal b.
ganglionic b.
gastric b.

NOTES

B

branch *(continued)*
- genital b.
- glandular b.
- gonadal b.
- hepatic b.
- iliac b.
- inferior temporal b.
- inguinal b.
- internal b.
- joint b.
- lateral calcaneal b.
- lateral nasal b.
- b. lesion
- lingual b.
- lingular b.
- lumbar b.
- major sinistral b.
- mammary b.
- marginal mandibular b.
- marginal tentorial b.
- mastoid b.
- medial cutaneous b.
- medial mammary b.
- mediastinal b.
- meningeal b.
- mental b.
- occipital b.
- omental b.
- orbital b.
- ovarian b.
- b. pad
- palmar b.
- palpebral b.
- pancreatic b.
- parietal b.
- parotid b.
- pectoral b.
- perforating b.
- pericardial b.
- petrosal b.
- pharyngeal b.
- phrenicoabdominal b.
- posterior basal b.
- pterygoid b.
- pubic b.
- recurrent meningeal b.
- renal b.
- right b.
- saphenous b.
- sectorial b.
- sinoatrial nodal b.
- splenic b.
- sternal b.
- stylohyoid b.
- subscapular b.
- superficial b.
- superior cervical cardiac b.
- superior labial b.
- superior laryngeal nerve external b.
- suprahyoid b.
- sympathetic b.
- temporal b.
- thoracic cardiac b.
- thymic b.
- tonsillar b.
- tracheal b.
- tubal b.
- ulnar b.
- ureteral b.
- ureteric b.
- zygomatic b.
- zygomaticofacial b.
- zygomaticotemporal b.

branched
- b. calculus
- b. vascular graft

branchial
- b. anomaly
- b. cartilage
- b. cyst
- b. fistula
- b. sinus

branching
- b. canal
- b. morphogenesis
- b. tubule formation

branchiogenous cyst
branchiomeric muscle
Brandt-Andrews maneuver
Brand tendon transfer technique
Brantigan procedure
Brantigan-Voshell procedure
Brasdor method
brassy body
Braun
- B. anastomosis
- B. procedure
- B. shoulder tenotomy

Braune
- B. canal
- B. muscle

Braun-Jaboulay gastroenterostomy
Braun-Wangensteen graft
brawny
- b. arm
- b. induration

breach
- serosal b.

breakdown
- anastomotic b.
- epithelial b.
- muscle b.
- sepsis-induced muscle b.

break point
breast
- b. abscess

accessory b.
adenoma of b.
b. approach thyroidectomy
b. augmentation
b. biopsy
b. biopsy tissue
b. bone
b. calcification
b. cancer
B. Cancer Detection Demonstration Project
b. cancer-related mutation
b. cancer risk
b. cancer risk prediction
b. cancer-specific survival (BCSS)
b. carcinoma
comedo carcinoma of b.
b. conservation therapy (BCT)
b. contour
b. cyst
b. cyst aspiration
b. discharge
B. Imaging Reporting and Data System (BIRADS)
b. incision
b. irradiation
b. lymphatic mapping
male b.
b. metastasis
b. mucocele
b. parenchyma
b. preservation
b. reconstruction
b. resection
b. size
b. skin envelope
b. stimulation contraction test
supernumerary b.

breast-conserving
b.-c. method
b.-c. procedure
b.-c. surgery
b.-c. technique
b.-c. therapy

breast-lift mastopexy
breast-milk jaundice
breast-preservation therapy
breast-sparing mastectomy
breath
b. excretion test
b. stacking

breathing
apneustic b.
Biot b.
b. circuit
continuous positive pressure b. (CPPB)
intermittent positive pressure b. (IPPB)
b. lung
b. method
negative inspiratory b.
pattern of b.
positive-negative pressure b. (PNPB)
sign mechanism for ventilator b.
spontaneous b.
work of b. (WOB)

Brecher-Cronkite
B.-C. method
B.-C. technique

Brecher new methylene blue technique
breech
b. extraction
b. head

bregma
bregma-mentum projection
bregmatic fontanelle
bregmatolambdoid arc
bregmatomastoid
b. suture
b. suture technique

Brenner
B. gastrojejunostomy technique
B. operation

brephoplastic graft
Breschet
B. bone
B. canal
B. hiatus

Brescia-Cimino
B.-C. A-V fistula
B.-C. graft

Breslow
B. classification
B. thickness

Brett-Campbell tibial osteotomy
Breuer-Hering inflation reflex
Breuerton view
breve
breves
brevia

NOTES

brevis
extensor carpi radialis b. (ECRB)
extensor digitorum b.
extensor pollicis b.
Bricker
B. conduit
B. operation
B. procedure
B. ureteroileostomy
Brickner position
bridge
adhesive resin-bonded b.
colostomy b.
conjugation b.
extension b.
fascial b.
Gaskell b.
b. graft
loop ostomy b.
membrane b.
mucosal b.
mylohyoid b.
B. operation
b. organ transplantation
b. pedicle flap
b. pedicle flap operation
b. plate fixation
retention suture b.
b. suture
suture b.
bridge-like
b.-l. lesion
b.-l. septum
bridging syndesmophyte
bridle
B. procedure
b. suture
b. suture technique
Brief Pain Inventory (BPI)
Briggs strabismus operation
Bright disease
brightness modulation
brim
pelvic b.
brine flotation method
Brinell hardness indenter point
Brisbane method
brisement therapy
Bristow-Helfet procedure
Bristow-May procedure
Bristow operation
brittle
b. nail
b. nail syndrome
broad
b. fascia
b. ligament hernia
b. uterine ligament
broadband attenuation
Broadbent registration point
Broadbent-Woolf four-limb Z-plasty
broadest muscle
broad-spectrum antibiotic
Broca
B. basilar angle
B. facial angle
B. pouch
B. visual plane
Brock
B. incision
B. infundibulectomy
B. operation
B. procedure
Brockenbrough
B. technique
B. transseptal commissurotomy
Brockhurst technique
Brockman incision
Brockman-Nissen wrist arthrodesis
Brödel bloodless line
Broders index of malignant tumors classification
Brodie bursa
Brodie-Trendelenburg tourniquet test
Brodi metaphysial abscess
Brodsky-Tullos-Gartsman approach
Broesike fossa
Bromage scale
bromide
bromination
Bromley foreign body operation
Brom repair
bronchi (*pl. of* bronchus)
bronchia (*pl. of* bronchium)
bronchial
b. adenocarcinoma
b. adenoma
b. artery
b. brush biopsy
b. brushing
b. carcinoma
b. fracture
b. gland
b. inflammation
b. inhalation challenge test
b. respiration
b. sleeve resection
b. tract
b. tree
b. vein
bronchial-associated lymphoid tissue
bronchiales
bronchiogenic
bronchiolar adenocarcinoma

bronchiole
respiratory b.
terminal b.
bronchioli (*pl. of* bronchiolus)
bronchiolitis
obliterative b.
bronchioloalveolar
b. adenocarcinoma
b. carcinoma
bronchiolopulmonary
bronchiolus, pl. **bronchioli**
bronchiomediastinalis
bronchiorum
bronchitis
bronchium, pl. **bronchia**
bronchoalveolar
b. carcinoma
bronchobiliary fistula
bronchocavernous respiration
bronchoconstriction
bronchodilatation
bronchodilation
bronchoesophageal
b. fistula
b. muscle
bronchoesophageus
bronchoesophagoscopy
bronchogenic adenocarcinoma
bronchomediastinal trunk
bronchoplasty
balloon b.
bronchopleural
b. fistula
b. leak squeak
bronchopleurocutaneous fistula (BPCF)
bronchopneumonia
sequestration b.
bronchoprovocation test
bronchopulmonale
bronchopulmonales
bronchopulmonary
b. dysplasia (BPD)
b. fistula
b. foregut malformation
b. segment
bronchorrhaphy
bronchoscope-guided intubation
bronchoscopic
b. needle biopsy
b. photodynamic therapy
bronchoscopy
b. anesthetic technique
fiberoptic b.
flexible fiberoptic b.
rigid b.
ultrasound-guided b.
bronchospasm
exercise-induced b.
induced b.
bronchospirography
bronchospirometry
bronchostomy
bronchotomy
bronchotracheal
bronchovesicular respiration
bronchus, pl. **bronchi**
ectatic b.
intermediate b.
lobar b.
right main b.
segmental b.
stem b.
Bronson foreign body removal operation
Brooke ileostomy
Brooks-Jenkins atlantoaxial fusion technique
Brooks-Seddon transfer technique
Brooks technique
Brooks-type fusion
Broomhead medial approach
Brophy operation
Broström
B. injection technique
B. procedure
Broström-Gould foot procedure
brow
b. fixation
b. position
brow-anterior position
brow-down position
browlift
brown
b. adipose tissue
b. atrophy
b. dietary method for colon preparation
b. fat tumor
b. knee approach
b. knee joint reconstruction
b. lateral approach
b. technique
b. and Wickham pressure profile method

NOTES

Brown-Beard technique
brown-black lesion
Brown-Brenn technique
Brown-Dodge method
Browning vein
Brown-McHardy pneumatic mercury bougie dilation
Brown-Wickham technique
brow-posterior position
brow-up position
B-RTO
balloon-occluded retrograde transvenous obliteration
Bruce bundle
Bruch membrane
Bruger
cul-de-sac of B.
Bruhat
B. laser fimbrioplasty
B. technique
Bruhn method
bruit
peripheral b.
Bruner approach
Brunner
B. gland
B. modified incision
B. palmar incision
Brunn nest
Brunschwig operation
Bruser
B. knee approach
B. lateral approach
B. skin incision
B. technique
brush
b. biopsy
b. cytology
b. technique filling
brush-border
b.-b. membrane
b.-b. membrane vesicle
brushing
bronchial b.
brusque dilatation of esophagus
bruxism
Bryan
B. arthroplasty
B. procedure
Bryan-Morrey
B.-M. elbow approach
B.-M. extensive posterior approach
B.-M. technique
Bryant operation
BSA
body surface area
BTD
bolus thermodilution
bubble oxygenation
bubbly bone lesion
bucca, pl. **buccae**
buccal
b. artery
b. aspect
b. branch
b. cavity
b. drug administration
b. fat pad
b. mucosal flap
b. nerve
b. ostectomy
b. restoration
b. smear
b. space
b. space abscess
b. space infection
b. surface
b. transmucosal delivery
b. vein
buccalis
buccinator
b. artery
b. crest
b. muscle
b. nerve
b. node
b. plication
b. space
buccinatorius
buccolingual (BL)
b. plane
b. relation
bucconeural duct
buccoocclusal line angle
buccopharyngea
buccopharyngeal
b. approach
b. fascia
b. space
buccopharyngeus
Buck
B. fascia
B. method
bucket-handle
b.-h. fracture
b.-h. incision
b.-h. tear
Buck-Gramcko
B.-G. pollicization
B.-G. technique
buckle fracture
Budd-Chiari
B.-C. syndrome
B.-C. syndrome with Behçet disease

B.-C. syndrome without Behçet disease
Budin-Chandler method
Budinger blepharoplasty operation
Bugg-Boyd technique
Buie position
built-in angulation
Buist method
bulb
b. deformity
duodenal b.
jugular venous b.
olfactory b.
Rouget b.
b. suction
bulbar
b. cephalic pain tractotomy
b. sheath fascia
bulbocavernosus
b. fat flap
b. fat pad
b. muscle
bulboid
bulbospongiosus
bulbourethral
b. gland
bulbourethralis
bulbous internal auditory canal
bulb-tip retrograde study
bulge
gastric b.
bulk
b. pack technique
tumor b.
bulkhead method
bulla, pl. **bullae**
ethmoid b.
bulldog head
bullectomy
transaxillary apical b.
bullet
b. trajectory
b. wound
bullous
b. edema
b. granulomatous inflammation
b. skin lesion
bull's eye macular lesion
bumper fracture
bunching
b. maneuver
b. suture technique
Buncke technique
bundle
anterior ground b.
anteromedial b.
arcuate nerve fiber b.
Arnold b.
atrioventricular b.
A-V b.
Bachmann b.
b. bone
Bruce b.
cingulum b.
coherent b.
commissural b.
Drualt b.
fiber b.
b. fiber
fiberoptic b.
Gierke respiratory b.
Held b.
Helweg b.
His b.
Hoche b.
IG b.
image guide b.
inferior arcuate b.
intercostal b.
intermediate b.
b. of Itis
James b.
Keith b.
Kent b.
Kent-His b.
Killian b.
Krause respiratory b.
lateral ground b.
LG b.
light guide b.
Lissauer b.
Loewenthal b.
maculopapillary b.
maculopapular b.
Mahaim b.
main b.
master IG b.
Meynert retroflex b.
microfilament b.
Monakow b.
neovascular b.
nerve fiber b.
neurovascular b.
olfactory b.

NOTES

bundle *(continued)*
olivocochlear b.
papillomacular nerve fiber b.
paracentral nerve fiber b.
Pick b.
posterior longitudinal b.
posterolateral b.
precommissural b.
predorsal b.
principal fiber b.
Rathke b.
Schütz b.
sensory nerve fiber b.
solitary b.
b. of Stanley Kent
superior arcuate b.
superior gluteal neurovascular b.
Thorel b.
Türck b.
vascular b.
Vicq d'Azyr b.
bundle-branch
b.-b. block
b.-b. reentrant tachycardia
b.-b. reentry
Bunge amputation
bunion
b. deformity
b. formation
bunionectomy
Akin b.
Austin b.
chevron b.
DuVries-Mann modified b.
Hauser b.
Joplin b.
Keller b.
Kreuscher b.
Lapidus b.
Ludloff b.
Mayo-Heuter b.
McBride b.
Peabody-Mitchell b.
Reverdin b.
Reverdin-Laird b.
Reverdin-McBride b.
Silver b.
tailor b.
tricorrectional b.
Wilson b.
bunk-bed fracture
Bunnell
B. atraumatic technique
B. modification of Steindler flexorplasty
B. opponensplasty
B. stitch
B. suture technique
B. tendon repair
B. tendon transfer technique
Bunnell-Williams procedure
Bunyavirus infection
buprenorphine narcotic analgesic therapy
Burch
B. bladder suspension
B. bladder suspension method
B. bladder suspension procedure
B. bladder suspension technique
B. colposuspension
B. colpourethropexy
B. eye evisceration operation
B. iliopectineal ligament urethrovesical suspension
B. laparo
B. modification
Burdach tract
burden
tumor b.
Burger technique for scapulothoracic disarticulation
Burgess
B. below-knee amputation
B. method
B. technique
Burhenne biliary duct stone extraction
bur hole
bur-hole placement
buried
b. flap
b. mass far-and-near suture technique
b. penis
Burkhalter
B. modification of Stiles-Bunnell technique
B. transfer technique
Burkhalter-Reyes method of phalangeal fracture
burn
b. boutonnière deformity
b. classification
corneal alkali b.
b. débridement
first-degree b.
full-thickness b.
b. injury
irrigation b.
partial-thickness b.
plaster cast application b.
radiation b.
b. scar carcinoma
second-degree b.
superficial b.
third-degree b.

burned
body surface b.
Burnet-Talmadge-Lederberg theory of antibody formation
Burnett syndrome
burn-induced muscle proteolysis
burning
b. dysesthesia
b. feet syndrome
b. pain
burn-out procedure
Burns-Haney incision
Burns space
Burow
B. flap operation
B. quantitative method
B. triangle
B. vein
Burrows technique
bursa, pl. **bursae**
Achilles b.
b. achillis
anserine b.
anterior tibial b.
bicipitoradial b.
b. bicipitoradialis
Boyer b.
Brodie b.
Calori b.
coracobrachial b.
deep infrapatellar b.
Fleischmann b.
gluteofemoral b.
iliac b.
iliopectineal b.
infrahyoid b.
infraspinatus b.
intermuscular gluteal b.
intrapatellar b.
ischial b.
laryngeal b.
medial malleolar subcutaneous b.
b. of Monro
b. mucosa
omental b.
ovarian b.
pharyngeal b.
prepatellar b.
radial b.
retrocalcaneal b.
retrohyoid b.
subacromial b.
subcoracoid b.
subcutaneous acromial b.
subcutaneous calcaneal b.
subcutaneous infrapatellar b.
subcutaneous olecranon b.
subdeltoid b.
subfascial prepatellar b.
subhyoid b.
sublingual b.
subscapular b.
subtendinous iliac b.
subtendinous prepatellar b.
suprapatellar b.
synovial b.
tibial intertendinous b.
triceps b.
trochanteric b.
trochlear synovial b.
ulnar b.
bursa-equivalent tissue
bursal
b. flap
b. projection
b. sac
b. tissue
bursectomy
burst fracture
bursting dislocation
burst-type laceration
Burton line
Burwell-Scott modification of Watson-Jones incision
Buschke-Löwenstein tumor
Butchart staging classification
Butler
B. fifth toe operation
B. procedure to correct overlapping toes
butterfly
b. flap
b. fracture
b. fracture fragment
b. patch
b. pattern
buttocks pad
button
b. abscess
belly b.
b. one-step gastrostomy
stoma b.
b. suture technique

NOTES

buttonhole
b. approach
b. deformity
b. fracture
b. iridectomy
b. operation
b. puncture technique for hemodialysis needle insertion
b. skin incision
b. suture technique
Buxton bolus suture technique
Buzzard maneuver
Buzzi operation
BVI
blood vessel invasion
Byers flap
bypass
Alden loop gastric b.
b. anesthesia
aortofemoral b.
aortoiliac b.
aortorenal b.
Aria coronary b.
axilloaxillary b.
axillobifemoral b.
axillofemoral b.
axillounifemoral b.
biliary enteric b.
biliointestinal b. (BIB)
biliopancreatic b. (BPB)
bowel b.
cardiac b. (CBP)
cardiopulmonary b. (CPB)
carotid artery b.
carotid-subclavian b.
carotid-subclavian artery b.
cervical-to-MCA b.
CFA-SFA b.
coronary artery b.
end-to-end jejunoileal b.
end-to-side jejunoileal b.
exclusion b.
extraanatomic b.
extracorporeal venous b.
extracranial-intracranial b.
b. failure
femoral-popliteal artery b.
femoral-tibial-peroneal b.
femorodistal b.
femoropopliteal b.
gastric b.
gastric loop b.
b. graft catheterization
Greenville gastric b.
Griffen Roux-en-Y b.
Hallberg biliointestinal b.
hand-assisted laparoscopic gastric b.
hepatorenal b.
ileojejunal b.
infrainguinal b.
infrapopliteal b.
jejunoileal b. (JIB)
laparoscopic gastric b.
left atrium-to-femoral artery circulatory b.
Litwak aortic b.
long-limb gastric artery b.
loop gastric b.
lower-extremity b.
lymphaticovenous b.
b. method
minimally invasive direct coronary artery b. (MIDCAB)
nonanatomic renal b.
obturator b.
off-pump coronary artery b. (OPCAB)
b. operation
operative biliary b.
palliative b.
pancreatic b.
partial ileal b.
Payne-DeWind jejunoileal b.
petrous-to-supraclinoid b.
primary antecubital jump b. (PAJB)
b. procedure
Roux-en-Y biliary b.
Roux-en-Y gastric b.
saphenous ICA b.
saphenous vein b.
Scopinaro pancreaticobiliary b.
Scott jejunoileal b.
Silastic ring vertical-banded gastric b. (SRVGB)
simple b.
in situ b.
subclavian-subclavian b.
superficial temporal artery-to-MCA b.
b. surgery
b. technique
b. tract
transected vertical gastric b.
venovenous b. (VVB)
venovenous extracorporeal b.
vertical gastric b.
Byrd-Drew method
Byron
B. Smith ectropion operation
B. Smith lazy-T correction
Bywaters lesion
Byzantine arch palate

C
C graft
C sliding osteotomy
CA 19-9
carbohydrate antigen 19-9
CABG
coronary artery bypass graft
redo CABG
cable wire suture technique
Cabot-Nesbit orchiopexy
Cabot trumpet valve
Cabral coronary reconstruction
cachexia
cancer c.
muscle c.
CACI
computer-assisted controlled infusion
CACT
celite-activated clotting time
CAD
cadaver donor
cadaver
c. donor (CAD)
c. renal preservation
cadaveric
c. donor
c. donor hepatectomy
c. hand transplant
c. whole organ transplant
CAF
coronary artery fistula
caffeine and halothane contracture test (CHCT)
cage
thoracic c.
Cairns
C. maneuver
C. operation
C. trabeculectomy
Cajal
C. gold-sublimate method
C. uranium silver method
Calandriello procedure
calcanea
calcaneal
c. apophysitis
c. arterial network
c. artery
c. avulsion fracture
c. bone
c. displaced fracture
c. fracture reduction
c. inclination angle
c. L osteotomy
c. process
c. region
c. spur syndrome
c. stance position
c. sulcus
c. tendon
c. tenodesis
c. tuber
c. tubercle
calcaneal-second metatarsal angle inclination angle
calcanean tendon
calcanei (*pl. of* calcaneus)
calcaneoastragaloid
calcaneocavovarus deformity
calcaneocavus
c. deformity
calcaneocuboid articulation
calcaneofibular
calcaneonavicular bar resection
calcaneoscaphoid
calcaneotibial fusion
calcaneovalgus deformity
calcaneovarus deformity
calcaneum
calcaneus, pl. **calcanei**
calcar
calcareous
c. artery
c. infiltration
c. metastasis
calcarina
calcarine
c. artery
calces (*pl. of* calx)
calcific aortic stenosis
calcification
breast c.
clustered c.
clustered c.
focal c.
intratumoral c.
c. line
linear c.
multiple c.
subependymal brain c.
c. zone
calcified
c. gallbladder
c. granulomatous inflammation
c. lesion
c. liver metastasis
c. renal mass
calcifying metastasis
calciotraumatic line
calcipexy

calcis
calcitonin
calcitriol supplementation
calcium
c. carbonate supplementation
c. entry blocker
c. pyrophosphate deposition disease
c. sensor
calcium-sensing receptor
calculous
c. cholecystitis
c. formation
c. gallbladder
calculus, pl. **calculi**
alvine c.
apatite c.
bile duct c.
biliary c.
bladder c.
blood c.
branched c.
caliceal diverticular c.
cat's eye c.
cerebral c.
cholesterol c.
combination c.
common duct c.
coral c.
cystine c.
decubitus c.
dendritic c.
ductal c.
encysted c.
fibrin c.
gallbladder c.
gastric c.
hard c.
hemic c.
hepatic duct c.
impacted c.
infection c.
intestinal c.
matrix c.
c. migration
mulberry c.
nephritic c.
oxalate c.
pancreatic c.
pleural c.
pocketed c.
preputial c.
primary renal c.
prostatic c.
renal c.
secondary renal c.
staghorn c.
struvite c.
urethral c.
urinary c.
vesical c.
weddellite c.
whewellite c.
Caldwell-Coleman flatfoot technique
Caldwell-Luc
C.-L. approach
C.-L. incision
C.-L. operation
C.-L. window procedure
Caldwell-Moloy
C.-M. classification
C.-M. method
Caldwell projection
calf, pl. **calves**
c. bone
Calhoun-Hagler lens extraction operation
calibrated electrical stimulation
calibration
c. curve
oscillometric c.
c. overshoot
caliceal
c. abnormality
c. diverticular calculus
c. diverticulum
c. extension
c. fornix
c. infundibulum
c. nephrostolithotomy
calicectasis
calicectomy
calices (*pl. of* calix)
caliciform
calicine
calicoplasty
calicotomy
caliectasis
caliectomy
caligation
calioplasty
caliorrhaphy
caliotomy
calix, pl. **calices**
major c.
minor c.
c. puncture
Callahan
C. approach
C. extension of cervical injury
C. fusion technique
C. operation
C. root canal filling method
Callander amputation
Callender cell-type classification
callosal disconnection syndrome
callosomarginal artery

callosotomy
corpus c.
callous formation
callus
fracture c.
irritation c.
Calori bursa
caloric
c. expenditure
c. irrigation
calorimetry
Calot triangle
calvaria, pl. **calvariae**
calvarial free bone graft
calves (*pl. of* calf)
calx, pl. **calces**
calyceal fistula
calycectomy
calyces (*pl. of* calyx)
calyciform
calycine
calycle
calycoplasty
calycotomy
calyoplasty
calyorrhaphy
calyotomy
calyx, pl. **calyces**
CAM
cystic adenomatoid malformation
Cambridge classification
cameral fistula
Cameron femoral component removal
Camey
C. enterocystoplasty
C. enterocystoplasty urinary diversion
C. ileocystoplasty
C. I, II operation
C. procedure
Camino catheter technique
Camitz technique
Campbell
C. interpositional arthroplasty
C. onlay bone graft
C. osteotomy
C. posterior shoulder approach
C. posterolateral approach
C. resection arthroplasty
C. technique
C. triceps reflection
Campbell-Akbarnia procedure
Campbell-Goldthwait procedure
Camper
C. chiasm
C. fascia
C. ligament
C. line
C. plane
Camp-Gianturco method
Campodonico
C. canal
C. operation
campotomy
camptomelic syndrome
***Campylobacter* infection**
***Campylobacter*-like organism biopsy**
Canadian Cardiovascular Society classification
canal
abdominal c.
accessory palatine c.
accessory root c.
acoustic c.
additional c.
adductor c.
Alcock c.
alimentary c.
alveolar c.
anal c.
anterior condylar c.
anterior semicircular c.
anterior vertical c.
antropyloric c.
c. of Arantius
Arnold c.
atrioventricular c.
auditory c.
auxiliary c.
basipharyngeal c.
bayonet c.
bayonet-curved c.
Bernard c.
Bichat c.
birth c.
blunderbuss apical c.
bony semicircular c.
Böttcher c.
branching c.
Braune c.
Breschet c.
bulbous internal auditory c.
Campodonico c.
caroticoclinoid c.

NOTES

canal *(continued)*
caroticotympanic c.
carotid c.
cartilage c.
caudal c.
central c.
cervical c.
cervicoaxillary c.
ciliary c.
Cloquet c.
collateral pulp c.
common c.
condylar c.
cortical bone primary c.
Cotunnius c.
cranial c.
craniopharyngeal c.
crural c.
C-shaped c.
c. curvature
curved c.
c. of Cuvier
c. débridement
defalcated root c.
deferent c.
dehiscent mandibular c.
dental c.
dentinal c.
dilacerated c.
diploic c.
Dorello c.
Dupuytren c.
ear c.
endocervical c.
ethmoid c.
external auditory c.
facial c.
fallopian c.
femoral c.
Ferrein c.
filling c.
Fontana c.
furcation c.
galactophorous c.
Gartner c.
gastric c.
gubernacular c.
Guyon c.
Hannover c.
haversian c.
Hensen c.
c. of Hering
Hirschfeld c.
His c.
horizontal c.
Hovius c.
Hoyer c.
Huguier c.
humeral c.
Hunter c.
hyaloid c.
hypoglossal c.
identifying c.
incisal c.
incisive c.
infraorbital c.
inguinal c.
c. innominate osteotomy
inoperable c.
interdental c.
interfacial c.
internal auditory c.
intramedullary c.
c. irrigation
Kovalevsky c.
lacrimal c.
Lambert c.
large c.
lateral c.
Lauth c.
locating c.
longitudinal c.
Löwenberg c.
lumbar c.
lumbosacral c.
lymphatic c.
mandibular c.
maxillary c.
medullary c.
mental c.
mesiobuccal c.
musculotubal c.
nasal c.
nasolacrimal c.
neural c.
neurenteric c.
Nuck c.
nutrient c.
c. obturation
obturator c.
optic c.
orbital c.
overfilled c.
palatine c.
palatomaxillary c.
palatovaginal c.
pancreatobiliary c.
partial atrioventricular c.
parturient c.
pelvic c.
perivascular c.
persistent common atrioventricular c.
Petit c.
pharyngeal c.
pleuroperitoneal c.

Got a Good Word for STEDMAN'S?

Help us keep STEDMAN'S products fresh and up-to-date with new words and new ideas! How can we make your STEDMAN'S product the best medical word reference possible for you?

Do we need to add or revise any items? Is there a better way to organize the content?

Be specific! Fill in the lines below with your thoughts and recommendations and FAX the page to **ATTENTION STEDMANS, 410.528.4153**.

You are our most important contributor, and we want to know what's on your mind. Thanks!

Please tell us a little bit about yourself:

Name/Title: ______________________

Company: ______________________

Address: ______________________

City/State/Zip: ______________________

Day Telephone No.: (   ) ______________________

E-mail Address: ______________________

TERMS YOU BELIEVE ARE INCORRECT:

Appears as:	Suggested revision:
____________	____________
____________	____________
____________	____________

NEW TERMS/WORDS YOU WOULD LIKE US TO ADD:

____

____

Other comments:

____

____

____

May we quote you? ☐ Yes ☐ No

All done? Great, just FAX this page to the attention of STEDMAN'S at 410.528.4153 or MAIL the page to us at:

ATTN: STEDMAN'S
Lippincott Williams & Wilkins
P.O. Box 17344
Baltimore, MD 21298-9595

OR enter your information ONLINE at **www.stedmans.com**

Thanks again!

SURG 738318

170990-B-04 1 5/23/02, 7:00 AM

posterior vertical c.
pterygoid c.
pterygopalatine c.
pudendal c.
pulmoaortic c.
pulp c.
pyloric c.
radicular c.
c. resonance response
Rivinus c.
root c.
ruffed c.
sacral c.
Santorini c.
Schlemm c.
scleral c.
semicircular c.
sickle-shaped c.
Sondermann c.
sphenopalatine c.
spinal c.
Stensen c.
c. of Stilling
straight c.
subsartorial c.
Sucquet c.
Sucquet-Hoyer c.
supplementary c.
supraciliary c.
supraoptic c.
supraorbital c.
talar c.
tarsal c.
temporal c.
tensor tympani c.
Tourtual c.
tympanic c.
type I–IV c.
uniting c.
urogenital c.
uterovaginal c.
Van Hoorne c.
Velpeau c.
ventricular c.
Verneuil c.
vertebral c.
c. of Vesalius
vesicourethral c.
vestibular c.
vidian c.
Volkmann c.
vomerine c.
vomerobasilar c.
vomerorostral c.
vomerovaginal c.
Walther c.
Wirsung c.
zipped c.
Zuckerkandl perforating c.
zygomaticofacial c.
zygomaticotemporal c.

Canale
C. osteotomy
C. technique

canales (*pl. of* canalis)

canalicular
c. duct
c. laceration
c. sphincter

canaliculi (*pl. of* canaliculus)

canaliculodacryocystostomy

canaliculodacryorhinostomy

canaliculorhinostomy

canaliculus, pl. **canaliculi**
auricular c.
biliary c.
lacrimal c.
mastoid c.
c. rod and suture
tympanic c.
c. vein
vestibular c.

canalis, pl. **canales**

canalith
free-floating c.
c. repositioning procedure

canalization

canaloplasty

canal/wall-up technique

cancellectomy

cancellous
c. chip bone graft
c. and cortical bone graft
c. insert graft
c. tissue

Cancell therapy

cancer
American Joint Committee on C. (AJCC)
ampullary c.
appendiceal c.
biliary tract c.
c. body
breast c.

NOTES

cancer *(continued)*
c. cachexia
clinically node-negative breast c.
colloid c.
colon c.
colorectal c. (CRC)
digestive glandular c.
ductal c.
early gastric c.
endobronchial c.
endometrial c.
esophageal c.
esophagogastric c.
European Organization for Research and Treatment of C. (EORTC)
extrahepatic bile duct c.
familial breast c.
familial colon c. (FCC)
gallbladder c.
gastric c.
c. genetics
C. Genetics Network
glandular c.
hard palate c.
hepatocellular c.
hereditary breast c.
hereditary nonpolyposis colon c. (HNPCC)
high-risk papillary c.
intraductal c.
c. invasion
invasive breast c.
invasive ductal c.
islet cell c.
c. juice
c. lesion
life-threatening c.
localized prostate c.
low rectal c.
low-risk papillary c.
lung c.
Merkel cell c.
metastatic colorectal c.
nasal cavity c.
neuroendocrine c.
node-positive breast c.
nonpalpable invasive breast c.
obstructing colorectal c.
obstructive esophagogastric c.
ovarian c.
c. pain
pancreas c.
pancreatic head c.
papillary c.
penile c.
perforated c.
periampullary c.
peritoneal c.
postgastrectomy c.
primary c.
prostate c.
proximal gastric c.
QUART procedure for breast c.
rectal c.
rectum c.
resectable periampullary c.
soft-palate c.
c. status
C. Surveillance Program
c. susceptibility syndrome
suture line c.
thyroid c.
Union Internationale Contre le C. (UICC)
unresectable periampullary c.
urologic system c.
Whitmore-Jewett classification for staging of prostate c.
W-J classification for staging of prostate c.
young onset c.

cancer-causing gene

cancerization
field c.

candela lithotripsy

***Candida* infection**

candidal infection

candidemia

canina

canine
c. fossa
c. teeth

caninus

Cannon point

cannulated nail

cannulation
bile duct c.
biliary c.
c. of the biliary tree
duct c.
endoscopic retrograde c.
endoscopic transpapillary c.
ERCP c.
ex vivo c.
intravenous c.
percutaneous arterial c.
peripheral venous c.
postsphincterotomy ERCP c.
retrograde c.
selective ductal c.
transpapillary c.
unilateral pedicle c.
vascular c.

cannulization

canonical
c. correlation
c. univariate parameter
canthal
canthectomy
canthi (*pl. of* canthus)
cantholysis
canthomeatal line
canthopexy
canthoplasty
Agnew c.
Ammon c.
Imre lateral c.
canthorrhaphy
Elschnig c.
canthotomy
external c.
lateral c.
canthus, pl. **canthi**
external c.
internal c.
lateral c.
medial c.
cantilevered bone graft
Cantlie line
Cantwell-Ransley
C.-R. epispadias repair
C.-R. urethroplasty
cap
corneal c.
duodenal c.
fibrous c.
metanephric c.
phrygian c.
capacity
demand minimum functional c. (DMFC)
exercise c.
forced expiratory c.
functional residual c. (FRC)
knot holding c. (KHC)
maximum breathing c. (MBC)
single-breath diffusing c.
treadmill exercise c.
vital c.
CAPD
continuous ambulatory peritoneal dialysis
Capello technique
Capener lateral rhachotomy
Cape Town technique
capillaroscopy
nail-fold c.
capillary
c. angioma
c. arteriole
c. dilation
c. drainage
c. endothelium
c. fracture
c. hemangioma
c. hyperfiltration
c. malformation
c. vein
c. wedge pressure
capillus, pl. **capilli**
capita (*pl. of* caput)
capital
c. femoral epiphysis
c. fragment
c. operation
capitate
c. bone
c. fracture
capitation
capitatum
capitellar fracture
capitellocondylar total elbow arthroplasty
capitellum
capitis
capitonnage suture technique
capitopedal
capitular
c. epiphysis
c. joint
capitulum, pl. **capitula**
capnograph
capnography
spectral edge frequency c.
capnometry
volumetric c.
capping technique
CAPRI
Cardiopulmonary Research Institute
CAPRI program
capstan knot
capsula, pl. **capsulae**
capsular
c. branch
c. dissection
c. exfoliation syndrome
c. fixation
c. flap pyeloplasty
c. imbrication

NOTES

C

capsular *(continued)*
c. incision
c. interposition arthroplasty
c. invasion
c. ligament
c. shift procedure
c. space
c. support tissue
capsulare
capsule
adipose c.
adrenal c.
articular c.
atrabiliary c.
Bonnet c.
cricothyroid articular c.
Crosby c.
Crosby-Kugler biopsy c.
external c.
extreme c.
fatty renal c.
fibrous articular c.
c. flap technique
c. forceps technique
Gerota c.
Glisson c.
glissonian c.
glomerular c.
hepatic c.
joint c.
liver c.
Müller c.
pancreatic c.
suprarenal c.
Tenon c.
tumor c.
capsulectomy
capsulitis
adhesive c.
glenohumeral adhesive c.
capsuloplasty
Zancolli c.
capsulorrhaphy
Boyd-Sisk posterior c.
duToit-Roux staple c.
medial c.
pants-over-vest c.
posterior c.
Rockwood posterior c.
Roux-duToit staple c.
staple c.
Tibone posterior c.
capsulotomy
anterior c.
Castroviejo c.
Curtis PIP joint c.
Darling c.
dorsal transverse c.
dorsolateral and medial c.
posterior c.
renal c.
triangular c.
T-shaped c.
Vannas c.
Verhoeff-Chandler c.
capture
c. cross-section
pacemaker c.
Capuron point
caput, pl. **capita**
carbohydrate antigen 19-9 (CA 19-9)
carbon
c. dioxide (CO_2)
c. dioxide concentration
c. dioxide dissociation curve
c. dioxide elimination ($VECO_2$)
c. dioxide fixation
c. dioxide laser plaque ablation
c. dioxide pressure
c. dioxide response
c. gelatin mass
c. monoxide (CO)
c. tetrachloride-induced liver regeneration
carbonate
carbonization
carbuncle
kidney c.
carcinoembryonic antigen (CEA)
carcinogenesis
foreign body c.
carcinoid
nonappendiceal c.
c. tumor
c. valve disease
carcinoma
acinous cell c.
adenocystic c.
adenoid cystic c.
adenoid squamous cell c.
adenosquamous c.
adnexal c.
adrenal c.
adrenocortical c.
aldosterone-producing c.
alveolar cell c.
ameloblastic c.
ampullary c.
anaplastic c.
anorectal c.
apocrine c.
basal cell c.
basosquamous cell c.
benign-acting renal cell c.
betel c.
bile duct c.

bilharzial c.
biliary c.
bladder c.
Borrmann type I-IV c.
breast c.
bronchial c.
bronchioloalveolar c.
bronchoalveolar c.
burn scar c.
cecal c.
cerebriform c.
cervical c.
chimney-sweep's c.
cholangitis c.
choroid plexus c.
clay pipe c.
clear cell hepatocellular c.
colloid c.
colon c.
colonic c.
colorectal c.
columnar cuff c.
comedo c.
corpus c.
cortisol-producing c.
cribriform c.
cutaneous metastatic breast c.
cylindrical c.
dendritic c.
differentiated thyroid c.
disseminated c.
duct c.
ductal c.
Dukes classification of c.
dye worker's c.
eccrine c.
Edmondson grading system for hepatocellular c.
embryonal cell c.
encephaloid gastric c.
c. en cuirasse
endometrial c.
epidermoid c.
esophageal c.
ethmoid sinus c.
excavated gastric c.
exophytic c.
extrahepatic abdominal c.
fallopian tube c.
false cord c.
follicular c.
gallbladder c.
gastric c.
gastric stump c.
gastrointestinal c.
gelatinous c.
genital c.
glandular c.
glottic c.
granulosa cell c.
gynecological c.
hepatic cell c.
hepatocellular c. (HCC)
hereditary nonpolyposis colon c. (HNPCC)
hilar c.
hypernephroid c.
infantile embryonal c.
infiltrating ductal c.
infiltrating lobular c.
infiltrative c.
inflammatory breast c.
insular c.
intraductal c.
intraepidermal c.
intraepithelial nonkeratizing c.
invasive breast c.
invasive ductal c.
invasive lobular c.
Japanese Classification for Gastric C. (JCGC)
juvenile embryonal c.
Kulchitsky cell c.
large cell c.
laryngeal c.
leptomeningeal c.
lobular c.
lung c.
maxillary sinus c.
medullary c.
meibomian gland c.
melanotic c.
meningeal c.
Merkel cell c.
metastatic colorectal c.
metastatic prostatic c.
metastatic renal cell c.
microinvasive c.
micropapillary c.
microscopic multifocal medullary c.
microtrabecular hepatocellular c.
morpheaform basal cell c.
mucoepidermal c.
mucoepidermoid c.

NOTES

carcinoma *(continued)*
napkin-ring c.
nasopharyngeal c.
neuroendocrine skin c.
oat cell c.
orofacial c.
oropharyngeal c.
ovarian c.
Paget c.
pancreatic c.
papillary gastric c.
parathyroid c.
parotid c.
penile c.
periampullary c.
pharyngeal wall c.
polypoid superficial gastric c.
prickle cell c.
primary bile duct c.
primary intraosseous c.
prostatic c.
pure insular c.
radiation-induced c.
rectal c.
rectosigmoid c.
renal cell c.
renal pelvis c.
resectable c.
salivary duct c.
salivary gland c.
scar c.
schistosomal bladder c.
schneiderian c.
sigmoid colon c.
signet-ring cell c.
sinonasal c.
c. in situ (CIS)
small cell lung c.
small round cell c.
spindle cell c.
splenic flexure c.
sporadic renal cell c.
stage B, C c.
c. stage irresectable
string cell c.
swamp c.
terminal duct c.
testicular c.
thymic c.
thyroid c.
transitional cell c.
tuberous sclerosis-associated renal cell c.
tubular c.
c. of uncertain primary site
undifferentiated squamous cell c.
urachal c.
ureteral c.
urethral c.
urothelial c.
uterine papillary serous c.
vaginal c.
vulvar c.
vulvovaginal c.
wolffian duct c.
yolk sac c.

carcinomatosis
diffuse c.
peritoneal c.

carcinosarcoma

card
Memorial Pain Assessment C. (MPAC)

cardia
gastric c.

cardiac
c. anesthesia
c. anesthetic
c. anomaly
c. arrest
c. bypass (CBP)
c. catheterization
c. compression
c. decompression
c. defibrillation
c. dilatation
c. dilation
c. event
c. examination
c. fibrillation
c. fibrous skeleton
c. herniation
c. impression
c. index (CI)
c. irradiation
c. lymphatic ring
c. mass
c. massage
c. metastasis
c. muscle wrap
c. output (CO)
c. patch
c. perforation
c. plexus
c. position
c. resuscitation
c. retransplantation
c. rhabdomyoma
c. rupture
c. segment
c. surgery
c. symphysis
c. transplantation
c. tumor
c. tumor plop

c. valvular malformation
c. vein
cardiacum
cardiacus
cardiae
achalasia c.
cardiectomy
cardinal
c. ligament
c. point
c. position
cardioesophageal relaxation
cardiogenic shock
cardiohepatic angle
cardiologist
interventional c.
cardiomyopathy
ischemic c.
underlying c.
cardiomyoplasty
dynamic c.
cardiomyotomy
Heller c.
laparoscopic c.
stomach c.
videolaparoscopic c.
cardioomentopexy
cardiopericardiopexy
Beck c.
cardiopexy
cardiophrenic angle mass
cardioplasty
Belsey Mark IV c.
cardioplegia
cardioplegic solution
cardiopressor reflex
cardioprotective effect
cardiopulmonary
c. bypass (CPB)
c. complication
c. manifestation
C. Research Institute (CAPRI)
c. resuscitation (CPR)
cardiorespiratory
c. complication
c. endurance (CRE)
cardiorrhaphy
cardiothoracic surgery
cardiotomy
cardiotoxic
c. effect
c. myolysis
cardiovalvotomy
cardiovalvulotomy
cardiovascular
c. adverse effect
c. anesthesia
c. complication
c. disease
c. imaging technique
c. malformation
c. patch graft
c. pressure
c. stability
c. surgery
cardiovasculorenal
cardioversion
cardiovert
care
medical c.
monitored anesthesia c. (MAC)
respiratory c.
tertiary c.
trauma c.
Carey Ranvier technique
caries classification
carina, pl. **carinae**
carinate abdomen
carinatum
carious
c. pulp exposure
c. restoration margin
Carlo Traverso maneuver
C-arm fluoroscopy
Carmody-Batson operation
carnea
Carnesale
C. acetabular extensile approach
C. hip approach
C. technique
Carnesale-Stewart-Barnes hip dislocation classification
carnosa
Caroli
C. syndrome
C. type I distal bile duct stricture
Carolinas
C. Laparoscopic Advanced Surgery Program (CLASP)
C. Laparoscopic Advanced Surgery Program procedure
Caroli-Sarles classification
carotica
carotici

NOTES

caroticoclinoid
c. canal
c. foramen
c. ligament
caroticotympanic
c. artery
c. canal
c. nerve
caroticum
caroticus
carotid
c. ablative procedure
c. angioplasty
c. angioplasty with stenting
c. arterial blood flow
c. artery atherosclerotic stenosis
c. artery bifurcation
c. artery bypass
c. artery compression
c. artery disease
c. artery dissection
c. artery occlusion
c. artery stump pressure
c. atherosclerosis
c. body
c. body tumor
c. canal
c. circulation
c. clamping
c. duplex ultrasonography
c. ejection time
c. endarterectomy (CEA)
external c.
c. foramen
c. ganglion
c. groove
c. injury
c. plaque
c. preservation
c. preservation technique
c. sheath
c. sinus
c. sinus branch
c. siphon
c. space
c. stenting
c. sulcus
c. surgery
c. transposition
c. triangle
c. tubercle
c. venous plexus
carotid-basilar anastomosis
carotid-cavernous sinus fistula
carotid-dural fistula
carotid-subclavian
c.-s. artery bypass
c.-s. bypass
carotid-vertebral
c.-v. anastomosis
c.-v. vein bypass graft
carotidynia
carpal
c. artery
c. bone stress fracture
c. boss
c. compression test
c. region
c. synovectomy
carpectomy
distal-row c.
Omer-Capen c.
proximal-row c.
Carpentier
C. annuloplasty
C. tricuspid valvuloplasty
Carpentier-Edwards
C.-E. stented bovine pericardial valve
C.-E. stented porcine xenograft valve
carpet lesion
carpet-like polyposis
carpi (*pl. of* carpus)
carpocarpal
carpometacarpal
c. arthroplasty
c. articulation
c. fracture-dislocation
c. joint dislocation
c. joint fracture
carpometacarpeae
carpopedal
Carpue method
carpus, pl. **carpi**
Carrel
C. operation
C. suture technique
C. treatment
Carrell
C. fibular substitution technique
C. resection
carrier
c. fluid
mutation c.
c. status
Carroll arthroplasty
CARS
compensatory antiinflammatory response syndrome
Carstan reverse wedge osteotomy
Cartam-Treander reverse wedge osteotomy
Carter operation
cartilage
alar c.

annular c.
arthrodial c.
articular c.
arytenoid c.
auricular c.
basilar c.
branchial c.
c. canal
connecting c.
corniculate c.
costal c.
cricoid c.
cuneiform c.
diarthrodial c.
ensiform c.
epiglottic c.
falciform c.
c. flap
c. graft
hypsiloid c.
c. inflammation
interosseous c.
intervertebral c.
intraarticular c.
intrathyroid c.
investing c.
Jacobson c.
Luschka c.
mandibular c.
c. matrix
meatal c.
Meckel c.
Meyer c.
Morgagni c.
c. overgrowth
quadrangular c.
Reichert c.
Santorini c.
Seiler c.
semilunar c.
sesamoid c.
sternal c.
sternum c.
supraarytenoid c.
thyroid c.
tracheal c.
triangular c.
triquetrous c.
triticeal c.
uniting c.
vomeronasal c.
Weitbrecht c.
Wrisberg c.
xiphoid c.
Y c.

cartilagines (*pl. of* cartilago)
cartilagineus
cartilaginis
cartilaginous
c. growth plate disorder
c. loose body
c. part of skeletal system
c. septum
c. tissue
cartilago, pl. **cartilagines**
cartwheel fracture
caruncle
Morgagni c.
Santorini major c.
Santorini minor c.
urethral c.
caruncula, pl. **carunculae**
hymenal c.
sublingual c.
caryothecae
Casanellas lacrimal operation
cascade
coagulation c.
caseated tissue
caseating granulomatous inflammation
caseation
c. necrosis
tuberculous c.
case-by-case approach
caseous
c. abscess
c. inflammation
Casey operation
CaSki cell line
Caspari repair
CASS
coronary artery surgery study
Casselberry position
Casser perforated muscle
cast
c. application
c. immobilization
c. removal
Castaneda procedure
Castellani point
Casten classification
Castle procedure
castrate

NOTES

castration
female c.
functional c.
male c.
parasitic c.
Castroviejo
C. capsulotomy
C. iridectomy
C. keratectomy
C. minikeratoplasty
C. operation
C. radial iridotomy
Castroviejo-Scheie cyclodiathermy operation
catabolic condition
cataract
c. aspiration
c. extraction
c. extraction operation
flap operation c.
c. formation
hard c.
c. irradiation
irradiation c.
c. mask ring
c. procedure
radiation c.
reduplication c.
ring-form congenital c.
ring-shaped c.
Soemmerring ring c.
soft c.
c. surgery
catarrhal
c. inflammation
c. marginal ulceration
catastrophe
intraabdominal c.
catastrophic
c. event
c. illness
catastrophizing subscale
catecholamine-resistant hypotension
caterpillar flap
catheter
c. ablation
c. balloon valvuloplasty
c. dilation
c. drainage
c. embolectomy
c. embolism
c. entrapment
c. exchange
c. fixation
c. fragment
c. insertion
c. instability
c. introduction method
c. kinking
c. knotting
c. malposition
c. manipulation
c. mapping
c. obstruction
c. patency
c. position
c. sepsis
c. site
c. specimen
c. tip placement
c. toe
c. tunnel
c. tunnel infection
catheter-directed
c.-d. fenestration
c.-d. interventional procedure
catheter-guided
c.-g. biopsy
c.-g. endoscopic intubation
catheter-induced pulmonary artery hemorrhage
catheterizable stoma
catheterization
antegrade c.
arterial c.
bile duct c.
bladder c.
bypass graft c.
cardiac c.
central venous c.
chronic c.
clean intermittent c.
combined heart c.
coronary sinus c.
cystic duct c.
diagnostic cardiac c.
in-and-out c.
intermittent c.
interventional cardiac c.
Judkins-Sones technique of cardiac c.
left heart c.
long-term epidural c.
percutaneous transhepatic cardiac c.
portal vein c.
pulmonary artery c.
retrograde c.
right heart c.
Seldinger cystic duct c.
selective c.
subclavian vein c.
c. technique
thoracic epidural c.
transfemoral venous c.
transhepatic c.
transnasal bile duct c.

transpapillary c.
transseptal left heart c.
transvaginal fallopian tube c.
transvaginal tubal c.
umbilical artery c.
umbilical vein c.
ureteral c.
urinary c.

catheterize
catheter-securing technique
catholysis
cation
c. exchange
cat's eye calculus
Cattell operation
Cattell-Warren pancreaticojejunostomy
Catterall classification
cauda, pl. **caudae**
c. epididymis
c. equina compression
c. equina syndrome
caudad
caudal
c. anesthesia
c. angulation
c. block
c. canal
c. corner
c. direction
c. dysplasia sequence
c. epidural anesthetic technique
c. fragment
c. lamina resection
c. ligament
c. pancreatic artery
c. pancreaticojejunostomy
c. retinaculum
c. sac
c. translation
c. transtentorial herniation
c. transverse fissure
c. vertebra
caudale
caudalis
caudate
c. body
c. branch
c. lobe
c. process
caudati
caudatus
caudocephalad
causalgia
genitofemoral c.
cause
cholestatic c.
definite c.
definitive c.
idiopathic c.
pathologic c.
underlying c.
cause-effect relationship
cause-specific mortality
cauterant
cauterization
bipolar c.
Bovie c.
phenol c.
unipolar c.
cauterize
cautery
c. conization
hook c.
c. incision
insulated c.
looped c.
c. operation
pure cutting c.
snare c.
wet field c.
cava (*pl. of* cavum)
caval
c. drainage
c. fold
c. insertion
cave
c. hip approach
c. knee approach
Meckel c.
trigeminal c.
caverna, pl. **cavernae**
cavernosa
cavernosal alpha blockade technique
cavernosi
cavernosorum
cavernosus
cavernous
c. angioma
c. body
c. groove
c. hemangioma
c. malformation
c. nerve
c. nerve-sparing prostatectomy

NOTES

C

cavernous *(continued)*
c. plexus
c. respiration
c. sinus fistula
c. sinus syndrome
c. venous sinus
Cave-Rowe shoulder dislocation technique
CAVH
continuous arteriovenous hemofiltration
cavitary
c. lung lesion
c. small-bowel lesion
cavitas, pl. **cavitates**
cavitating
c. inflammation
c. metastasis
cavitation
collapse c.
pulmonary c.
stable c.
transient c.
cavity
abdominal c.
abdominopelvic c.
c. access
access c.
acetabular c.
alveolar c.
amniotic c.
articular c.
artificial classification c.
axial surface c.
biopsy c.
body c.
buccal c.
chorionic c.
c. classification
complex c.
compound c.
cotyloid c.
cranial c.
cystic c.
c. débridement
dental c.
distal c.
DO c.
endodontic c.
endolymphatic c.
endometrial c.
epidural c.
exocelomic c.
fissure c.
frontal sinus c.
gingival c.
glenoid c.
greater peritoneal c.
idiopathic bone c.
incisal c.
inferior laryngeal c.
inflammatory c.
infraglottic c.
intermediate laryngeal c.
intracranial c.
intraperitoneal c.
joint c.
labial c.
laser c.
lesser peritoneal c.
c. line angle
lingual c.
c. lining
c. lining agent
lung c.
c. margin
marrow c.
mastoid c.
maxillary sinus c.
Meckel c.
medullary c.
miniature uterine c.
nasal c.
nephrotomic c.
nonseptate c.
occlusal c.
open c.
optic papilla c.
oral c.
orbital c.
pelvic c.
perilymphatic c.
peritoneal c.
pharyngonasal c.
pit and fissure c.
pleural c.
postexcision c.
c. preparation
c. preparation base
prepared c.
c. primer
proximal c.
pulmonary c.
pulp c.
residual cystic c.
retroperitoneal c.
Retzius c.
saclike c.
c. seal
seroma c.
sinonasal c.
sinus c.
smooth surface c.
Stafne idiopathic bone c.
subarachnoid c.
subdural c.
subglottic c.

superior laryngeal c.
synovial c.
syringohydromyelic c.
c. test
thoracic c.
c. toilet
trigeminal c.
tympanic c.
uterine c.
vitreous c.
c. wall
wound c.

cavoatrial shunt
cavohepatic junction
cavopulmonary anastomosis
cavotomy
infrahepatic c.
cavovarus deformity
cavum, pl. **cava**
inferior vena cava (IVC)
inferior vena c. (IVC)
infrahepatic inferior vena cava
infrarenal cava
retrohepatic inferior vena cava
Spencer plication of vena cava
superior vena c.
suprahepatic inferior vena cava (SHVC)
suprahepatic vena cava
cavus deformity
Cawthorne
C. destruction
C. operation
Cawthorne-Day procedure
CBD
common bile duct
CBDS
common bile duct stone
CBF
cerebral blood flow
CBP
cardiac bypass
CBT
cognitive behavior treatment
CCD
central core disease
CCM
critical care medicine
CCS
celiac artery compression syndrome
Clinical Classification System
CCSG
Children's Cancer Study group
CDBR computerized diaphragmatic breathing retraining10000
computerized diaphragmatic breathing retraining
CDH
congenital diaphragmatic hernia
C-D screw modification
CEA
carcinoembryonic antigen
carotid endarterectomy
CEA level
serum CEA
ceanothus extract
CEAP
clinical manifestations, etiologic factors, anatomic involvement, pathophysiologic features
CEAP classification
ceca (*pl. of* cecum)
cecal
c. appendix
c. artery
c. bascule
c. carcinoma
c. colonoscopy
c. deformity
c. distention
c. diverticulitis
c. fold
c. foramen
c. hernia
c. imbrication procedure
c. intussusception
c. ligation and puncture (CLP)
c. recess
c. serosa
c. volvulus
cecales
cecectomy
ceci
Cecil
C. procedure
C. urethroplasty
cecocolostomy
cecocystoplasty
cecofixation
cecoileostomy
cecopexy
cecoplication
cecoproctostomy

NOTES

cecorrhaphy
cecosigmoidostomy
cecostomy
- percutaneous catheter c.
- tube c.

cecotomy
cecoureterocele
cecum, pl. **ceca**
Cedars-Sinai classification
ceiling analgesia
Celermajer method
Celestin procedure
celiac
- c. alcohol ablation
- c. arterial system
- c. artery
- c. artery aneurysm
- c. artery compression syndrome (CCS)
- c. axis
- c. band syndrome
- c. branch
- c. crisis
- c. dimple
- c. ganglion
- c. gland
- c. infantilism
- c. lymph node metastasis
- c. nervous plexus
- c. nodal involvement
- c. ostium
- c. plexus block
- c. plexus block anesthetic technique
- c. plexus reflex
- c. rickets
- c. trunk
- c. tumor
- c. vessel

celiaca
celiacography
celiacomesenteric artery
celiacus
celiectomy
celiocentesis
celioenterotomy
celiogastrostomy
celiogastrotomy
celiohysterectomy
celiohysterotomy
celioma
celiomyomectomy
celiomyomotomy
celioparacentesis
celiorrhaphy
celiosalpingectomy
celiosalpingotomy
celioscopy
celiotomy
- exploratory c.
- formal c.
- c. incision
- mandatory c.
- negative c.
- staging c.
- vaginal c.

celite-activated clotting time (CACT)
cell
- Claudius c.
- c. collection
- Deiters c.
- ependymal c.
- epithelial c.
- epitympanic c.
- ethmoid c.
- follicular c.
- gut epithelial c.
- Hensen c.
- hypotympanic c.
- inflammation c.
- inflammatory c.
- irradiated melanoma c.
- islet c.
- Kirchner c.
- c. line
- lymphocyte c.
- malignant c.
- mastoid c.
- melanoma antigen reacting to T c. (MART)
- c. membrane
- mesothelial c.
- c. migration
- multipotential stem c.
- c. oxygenation
- packed red blood c.'s (PRBC)
- paranasal c.
- parenchymal c.
- petrous apex c.
- pharyngeal c.
- photosensitive c.
- pituitary tumor c.
- pulmonary epithelial c.
- retinal pigment epithelial c.
- rod c.
- Schwann c.
- c. separation technique
- stem c.
- tumor c.
- c. web
- white c.

cell-cell adhesion
cell-extracellular matrix adhesion
cellophane tape method
cellula, pl. **cellulae**

cellular
c. biology
c. cooperation
c. damage
c. debris
c. immunity
c. infiltration
c. migration
c. nidus
c. polyp
c. xenograft rejection
c. xenotransplantation
cellularity
high c.
cellulocutaneous flap
cellulose-based membrane
celotomy
Celsus-Hotz operation
Celsus spasmodic entropion operation
cement
c. base
c. disease
c. interface
c. line
c. removal
c. substance
c. technique
cemental
c. lesion
c. line
c. repair
cementation
final c.
trial c.
cement-bone interface
cemented total hip arthroplasty
cementification
cementing line
cementless
c. technique
c. total hip arthroplasty
cementoid tissue
cementoma
cementum
c. fracture
c. pain
center
ambulatory surgery c.
C. for Disease Control HIV infection classification
limbic c.
tertiary trauma c.
urban trauma c.
centesis
centra (*pl. of* centrum)
central
c. c.
c. anesthetic technique
c. anticholinergic syndrome
c. approach
c.-bearing point
c. bis
c. block
c. bone
c. canal
c. carbon dioxide ventilatory response
c. chemoreflex loop
c. cone technique reduction
c. cord syndrome
c. core disease (CCD)
c. dislocation
c. excitatory state
c. extensor mechanism
c. fibroelastic core
c. fibrous body
c. fixation
c. fracture
c. fusion
c. heel pad syndrome
c. hepatectomy
c. hepatic gunshot wound
c. herniation
c. hyperalimentation
c. illumination
c. incisor teeth
c. iridectomy
c. lesion
c. line infection
c. nervous system
c. nervous system disease
c. nervous system malformation
c. nervous system manifestation
c. nervous system tuberculosis
c. pain
c. palmar space
c. perineum tendon
c. physiolysis
c. pontine myelinolysis
c. posterior-anterior pressure
c. poststroke pain (CPSP)
c. ray amputation
c. respiration

NOTES

central *(continued)*
c. retinal artery
c. sensitization
c. slip sparing technique
c. stellate laceration
c. sulcal artery
c. systemic-to-pulmonary shunt
c. tegmental tract
c. tendon
c. tendon diaphragm
c. vein
c. venous access
c. venous alimentation
c. venous cannulation anesthetic technique
c. venous catheterization
c. venous hypercarbia
c. venous pressure (CVP)
c. venous pressure monitoring
c. vision
c. yellow point
c. zone inflammation
centrales
centralis
centralization
Bayne-Klug c.
Bora c.
Manske-McCarroll-Swanson c.
tendon c.
centration
centric
c. fusion
c. jaw relation
c. occluding relation
c. occluding relation record
point c.
c. position
c. relation occlusion
centriciput
centrifugalization
centrifugal nerve
centrifugation
centrifuged
centrilobular
c. lesion
c. necrosis
c. pancreatitis
centriole
distal c.
proximal c.
centripetal nerve
centroneuroaxis anesthesia
centrum, pl. **centra**
cephalad
c. corner
c. direction
c. fragment
c. translation
cephaladly
cephalalgia
coital c.
cephalic
c. arterial ramus
c. index
c. tetanus
c. triangle
c. vein
c. vein graft
cephalica
cephalin-cholesterol flocculation
cephalization
cephalocaudal axis
cephalocele
occipital c.
oral c.
cephalocentesis
cephalodactyly
cephalomedullary nail fracture
cephalometric
c. correction
c. landmark
cephalopelvic disproportion
cephalopharyngeus
cephalorrhachidian index
cephalothoracic
cephalotrigonal technique
ceramic restoration
ceramometal
c. restoration
ceratectomy
ceratocricoid
c. ligament
c. muscle
ceratocricoideum
ceratocricoideus
ceratopharyngeus
cerclage
c. operation
c. wire fixation
cerebellar
c. artery
c. ectopia
c. hematoma
c. hemisphere
c. hemorrhage
c. vein
cerebelli
cerebellomedullaris
cerebellomedullary
c. cistern
c. malformation syndrome
cerebellopontine
c. angle approach
c. angle cistern
c. angle syndrome
cerebellorubral tract

cerebellothalamic tract
cerebra (*pl. of* cerebrum)
cerebral
c. abscess
c. angioma
c. aqueduct compression
c. arteriovenous malformation
c. artery
c. blood
c. blood flow (CBF)
c. calculus
c. circulation
c. circulation time
c. death
c. decompression
c. decortication
c. edema
c. event
c. fornix
c. hemicorticectomy
c. hemisphere
c. hemorrhage
c. hernia
c. herniation
c. index
c. injury
c. lesion
c. metabolic rate (CMR)
c. metastasis
c. palsy pathological fracture
c. perfusion
c. perfusion pressure
c. protection
c. protective therapy
c. radiation necrosis (CRN)
c. respiration
c. revascularization
c. sinus
c. spinal fluid drainage
c. sulcus
c. vascular malformation
c. vein
cerebrale
cerebral-sacral loop
cerebration
cerebri
cerebriform carcinoma
cerebrospinal
c. fluid (CSF)
c. fluid-brain barrier
c. fluid fistula
c. fluid outflow
c. fluid pressure (CSFP)
c. index
cerebrotendinous xanthomatosis
cerebrotomy
cerebrovascular
c. accident
c. complication
c. disease
c. event
c. malformation
cerebrum, pl. **cerebra**
cerecloth
cereolus, pl. **cereoli**
certified registered nurse anesthetist (CRNA)
cervical
c. acceleration-deceleration syndrome
c. adenocarcinoma
c. adenopathy
c. amputation
c. anastomosis
c. anesthesia
c. anomaly
c. approach
c. aspiration
c. branch
c. canal
c. carcinoma
c. carcinoma stimulation
c. compression syndrome
c. condyloma
c. cone biopsy
c. conization
c. corpectomy
c. decompression surgery
c. dilation
c. diskectomy
c. disk excision
c. disk surgery
c. diverticulum
c. esophagogastrostomy
c. esophagoplasty
c. esophagostomy
c. esophagotomy
c. esophagus
c. extension strength
c. fistula
c. flap
c. fusion syndrome
c. general rotation
c. gland

NOTES

cervical *(continued)*
c. immobilization
c. incision
c. infection
c. inflammation
c. insemination
c. instability
c. interbody fusion
c. laceration
c. leakage
c. lesion
c. ligament
c. line
c. loop
c. manipulation
c. metastasis
c. midline disk herniation
c. nerve root injection
c. node dissection
c. osteotomy
c. perivascular sympathectomy
c. pleura
c. plexus
c. plexus block
c. plexus block anesthetic technique
c. position
c. rib
c. rotator muscle
c. screw insertion technique
c. segment
c. sinus
c. soft tissue
c. spine fracture
c. spine internal fixation
c. spine kyphotic deformity
c. spine laminectomy
c. spine posterior fusion
c. spine screw-plate fixation
c. spine stabilization
c. spine stabilization procedure
c. splanchnic nerve
c. spondylitic myelopathy
c. spondylotic myelopathy fusion technique
c. spondylotic myelopathy vertebrectomy
c. stenosis
c. stump
c. suture
c. thymectomy
c. transformation zone
c. triangle
c. tumor
c. ulcer
c. ultrasound
c. vein
c. vertebra
c. vessel compression

cervicale
cervicales
cervicalia
cervicalis
cervicalium
cervical-to-MCA bypass
cervicectomy
cervices (*pl. of* cervix)
cervicis
cervicoaxillary canal
cervicobrachial
cervicofacial
cervicogenic headache
cervicomedullary
c. deformity
c. junction compression

cervicooccipital
cervicoplasty
cervicothoracic
c. approach
c. ganglion
c. junction stabilization
c. junction surgery
c. pedicle anatomy
c. sympathectomy
c. transition

cervicothoracicum
cervicotomy
cervicotrochanteric displaced fracture
cervicovaginal
c. artery
c. fistula
c. infection

cervicovaginalis
cervicovesical
cervix, pl. **cervices**
implant c.

cesarean
c. delivery
c. hysterectomy
c. operation
c. resection
c. section (C-section)
c. section incision

cesium irradiation
CFA
common femoral artery

CFA-SFA
common femoral artery-superficial femoral artery
CFA-SFA bypass

C-form osteotomy
CHADD
controlled heat-aided drug delivery

Chadwick-Bentley classification

chain
lymphatic c.
obturator lymphatic c.
recurrent nerve lymphatic c.
c. suture technique
chain-of-lakes
c.-o.-l. deformity
c.-o.-l. filling defect
c.-o.-l. sign
challenge
methacholine bronchoprovocation c.
Chamberlain
C. mediastinoscopy
C. procedure
chamber rupture
Chambers
C. osteotomy
C. procedure
chamfer preparation
Chance
C. fracture thoracolumbar spine
C. vertebral fracture
chancre
hard c.
mixed c.
monorecidive c.
c. redux
soft c.
chancriform
chancroid
Chandler
C. hip fusion
C. iridectomy
C. vitreous operation
Chandler-Verhoeff
C.-V. lens extraction
C.-V. operation
Chang aniline-acid fuchsin method
change
aging degenerative c.
degenerative c.
diffuse c.
fibrocystic c.
fractional area c. (FAC)
hemodynamic c.
Hürthle cell c.
ischemic mesenteric c.
metabolic c.
mitral valve prolapse, aortic anomalies, skeletal c.s, and skin c.'s (MASS)
motor c.
multifocal c.
muscular c.
nail c.
neurocognitive c.
parenchymal c.
physiologic c.
c. point
postradiation c.
postsurgical motor c.
postthoracotomy c.
sepsis-induced metabolic c.
surgical c.
Chang-Miltner incision
channel
c. and core biopsy
open venous c.
c. shoulder pin technique
venous c.
Chaput
C. anal operation
C. fracture
C. operation
characteristic
clinical c.
heterogeneity c.
histologic c.
pathologic c.
c. radiation
Charcot
C. triad
C. triangle
charged-particle irradiation
Charles
C. lensectomy
C. operation
C. procedure
Charnley
C. compression
C. compression arthrodesis
C. compression-type knee fusion
C. incision
C. total hip arthroplasty
Charrière scale
Charters
C. method
C. technique
char-zone depth
chasm
Chassaignac
C. space
C. tubercle

NOTES

Chassar
C. Moir-Sims procedure
C. Moir sling procedure
Chauffard point
chauffeur fracture
Chaussier line
Chaves-Rapp muscle transfer technique
Chayes method
CHCT
caffeine and halothane contracture test
Cheatle
C. slit
C. syndrome
Cheatle-Henry hernia
checklist
Rotterdam Symptom C.
checkrein
c. deformity
c. procedure
cheek
c. advancement flap
c. bone
c. muscle
c. rotation flap
cheesy necrosis
cheilectomy
Garceau c.
Mann-Coughlin-DuVries c.
Sage-Clark c.
cheilion
cheiloangioscopy
cheiloplasty
cheilorrhaphy
cheilostomatoplasty
cheilotomy
cheiroplasty
chemexfoliation
chemical
c. disinfection
c. exchange
c. exposure
c. hemostasis
c. litholysis
c. matrixectomy
c. peritonitis
c. sedation
c. shift misregistration
c. splanchnicectomy
c. sympathectomy
c. thrombectomy
c. vapor sterilization
chemicocautery
chemoactivation
chemoattraction
fibroblast c.
chemocautery
chemocoagulation
chemoembolization
arterial c.
intraarterial c.
transarterial c.
chemolysis
intrarenal c.
chemoneurolysis
glycerol c.
percutaneous retrogasserian glycerol c.
chemonucleolysis
chymopapain c.
double-needle c.
chemopallidectomy
chemopallidothalamectomy
chemopallidotomy
chemoprevention
c. agent
medical c.
chemopreventive agent
chemoprophylaxis
chemoradiation
chemoradiotherapy
c. effect
preoperative c.
chemoreflex
chemosensitive
chemosterilization
chemostimulation
chemosurgery
chemosurgical gingivectomy
chemotactic property
chemothalamectomy
chemothalamotomy
chemotherapeutic
c. scheme
c. treatment
chemotherapist
chemotherapy
adjunctive c.
adjuvant c.
combination c.
concurrent c.
induction c.
infusional c.
initial systemic c.
intraarterial c. (IAC)
intraperitoneal hyperthermic c. (IPHC)
intravesical c.
postoperative c.
postoperative systemic c.
preoperative induction c.
preoperative systemic c.
c. protocol
second-line c.
systemic c.

Cherney
C. lower transverse abdominal incision
C. suture technique
Chernez incision
cherry angioma
Cherry-Crandall procedure
cherry-picking procedure
chessboard graft
chest
c. compression
c. examination
flail c.
flat c.
c. index
c. lesion
c. physical therapy
pneumonectomy c.
c. port
stove-in c.
c. tube drainage (CTD)
c. tube output (CTO)
c. wall
c. wall compliance
c. wall fixation
c. wall invasion
c. wall stabilization
c. x-ray
Chester-Winter procedure
chevron
c. bunionectomy
c. hallux valgus correction
c. incision
c. laceration
c. osteotomy
c. technique
chevron-shaped incision
chewing method
chew-in technique
Cheyne operation
Cheyne-Stokes respiration
Chiari
C. anomaly
C. innominate osteotomy
C. I–III malformation
C. II syndrome
C. technique
Chiari-Salter-Steel pelvic osteotomy
chiasm
Camper c.
chiasma, pl. **chiasmata**
c. formation
chiasmal
c. compression
c. lesion
c. metastasis
chiasmapexy
chiasmata (*pl. of* chiasma)
chiasmatic
c. cistern
c. cisterna
c. groove
c. sulcus
chiasmatis
Chicago classification
chicken fat clot
Chiene incision
Chiffelle and Putt method
Child
C. class A, B, C
C. classification of cirrhosis
C. esophageal varix classification
C. hepatic dysfunction classification
C. hepatic risk criteria classification
C. liver disease classification
C. operation
C. pancreaticoduodenostomy
C. radical pancreatectomy
childbirth
Bradley method of prepared c.
Kitzinger method of c.
childhood thyroid irradiation
Child-Phillips bowel plication
Child-Pugh classification
children
faces rating scale for c.
children's
C. Cancer Study Group
C. coma scale
Childress ankle fixation technique
Child-Turcotte hepatic surgery classification
chiloplasty
chilostomatoplasty
chimera
radiation c.
chimerism
chimney-sweep's carcinoma
chin
c. augmentation
double c.
c. elevation

NOTES

chin *(continued)*
c. muscle
c. position
Chinese flap
CHIP
Coping with Health, Injuries, and Problems
CHIP scale
chip
bone c.
c. fracture
c. graft
chiroplasty
chiropractic treatment of fracture
chisel fracture
chlamydial infection
***Chlamydia trachomatis* infection**
chloramine-T technique
chloranilate method
chlormerodrin accumulation test
Cho
C. anterior cruciate ligament reconstruction
C. tendon technique
choana, pl. **choanae**
chocolate cyst
cholangiectasis
cholangiocarcinoma
hilar c.
cholangioenterostomy
cholangiofibroma
cholangiofibrosis
cholangiogastrostomy
cholangiogram
common duct c.
false-negative c.
intraoperative c. (IOC)
preoperative retrograde c.
retrograde c.
cholangiographic
c. interpretation
c. technique
cholangiography
completion c.
drip-infusion c.
endoscopic retrograde c.
infusion c.
intraoperative dynamic c.
magnetic resonance imaging c.
MRI c.
operative c. (OC)
percutaneous transhepatic c. (PTC)
cholangiohepatitis
Oriental c.
recurrent pyogenic c. (RPC)
cholangiointrahepatic
cholangiole
cholangioma
cholangiopancreatography
endoscopic retrograde c. (ERCP)
magnetic resonance c.
cholangiopancreatoscopy
peroral c.
cholangioplasty
cholangioscopy
intraductal c.
percutaneous transhepatic c.
peroral c.
cholangiostomy
cholangiotomy
cholangitis
c. carcinoma
primary sclerosing c.
recurrent pyogenic c.
cholecyst
cholecystectasia
cholecystectomy
combined laparoscopic splenectomy and c.
laparoscopic c. (LC)
laparoscopic laser c. (LLC)
laser laparoscopic c. (LLC)
microlaparoscopic c.
minilaparoscopic c.
needlescopic laparoscopic c.
open c.
percutaneous c.
prophylactic c.
retrograde c.
surgical c.
three-trocar technique c.
transcylindrical c.
c. treatment
two-trocar laparoscopic c.
cholecystenteric fistula
cholecystenteroanastomosis
cholecystenterorrhaphy
cholecystenterostomy
cholecystenterotomy
cholecystic
cholecystis
cholecystitis
acalculous c.
acute acalculous c. (AAC)
acute calculous c.
asymptomatic c.
calculous c.
chronic c.
emphysematous c.
erythromycin-induced c.
follicular c.
gangrenous c.
gaseous c.
perforated c.
scleroatrophic c.
suppurative c.

typhoidal c.
uncomplicated acute c.
xanthogranulomatous c.
cholecystobiliary fistulization
cholecystocholangiography
cholecystocholedochal fistula
cholecystocholedocholithiasis
cholecystocolic fistula
cholecystocolonic fistula
cholecystocolostomy
cholecystoduodenal
c. fistula
c. ligament
cholecystoduodenocolic
c. fistula
c. fold
cholecystoduodenostomy
Jenckel c.
cholecystoendoprosthesis
endoscopic retrograde c.
cholecystoenterostomy
direct c.
cholecystogastrostomy
cholecystoileostomy
cholecystojejunostomy
cholecystokinin secretion
cholecystolithiasis
cholecystolithotomy
percutaneous c.
cholecystolithotripsy
cholecystomy
cholecystopaque
cholecystopexy
cholecystorrhaphy
cholecystoscopy
percutaneous transhepatic c.
cholecystostomy
laparoscopy-guided subhepatic c.
percutaneous c.
surgical c.
cholecystotomy
laparoscopic c.
transpapillary endoscopic c.
choledochal
c. basal pressure
c. cyst
c. cyst disease
c. fiberoscopic approach
c. region
c. sphincter
choledochal-colonic fistula
choledoch duct
choledochectomy
choledochendysis
choledochi
choledochocele
choledochocholedochostomy side-to-side anastomosis
choledochocolonic fistula
choledochoduodenal
c. fistula
c. fistulotomy
c. junction
c. junctional stenosis
choledochoduodenostomy
choledochoenteric fistula
choledochoenterostomy
choledochofiberoscopy
T-tube tract c.
choledochogastrostomy
choledochohepatostomy
choledochoileostomy
choledochojejunostomy
end-to-side c.
loop c.
retrocolic end-to-side c.
Roux-en-Y c.
choledocholith
choledocholithiasis
choledocholithotomy
choledocholithotripsy
choledochopancreatic ductal junction
choledochoplasty
choledochorrhaphy
choledochoscopy
Berci-Shore c.
cystic duct c.
jejunostomy tract c.
operative c.
postoperative c.
T-tube tract c.
choledochostomy
choledochotomy
c. incision
longitudinal c.
choledochous
choledochus
cholelith
cholelithiasis
cholelitholysis
cholelithotomy
cholelithotripsy
cholelithotrity
cholescintigraphy

NOTES

C

cholestasis
cholestatic
c. cause
c. cirrhosis
c. jaundice
cholesteatoma pearl
cholesterol
c. calculus
c. saturation index
c. solitaire
c. stone
CholesTrak test
Cholestron PRO test
cholicele
cholinergic
c. blockade
c. mechanism
c. tract
chondral
c. edge
c. fracture
c. fragment
chondrectomy
chondrification
chondritis
xiphisternal junction c.
chondrocostal
chondrodermatitis
nodular c.
chondroepiphysis
chondroglossus muscle
chondrolysis
posttraumatic c.
chondromalacia
chondromyofibroma
chondromyxofibroma
chondromyxoma
chondroosseous
chondroosteodystrophy
chondropharyngeus
chondrophyte
chondroplasty
abrasion c.
arthroscopic abrasion c.
chondroporosis
chondrosarcoma
chondrosteoma
chondrosternal
chondrosternoplasty
chondrotomy
chondroxiphoid ligament
chop amputation
Chopart
C. amputation
C. ankle dislocation
C. articulation
chorda, pl. **chordae**
chordae tendineae rupture
c. tympani
c. tympani nerve
chordal
c. rupture
c. shortening
chordee
chord incision
chordoblastoma
chordoplasty
chordotomy
chorioadenoma
chorioallantoic membrane
chorioamnionic infection
chorioangioma
chorioblastoma
choriocapillaris
choriocarcinoma
choriocele
chorioepithelioma
chorioma
chorion
chorionic
c. cavity
c. sac
c. villus biopsy
chorioretinitis
choristoblastoma
choristoma nest
choroid
c. plexus
c. plexus carcinoma
c. plexus papilloma
c. point
c. vein
choroidal
c. artery
c. hemangioma
c. hemorrhage
c. infiltration
c. lesion
c. metastasis
c. neovascularization
c. neovascular membrane
c. ring
c. rupture
choroidea
choroidectomy
choroideus
choroiditis
choroidocapillaris
Chow technique
Chrisman-Snook
C.-S. ankle technique
C.-S. procedure
C.-S. reconstruction
chromaffin
c. body
c. tissue

chromate method
chromatic lens aberration
chromatin
c. condensation
c. pattern
chromatinic body
chromatography
gas c.
chrome alum hematoxylin-phloxine method
chromic
chromocystoscopy
chromogenic method
chromohydrotubation
chromolytic method
chromopertubation
chromoscopy
chromotubation
chronic
c. allograft rejection
c. anoplasty treatment
c. appendicitis
c. atrial fibrillation
c. catheterization
c. cholecystitis
c. course
c. digestive bleeding
c. Epstein-Barr virus infection
c. extrinsic alveolitis
c. graft-versus-host disease
c. hemolysis
c. hyperparathyroid state
c. hyperventilation syndrome
c. inflammatory demyelinating polyradiculoneuropathy (CIDP)
c. intestinal failure
c. jejunal inflammation
c. liver disease
c. motor disturbance
c. multisystem disorder
c. nonmalignant
c. obstructive pulmonary dysfunction
c. opioid analgesic therapy (COAT)
c. pain
c. pancreatitis
c. paroxysmal hemicrania (CPH)
c. presentation
c. reflux symptom
c. renal failure (CRF)
c. sinusitis
c. subareolar abscess
c. subcutaneous infusion
c. subdural hematoma
c. thrombosis
c. transplant rejection
c. ulcerative colitis (CUC)
Chuinard-Peterson ankle fusion
chylangioma
chyle
c. cistern
c. cyst
c. fistula
c. vessel
chyli
chylifera
chyliform ascites
chylocyst
chyloma
chyloperitoneum
chylothorax
chylous
c. ascites
c. ascitic fluid
c. effusion
c. hydrotherapy
c. leak
c. leakage
chyme
chymopapain chemonucleolysis
CI
cardiac index
normal CI
supranormal CI
Ciaccio method
Cibis
C. liquid silicone procedure
C. operation
cicatrectomy
cicatrices (*pl. of* cicatrix)
cicatriceum
cicatricial
c. kidney
c. mass
c. stricture
c. tissue
cicatricotomy
cicatrix, pl. **cicatrices**
cicatrizant
cicatrization
CIDP
chronic inflammatory demyelinating polyradiculoneuropathy
Cierny-Mader technique

NOTES

cilia
ciliare
ciliares
ciliaris
ciliarotomy
ciliary
c. artery
c. body
c. body band
c. canal
c. ganglion
c. ganglion root
c. injection
c. ligament
c. nerve
c. procedure
c. process
c. ring
c. vein
c. zone
c. zonule
ciliectomy
ciliodestructive surgery
cilioretinal artery
ciliotomy
ciliovitrectomy block
Cimino-Brescia arteriovenous fistula
Cimino fistula
cinching operation
Cincinnati
C. incision
C. technique
cinedefecography
cine-esophagoscopy
cinefluoroscopic method
cinefluoroscopy
valve c.
cinegastroscopy
cinereum
cine view
cingula (*pl. of* cingulum)
cingulate
c. cortex
c. herniation
c. sulcus
cingulectomy
cingulotomy
rostral c.
cingulum, pl. **cingula**
c. bundle
cingulumotomy
circinate exudate
circle
c. absorption anesthesia
arterial cerebral c.
articular vascular c.
Bain c.
closed c.
c. dissipation
Huguier c.
c. loop biliary drainage
Pagenstecher c.
pediatric c.
semiclosed c.
c. straight cutting
c. system
vascular c.
c. of Willis
c. wire nephrostomy
circuit
anesthesia breathing c.
anesthetic c.
breathing c.
extracorporeal cardiopulmonary c.
feedback reduction c.
low-flow c.
ventilation c.
circuitry
intrinsic c.
circular
c. anastomosis
c. cherry-red lesion
c. fold
c. griseotomy
c. incision
c. myotomy
c. open amputation
c. pharyngeal muscle
c. suture
c. suture technique
c. venous sinus
circulares
circularis
circulating
c. air pocket
c. blood
c. hormone
c. MEN I-specific growth factor
circulation
airway, breathing, and c. (ABC)
allantoic c.
c. aneurysm
arterial c.
assisted c.
bile acid c.
carotid c.
cerebral c.
collateral abdominal c.
collateral arterial c.
collateral mesenteric c.
compensatory c.
conjunctival c.
coronary collateral c.
cutaneous collateral c.
derivative c.
ductal-dependent pulmonary c.

enterohepatic c.
episcleral c.
extracorporeal c. (ECC)
extracranial carotid c.
femoral c.
fetal c.
fetoplacental c.
hepatic c.
hyperdynamic c.
hypophyseal portal c.
hypothalamic-hypophysial portal c.
intracranial c.
left dominant coronary c.
mesenteric c.
perichondral c.
peripheral c.
persistent fetal c.
placental c.
portal-collateral c.
portal-hypophysial c.
portosystemic collateral c.
posterior fossa c.
pulmonary c.
c. rate
retinal c.
sludging of c.
spinal cord c.
systemic venous c.
thalamic c.
thebesian c.
c. time
umbilical c.
uteroplacental c.
venous c.
c. volume
circulator fold
circulatory
c. arrest
c. arrest anesthetic technique
c. arrest procedure
c. decompensation
c. overload
circulus, pl. **circuli**
circumalveolar fixation
circumanales
circumanal gland
circumareolar
c. incision
c. mastopexy
c. quadrant
circumaxillary
circumbulbar
circumcise
circumcision suture technique
circumcorneal injection
circumcostal gastropexy
circumduction maneuver
circumference
fetal head c.
circumferentia
circumferential
c. esophageal reconstruction
c. esophagomyotomy
c. fibrocartilage
c. fracture
c. implantation
c. incision
c. mesorectal excision
c. mobilization
c. mucosal dissection
c. strip
c. venolysis
c. wire-loop fixation
circumferentially ligated
circumflex
c. femoral artery
c. humeral artery
c. iliac artery
c. nerve
c. scapular artery
c. vein
circumintestinal
circumlental space
circumlimbal incision
circumlinear incision
circummandibular fixation
circummesencephalic cistern
circumocular
circumorbital
circumrenal
circumscribed
c. inflammation
c. mass
circumscribing incision
circumumbilical
c. incision
c. pyloromyotomy
circumvallate papilla
circumvascular
circumzygomatic fixation
cirrhosis
Child classification of c.
cholestatic c.

NOTES

cirrhosis *(continued)*
end-stage c.
primary biliary c.
cirrhotic
c. liver
c. liver parenchyma
c. liver remnant
cirsectomy
cirsodesis
cirsotomy
CIS
carcinoma in situ
cistern
basal c.
cerebellomedullary c.
cerebellopontine angle c.
chiasmatic c.
chyle c.
circummesencephalic c.
interpeduncular c.
lumbar c.
mesencephalic c.
Pecquet c.
perimesencephalic c.
pontine c.
prepontine c.
quadrigeminal c.
subarachnoid c.
suprasellar subarachnoid c.
sylvian c.
cisterna, pl. **cisternae**
ambient c.
chiasmatic c.
cylindrical confronting c.
perinuclear c.
subsarcolemma c.
terminal c.
cisternal
c. herniation
c. puncture
citrate intoxication
Civinini
C. ligament
C. process
CKC
cold knife cone
2C-L
two-chamber longitudinal
2C-L image
Clado
C. anastomosis
C. band
C. ligament
C. point
Clagett
C. closure
C. operation
Clagett-Barrett esophagogastrostomy
clam
c. enterocystoplasty
c. ileocystoplasty
clamp-and-sew technique
clamping
aortic c.
blind c.
carotid c.
portal triad c.
selective vascular c. (SVC)
clamshell
c. closure
c. incision
c. technique
c. thoracotomy
Clancy
C. cruciate ligament reconstruction
C. ligament technique
C. patellar tendon graft
CLAP
contact laser ablation of prostate
Clapton line
Clark
C. level
C. transfer technique
Clark-Collip method
Clark-Southwick-Odgen modification
CLASP
Carolinas Laparoscopic Advanced Surgery Program
CLASP procedure
clasped thumb deformity
classic
c. abdominal Semm hysterectomy
c. DSRS technique
c. multiple organ failure syndrome
classical
c. cesarean section
c. Judd-Mayo overlap midline incisional hernioplasty
c. subtotal resection
c. transverse incision
classification
Ackerman-Proffitt c. of malocclusion
Acosta c.
acromioclavicular injury c.
Aitken epiphysial fracture c.
AJCC TNM tumor c.
Allman acromioclavicular injury c.
Alonso-Lej c.
American Association for Surgery of Trauma Organ Injury Scale c.
American Heart Association c.
American Society of Anesthesiologists c.
Anderson-D'Alonzo odontoid fracture c.

Anderson modification of Berndt-Harty c.
Angle malocclusion c.
Ann Arbor c.
AO c.
Arneth c.
Ashhurst-Bromer ankle fracture c.
Astler-Coller A, B1, B2, C1, C2 c.
Astler-Coller modification of Dukes c.
Bado c.
Bailyn c.
Banff c.
Bauer-Jackson c.
Baume c.
Bennett c.
Bergey c.
Berndt-Harty c.
Bethesda System for Pap smear c.
Binet system of c.
BIRADS c.
Bishop c.
bismuth benign bile duct stricture c.
bismuth bile duct stricture type I-V c.
Black c.
bladder carcinoma c.
Borrmann gastric cancer c.
Borrmann gastric cancer typing systems (types I–IV) c.
Bosniak c.
Boyd c.
Boyd-Griffin trochanteric fracture c.
Breslow c.
Broders index of malignant tumors c.
burn c.
Butchart staging c.
Caldwell-Moloy c.
Callender cell-type c.
Cambridge c.
Canadian Cardiovascular Society c.
caries c.
Carnesale-Stewart-Barnes hip dislocation c.
Caroli-Sarles c.
Casten c.
Catterall c.
cavity c.
CEAP c.
Cedars-Sinai c.
Centers for Disease Control HIV infection c.
Chadwick-Bentley c.
Chicago c.
Child esophageal varix c.
Child hepatic dysfunction c.
Child hepatic risk criteria c.
Child liver disease c.
Child-Pugh c.
Child-Turcotte hepatic surgery c.
clean-contaminated operative wound c.
clean operative wound c.
cleft palate c.
clinical pathologic c.
Codman c.
Cohen-Rentrop c.
Colonna hip fracture c.
Colton c.
contaminated operative wound c.
Cori c.
Correa c.
Couinaud c.
Croften c.
Crowe c.
Cummer c.
Dagradi esophageal variceal c.
Danis-Weber ankle injury c.
DeBakey c.
de Groot c.
DeLee c.
Denis Browne spinal fracture c.
denture c.
Denver c.
Dexter-Grossman c.
Diamond c.
Dias-Tachdijian physical injury c.
dichotomous c.
Dickhaut-DeLee discoid meniscus c.
dirty operative wound c.
Dripps c.
Duane c.
Dubin-Amelar varicocele c.
Dukes c.
Dyck-Lambert c.
Eckert-Davis c.
Edmondson-Steiner c.
Efron jackknife c.
El-Ahwany humeral supracondylar fracture c.
Ellis c.

C

NOTES

classification *(continued)*
Enna c.
Enneking c.
Epstein hip dislocation c.
Epstein-Thomas c.
Essex-Lopresti calcaneal fracture c.
Evans intertrochanteric fracture c.
FAB c.
Federation of Gynecology and Obstetrics c.
Fielding femoral fracture c.
Fielding-Magliato subtrochanteric fracture c.
Flatt c.
Foucher epiphysial injury c.
fracture c.
Fränkel neurologic deficit c.
Franz-O'Rahilly c.
Fredrickson hyperlipoproteinemia c.
Fredrickson-Levy-Lees c.
Freeman calcaneal fracture c.
French-American-British c.
Frykman distal radius fracture c.
Frykman radial fracture c.
Fukunaga-Hayes unbiased jackknife c.
functional capacity c.
Garden femoral neck fracture c.
Gartland humeral supracondylar fracture c.
Gartland Universal radial fracture c.
gastric mucosal pattern c.
Gell and Coombs c.
Goldman c.
Grantham femur fracture c.
Greenfield spinocerebellar ataxia c.
Gustilo-Anderson open fracture c.
Gustilo puncture wound c.
Haggitt c.
Halverson c.
Halverson-McVay hernia c.
Hannover c.
Hansen fracture c.
Hara gallbladder inflammation c.
Hardcastle tarsometatarsal joint injury c.
Hawkins talar fracture c.
Henderson c.
Hepatitis Activity Index c.
Herring lateral pillar c.
Hinchey diverticulitis grade c.
HIV c.
Hoaglund-States c.
Hohl-Luck tibial plateau fracture c.
Hohl-Moore c.
Hohl tibial condylar fracture c.
Holdsworth spinal fracture c.
House-Brackmann c.
Hughston c.
human immunodeficiency virus c.
Hunt and Kosnik c.
Ideberg glenoid fracture c.
immunologic c.
Ingram-Bachynski hip fracture c.
Insall patellar injury c.
International cancer of cervix c.
International C. of Diseases, Adapted for Use in the United States (ICDA)
International Federation of Gynecology and Obstetrics c.
international stage c.
Isaacson c. (IC)
Jansky c.
Japanese cancer c.
Jeffery radial fracture c.
Jensen c.
Jewett and Whitmore c.
Johner-Wruhs tibial fracture c.
Jones-Barnes-Lloyd-Roberts c.
Kajava c.
Kalamchi c.
Karnofsky rating scale c.
Kasugai c.
Kauffman-White c.
Keil tumor cell c.
Keith-Wagener c.
Keith-Wagener-Barker c.
Kelami c.
Kellam-Waddel c.
Kennedy c.
Kernohan system of glioma c.
KESS constipation scoring system c.
Key-Conwell pelvic fracture c.
Kiel c.
Kilfoyle humeral medial condylar fracture c.
Killip-Kimball heart failure c.
Kocher c.
KWB c.
Kyle-Gustilo c.
Kyle-Gustilo-Premer c.
Lagrange humeral supracondylar fracture c.
Lancefield c.
Lanza scale for drug-induced mucosal damage c.
Lauge-Hansen ankle fracture c.
Lauren gastric carcinoma c.
Le Fort c.
Leishman c.
Lennert c.
Letournel-Judet acetabular fracture c.

Leung thumb loss c.
Levine-Harvey c.
Lindell c.
Linell-Ljungberg c.
Lloyd-Roberts-Catteral-Salamon c.
Loesche c.
Lown c.
Lukes and Butler Hodgkin disease c.
Lukes-Collins c.
MacCallan c.
Macewen c.
MacNichol-Voutsinas c.
Mallampati oropharyngeal c.
Mallampati pharyngeal visibility c.
Marseille pancreatitis c.
Mason radial head fracture c.
Mast-Spieghel-Pappas c.
Masuka modified thymic carcinoma c.
Mathews olecranon fracture c.
Mayo carpal instability c.
Mayo rheumatoid elbow c.
McNeer c.
Melone distal radius fracture c.
Meyers-McKeever tibial fracture c.
microinvasive carcinoma c.
Milch condylar fracture c.
Milch elbow fracture c.
Milch humeral fracture c.
Ming gastric carcinoma c.
Minnesota EKG c.
Moore tibial plateau fracture c.
morphologic c.
Moss c.
Mueller femoral supracondylar fracture c.
Mueller tibial fracture c.
multiaxial c.
Munro and Parker laparoscopic hysterectomy c.
Nalebuff c.
Neer femur fracture c.
Neer-Horowitz humeral fracture c.
Neer shoulder fracture c.
Newman radial neck and head fracture c.
New York Heart Association heart disease c.
Nicoll c.
Niemeier c.
Nyhus c.
Ogden epiphysial fracture c.
Ogden knee dislocation c.
O'Rahilly limb deficiency c.
ordinal c.
Orthopaedic Trauma Association c.
Outerbridge c.
Paley c.
Papavasiliou olecranon fracture c.
Paris c.
Pauwels femoral neck fracture c.
Pell and Gregory c.
Pennal c.
Pipkin femoral fracture c.
Pipkin posterior hip dislocation c.
Pipkin subclassification of Epstein-Thomas c.
Poland epiphysial fracture c.
Poland physical injury c.
Potter c.
Pugh c.
Pugh-Child bleeding esophageal varices grading scale c.
Pulec and Freedman c.
Quénu-Küss tarsometatarsal injury c.
Quinby pelvic fracture c.
Rai c.
Ranawat c.
Ranson acute pancreatitis c.
Rappaport c.
Rentrop c.
Riseborough-Radin intercondylar fracture c.
Rockwood acromioclavicular injury c.
Rockwood clavicular fracture c.
Rosenthal nail injury c.
round-robin c.
Rowe calcaneal fracture c.
Rowe-Lowell hip dislocation c.
Rowe-Lowell system for fracture-dislocation c.
Ruedi-Allgower c.
Runyon c.
Russe c.
Russell-Taylor c.
Rüter c.
Rutkow-Robbins-Gilbert c.
Rutledge extended hysterectomy c.
Rye Hodgkin disease c.
Sage-Salvatore acromioclavicular joint injury c.

C

NOTES

classification *(continued)*
- Saha shoulder muscle c.
- Sakellarides calcaneal fracture c.
- Salter epiphysial fracture c.
- Salter-Harris epiphysial fracture c.
- Santiani-Stone c.
- Sassouni c.
- Savary-Mille grading scale c.
- scalar c.
- Schatzker tibial plateau fracture c.
- Scheie c.
- Schuknecht c.
- Schwarz c.
- Seattle c.
- Seddon c.
- Seinsheimer femoral fracture c.
- sentence c.
- Severin c.
- Shaffer-Weiss c.
- Shaher-Puddu c.
- Shelton femoral fracture c.
- Singh osteoporosis c.
- Siurala c.
- Skinner c.
- Snyder c.
- Solcia c.
- Sonnenberg c.
- Sorbie calcaneal fracture c.
- Spaulding c.
- Speed radial head fracture c.
- Spetzler-Martin c.
- Stark c.
- Steinbrocker c.
- Suda type I, II, III papilla c.
- Sunderland nerve injury c.
- Swanson c.
- Sydney system gastritis c.
- Tachdjian c.
- Tessier c.
- Thomas c.
- Thompson-Epstein femoral fracture c.
- Three Color Concept of wound c.
- thrombolysis in myocardial infarction c.
- Tile c.
- TIMI c.
- TNM carcinoma c.
- tongue thrust c.
- Torg c.
- Torode-Zieg c.
- Toronto pelvic fracture c.
- Tronzo intertrochanteric fracture c.
- Tscherne c.
- Tscherne-Gotzen tibial fracture c.
- tumor, node, metastasis carcinoma c.
- UICC tumor c.
- Vaughan Williams antiarrhythmic drug c.
- Veau c.
- Venn-Watson c.
- Visick dysphagia c.
- Vostal radial fracture c.
- Wagener-Clay-Gipner c.
- Wagner c.
- Walter Reed c.
- Walter Reed c. for HIV infection
- Warren-Marshall c.
- Wassel thumb duplication c.
- Watanabe discoid meniscus c.
- Watson-Jones tibial fracture c.
- Watson-Jones tibial tubercle avulsion fracture c.
- Weber-Danis ankle injury c.
- Weber physical injury c.
- Weiland c.
- Weissman c.
- White c.
- Whitehead c.
- WHO gastric carcinoma c.
- Wiberg patellar c.
- Wiley-Galey c.
- Wilkins radial fracture c.
- Winquist femoral shaft fracture c.
- Winquist-Hansen femoral fracture c.
- Winter c.
- Wolfe breast carcinoma c.
- Woofry-Chandler c. of Osgood-Schlatter lesion
- World Health Organization c.
- Yacoub and Radley-Smith c.
- Young pelvic fracture c.
- Zickel c.
- Zlotsky-Ballard acromioclavicular injury c.
- Zollinger c.

claudication

Claudius
- C. cell
- C. fossa

Clausen method

claustra

claustral

claustrum, pl. **claustra**

clavi (*pl. of* clavus)

clavicectomy

clavicle
- c. excision

clavicula, pl. **claviculae**

clavicular
- c. birth fracture
- c. branch
- c. epiphysis
- c. facet

c. fracture aneurysm
c. incision
clavicularis
claviculectomy
clavipectoral fascia
clavipectoralis
clavus, pl. **clavi**
clawfoot deformity
clawhand deformity
clawing deformity
clawtoe deformity
clay pipe carcinoma
clay-shoveler fracture
Clayton
C. forefoot arthroplasty
C. procedure
C. procedure with panmetatarsal head resection
Clayton-Fowler technique
C-LDP
complete laparoscopic distal pancreatectomy
clean
c. contaminated surgery
c. intermittent catheterization
c. intermittent self-catheterization
c. operation
c. operative wound classification
clean-catch collection method
clean-contaminated
c.-c. operation
c.-c. operative wound classification
cleaning solution
cleansing
bowel c.
clear
c. cell hepatocellular carcinoma
c. cell hidradenoma
c. effluent
c. fluid
c. liquid diet
c. otorrhea
clearance
elimination c.
lactate c.
oncologic c.
c. technique
Cleasby iridectomy operation
cleavage
c. fracture
c. lesion
c. line
c. plane
cleft
anal c.
c. closure
corneal c.
facial c.
c. hand deformity
Larrey c.
c. lip
c. lip deformity
natal c.
c. nose
oblique facial c.
c. palate
c. palate classification
pudendal c.
residual c.
soft-palate c.
subdural c.
urogenital c.
cleidocostal
cleidocranial
cleidoepitrochlearis
cleidomastoideus
cleido-occipitalis
cleidotomy
Cleveland
C. Clinic weighted scale of endoscopic procedure
C. procedure
Cleveland-Bosworth-Thompson technique
clidal
clidocostal
clidocranial
clinch knot
clinic
dialysis c.
outpatient dialysis c.
clinical
c. acute pancreatitis
c. characteristic
C. Classification System (CCS)
c. correlation
c. defect
c. deterioration
c. diagnosis
c. encephalopathy
c. evaluation
c. evidence
c. examination
c. followup

NOTES

clinical *(continued)*
c. geneticist
c. implication
c. improvement
c. indication
c. intestinal transplantation
c. manifestation
c. manifestations, etiologic factors, anatomic involvement, pathophysiologic features (CEAP)
c. outcome
c. parameter
c. pathologic classification
c. pathology
c. picture
c. presentation
c. principle
c. problem
c. response
c. spectroscopy
c. suspicion
c. syndrome
clinically
c. node-negative breast cancer
c. silent rhabdomyoma
clinician
nonsurgical c.
surgical c.
clinicopathologic
c. correlation
c. data
c. feature
Clinitron air-fluidized therapy
clinoidectomy
anterior extradural c.
extradural c.
clinoideus
clinoid process
clip
c. application
c. graft
c. occlusion
c. placement
c. technique
clip-induced bile duct stricture
clitoral recession
clitoridectomy
clitoridis
clitoris, pl. **clitorides**
clitoroplasty
clitorovaginoplasty
clival
clivus, pl. **clivi**
Blumenbach c.
c. canal line
c. metastasis
c. syndrome
CLO
C. biopsy
C. test
cloaca, pl. **cloacae**
cloacal
c. formation
c. malformation
c. membrane
clock
around the c. (ATC)
clockwise
c. direction
c. rotation
clomiphene fetal malformation
clonal
c. deletion
c. expansion
C-loop intraocular lens
Cloquet
C. canal
C. canal remnant
C. fascia
C. hernia
C. ligament
C. node
C. pseudoganglion
C. septum
close
c. c.
c. margin
c. monitoring
c. proximity
closed
c. anesthesia
c. anesthesia system
c. chest commissurotomy
c. chest thoracostomy
c. circle
c. circuit method
c. dislocation
c. flap amputation
c. head injury
c. hemorrhoidectomy
c. intramedullary osteotomy
c. irrigation
c. laparoscopy
c. manipulative maneuver
c. nail
c. patch test
c. pinning
c. reduction
c. reduction/chemical splinting
c. reduction and percutaneous fixation (CRPF)
c. skull fracture
c. soft tissue injury
c. suction drainage
c. surgery

c. transventricular mitral commissurotomy
c. tubule fixation technique
c. wedge osteotomy
closed-break fracture
closed-circuit
c.-c. anesthesia
c.-c. anesthetic technique
closed-eye surgery
closed-gloving technique
closed-loop
c.-l. automated delivery
c.-l. intestinal obstruction
closed-space infection
closed-system pars plana vitrectomy
closing
c. abductory wedge osteotomy
c. base wedge
c. base wedge osteotomy
c. pressure
c. ring of Winkler-Waldeyer
clostridial
c. infection
c. myonecrosis
closure
abdominal wall c.
abdominal wound c.
aponeurotic c.
auditory c.
Barsky cleft c.
Clagett c.
clamshell c.
cleft c.
colostomy c.
compression skull-cap c.
crowfoot c.
crural c.
delayed primary c.
direct c.
double-umbrella c.
epiphysial c.
exstrophy c.
fascial c.
c. of fistula
flask c.
floor-of-mouth c.
Fontan fenestration c.
forced-eye c.
general c.
glottic c.
Graham c.
Hartmann c.
ileostomy c.
incision c.
King ASD umbrella c.
latex c.
layered c.
Marlex c.
mastectomy c.
maxillary antrum c.
midline aponeurotic c.
muscularis tunnel c.
nonoperative c.
nonprosthetic c.
palatopharyngeal c.
pancreatic stump c.
percutaneous patent ductus arteriosus c.
premature airway c.
premature ductus arteriosis c.
c. pressure
primary c.
c. principle
retainer c.
scalloped c.
scalp c.
secondary c.
shoelace fasciotomy c.
single-layer continuous c.
sinus c.
skin c.
Smead-Jones c.
stoma c.
suture c.
sutureless colostomy c.
transcatheter c.
transmural c.
two-layer latex c.
umbrella c.
vacuum-assisted c. (VAC)
velopharyngeal c.
ventricular septal defect c.
visual c.
Von Langenbeck palatal c.
V-to-Y c.
watertight c.
wound c.
clot
afferent c.
agonal c.
antemortem c.
autologous c.
black blood c.
blood c.

NOTES

clot *(continued)*
chicken fat c.
c. colic
currant jelly c.
distal c.
evacuating c.
exogenous fibrin c.
c. extension
external c.
c. formation
fresh blood c.
friable c.
heart c.
internal c.
laminated c.
marantic c.
organized c.
passive c.
plastic c.
postmortem c.
c. propagation
proximal c.
c. regression
retraction of c.
c. retraction coagulation panel
Schede c.
sentinel blood c.
c. size
spider-web c.
stratified c.
washed c.
clothespin
c. H spinal fusion
clot-induced urinary tract obstruction
clotting
abnormal c.
c. abnormality
c. factor
graft c.
c. mechanism
c. parameter
c. time coagulation panel
cloudy
c. ascites
c. fluid
cloven-hoof fracture of finger
cloverleaf
c. condylar-plate fixation
c. skull
c. skull deformity
c. skull syndrome
Cloward
C. anterior spinal fusion
C. back fusion
C. cervical disk approach
C. fusion diskectomy
C. operation
C. procedure
C. technique
CLP
cecal ligation and puncture
clubbed
c. nail
c. penis
clubbing
nail c.
clubfoot deformity
clune
cluneal
clunium
cluster
c. headache
c. operation
c. reduction
repetitive c.
c. tic syndrome
clustered
c. calcification
CMAP
compound muscle action potential
CMR
cerebral metabolic rate
CMV
controlled mechanical ventilation
cytomegalovirus
CMV colitis
CMV infection
CMV prophylaxis
CMV-associated ulceration
CMV-induced esophageal ulceration
CMV-positive donor
cnemial
cnemis
CO
carbon monoxide
cardiac output
CO_2
carbon dioxide
arterial partial pressure of CO_2
CO_2 elimination
CO_2 inhalation test
CO_2 pneumoperitoneum
coagula (*pl. of* coagulum)
coagulate
coagulating
c. diathermy
c. factor
coagulation
argon beam c.
bipolar c.
blood c.
Bovie c.
c. cascade
cold c.
c. defect

diffuse intravascular c.
c. disorder
disseminated intravascular c. (DIC)
electric c.
endoscopic microwave c.
endovascular c.
exogenous anticoagulant c.
c. factor
c. factor assay
c. factor transfusion
fibrinolysin c.
free-beam c.
heater-probe c.
infrared c.
laser c.
light c.
low-current monopolar c.
Meyer-Schwickerath light c.
microwave c.
monopolar c.
multipolar c.
c. necrosis
c. pathway
plasmin c.
c. profile
c. screen
sepsis-induced disseminated intravascular c.
tissue c.

coagulative
c. laser therapy
c. myocytolysis

coagulopathic disorder

coagulopathy
hypothermia-induced c.
hypothermia-related c.
uremia-related c.

coagulum, pl. **coagula**
c. formation
c. pyelolithotomy

Coakley suture technique

coalesce

coal-mining lensectomy

coapt

coaptation
end-to-side nerve c.
nerve c.
c. site
c. suture technique
urethral c.

coarct

coarctate

coarctation
c. of aorta
postductal c.
c. of pulmonary artery
c. repair
c. syndrome

coarctectomy

coarctotomy

coarticulation
anticipatory c.
backward c.
forward c.

COAT
chronic opioid analgesic therapy

coat
muscular c.
seromuscular c.

Coats white ring

coaxial
c. illumination
c. pressure

cobalt-60 moving strip technique

cobaltinitrite method

cobalt therapy

cobbler's suture technique

cobblestone appearance

Cobb scoliosis measuring technique

cobra-head anastomosis

cocaine anesthesia

cocaine-induced respiratory failure

cocainization

coccidian body

***Coccidioides* infection**

coccygea

coccygeae

coccygeal
c. body
c. cornua
c. dimple
c. fistula
c. foveola
c. ganglion
c. gland
c. horn
c. joint
c. muscle
c. nerve
c. plexus
c. vertebra
c. whorl

coccygealia

NOTES

coccygectomy
Lougheed-White c.
coccygei
coccyges (*pl. of* coccyx)
coccygeum
coccygeus
c. muscle
coccygotomy
coccyx, pl. **coccyges**
c. fracture
cochlea, pl. **cochleae**
cochlear
c. artery
c. duct
c. ganglion
c. lesion
c. nerve
cochleariform process
cochleosacculotomy
cochleostomy
cochleovestibular
c. approach
c. neurectomy
cocked-half flap
Cocke maxillectomy
Cockett procedure
Cockroft method
cocktail
lytic c.
cock-up deformity
codfish deformity
Codivilla
C. tendon lengthening technique
Codman
C. classification
C. incision
C. saber-cut shoulder approach
coefficient
octanol/water c.
coeliac
c. artery
c. axis
c. branch
coeliaci
co-eluted
coenzyme
ameliorating myocardial stunning liposomal c.
coexistence
coffee-grounds
c.-g. emesis
c.-g. vomitus
Coffey
C. incision
C. suspension
C. technique
C. ureterointestinal anastomosis
Coffey-Witzel jejunostomy technique
Cofield technique
Cogan syndrome
cognitive
c. anxiety subscale
c. behavior treatment (CBT)
C. Errors Questionnaire
cognitive-attitudinal factor inquiry
cognitive-behavioral therapy
cogwheel respiration
Cohen
C. antireflux procedure
C. cross-trigonal reimplantation
C. cross-trigonal technique
Cohen-Rentrop classification
coherent bundle
coiled
c. intracranial aneurysm
c. spring appearance
c. spring sign
coiling
endovascular c.
coil-shaped varix
coin
c. biopsy
fracture en c.
c. lesion
coincidence correction
coinduction of anesthesia
coital cephalalgia
Coiter muscle
Colanis maneuver
Colcher-Sussman method
cold
c. abscess
c. application
c. coagulation
c. cone biopsy
c. conization
c. cup biopsy
c. defect
c. erythema
c. exposure
c. forceps ablation
c. gangrene
c. gas sterilization
c. gas sterilized
c. ischemia time
c. knife cone (CKC)
c. knife endoureterotomy
c. knife method
c. lesion
c. nodule
c. pressor test (CPT)
c. pressor testing maneuver
c. restraint stress
c. saline-induced paresthesia technique
c. snare ablation

c. snare excision
c. soak solution
c. spot

cold-cup resection

cold-knife conization

Cole
C. intubation procedure
C. osteotomy
C. sign
C. technique
C. tendon fixation

colectasia

colectomy
abdominal c.
hand-assisted laparoscopic c.
laparoscopic c.
laparoscopy-assisted c.
left c.
one-stage left c.
open c.
partial c.
prophylactic c.
restorative c.
subtotal c. (SC)
total c. (TC)
total abdominal c. (TAC)
transverse c.

Coleman
C. flatfoot technique
C. plasty

coleocele

coleoptosis

coleotomy

coli
adenomatous polyposis c. (APC)

colic
abdominal c.
appendiceal c.
appendicular c.
c. artery
bile duct c.
biliary c.
bilious c.
clot c.
common duct c.
Devonshire c.
episodic c.
c. epithelium
esophageal c.
flatulent c.
c. flexure
gallbladder c.
gallstone c.
hepatic c.
hysterical c.
c. impression
infantile c.
intestinal c.
kidney c.
lead c.
mucous c.
nephritic c.
c. omentum
Painter c.
pancreatic c.
c. patch
c. patch esophagoplasty
c. plexus
psychogenic c.
renal c.
saturnine c.
spasmodic c.
c. sphincter
ureteral c.
c. vein
vermicular c.

colica

colici

colicky pain

coliform urinary infection

coliplication

colipuncture

colitis
amebic c.
chronic ulcerative c. (CUC)
CMV c.
cytomegalovirus c.
granulomatous c.
ischemic c.
c. perineal complication
radiation-induced c.
ulcerative c. (UC)

colla (*pl. of* collum)

collagen
c. accumulation
c. injection
c. production
c. staining method
c. synthesis

collagenase level

collagenous
c. sprue
c. tissue
c. trabecular ring

NOTES

collapse
abrupt hemodynamic c.
bone graft c.
c. cavitation
hemodynamic c.
collar
c. bone
c. incision
collar-bone appearance
collar-button
c.-b. abscess
c.-b. appearance
c.-b. ulceration
collar-button-like ulcer
collateral
c. abdominal circulation
c. arterial circulation
c. digital artery
c. ligament
c. ligament rupture
c. mesenteric circulation
portal c.
portal-systemic c.
pulmonary c.
c. pulp canal
c. respiration
c. vein
venous c.
c. vessel
collaterale
collateralization
ventilation c.
collecting duct
collection
abdominal air c.
abdominal fluid c.
air c.
arterial blood c.
cell c.
duodenal fluid c.
encysted intraabdominal c.
expired air c.
extraaxial fluid c.
extracerebral fluid c.
fluid c.
gas c.
globular c.
gravitational particle c.
infected c.
intraglandular fluid c.
isokinetic c.
pancreatic fluid c.
periarticular fluid c.
pericholecystic fluid c.
perinephric fluid c.
pleural fluid c.
posttraumatic subcapsular hepatic fluid c.
pus c.
quantitative stool c.
saccular c.
urine specimen c.
Colles
C. fascia
C. fracture
C. ligament
C. space
colli artery
colliculectomy
colliculitis
colliculus, pl. **colliculi**
facial c.
seminal c.
Collier tract
Collin-Beard operation
Collis
C. antireflux operation
C. broken femoral stem technique
C. gastroplasty
C. gastroplasty procedure
C. repair
Collis-Dubrul femoral stem removal
Collis-Nissen
C.-N. esophageal lengthening procedure
C.-N. fundoplication
C.-N. fundoplication method
C.-N. fundoplication procedure
C.-N. fundoplication technique
C.-N. gastroplasty
collodion
flexible c.
hemostatic c.
c. membrane
styptic c.
collodium
colloid
c. body
c. cancer
c. carcinoma
c. cyst
c. formation
c. goiter
c. material
c. osmotic pressure (COP)
c. solution
c. theory of narcosis
colloidal osmotic pressure
collum, pl. **colla**
coloanal
c. anastomosis
c. resection
coloboma anomaly
colobronchial fistula
colocentesis
colocholecystostomy

colocolic
c. anastomosis
c. intussusception
colocolonic anastomosis
colocolostomy
colocutaneous fistula
colocystoplasty
seromuscular c.
coloendoanal anastomosis
cologastrocutaneous fistula
colohepatopexy
coloileal
c. fistula
cololysis
colon
ascending c.
c. cancer
c. carcinoma
c. conduit
descending c.
distended c.
c. epithelium
c. flexure
giant c.
haustration of c.
iliac c.
c. incarceration
lead-pipe c.
normal c.
c. obstruction
c. perforation
c. polyp
c. problem
c. procedure
pulled-down c.
c. and rectal surgery
c. resection
sigmoid c.
spastic c.
spike burst on electromyogram of c.
transverse c.
c. tumor
colonic
c. abscess
c. adenocarcinoma
c. adenoma
c. air
c. carcinoma
c. dilation
c. distention
c. diverticular hemorrhage
c. esophagoplasty
c. explosion
c. fistula
c. foreign body
c. inertia
c. infiltration
c. intussusception
c. J-pouch
c. lavage
c. lavage solution
c. lesion identification
c. loop
c. mass
c. mesenteric plexus
c. metastasis
c. mobilization
c. mucosal line
c. neoplasm
c. obstruction
c. patch
c. perforation
c. pouch
c. pouch anal anastomosis
c. resection
c. tattooing
c. vascular lesion
colonization
concomitant c.
c. infection
colonizing organism
Colonna
C. hip fracture classification
C. trochanteric arthroplasty
Colonna-Ralston
C.-R. ankle approach
C.-R. incision
C.-R. medial approach
colonoscopic
c. appendectomy
c. biopsy
c. examination
c. polypectomy
c. removal
colonoscopy
cecal c.
complete c.
c. complication
diagnostic c.
emergency c.
high-magnification c.
incomplete c.
pediatric c.

NOTES

colonoscopy *(continued)*
c. per rectum
c. per stoma
real-time c.
c. screening
splenic flexure c.
stomal c.
tandem c.
therapeutic c.
total c.
upper endoscopy and c.
virtual c.
colonoscopy-related
c.-r. emphysema
c.-r. incarceration
colonostomy
colony
c. culture
c. formation
colopexostomy
colopexotomy
colopexy
coloplasty
c. pouch
c. procedure
coloplication
coloproctostomy
coloptosis
colopuncture
color
c. aberration
c. duplex ultrasonography
c. fusion
c. imaging
c. saturation
colorectal
c. adenocarcinoma
c. adenoma
c. anastomosis
c. biopsy
c. bleeding
c. cancer (CRC)
c. cancer endoscopy
c. cancer resection
c. carcinoma
c. disease
c. disorder
c. distention pain
c. fistula
c. hemorrhage
c. metastasis
c. mucosa
c. operation
c. pathology
c. physiology
c. polyp
c. primary
c. primary tumor
c. segment
c. septum
c. specimen
c. surgeon
c. surgery
colorectostomy
Colored Visual Analogue Scale (CVAS)
colorrhaphy
colosigmoidostomy
colosigmoid resection
colostomy
blowhole decompressing c.
c. bridge
c. closure
continent c.
decompression c.
descending loop c.
Devine c.
diverting loop c.
diverting proximal c.
divided-stoma c.
double-barrel c.
dry c.
end c.
end-loop c.
end-sigmoid c.
exteriorization c.
fecal diversion c.
Hartmann c.
ileoascending c.
ileosigmoid c.
ileotransverse c.
initial c.
juxta-anal c.
Lazaro da Silva technique c.
loop transverse c.
Mikulicz c.
permanent end c.
c. pyloric autotransplantation
resective c.
sigmoid end c.
sigmoid-loop rod c.
c. soiling
c. takedown
temporary diverting c.
temporary end c.
terminal c.
transverse c.
transverse-loop rod c.
Turnbull c.
wet c.
colotomy
colovaginal fistula
colovesical fistula
colpectomy
skinning c.

colpocleisis
Latzko partial c.
Le Fort partial c.
colpocystoplasty
colpocystotomy
colpocystoureterotomy
colpocystourethropexy
colpohysterectomy
colpohysteropexy
colpohysterotomy
colpomicroscopy
colpomyomectomy
colpoperineopexy
abdominal-sacral c.
colpoperineoplasty
colpoperineorrhaphy
colpopexy
colpoplasty
colpopoiesis
colporectopexy
colporrhaphy
Goffe c.
posterior c.
colposcopic diagnosis
colposcopy
digital imaging c.
estrogen-assisted c.
colpostenotomy
colposuspension
Burch c.
laparoscopic needle c.
laparoscopic retropubic c.
colpotomy incision
colpoureterotomy
colpourethrocystopexy
retropubic c.
colpourethropexy
Burch c.
Coltart
C. calcaneotibial fusion
C. fracture technique
Colton classification
columellar
c. reconstruction
c. repair
column
anal c.
anterior c.
Bertin c.
lateral c.
posterior c.
rectal c.
renal c.
rugal c.
spinal c.
vaginal c.
variceal c.
vertebral c.
columnar
c. cuff carcinoma
c. epithelium
c. metaplasia
columnar-lined esophagus
coma
c. aberration
acute hepatic c.
alcoholic c.
apoplectic c.
barbiturate c.
c. dé passé
diabetic c.
electrolyte imbalance c.
c. grade
hepatic c.
hyperosmolar diabetic c.
hyperosmolar hyperglycemic nonketotic c.
insulin c.
irreversible c.
Kussmaul c.
metabolic c.
myxedema c.
c. scale
thyrotoxic c.
trance c.
uremic c.
c. vigil
Comberg foreign body operation
combination
c. calculus
c. chemotherapy
c. of isotonics technique
c. restoration
c. skin
c. surgery
combined
c. analysis
c. anterior and posterior approach
c. cavus deformity
c. chemoradiation therapy
c. defect
c. epidural-general anesthesia
c. flexion-distraction injury and burst fracture

NOTES

combined *(continued)*
- c. gastrointestinal resection
- c. heart catheterization
- c. hiatal hernia
- c. injuries
- c. laparoscopic splenectomy and cholecystectomy
- c. laparoscopic and thoracoscopic approach
- c. low cervical and transthoracic approach
- c. method
- c. organ resection
- c. presigmoid-transtransversarium intradural approach
- c. radial-ulnar-humeral fracture
- c. spinal-epidural anesthesia (CSEA)
- c. spinal-epidural anesthetic technique
- c. system disease
- c. transsylvian and middle fossa approach
- c. ureterolysis

comblike septum
combustion
- surgical drape c.

come-and-go anesthesia
comedo
- c. carcinoma
- c. carcinoma of breast
- c. extraction
- c. subtype

comedocarcinoma
comitans vein
commando
- c. operation
- c. procedure
- C. radical glossectomy

commensal organism
comminuted
- c. intraarticular fracture
- c. orbital fracture
- c. skull fracture

comminution
commissura, pl. **commissurae**
commissural
- c. bundle
- c. fusion
- c. lip pit
- c. myelorrhaphy
- c. myelotomy

commissure
- anterior labial c.
- posterior labial c.

commissurotomy
- balloon mitral c.
- Brockenbrough transseptal c.
- closed chest c.
- closed transventricular mitral c.
- mitral balloon c.
- percutaneous mitral balloon c.
- percutaneous transatrial mitral c.
- percutaneous transvenous mitral c.
- transventricular mitral valve c.

common
- c. annular ring
- c. annular tendon
- c. basal vein
- c. bile duct (CBD)
- c. bile duct exploration
- c. bile duct ligation
- c. bile duct stone (CBDS)
- c. canal
- c. carotid plexus
- c. cavity phenomenon
- c. duct calculus
- c. duct cholangiogram
- c. duct colic
- c. duct obstruction
- c. dural sac
- c. extensor tendon
- c. facial vein
- c. femoral artery (CFA)
- c. femoral artery-superficial femoral artery (CFA-SFA)
- c. flexor sheath
- c. hepatic artery
- c. hepatic duct
- c. iliac artery
- c. interosseous artery
- c. mode rejection ratio
- c. palmar digital artery
- c. peroneal artery
- c. peroneal nerve
- c. peroneal nerve syndrome
- c. plantar digital artery
- c. tendinous ring

commune
communes
communicans
communicantes
communicating
- c. artery
- c. branch
- c. fistula
- c. hematoma

communication
- microfistulous c.

communis
community-acquired infection
commutator
comorbid medical problem
compact
- c. bone
- c. substance

compacta

companion
c. artery
c. lymph node
comparative radiographic examination
comparison operation
compartment
c. compression syndrome
extraaxial c.
extracellular c.
extravascular c.
c. procedure
compartmental
c. pressure
c. radioimmunoglobulin therapy
c. volume
compartmentalization
compensation
c. reaction
c. technique
compensatory
c. antiinflammatory response syndrome (CARS)
c. basilar osteotomy
c. blood supply
c. circulation
c. deformity
c. head posture
c. regeneration
c. wedge
competing messages integration
compilation autogenous vein graft
complementary
c. and alternative medicine
c. balloon angioplasty
c. therapy
c. treatment
complement fixation
complement-induced lung injury
complete
c. adrenalectomy
c. anterior dislocation
c. atrioventricular dissociation
c. A-V dissociation
c. axillary dissection
c. bilateral deformity
c. blockage
c. circumferential mesorectal excision
c. colonoscopy
c. common peroneal nerve lesion
c. duplication
c. fistula
c. fracture
c. hemostasis
c. hernia
c. inferior dislocation
c. integration
c. internal hemipelvectomy
c. iridectomy
c. laparoscopic distal pancreatectomy (C-LDP)
c. lateral hemilaminectomy
c. left bundle-branch block
c. mesh excision
c. motor paraplegia
c. obstruction
c. posterior dislocation
c. pulpectomy
c. pulpotomy
c. resection
c. right bundle-branch block
c. rupture
c. skin-sparing mastectomy
c. sphincter relaxation
c. superior dislocation
c. surgical exploration
c. thymectomy
c. thyroidectomy
c. wrap Nissen operation
completion
c. cholangiography
c. thyroidectomy
complex
c. adrenal endocrine disorder
c. anorectal fistula
c. aortic disease
areolar c.
c. cavity
c. chest mass
c. dissection
epispadias-exstrophy c.
exstrophy-epispadias c.
fibrocystic c.
c. fracture
fusion c.
Ghon c.
c. gonadal endocrine disorder
growth plate c.
c. hepatojejunostomy
internal hemorrhoidal c.
c. intracranial aneurysm
juxtaglomerular c.
c. left ventricular outflow tract obstruction

NOTES

complex *(continued)*
limb-body wall c.
major histocompatibility c. (MHC)
c. pituitary endocrine disorder
plasmin-inhibitor c. (PIC)
c. regional pain syndrome (CRPS)
c. regional pain syndrome I, II
c. signal transduction
sling-ring c.
c. thyroid endocrine disorder
triangular fibrocartilage c. (TFCC)
tuberous sclerosis c.
vertebral subluxation c.
Xase c.

compliance
chest wall c.
dynamic c.
pulmonary c.
c., rate, oxygenation, and pressure (CROP)
c., rate, oxygenation, and pressure index

compliant bowel

complicated
c. diverticular disease
c. fracture

complication
abdominal c.
anastomotic c.
bacterial c.
benign pneumatic colonoscopy c.
bleeding c.
cardiopulmonary c.
cardiorespiratory c.
cardiovascular c.
cerebrovascular c.
colitis perineal c.
colonoscopy c.
concomitant obesity c.
deep abdominal c. (DAC)
delayed c.
diabetic c.
disease-related c.
endoscopy c.
extraabdominal infective c.
extraintestinal c.
feeding c.
gastroduodenal c.
gastrointestinal c.
gonadal c.
hematologic c.
hemorrhagic c.
hepatic c.
immunologic c.
infectious c.
infective extraabdominal c.
intraoperative c.
late c.
life-threatening c.
metabolic c.
neurologic c.
neurovascular c.
nonfatal c.
nonimmunologic c.
noninfective extraabdominal c.
obstetrical c.
operative site c.
opportunistic c.
oral c.
pancreatic c.
perioperative c.
postbiopsy vascular c.
postoperative respiratory c.
postsplenectomy c.
pregnancy c.
pulmonary c.
c. rate
recurrent thromboembolic c.
renal c.
respiratory c.
sclerotherapy c.
septic c.
stomal c.
surgery c.
thromboembolic c.
thrombotic c.
trocar wound site c.
urologic c.
vascular c.
venous-related c.
wound c.

component
allogenic blood c.
dominant c.
extensive intraductal c. (EIC)
intraductal c.
monoclonal c.

composita

composite
c. addition technique
c. flap
c. free tissue transfer
c. joint
c. pelvic resection
c. pelvic resection method
c. pelvic resection procedure
c. pelvic resection technique
c. resin restoration
c. rib graft
c. skin graft
c. tissue transplantation

compound
c. aneurysm
c. cavity
c. comminuted fracture
c. cyst

c. dislocation
c. flap
c. joint
c. muscle action potential (CMAP)
c. restoration
c. skull fracture
c. suture technique

compressed
c. body
c. fracture

compressible cavernous body

compression
c. anesthesia
anterior cord c.
anterior-posterior c.
anteroposterior c.
c. arthrodesis
axial c.
c. bandage
barrel-hooping c.
c. bone conduction
brainstem c.
c. button gastrojejunostomy
cardiac c.
carotid artery c.
cauda equina c.
cerebral aqueduct c.
cervical vessel c.
cervicomedullary junction c.
Charnley c.
chest c.
chiasmal c.
continuous c.
cord c.
c. cough
c. cyanosis
direct c.
disk c.
duodenal c.
duplex-guided c.
dynamic c.
early supraclavicular c.
elastic c.
esophageal c.
c. extension
external pneumatic calf c.
extrinsic bladder c.
c. fracture
gastric c.
gentle c.
head c.
image c.
c. injury
interfragmentary c.
intermittent pneumatic c.
intrinsic c.
ischemic c.
lateral c.
limbal c.
lower plexus c.
mechanical variceal c.
median nerve c.
c. molding
napkin-ring c.
nerve root c.
neurovascular cross c.
optic chiasm c.
optic tract c.
c. overload
c. paralysis
c. plate fixation
c. plating
pneumatic c.
prechiasmal c.
progressive c.
c. rod treatment
root c.
c. skull-cap closure
spinal cord c.
spot c.
static c.
c. strain
supraclavicular c.
suprascapular nerve c.
c. switch
c. syndrome
c. technique
c. test
c. testing
thecal sac c.
thoracic outlet c.
tissue c.
tracheal c.
uterine c.
variable-release c.
vascular c.
venous c.
vertebral c.
vertical c.
c. wiring

compression-evoked allodynia

compressor naris muscle

compromise
airway c.

NOTES

compromise *(continued)*
organ c.
renal c.
respiratory c.
visual c.
computed
c. tomography (CT)
c. tomography arterial portography (CTAP)
c. tomography-guided biopsy
c. tomography-guided selective drainage
c. tomography scan
c. tomography severity index (CTSI)
computer-assisted
c.-a. anesthesia
c.-a. continuous infusion anesthetic technique
c.-a. controlled infusion (CACI)
c.-a. design-controlled alignment method
c.-a. stereotactic surgery
c.-a. treatment
computer-controlled
c.-c. drug administration anesthetic technique
c.-c. infusion anesthetic technique
computerized
c. diaphragmatic breathing retraining (CDBR)
c. electronic endoscopy
c. image guidance
concatenation
concave abdomen
concealed
c. bypass tract
c. hemorrhage
c. hernia
c. penis
c. umbilical stoma
concentrate
platelet c.
concentration
ambient oxygen c.
approximate lethal c.
bactericidal c.
bilirubin c.
blood alcohol c.
carbon dioxide c.
end-tidal nitrogen c.
hazardous c.
inspiratory vapor c.
lethal c.
mass c.
maximal drug c.
maximum permissible c.
minimal alveolar c.
minimal anesthetic c. (MAC)
minimal bactericidal c.
minimum alveolar c. (MAC)
1-minimum alveolar c. (1-MAC)
minimum alveolar anesthetic c. (MAC)
minimum bactericidal c.
minimum detectable c.
minimum effective c. (MEC)
minimum effective analgesic c.
minimum lethal c.
minimum local analgesic c. (MLAC)
c. performance test
plasma c.
plasma endotoxin c.
plasma gastrin c.
plasma iron c.
plasma norepinephrine c.
plasma renin c.
plasma urea c.
predialysis plasma phosphate c.
prick-test c.
c. procedure
radioactive c.
renal vein renin c.
serum bactericidal c.
serum bilirubin c.
serum calcium c.
serum lithium c.
steroid c.
subanesthetic c.
substance c.
target plasma c. (TPC)
thyroid hormone serum c.
time of maximum c.
c. times time
total L-chain c.
total protein c.
concentration-effect relation
concentric
c. exercise
c. hernia
c. lesion
c. mastopexy
c. reduction
concept
C. ablation
concept formation
concertina-like fashion
concha, pl. **conchae**
nasal c.
sphenoidal c.
concharum
conchoidal
concomitant
c. acidosis
c. administration

c. antireflux surgery
c. bleeding
c. colonization
c. hepatectomy
c. median sternotomy
c. medication
c. obesity complication
c. spinal cord injury
c. therapy
concurrent
c. chemotherapy
c. DVT
c. hepatic laceration
c. medical condition
concussion
brain c.
spinal cord c.
condensation
amalgam c.
chromatin c.
filling material c.
gold foil c.
heavy c.
lateral c.
porcelain c.
pressure c.
resin c.
spatulation c.
vibration c.
warm c.
whipping c.
condenser point
condition
catabolic c.
concurrent medical c.
fibrocystic c.
gastrointestinal c.
genetic c.
medical systemic c.
predisposing c.
systemic c.
tumor-like bone c.
conditioning
interceptive c.
operant c.
c. program
semantic c.
c. therapy
conductance
skin c.
conduction
c. analgesia
c. anesthesia
compression bone c.
osteotympanic bone c.
conductivity
tissue c.
conduit
antirefluxing colonic c.
aortic c.
biliary c.
Bricker c.
colon c.
cutaneous appendiceal c.
ileal c.
ileocolic c.
intestinal c.
Koch c.
Mitrofanoff c.
Rastelli c.
respiratory syncytial virus c.
urinary c.
condylar
c. articulation
c. canal
c. emissary vein
c. femoral fracture
c. guidance inclination
c. hinge position
c. implant arthroplasty
c. process
c. process fracture
c. screw fixation
condylaris
condylarthrosis
condyle
c. cord
c. dissection
c. head
lateral c.
mandibular c.
medial c.
occipital c.
c. resection
condylectomy
DuVries plantar c.
mandibular c.
plantar c.
condylion
condylocephalic nail
condyloideum
condyloid process
condyloma, pl. **condylomata**
c. acuminatum

NOTES

condyloma *(continued)*
anal c.
cervical c.
flat c.
genital c.
giant c.
perianal c.
c. planus
pointed c.
vaginal c.
venereal c.
condylomatous
condylotomy
condylus
cone
c. biopsy
coned-down
c.-d. appearance of colon
c.-d. view
configuration
stellate c.
confirmation
histopathologic c.
intraoperative c.
tissue c.
confirmatory
c. axillary dissection
c. incision
confluence
hepatic venous c.
vein c.
venous c.
confluent inflammation
conformal radiation therapy
confrontation
c. method
c. testing
c. visual field test
congenital
c. above-elbow amputation
c. adrenal hyperplasia
c. aspiration pneumonia
c. below-elbow amputation
c. brain malformation
c. central hypoventilation syndrome
c. cerebral aneurysm
c. cervical instability
c. choledochal cyst
c. conotruncal anomaly
c. cystic adenomatoid malformation
c. cystic dilatation
c. depigmentation
c. diaphragmatic hernia (CDH)
c. diverticulum
c. duplication
c. esotropia
c. fracture
c. goiter
c. heart malformation
c. hip dislocation
c. HIV infection
c. instability
c. lens dislocation
c. lesion
c. nasal mass
c. postural deformity
c. pulmonary arteriovenous fistula
c. pyloric membrane
c. pyloric stenosis
c. renal mass
c. ring
c. ring syndrome
c. scapular elevation
c. splenomegaly
c. stippled epiphysis
c. tracheobiliary fistula
c. urethroperineal fistula
c. vascular malformation
congenitally altered anatomy
congestion
brain c.
flap c.
hepatic c.
sinusoidal c.
splanchnic c.
congestive
c. heart disease
c. heart failure
c. hepatomegaly
conglomerate mass
conglutinant
conglutination
congruent affect
coni (*pl. of* conus)
coniotomy
conization
cautery c.
cervical c.
cold c.
cold-knife c.
hot-knife c.
Hyam c.
laser cervical c.
LEEP c.
loop diathermy cervical c.
loop electrosurgical excision procedure c.
conjoined
c. anastomosis
c. nerve-root anomaly
c. tendon
conjoint tendon
conjugate
c. axis
c. foramen
c. point

conjugation bridge
conjunctiva, pl. **conjunctivae**
conjunctiva-associated lymphoid tissue
conjunctival
c. angioma
c. circulation
c. cul-de-sac
c. exudate
c. flap
c. fornix
c. hemorrhage
c. incision
c. injection
c. laceration
c. limbus
c. melanotic lesion
c. membrane
c. patch graft
c. ring
c. sac
conjunctiva-Müller muscle excision
conjunctiviplasty
conjunctivitis
conjunctivodacryocystorhinostomy
conjunctivodacryocystostomy
conjunctivoplasty
conjunctivorhinostomy
conjunctivo-Tenon flap
conjunctivus
Con-Lish polishing method
connecting cartilage
connection
atriopulmonary c.
connective
c. tissue
c. tissue activating peptide
c. tissue augmentation
c. tissue disease
c. tissue disorder
c. tissue graft
c. tissue massage
c. tissue membrane
c. tissue plasticity
Connell
C. incision
C. stitch
C. suture technique
Connolly
C. procedure
C. technique
Conn operation
conoid
c. process
c. tubercle
conotruncal anomaly
Conradi line
Conrad orbital blowout fracture operation
consciousness
conscious sedation
consecutive
c. amputation
c. aneurysm
c. dislocation
consent
informed c.
consequence
familial c.
psychologic c.
social c.
conservation
splenic c.
c. surgery
conservative
c. resection
c. surgery
c. surgical treatment
c. therapy
consideration
anesthetic c.
oncologic c.
technical c.
consolidation of lung
consonant-injection method
consonant position
consortial approach
constant
c. flow insufflation
c. vacuum
constipation
idiopathic c.
constitutive heterochromatin method
constrained
c. ankle arthroplasty
c. reconstruction
c. shoulder arthroplasty
constricting lesion
constriction
duodenopyloric c.
esophageal c.
pyloric c.
c. ring
constrictive pericarditis

NOTES

construct
AO dynamic compression plate c.
compression instrumentation posterior c.
double-rod c.
pedicle screw c.
segmental compression c.
TSRH double-rod c.
Wiltse system double-rod c.
Wiltse system H c.
Wiltse system single-rod c.
construction
Abbe vaginal c.
absolute c.
exocentric c.
ileal reservoir c.
ileostomy c.
loop ileostomy c.
McIndoe-Hayes c.
pelvic ileal reservoir c.
single denture c.
sphincteric c.
stent c.
tandem c.
Thiersch-Duplay urethral c.
U-pouch c.
vaginal c.
consumption
oxygen c.
peak exercise oxygen c.
splanchnic oxygen c.
contact
c. activation product
c. area point
c. dissolution therapy
c. illumination
c. laser ablation of prostate (CLAP)
C.Laser vaporization
c. manipulation
c. metastasis
c. method
contaminated operative wound classification
contamination
bacterial c.
fecal c.
gas c.
graft c.
gross fecal c.
hub c.
intraoperative c.
metastatic c.
postautoclave c.
content
abdominal c.
bile c.
bile-stained cyst c.
cyst c.
gastrointestinal c.
intestinal c.
luminal c.
mixed venous oxygen c.
platelet nucleotide c.
protein c.
tissue water c.
context-sensitive half-time
contiguity
solution of c.
contiguous loop
contiguum
per c.
continence
anal c.
short-term total c.
sphincteric c.
total c.
continent
c. colostomy
c. cutaneous appendicocystostomy
c. ileal pouch
c. ileostomy
c. urinary pouch
continua
continuity
bowel c.
digestive c.
gastrointestinal c.
gut c.
solution of c.
continuous
c. ambulatory peritoneal dialysis (CAPD)
c. arteriovenous hemofiltration (CAVH)
c. arteriovenous ultrafiltration
c. atrial fibrillation
c. bladder irrigation
c. catheter drainage
c. compression
c. distending airway pressure
c. endothelium
c. epidural anesthesia
c. gum technique
c. hyperthermic peritoneal perfusion
c. infusion anesthetic technique
c. intramucosal PCO_2 measurement
c. loop wiring
c. lumbar peridural anesthesia
c. mandatory ventilation
c. medical treatment
c. negative airway pressure
c. NG suction
c. on-line recording
c. positive airway pressure (CPAP)

c. positive pressure breathing (CPPB)
c. positive pressure ventilation (CPPV)
c. postoperative closed lavage
c. pull-through technique
c. renal replacement therapy
c. sanguineous perfusion
c. spinal anesthesia
c. spinal anesthetic technique
c. subcutaneous insulin injection
c. suture technique
c. venovenous hemodialysis (CVVHD)
c. venovenous hemofiltration

continuous-flow ventilation

continuous-wave
c.-w. laser ablation
c.-w. technique

continuum
per c.

contour
breast c.
corneal c.
intonation c.
c. line
lobulated c.
restoration c.
c. restoration
rounded c.

contoured
c. adduction trochanteric-controlled alignment method
c. anterior spinal plate technique

contouring
three-dimensional c.

contraangle

contraaperture

contraceptive
c. method
c. technique

contracted
c. kidney
c. pelvis

contractile
c. motility
c. ring
c. ring dysphagia

contractility

contraction
anal canal rhythmic c.
c. fasciculation
muscular c.
propagating clustered c. (PCC)
c. wave

contract-relax technique

contracture
Dupuytren c.
functional c.
Volkmann ischemic c.

contraindication

contralateral
c. axillary metastasis
c. carotid artery occlusion
c. groin exploration
c. ischemia
c. mobile cord
c. parathyroid gland
c. side
c. site
c. weakness

contralaterally

contrast
c. bath
blood oxygenation level-dependent c.
c. enema
c. injection
intravenous c.
IV c.
c. material
c. material instillation
c. medium
c. study
c. venography
c. visualization

contrast-enhanced
c.-e. computed tomography
c.-e. CT
c.-e. CT scan
c.-e. CT scanning

contrecoup
c. fracture

control
endoscopic c.
exsanguination tourniquet c.
extrahepatic c.
fluoroscopic c.
hemorrhage c.
inflow c.
intrahepatic c.
monitored anesthesia c.
outflow c.
Pringle vascular c.

NOTES

control *(continued)*
pronation c.
proximal vascular c.
tourniquet c.
transcriptional c.
vascular c.
c. of ventilation
x-ray c.
controlled
c. diaphragmatic respiration
c. expansion
c. fistula
c. heat-aided drug delivery (CHADD)
c. mechanical ventilation (CMV)
c. release anesthetic technique
c. release silver technology
c. rotational osteotomy
c. ventilation
c. water-added technique
control-mode ventilation
contusion
brain c.
corneal c.
myocardial c.
pulmonary c.
conus, pl. **coni**
convalescence
short-term c.
convenience
c. jaw relation
c. point
conventional
c. aortic aneurysmectomy
c. distal pancreatectomy
c. endarterectomy
c. method
c. operation
c. pancreatoduodenectomy
c. parameter
c. procedure
c. surgery
c. suturing
c. technique
c. thoracoplasty
convergence
c. facilitation
c. point
c. position
c. projection
convergent beam irradiation
converse
scalping flap of C.
conversion
above-knee amputation c.
extraglandular c.
pressure c.
converter
convex
c. condylar implant arthroplasty
c. fusion
c. nail
convexoconcave
convoluted
c. seminiferous tubule
convulsion
ether c.
convulsive therapy
Conyers technique
cooled-knife method
cooling
active core c.
external c.
passive tissue c.
topical c.
whole-body c.
Coomassie brilliant blue technique
Coonrad-Morrey total elbow arthroplasty
Coonrad total elbow arthroplasty
Coonse-Adams
C.-A. knee approach
C.-A. technique
Cooper
C. fascia
C. hernia
C. ligament
C. operation
C. reduction
C. syndrome
cooperation
cellular c.
coordination
hand-eye c.
co-oximetry
COP
colloid osmotic pressure
Cope
C. method
C. technique
Copeland
C. retinoscopy
C. technique
Copeland-Howard scapulothoracic fusion
coping
C. Strategies Questionnaire (CSQ)
C. with Health, Injuries, and Problems (CHIP)
C. with Health, Injuries, and Problems scale
copious
c. irrigation
c. peritoneal lavage
copper sulfate method
copper-wire
c.-w. arteriole

c.-w. artery
c.-w. reflex
coproporphyria
hereditary c.
copula
copular point
copulating pouch
coracoacromiale
coracoacromial ligament
coracobrachial
c. bursa
c. muscle
coracobrachialis
c. muscle
coracoclavicular
c. articulation
c. ligament
c. screw fixation
c. space
c. suture fixation
c. technique
coracoclaviculare
coracohumerale
coracohumeral ligament
coracoid
c. fracture
c. process
coracoideus
coral calculus
Corbin technique
cord
anterior c.
c. compression
condyle c.
contralateral mobile c.
false vocal c.
Ferrein c.
gangliated c.
genital c.
germinal c.
gonadal c.
lateral c.
nephrogenic c.
oblique c.
c. paralysis
presentation of c.
rete c.
spermatic c.
spinal c.
c. structure
tendinous c.
testicular c.
testis c.
c. traction syndrome
true vocal c.
umbilical c.
vocal c.
Weitbrecht c.
Willis c.
cordate pelvis
cordectomy
cordis
cordopexy
cordotomy
anterolateral c.
dorsal c.
open surgical c.
percutaneous c.
posterior column c.
spinothalamic c.
stereotactic c.
core
central fibroelastic c.
c. drilling procedure
c. hypothermia
c. needle biopsy
c. vitrectomy
corectomy
coreoplasty
corepexy
Cori classification
corium, pl. **coria**
corkscrew
c. appearance
c. maneuver
corn
hard c.
soft c.
web c.
cornea, pl. **corneae**
anterior c.
c. guttate lesion
corneal
c. abrasion
c. abscess
c. abscission
c. alkali burn
c. anesthesia
c. apex
c. arcus
c. astigmatism
c. blood staining
c. cap
c. cleft

NOTES

corneal *(continued)*
c. contour
c. contusion
c. curvature
c. dendrite
c. diameter
c. distortion
c. dystrophy
c. ectasia
c. edema
c. endothelium
c. epithelium
c. erosion
c. erysiphake
c. facet
c. filament
c. fissure
c. fistula
c. flap
c. foreign body
c. full-thickness
c. graft operation
c. graft step
c. guttering
c. incision
c. inlay
c. iron line
c. laceration
c. lamella
c. lamellar groove
c. leakage
c. lens
c. light reflex
c. limbus
c. luster
c. marginal furrow
c. meridian
c. mushroom
c. nebula
c. neovascularization
c. nerve
c. perforation
c. protrusion
c. punctate lesion
c. reflection
c. scarring
c. spot
c. staining test
c. stria
c. substance
c. surgery
c. thinning
c. tissue
c. transplant
c. transplantation
c. trauma
c. trepanation
c. ulceration
c. velum

corneoscleral
c. incision
c. laceration

corner
caudal c.
cephalad c.
c. fracture

corniculate
c. cartilage
c. process
c. tubercle

corniculum laryngis

cornification disorder

Corning method

cornu, pl. **cornua**
coccygeal cornua
cornua of hyoid bone
c. of hyoid bone
sacral cornua
styloid c.

cornual anastomosis

cornucopia
sinusoidal endothelium c.

corona, pl. **coronae**

coronal
c. angulation
c. oblique projection
c. plane
c. plane correction
c. plane deformity
c. plane deformity sagittal translation
c. pulp tissue
c. reconstruction
c. section
c. split fracture
c. suture

coronalis

coronarii

coronarius

coronary
c. angioplasty versus excisional atherectomy
c. artery angioplasty
c. artery anomaly
c. artery bypass
c. artery bypass graft (CABG)
c. artery disease
c. artery dissection
c. artery ectasia
c. artery fistula (CAF)
c. artery revascularization procedure
c. artery-right ventricular fistula
c. artery surgery study (CASS)
c. balloon angioplasty
c. bifurcation

c. bypass procedure
c. collateral circulation
c. endarterectomy
c. flow reserve technique
c. node
c. perfusion pressure
c. plexus
c. revascularization
c. ring
c. rotational ablation
c. rotational atherectomy
c. sinus catheterization
c. sinus perfusion system
c. sulcus
c. syndrome
c. thrombolysis
c. vein
c. venous pressure
c. vessel anatomy

coronoid
c. line
c. process
c. process fracture

coronoidectomy
coronoideus
coronoradicular stabilization
coroplasty
coroscopy
corotomy
corpectomy
anterior c.
cervical c.
median c.
c. model
vertebral body c.

corpora (*pl. of* corpus)
corporal biopsy
corporeal
c. aspiration
c. reconstruction
c. rotation procedure
c. sacrospinous suspension

corporectomy amputation
corporis
corporoplasty
incisional c.
modified Essed-Schroeder c.

corporotomy
corpus, pl. **corpora**
c. callosotomy
c. carcinoma
c. epididymis
c. luteum cyst
c. luteum hematoma

Correa classification
corrected sternal position
correction
adaptive c.
Allen c.
Alliston GE reflux c.
anterior c.
anteroposterior c.
aphakic c.
astigmatism c.
attenuation c.
Beckenbaugh c.
Bonferroni c.
Byron Smith lazy-T c.
cephalometric c.
chevron hallux valgus c.
coincidence c.
coronal plane c.
cubitus varus c.
dioptric c.
epicanthal c.
frontal plane c.
hallux varus c.
heparinase c.
Johnson-Spiegl hallux varus c.
King type IV curve posterior c.
Küstner uterine inversion c.
kyphosis c.
occlusal c.
oligosegmental c.
operative c.
optical c.
phalangeal malunion c.
protamine c.
rotational c.
Ruiz-Mora c.
scatter c.
scoliosis c.
secondary ptosis c.
skeletal c.
spectacle c.
speech c.
Steel c.
surgical c.
Tukey post-hoc c.
with c.
without c.
Yates c.

corrective therapy

NOTES

correlation
canonical c.
clinical c.
clinicopathologic c.
negative c.
positive c.
semilinear canonical c.
c. time
correlational method
Correra line
corresponding point
corridor
c. incision
c. procedure
Corrigan respiration
corrosion preparation
corrugator
c. cutis muscle
c. supercilii muscle
corset suspension
cortex, pl. **cortices**
adrenal c.
anterior c.
aspiration of c.
association c.
cingulate c.
ovarian c.
renal c.
suprarenal c.
vertebral body anterior c.
Corti
C. organ
cortical
c. activation
c. arch of kidney
c. area
c. artery
c. atrophy
c. biopsy
c. bone
c. bone graft
c. bone primary canal
c. destruction
c. dysplasia
c. fracture
c. fragment
c. hamartoma
c. implantation
c. incision
c. lateralization
c. lesion
c. mass
c. perforation
c. respiration
c. stimulation
c. strut graft
c. substance
c. tuber
corticalis
corticalosteotomy
corticectomy
cortices (*pl. of* cortex)
corticoadenoma
corticobulbar tract
corticocancellous bone graft
corticoid injection
corticomedullary demarcation
corticopontine tract
corticospinal
c. axon
c. tract
corticosteroid
depot c.
corticotomy
DeBastiani c.
percutaneous c.
cortisol-producing carcinoma
Cortrosyn stimulation test
Cosgrove mitral valve replacement
cosmesis
cosmetic
c. evaluation
c. outcome
c. problem
c. result
c. score
c. surgery
costa, pl. **costae**
costal
c. angle
c. cartilage
c. facet
c. groove
c. margin
c. notch
c. pit
c. pleura
c. process
c. respiration
c. surface
c. tuberosity
costale
costalis
costarum
costectomy
cost-effective alternative
Costen syndrome
costicartilage
costiform
costoaxillary vein
costocentral
costocervical
c. artery
c. trunk
costocervicalis

costochondral
c. articulation
c. joint
c. junction
costochondralis
costoclavicular
c. ligament
c. line
c. maneuver
c. space
costoclaviculare
costocolic ligament
costocoracoid
costodiaphragmatic recess
costodiaphragmaticus
costoinferior
costomediastinal
c. recess
c. sinus
costomediastinalis
costophrenic septal line
costoscapular
costoscapularis
costosternal
costosternoplasty
costosuperior
costotomy
costotransversaria
costotransversarium
costotransverse
c. foramen
c. joint
c. ligament
costotransversectomy
Seddon dorsal spine c.
c. technique
costoversion thoracoplasty
costovertebrales
costovertebral joint
costoxiphoideum
costoxiphoid ligament
cotransplantation
Cotrel-Dubousset fixation
Cotte
C. operation
C. presacral neurectomy
Cotting toenail operation
cotton
c. ankle fracture
c. cartilage graft
c. reduction
cottonloader position
cotton-wool
c.-w. exudate
c.-w. patch
c.-w. separation
cotunnii
Cotunnius
C. aqueduct
C. canal
C. space
cotyle
cotylica
cotyloid
c. cavity
c. joint
c. ligament
cotyloideum
cough
compression c.
c. CPR technique
extrapulmonary c.
c. fracture
coughing
expulsive c.
cough-pressure transmission ratio
Couinaud
C. classification
C. nomenclature
coulometric titration
coumadinization
Councilman lesion
Counsellor-Davis artificial vagina operation
Counsellor-Flor modification of McIndoe technique
count
blood cell c.
ex vivo c.
posttetanic c.
counterbalance
counterclockwise
c. direction
c. rotation
countercurrent
c. extraction
c. heat exchanger
c. mechanism
counterincision
counterirritation
counteropening
counterpulsation
balloon c.
enhanced external c.

NOTES

counterpulsation *(continued)*
intraaortic balloon c.
intraarterial c.
percutaneous intraaortic balloon c.
counterpuncture
countersinking osteotomy
countersink screw head
counterstimulation
countertraction
coup injury
coupling head
course
chronic c.
intrahepatic c.
postoperative c.
Courvoisier
C. gastroenterostomy
C. incision
Couvelaire
C. ileourethral anastomosis
C. incision
Coventry
C. distal femoral osteotomy
C. vagal osteotomy
cove plane
Cowen-Loftus toe-phalanx transplantation
cow face
cowl muscle
Cowper
C. gland
C. ligament
COX-2
cyclooxygenase enzyme
COX-2 inhibitor
coxa, pl. **coxae**
coxal bone
coxale
Cox Maze III procedure
coxofemoral articulation
coxsackievirus A, B virus
Cozen-Brockway
C.-B. technique
C.-B. Z-plasty
CPAP
continuous positive airway pressure
CPB
cardiopulmonary bypass
CPH
chronic paroxysmal hemicrania
C-plasty
CPPB
continuous positive pressure breathing
CPPV
continuous positive pressure ventilation
CPR
cardiopulmonary resuscitation
simultaneous compression-ventilation CPR
CPS
cumulative pain score
CPSP
central poststroke pain
CPT
cold pressor test
current perception threshold
Cracchiolo
C. forefoot arthroplasty
C. procedure
Cragg endoluminal graft
Craigie tube method
cramp
abdominal c.
Crampton
C. line
C. test
crania (*pl. of* cranium)
craniad
cranial
c. base
c. bone
c. canal
c. cavity
c. duplication
c. epidural space
c. extension
c. fontanelle
c. fracture
c. index
c. insufflation
c. irradiation
c. nerve
c. nerve dissection
c. nerve (I–XII)
c. nerve manipulation
c. nerve rhizotomy
c. osteopetrosis
c. osteosynthesis
c. pin
c. suture
c. vault
c. venous sinus
craniales
cranialis
craniamphitomy
craniectomy
endoscopic strip c.
keyhole-shaped c.
linear c.
partial-thickness c.
retromastoid suboccipital c.
cranii
cranio-aural
craniocele
craniocerebral

craniofacial
c. anomaly
c. axis
c. deformity
c. fixation
c. malformation
c. notch
c. osteotomy
c. reconstruction
c. reconstructive surgery
c. resection
c. suspension wiring
craniomeningocele
craniometric point
cranio-orbital surgery
craniopathy
craniopharyngeal
c. canal
c. duct
craniopharyngioma
ectopic c.
cranioplasty
aluminum c.
metallic c.
tantalum c.
craniopuncture
craniorrhachidian
craniosacral outflow
cranioscopy
craniosinus fistula
craniospinal
c. irradiation
c. space
craniosynostosis
craniotomy
attached c.
awake c.
bifrontal c.
c. defect
detached c.
endoscopic frontal c.
frontal c.
frontotemporal c.
left frontal c. (LFC)
open stereotactic c.
osteoplastic c.
pterional c.
right temporoparietal c.
stereotactic c.
supratentorial c.
Yasargil c.
craniotonoscopy
craniotrypesis
craniotympanic
cranium, pl. **crania**
crash technique
crassum
crater formation
Crawford
C. graft inclusion technique
C. incision
C. method
C. sling operation
Crawford-Adams cup arthroplasty
Crawford-Marxen-Osterfeld technique
craze line
CRBSI
CRC
colorectal cancer
CRC resection
sporadic CRC
CRE
cardiorespiratory endurance
crease
digital flexion c.
flexion c.
inframammary c.
midline abdominal c.
palmar c.
skin c.
torso c.
c. wound
creation
kyphosis c.
lordosis c.
McIndoe vaginal c.
Politano-Leadbetter tunnel c.
tunnel c.
Credé
C. maneuver
C. method
Creech
C. aortoiliac graft
C. technique
creeping fat
Crego
C. femoral osteotomy
C. tendon transfer technique
cremasteric
c. fascia
c. muscle
c. reflex
c. vein
cremasterica

C

NOTES

cremaster muscle
crena, pl. **crenae**
Creola body
crescent
articular c.
c. body
c. corneal graft
glomerular c.
c. mastopexy
c. operation
sublingual c.
crescentic
c. calcaneal osteotomy
c. rupture
Crespo operation
crest
articular c.
buccinator c.
conchal c.
deltoid c.
endoalveolar c.
ethmoidal c.
external occipital c.
falciform c.
frontal c.
iliac c.
infratemporal c.
inguinal c.
intermediate sacral c.
internal occipital c.
interosseous c.
intertrochanteric c.
lacrimal c.
nasal c.
obturator c.
pubic c.
sacral c.
supinator c.
supraventricular c.
terminal c.
tibial c.
trochanteric c.
urethral c. of male
vestibular c.
CRF
chronic renal failure
Cribier method
cribriform
c. area
c. carcinoma
c. fascia
c. plate
status c.
c. subtype
cribrosa
cribrous lamina
cribrum, pl. **cribra**
cricoarytenoid
c. ligament
c. muscle
cricoarytenoideus
cricoesophageal tendon
cricohyoidepiglottopexy
cricoid
c. cartilage
c. myotomy
c. pressure
c. pressure anesthetic technique
c. ring
stenotic c.
c. yoke
cricoidea
cricoideae
cricomyotomy
cricopharyngeal
c. dilatation
c. myotomy
cricopharyngeus muscle
cricothyroid
c. artery
c. articular capsule
c. articulation
c. joint
c. ligament
c. membrane
c. muscle
cricothyroidea
cricothyroidei
cricothyroideum
cricothyroideus
cricothyroidotomy
cricotracheal
c. ligament
c. membrane
c. resection
cricotracheale
cricotracheotomy
cricovocal membrane
Crile-Matas operation
Crippa lead tetraacetate method
crisscrossing abdominal wall incisions
Critchett operation
criterion, pl. **criteria**
AMES criteria
Dawson criteria
Harvard criteria
MACIS criteria
observer-dependent criteria
organ failure criteria
Ranson pancreatitis criteria
standard organ failure criteria
critical
c. care anesthesiology
c. care medicine (CCM)
c. closing pressure

c. illumination
c. mass
CRN
cerebral radiation necrosis
CRNA
certified registered nurse anesthetist
Crock encircling operation
Croften classification
Crohn disease
Cronkhite-Canada syndrome
CROP
compliance, rate, oxygenation, and pressure
Crosby
C. capsule
C. reduction
Crosby-Kugler
C.-K. biopsy capsule
C.-K. capsule for biopsy
cross
c. flap
c. infection
c. section
cross-arch fulcrum line
crossarm flap
crossbar
c. stomach deformity
cross-bracing, crossbracing
cross-clamping, crossclamping
aortic c.-c.
infrarenal aortic c.-c.
thoracic aortic c.-c. (TACC)
cross-consonant injection method
crossed
c. anesthesia
c. extension reflex
c. extensor reflex
c. fixation
c. pyramidal tract
cross-facial, crossfacial
c.-f. nerve graft
c.-f. nerve graft anastomosis
c.-f. technique
cross-finger flap
crosshatch incision
cross-leg flap
crosslink plate size
cross-lip
c.-l. flap
c.-l. pedicle flap
cross-modality matching
crossover
femorofemoral c.
FF c.
c. toe deformity
crosspin
cross-polarization photography
crossreact
crossreactivity
cross-section
capture c.-s.
c.-s. technique
cross-sectional
c.-s. method
c.-s. projection
cross-table lateral projection
cross-tolerance
cross-trigonal repair
cross-tunneling incision
cross-vector A scan
crotaphion
crotaphytico-buccinatorius
croup
postextubation c.
croupous
c. inflammation
c. membrane
Crouzon
C. disease
C. syndrome
Crowe
C. classification
C. pilot point
crowfoot closure
crowing inspiration
crown
c. fracture
c. inclination
c. restoration
C. suture technique
crown-contouring method
crown-root fracture
Crozat therapy
CRPF
closed reduction and percutaneous fixation
CRPS
complex regional pain syndrome
crucial
c. anastomosis
c. incision
cruciate
c. anastomosis

NOTES

C

cruciate *(continued)*
- c. eminence
- c. four-strand suture
- c. incision
- c. ligament reconstruction
- c. muscle

cruciatus
cruciform
- c. eminence
- c. ligament
- c. suture technique

crunch-stick anastomosis
cruor
crura (*pl. of* crus)
crural
- c. arch
- c. area
- c. canal
- c. closure
- c. fascia
- c. fossa
- c. hernia
- c. repair
- c. ring
- c. septum
- c. sheath

cruralis
cruris
crurotomy
crus, pl. **crura**
- ampullary crura
- anterior c.
- lateral c.
- medial c.
- c. muscle
- posterior c.

crush
- c. fracture
- c. injury
- c. preparation
- c. syndrome

crushed
- c. eggshell fracture
- c. tissue

crushing
- c. anastomosis
- oval-shaped c.
- c. technique

crusotomy
Crutchfield reduction technique
Cruveilhier
- C. fascia
- C. fossa
- C. plexus
- C. ulcer

Cruveilhier-Baumgarten anomaly
cryoablation
- encircling c.
- laparoscopically guided c.

cryoanalgesia
cryoanesthesia
cryoapplication
cryo-assisted resection
cryocautery
cryocoagulation
cryoconization
cryoelectron microscopy
cryoextraction operation
cryogenic ablation
cryohypophysectomy
Cryolife Single Step dilution method
cryolysis
cryopallidectomy
cryopexy
- barrage c.
- double freeze-stalk c.
- double freeze-thaw c.

cryopreserved
- c. aortic homograft
- c. extrapelvic ovarian transplantation
- c. heart-valve allograft
- c. tissue banking

cryoprostatectomy
cryopulvinectomy
cryoretinopexy
cryoscopy
cryostat
- c. section
- c. tissue

cryosurgery
cryosurgical
- c. ablation
- c. technique

cryothalamectomy
cryotherapy operation
crypt
- c. abscess
- anal c.
- c. atrophy
- enamel c.
- c. epithelium
- ileal c.
- Lieberkühn c.
- Morgagni c.
- tonsillar c.

crypta, pl. **cryptae**
cryptectomy
cryptococcal infection
Cryptococcus **infection**
cryptogenic infection
cryptorchidectomy
cryptorchidopexy
cryptorchid testis

cryptorchism
cryptosporidial infection
crystalline lens equator
crystallized trypsin
crystalloid
c. cardioplegic solution
Reinke c.
Csapody orbital repair operation
CSEA
combined spinal-epidural anesthesia
C-section
cesarean section
lower uterine segment transverse C-section
LUST C-section
CSF
cerebrospinal fluid
blood-tinged CSF
CSF pressure
CSFP
cerebrospinal fluid pressure
C-shaped
C-s. canal
C-s. scalp flap
CSQ
Coping Strategies Questionnaire
CT
computed tomography
appendiceal CT
contrast-enhanced CT
helical CT
CT portography
CT scan
CT scan-guided needle aspiration
CT scanning
CT volumetry
4C-T
four-chamber transverse
4C-T image
5C-T
five-chamber transverse
5C-T image
CTAP
computed tomography arterial portography
CTD
chest tube drainage
mediastinal CTD
CT-directed needle aspiration
CT-guided
CT-g. fine-needle aspiration
CT-g. liver biopsy
CT-g. needle-aspiration biopsy
CT-g. selective drainage
CT-g. stereotactic evacuation
CTL
cytolytic T-cell
CTL immunity
CTL immunity against melanoma
CTL-inducing peptide antigen
CTO
chest tube output
CTSI
computed tomography severity index
Cubbins
C. arthroplasty
C. incision
C. open reduction
C. shoulder approach
C. shoulder dislocation technique
cubitales
cubitus, pl. **cubiti**
c. valgus deformity
c. varus correction
cuboid bone
cuboidei
cuboideum
CUC
chronic ulcerative colitis
cue exposure
cuff
c. abscess
aortic c.
denuded rectal c.
distal vein c.
gastric c.
c. malfunction
musculotendinous c.
rectal muscle c.
c. resection
rotator c.
suprahepatic c.
c. suspension
c. tear arthropathy
c. tear arthroplasty
vaginal c.
vein c.
Cuignet method
cuirasse
carcinoma en c.
cuirass ventilation
cular subvalvular aortic stenosis
Culcher-Sussman technique

NOTES

cul-de-sac
c.-d.-s. of Bruger
conjunctival c.-d.-s.
c.-d.-s. of Douglas
c.-d.-s. fluid
glaucomatous c.-d.-s.
greater c.-d.-s.
Gruber c.-d.-s.
lesser c.-d.-s.
c.-d.-s. mass
ocular c.-d.-s.
ophthalmic c.-d.-s.
optic c.-d.-s.
rectouterine c.-d.-s.
culdoplasty
Halban c.
Marion-Moschcowitz c.
McCall c.
culdoscopy
culdotomy
culprit
c. lesion
c. lesion angioplasty
Culp spiral flap pyeloplasty
culture
colony c.
fibroblast c.
c. medium
cultured epithelial autograft
culturing technique
cumarin necrosis
Cummer classification
cumulative
c. operative morbidity
c. operative mortality
c. pain score (CPS)
c. score
c. trauma disorder
cuneatus
cuneiform
c. bone
c. cartilage
c. osteotomy
c. tubercle
cuneiforme
cuneocerebellar tract
cuneonavicular
cunnus
cup
c. arthroplasty
c. insemination
optic c.
cup-and-ball osteotomy
cup-and-cone method
cup-cement interface
cup-patch technique
Cupper-Faden operation
Cüppers method of pleoptics
Cupper suture technique
cuprophane membrane
cup-to-disc ratio
cupula, pl. **cupulae**
pleural c.
cupular blind sac
cupulolithiasis
curability
curage
curare
curarization
curative
c. intent
c. potential
c. procedure
c. radical total gastrectomy
c. resection
c. sphincter-saving operation
curative-intent
c.-i. operation
c.-i. procedure
c.-i. surgery
curb tenotomy
curettage
dilatation and c. (D&C)
dilation and c. (D&C)
endocervical c. (ECC)
endometrial c.
fractional dilation and c.
periapical c.
soft-tissue c.
suction c.
curettement
curioscopy
curlicue ureter
currant jelly clot
current
amplitude-summation interferential c.
demarcation c.
Limoge c.
membrane c.
c. perception threshold (CPT)
saturation c.
curse
Ondine c.
Curth-Maklin cornification disorder
Curtin
C. incision
C. plantar fibromatosis excision
Curtis
C. PIP joint capsulotomy
C. technique
Curtis-Fisher knee technique
curvatura, pl. **curvaturae**
curvature
c. aberration
anterior corneal c.
canal c.

corneal c.
greater c.
lesser c.
curve
accommodation c.
area under c. (AUC)
articulation c.
calibration c.
carbon dioxide dissociation c.
discrimination c.
displacement c.
dissociation c.
dose-effect c.
dose-response c.
elimination c.
hemoglobin-oxygen dissociation c.
indicator-dilution c.
intracardiac pressure c.
load-deflection c.
load-deformation c.
load-displacement c.
oxygen dissociation c.
oxygen-hemoglobin dissociation c.
oxyhemoglobin dissociation c.
pressure-natriuresis c.
pressure-volume c.
strength-duration c.
survival c.
time-concentration c.
Traube-Hering c.
whole-body titration c.
curved
c. approach
c. canal
c. end-to-end anastomosis
c. flank position
c. incision
c. radiolucent line
curved-needle surgeon knot
curvilinear incision
Cushieri maneuver
Cushing
C. operation
C. pressure response
C. reflex
C. suture technique
cushioning suture technique
Cusick operation
Cusick-Sarrail ptosis operation
cusp
c. fenestration
c. plane
c. restoration
valve c.
cusp-fossa relation
cuspid
cuspid-molar position
Custodis nondraining procedure
cut
c. end
c. point
sector c.
semilunate c.
c. surface
cutaneobiliary fistula
cutaneomucosal
cutaneomucosus
cutaneomucous muscle
cutaneomucouveal syndrome
cutaneous
c. appendiceal conduit
c. bacterial infection
c. burn injury
c. cervical nerve
c. collateral circulation
c. forearm flap
c. gangrene
c. gland
c. graft-versus-host disease
c. graft-versus-host reaction
c. heat loss
c. hemorrhoid
c. ileocystostomy
c. innervation
c. lesion
c. loop ureterostomy
c. malformation
c. manifestation
c. melanoma
c. metastasis
c. metastatic breast carcinoma
c. muscle
c. suture technique
c. tissue
c. vesicostomy
c. viral infection
cutaneus
cutback anoplasty
cutback-type vaginoplasty
cutdown
c. access
c. incision
c. technique
venous c.

C

NOTES

cuticular
c. membrane
c. stitch
c. suture technique
cuticularization
cutin
cutis
c. graft
Cutler-Beard
C.-B. bridge flap
C.-B. operation
Cutler-Ederer method
Cutler operation
cutoff
anesthetic c.
cutting
circle straight c.
c. needle biopsy
section c.
ultrasonic c.
Cuvier
canal of C.
CVAS
Colored Visual Analogue Scale
CVP
central venous pressure
intraoperative CVP
CVP line
CVVHD
continuous venovenous hemodialysis
cyanoacrylate retinopexy
cyanogen bromide method
cyanosis
compression c.
shunt c.
cyanotic induration
cyclarthrodial
cyclarthrosis
cyclectomy
cyclic
c. fasting motility
c. pain
c. respiration
c. vertigo
cyclicotomy
cyclitic membrane
cyclocryopexy
cyclodestructive procedure
cyclodiathermy operation
cycloelectrolysis
cyclooxygenase enzyme (COX-2)
cyclophotocoagulation
Nd:YAG c.
transpupillary c.
cyclopropane
cyclops
C. formation
C. procedure
cycloscopy
cyclotomy
cylicotomy
cylinder
hilar c.
c. retinoscopy
cylindrical
c. carcinoma
c. confronting cisterna
c. osteotomy
cylindroadenoma
cylindroid aneurysm
cylindroma
cylindromatous lesion
cylindrosarcoma
cyma line
cyst
air c.
amebic c.
anterior c.
arachnoid c.
c. aspiration
Baker c.
benign liver c.
benign subcutaneous c.
blue dome breast c.
brachial cleft c.
branchial c.
branchiogenous c.
breast c.
chocolate c.
choledochal c.
chyle c.
colloid c.
compound c.
congenital choledochal c.
c. content
corpus luteum c.
daughter c.
dermoid c.
double unilateral c.'s
duplication c.
echinococcal liver c.
echinococcus c.
enteric c.
enterogenous c.
epidermal inclusion c.
epidermoid c.
epithelial c.
c. fenestration
follicular c.
ganglion c.
gastric duplication c.
granddaughter c.
hepatic parasitic c.
hydatic liver c.
hydatid c.
hyperplastic c.

intraluminal c.
involution c.
laryngeal c.
mesenteric c.
milk-filled c.
mother c.
multilocular c.
myoid c.
nabothian c.
old posterior c.
omental c.
ovarian dermoid c.
pancreatic c.
parasitic c.
pilonidal c.
posterior c.
preauricular c.
primordial c.
Rathke pouch c.
renal c.
residual c.
retention c.
sacrococcygeal c.
Sampson c.
sebaceous c.
splenic c.
sublingual c.
theca-lutein c.
thymic c.
thyroglossal duct c.
Tornwaldt c.
unilocular c.
vitellointestinal c.
c. wall
wolffian c.
young c.

cystadenocarcinoma
bile duct c.
mucinous c.
papillary c.
pseudomucinous c.
serous c.

cystadenofibroma

cystadenoma
ductal c.
hyperplastic c.
thyroid c.

cystauchenotomy

cystectomy
Bartholin c.
ovarian c.
partial c.
pilonidal c.
radical c.
salvage c.
total c.
vulvovaginal c.

cysteic acid method

cystenterostomy
direct c.
endoscopic c.

cystgastrostomy
endoscopic c.
surgical c.

cystic
c. acute inflammation
c. adenocarcinoma
c. adenomatoid malformation (CAM)
c. artery
c. bone lesion
c. cavity
c. chronic inflammation
c. dilatation
c. dilation
c. duct
c. duct catheterization
c. duct choledochoscopy
c. duct-infundibulum junction
c. duct stump leak
c. granulomatous inflammation
c. hidradenoma
c. kidney
c. kidney disease
c. lymphoepithelial AIDS-related lesion
c. mass
c. medial necrosis
c. metastasis
c. node
c. polyp
c. puncture
c. structure

cystica

cysticercal infection

cystici

cysticolithectomy

cysticolithotripsy

cysticorrhaphy

cysticotomy

cysticus

cystides (*pl. of* cystis)

cystidoceliotomy

cystidolaparotomy

NOTES

cystidotrachelotomy
cystine calculus
cystis, pl. **cystides**
cystitis
interstitial c.
schistosomal c.
cystoadenoma
cystocarcinoma
cystocele repair
cystochromoscopy
cystocolostomy
cystodiaphanoscopy
cystoduodenal ligament
cystoduodenostomy
endoscopic c.
pancreatic c.
cystoenterocele
cystoenterostomy
cystoepithelioma
cystofibroma
cystogastric fistula
cystogastrostomy
endoscopic c.
cystography
cystoid body
cystojejunostomy
Roux-en-Y c.
cystolateral pancreatojejunostomy
cystolith
cystolithectomy
cystolithiasis
cystolithic
cystolitholapaxy
cystolithotomy
cystolysis
cystoma
cystometrography
cystometry
cystopanendoscopy
cystopericystectomy
cystopexy
cystoplasty
augmentation c.
Gil-Vernet ileocecal c.
human lyophilized dura c.
ileocecal c.
nonsecretory sigmoid c.
sigmoid c.
cystoproctostomy
cystoprostatectomy
cystoprostatourethrectomy
cystoprostatovesiculectomy
cystorectostomy
cystorrhaphy
cystosarcoma phyllode
cystoscopic electrohydraulic lithotripsy
cystoscopy
percutaneous fetal c.
steerable c.
virtual c.
cystostomy
trocar c.
cystotomy
suprapubic c.
cystotrachelotomy
cystourethrocele
cystourethrography
cystourethropexy
obturator shelf c.
Pereyra-Raz c.
vaginal c.
cystourethroplasty
Kropp c.
Leadbetter c.
cystourethroscopy
dynamic c.
cytobrush biopsy
cytochrome
myocardial c.
cytoid body
cytokeratin immunostain
cytokine
inflammatory c.
c. network
c. receptor inhibitor
cytologic
c. abnormality
c. biopsy
c. diagnosis
c. evaluation
c. examination
c. feature
c. result
c. specimen
c. study
c. washing
cytological assessment
cytology
abnormal c.
aspiration biopsy c.
brush c.
endometrial c.
endoscopic brush c.
endoscopic fine-needle aspiration c.
endoscopic ultrasonography-guided c.
equivocal pancreatic c.
EUS-guided c.
c. examination
exfoliative c.
fine-needle aspiration c.
gastric c.
guided-needle aspiration c.
intraoperative touch prep c.
needle aspiration c.
negative c.

negative peritoneal c. (NPC)
nipple aspiration c.
oral cavity c.
peritoneal c.
positive c.
positive peritoneal c. (PPC)
salvage c.
c. sample
c. specimen
cytolytic T-cell (CTL)
cytomegalovirus (CMV)
c. colitis
c. infection
c. prophylaxis
cytomegalovirus-positive donor
cytoplasm
cytoplasmic membrane
cytopreparation
cytoreductive surgery
cytospin collection fluid
cytotoxicity
Czermak pterygium operation
Czerny
C. operation
C. suture technique
Czerny-Lembert suture technique

NOTES

D
D chromosome ring syndrome
D line
D point
D2
D2 dissection
D2 lymphadenectomy
D2 resection
DAC
deep abdominal complication
dacryoadenectomy operation
dacryocyst
dacryocystectomy operation
dacryocystocele
dacryocystoethmoidostomy
dacryocystorhinostomy
dacryocystorhinotomy operation
dacryocystostomy operation
dacryon
dacryorhinocystostomy
dacryorhinocystotomy
dacryostenosis
dacryostomy
Arroyo d.
Arruga d.
Dupuy-Dutemps d.
Kuhnt d.
Rowinski d.
dactylomegaly
dactyloscopy
dacuronium
Dagradi esophageal variceal classification
Dahlman diverticulum excision
Dailey operation
Daines-Hodgson anastomosis
Dakin-Carrel treatment
Dale-Laidlaw clotting time method
Dalgleish operation
Dallas operation
damage
anterior cervical surgery vocal cord d.
cellular d.
end-organ d.
endothelial d.
irradiation d.
liver d.
nervous d.
obturator nerve d.
postsurgical nervous d.
projection fiber d.
radiation d.
soft-tissue d.
subretinal d.
sun and chemical combination d.
damaged parenchyma
Damian graft procedure
Damus-Kaye-Stansel (DKS)
D.-K.-S. operation
D.-K.-S. procedure
Damus-Stansel-Kaye procedure
DANA
designed after natural anatomy
Dana
D. operation
D. posterior rhizotomy
Dana-Farber Cancer Institute
Dandy
D. maneuver
D. myocutaneous scalp flap
D. operation
Dandy-Walker
D.-W. deformity
D.-W. malformation
D.-W. syndrome
Dane method
Danforth fetal operation
Dangel slip knot
danger space
Daniel iliac bone graft
Danielson method
Danis-Weber
D.-W. ankle injury classification
D.-W. fracture
Danus-Fontan procedure
Danus-Stanzel repair
Dardik umbilical graft
DA receptor
dark-field
d.-f. examination
d.-f. illumination
d.-f. microscopy
dark-ground illumination
Darling capsulotomy
Darrach
D. procedure
D. resection
Darrach-McLaughlin shoulder technique
darting incision
dartos
d. fascia
d. muscle
d. pouch procedure
Das
D. Gupta procedure
D. Gupta scapular excision
D. Gupta scapulectomy

D

dashboard
d. dislocation
d. fracture
data
bacteriologic d.
clinicopathologic d.
followup d.
histopathologic d.
manometric d.
on-line d.
ultrasonographic d.
Datta procedure
datum plane
Daubenton
D. angle
D. line
D. plane
d'Aubigne
d. femoral reconstruction
d. resection reconstruction
daughter cyst
Davey-Rorabeck-Fowler decompression technique
Daviel operation
Davis
D. drainage technique
D. fusion
D. intubated ureterostomy
D. intubated ureterotomy
D. muscle-pedicle graft
Davis-Geck blepharoplasty
Davis-Kitlowski procedure
Davydov procedure
DAWG
demucosalized augmentation with gastric segment
DAWG procedure
Dawson criteria
day
d. care surgical unit (DCSU)
postoperative d. (POD)
posttransplant d.
day-case operation
DBP
diastolic blood pressure
D&C
dilatation and curettage
dilation and curettage
DCIS
ductal carcinoma in situ
focal DCIS
multifocal-extensive DCIS
residual DCIS
DCS
dorsal column stimulation
DCSU
day care surgical unit
DCT
deceleration time
D-D
duct-to-duct
D-D anastomosis
D-dimer
D&E
dilatation and evacuation
dilation and evacuation
de
de Grandmont operation
de Groot classification
de Lapersonne operation
de Mussy point
de novo lesion
de novo needle-knife technique
de Quervain fracture
de Quervain stenosing tenosynovitis release
de Quervain syndrome
de Quervain tenosynovitis
de Vincentiis operation
dead
d. space
d. space:tidal volume ratio
d. tract
deafferentation
d. pain
d. pain syndrome
de-airing procedure
Dean and Webb titration
dearterialization
hepatic d.
death
brain d.
cerebral d.
intraoperative d.
noncancer d.
perioperative d.
postoperative d.
trauma-related d.
tumor-related d.
vascular disease d.
Deaver incision
DeBakey
D. classification
D. graft
DeBakey-Creech aneurysm repair
DeBakey-type aortic dissection
DeBastiani corticotomy
Debeyre-Patte-Elmelik rotator cuff technique
debility
debouch
débouchement
Debove membrane
débridement
autolytic d.

burn d.
canal d.
cavity d.
diagnostic arthroscopy and d.
enzymatic d.
exploration and d.
operative d.
root canal d.
surgical d.
tangential d.

debris
cellular d.
valve d.

debt
oxygen d.

debubbling procedure

debulking
d. operation
ovarian carcinoma d.
d. procedure
d. surgery
surgical d.
d. of tumor

decalcification

decannulation

decapsulation

decayed, extracted, and filled

deceleration time (DCT)

decentration of contact lens

decerebration
bloodless d.

decerebrize

dechondrification

decidua

decidual membrane

deciduous

decimal reduction time

declamping
d. phenomenon
d. shock

declination angle

decompensated liver disease

decompensation
circulatory d.
hepatic d.
d. injury
vascular d.

decompress

decompression
anterior retroperitoneal d.
bone graft d.
cardiac d.
cerebral d.
d. colostomy
endoscopic biliary d.
extensive posterior d.
d. fasciotomy
gaseous d.
gastric d.
d. incision
internal d.
d. jejunostomy
d. laminectomy
microvascular d. (MVD)
nerve d.
orbital d.
paraclavicular thoracic outlet d.
pericardial d.
portal d.
posterior fossa d.
retroperitoneal d.
d. rhachotomy
Rowbotham orbital d.
selective portal d.
spinal d.
suboccipital d.
subtemporal d.
surgical portal d.
d. technique
transduodenal endoscopic d.
trigeminal d.
tube d.
variceal d.
vein d.
vertebral body d.

decompressive
d. laminectomy
d. surgery

deconditioned exercise response

decontamination
selective bowel d.

deconvolution

decortication
arterial d.
cerebral d.
laparoscopic cyst d.
renal cyst d.
reversible d.
d. technique

decrease
hypoxic ventilatory d.

decreased
d. afterload

D

NOTES

decreased *(continued)*
d. preload
d. respiration
decubital gangrene
decubitus
d. calculus
d. position
d. view
decussation
dorsal tegmental d.
Forel d.
fountain d.
Held d.
Meynert d.
motor d.
oculomotor d.
optic d.
pyramidal d.
rubrospinal d.
tectospinal d.
ventral tegmental d.
Wernekinck d.
dedolation
de-endothelialization
de-endothelialized
deep
d. abdominal complication (DAC)
d. anal sphincter
d. anterior neck
d. anterior wall
d. articular aorta
d. articulation test
d. auricular artery
d. brachial artery
d. cardiac plexus
d. cervical artery
d. cervical fascia
d. cervical vein
d. chest therapy
d. circumflex iliac artery-iliac crest flap
d. circumflex inguinal artery
d. crural arch
d. delayed infection
d. Doppler velocity interrogation
d. epigastric artery
d. femoral artery
d. forearm
d. hypothermia
d. hypothermic circulatory arrest (DHCA)
d. iliac dissection
d. infrapatellar bursa
d. inguinal ring
d. interloop abscess
d. lamina
d. liver tract
d. lymphatic vessel
d. orbit
d. palmar arch
d. palmar branch
d. penis
d. perineal pouch
d. perineal space
d. peroneal nerve
d. petrosal nerve
d. plantar branch
d. postanal anorectal space
d. profunda brachial artery
d. temporal artery
d. temporal nerve
d. tumor
d. vein thrombosis
d. venous thrombosis (DVT)
d. venous thrombosis prophylaxis
d. venous thrombus
d. wound infection
deep-gastric
d.-g. longitudinal (DG-L)
d.-g. transverse (DG-T)
de-epicardialization
de-epithelialization
de-epithelialized
d.-e. rectus abdominis muscle (DRAM)
d.-e. rectus abdominis muscle flap
deep-seated fungal infection
defalcated root canal
Defares rebreathing method
defecation
d. score
sense of d.
defect
aponeurotic d.
atrial septal d.
atrioventricular canal d.
atrioventricular septal d.
bandeau d.
chain-of-lakes filling d.
clinical d.
coagulation d.
cold d.
combined d.
craniotomy d.
dentinoenamel d.
diaphragmatic d.
direct d.
fascial d.
filling d.
frondlike filling d.
hernia d.
hot d.
iatrogenic hernia d.
indirect d.
mass d.
napkin-ring d.

neural tube d.
oromandibular d.
osteoarticular d.
osteochondral d.
parietal d.
perineal d.
peritoneal d.
pinpoint gastric mucosal d.
postinjury immunologic d.
postresection d.
Rastelli type A, B, C classification of atrioventricular septal d.
repairable parietal d.
septal d.
slitlike d.
surgical d.
tumor d.
ventilation d.
ventilation/perfusion d.
ventricular septal wound d.

defense

deferens

deferent
d. canal
d. duct

deferentectomy

deferential
d. artery
d. plexus

deferentialis

deferentis

deferred shock

defibrillation
cardiac d.
d. shock
d. threshold

deficiency
protein-C d.

deficit
base d. (BD)
neurologic d.
neuropsychological d.
normal base d.
transient neurologic d.

defined sterilization

definite cause

definitive
d. cause
d. local therapy
d. method
d. resection
d. stabilization
d. surgery
d. tracheostomy
d. treatment

deflation
targeted lobar d.

deformation

deformity
abduction d.
acetabular protrusio d.
acquired d.
adduction d.
adduction-internal rotation d.
adductovarus d.
Åkerlund d.
d. analysis
Andy Gump d.
angel-wing d.
d. angle
angular d.
angulation d.
Arnold-Chiari d.
back-knee d.
bell-clapper d.
bifid thumb d.
bird-beak d.
bony d.
boutonnière d.
bowing d.
bowleg d.
bulb d.
bunion d.
burn boutonnière d.
buttonhole d.
calcaneocavovarus d.
calcaneocavus d.
calcaneovalgus d.
calcaneovarus d.
cavovarus d.
cavus d.
cecal d.
cervical spine kyphotic d.
cervicomedullary d.
chain-of-lakes d.
checkrein d.
clasped thumb d.
clawfoot d.
clawhand d.
clawing d.
clawtoe d.
cleft hand d.
cleft lip d.
cloverleaf skull d.

NOTES

deformity *(continued)*

clubfoot d.
cock-up d.
codfish d.
combined cavus d.
compensatory d.
complete bilateral d.
congenital postural d.
coronal plane d.
craniofacial d.
crossbar stomach d.
crossover toe d.
cubitus valgus d.
Dandy-Walker d.
dentofacial d.
duodenal bulb d.
elevatus d.
equinovalgus d.
equinus d.
Erlenmeyer flask d.
eversion-external rotation d.
extension d.
facial d.
finger d.
fishtail d.
fixed d.
flat back d.
flexion d.
flexion-internal rotational d.
foot d.
funnel chest d.
garden spade d.
genu valgum d.
genu varum d.
gibbous d.
gingival d.
gooseneck d.
gross d.
Haglund d.
hallux valgus d.
hammertoe d.
hand d.
hatchet-head d.
Hill-Sachs d.
hindbrain d.
hindfoot d.
hip d.
hockey-stick d.
hook-nail d.
hourglass d.
humpback d.
hyperextension d.
internal rotation d.
intrinsic minus d.
intrinsic plus d.
joint d.
J-sella d.
keyhole d.
Kirner d.
kleeblatschädel d.
Klippel-Feil d.
knock-knee d.
kyphotic d.
lanceolate d.
limb d.
lobster-claw d.
lumbar spine kyphotic d.
Madelung d.
mallet finger d.
mallet toe d.
Michel d.
Mondini d.
nasal d.
one-plane d.
opera-glass d.
parachute d.
pectus carinatum d.
pectus excavatum d.
pencil-in-cup d.
penile d.
pes planus d.
phrygian cap d.
pigeon-breast d.
ping-pong ball d.
plantar flexion-inversion d.
posttraumatic spinal d.
postural d.
protrusio d.
pseudoboutonnière d.
rat-tail d.
recurvatum angulation d.
rotational d.
round back d.
round shoulder d.
sabre-shin d.
saddle-nose d.
sagittal d.
shepherd's crook d.
silver-fork d.
skeletal d.
spastic thumb-in-palm d.
spinal coronal plane d.
spine d.
spinning-top d.
splayfoot d.
splenic vein d.
split-hand d.
split-nail d.
spondylitic d.
Sprengel d.
S-shaped d.
subcondylar d.
supination d.
swan-neck finger d.
talipes cavus d.
thoracic spine kyphotic d.

thoracic spine scoliotic d.
three-plane d.
thumb d.
thumb-in-palm d.
trefoil d.
triphalangeal thumb d.
turned-up pulp d.
two-plane d.
ulnar deviation d.
ulnar drift d.
valgus d.
varus hindfoot d.
Velpeau d.
volar angulation d.
Volkmann clawhand d.
whistling d.
Whitehead d.
windblown d.
windsock d.
windswept d.
wrist d.
Zancolli procedure for clawhand d.
zig-zag compensatory d.
Z-type d.
deformity-instability
spinal d.-i.
DEFT
driven equilibrium Fourier transform
DEFT technique
defunctionalization
defunctioning loop ileostomy
Dega pelvic osteotomy
degasified distilled water
degenerated fibroadenolipoma
degenerating otoconia
degeneration
aberrant third nerve d.
age-related macular d.
malignant d.
degenerative
d. change
d. discogenic end-plate disease
d. encephalopathy
d. inflammation
d. mitral valve insufficiency
degloving procedure
degradation
intracellular protein d.
d. product
protein d.
degrade
degree of inspiration
dehiscence
abdominal incision d.
anastomotic d.
Roux limb stump d.
scar d.
staple line d.
stump d.
suture line d.
total d.
wound d.
dehiscent mandibular canal
dehydration fever
dehydrogenation
Deisting prostatic dilation technique
Deiter operation
deiterospinal tract
Deiters cell
Dejerine-Roussy syndrome
DeKlair operation
delay
fixation d.
d. line
delayed
d. complication
d. direct coloanal anastomosis
d. expansion
d. femoral osteotomy
d. flap
d. fracture union
d. gastric emptying
d. graft
d. hyperacute transplant rejection
d. onset muscle soreness (DOMS)
d. open reduction
d. pneumothorax
d. primary closure
d. primary repair
d. primary suture technique
d. resuscitation
d. urination
Delbet splint for heel fracture
DeLee
D. classification
D. maneuver
deletion
clonal d.
deliberate
d. hypotension (DH)
d. hypotension anesthetic technique
delimiting keratotomy
delineating

NOTES

D

delirium
emergence d.
delivery
buccal transmucosal d.
cesarean d.
closed-loop automated d.
controlled heat-aided drug d. (CHADD)
epidural d.
spinal d.
transmucosal d.
vacuum extractor d.
vaginal birth after cesarean d.
Dellepiane hysterectomy
Deller modification
Delorme
D. rectal prolapse operation
D. thoracoplasty
delta
portal d.
deltoid
d. branch
d. crest
d. eminence
d. flap
d. muscle
deltoidea
deltoideus
deltoid-splitting
d.-s. incision
d.-s. shoulder approach
deltopectoral
d. approach
d. fascia
d. flap
d. groove
d. incision
d. sulcus
Del Toro operation
deltoscapular flap
demand-adapted administration anesthetic technique
demand minimum functional capacity (DMFC)
demarcation
corticomedullary d.
d. current
d. potential
demineralization
bony d.
demonstration
angiographic d.
Demours membrane
demucosalized
d. a. w. g. s. augmentation with gastric segment (DAWG)
demyelinating lesion
demyelination
autoimmune d.
axonal d.
intramedullary d.
DeMyer system of cerebral malformation
dendriform
dendrite
corneal d.
dendritic
d. calculus
d. carcinoma
d. lesion
dendrocytoma
denervate
denervation
d. disease
extrinsic d.
d. hypersensitivity
Krause d.
law of d.
d. potential
preganglionic sympathetic d.
sinoaortic d.
dengue hemorrhagic fever infection
Denham external fixation
Denis
D. Browne spinal fracture classification
D. Browne urethroplasty technique
denitrogenation
Denker sinus operation
Dennie line
Dennie-Morgan line
Dennis-Brooke ileostomy
Dennis technique
Dennis-Varco pancreaticoduodenostomy
Denonvilliers
D. aponeurosis
D. fascia
D. ligament
dens
d. anterior screw fixation
d. fracture
pit of atlas for d.
densa
dense
d. adhesion
d. body
d. brain mass
d. nature
density
raspberry-like d.
vapor d.
density-dependent repair
dental
d. anatomy
d. anesthesia

d. anomaly
d. arch expansion
d. articulation
d. canal
d. cavity
d. fenestration
d. fistula
d. index
d. infection
d. nerve
d. polyp
d. prosthetic laboratory procedure
d. psychosedation
d. pulp extirpation
d. puncture
d. restoration
d. sac
d. sinus tract
d. surgery
d. trepanation
d. trephination
d. tubercle
d. wedge

dentate
d. fracture
d. line
d. margin
d. suture

dentatectomy
dentatothalamic tract
denticulate ligament
denticulatum
dentin
d. crystal alteration
d. pain

dentinal canal
dentinoenamel
d. defect
d. membrane

dentis
dentoalveolaris
dentoalveolar joint
dentofacial
d. anomaly
d. deformity
d. surgery

denture
d. classification
d. foundation
d. foundation area
d. foundation surface
d. space

denudation
endothelial d.
interdental d.

denuded
d. bowel
d. connective tissue
d. furcation
d. rectal cuff

Denver classification
Depage incision
Depage-Janeway
D.-J. gastrostomy
D.-J. gastrotomy

DePalma modified patellar technique
dependency
ventilator d.

dependent drainage
depigmentation
congenital d.

depigmented lesion
depilation
deplasmolysis
deployment
stent d.

depolarization block
depolarizing
d. block
d. relaxant

deposition
abdominal iron d.

depot corticosteroid
depressant
depressed
d. lesion
d. side
d. skull fracture
d. type

depression
d. fracture
Hamilton Rating Scale for D.
inspiratory rib cage d.
respiratory d.
twitch d.
ventilatory d.

deprivation amblyopia
depth
d. of anesthesia
d. of anesthesia monitoring
anesthetic d.
d. caliper-meter stick method
char-zone d.

NOTES

D

depth *(continued)*
d. of insertion (DOI)
d. pulse technique
derby hat fracture
Derby operation
derivation
derivative circulation
dermabrasion
dermal
d. fasciectomy
d. fat-free flap
d. fat-free tissue transfer
d. fat pedicle flap
d. fibroblast
d. graft
d. injection
d. lesion
d. loss
d. lymphatics
d. pouch
d. pouch reconstruction
d. route of injection
d. sinus tract
d. suture technique
dermatica
dermatoalloplasty
dermatoautoplasty
dermatocele
dermatofibroma
dermatofibrosarcoma
dermatoheteroplasty
dermatohomoplasty
dermatologic
d. disorder
d. problem
dermatolysis
dermatomal level of analgesia
dermatome
d. mapping
trigeminal d.
dermatomyoma
dermatophyte fungal infection
dermatoplasty
dermatoscopy
dermatosis
dermatoxenoplasty
dermis patch graft
dermodesis
resection d.
dermoid cyst
dermoidectomy
dermolipoma
dermolysis
dermoplasty
dermovascular
derotation
derotational osteotomy
DES
diffuse esophageal spasm
desaturation
arterial oxygen d.
jugular bulb oxyhemoglobin d.
oxygen d.
red d.
Desault wrist dislocation
Descemet
D. membrane
D. membrane detachment
descending
d. anterior branch
d. aortic aneurysm
d. artery of knee
d. colon
d. genicular artery
d. genicular vein
d. loop colostomy
d. mesocolon
d. nerve
d. palatine artery
d. posterior branch
d. scapular artery
d. technique
Descot fracture
Descriptor Differential Scale of Pain Intensity
desensitization with towel rubbing
desiccation
electrosurgical d.
mucous d.
designated blood donation
designed after natural anatomy (DANA)
Desjardins point
Desmarres operation
desmocytoma
desmoid lesion
desmoplastic
d. medulloblastoma
d. trichilemmoma
desmopressin
desmotomy
destruction
bone d.
bony element d.
bony necrosis and d.
Cawthorne d.
cortical d.
moth-eaten bone d.
mucosal d.
progressive parenchymal d.
destructive
d. bone lesion
d. interference technique
desyndactylization
Weinstock d.

detached
d. cranial section
d. craniotomy
detachment
Descemet membrane d.
exudative retinal d.
traction d.
detection
pancreatic fungal d.
d. threshold
detector response
deterioration
aortic wall d.
clinical d.
determinant
prognostic d.
detritus
tissue d.
detrusor
d. areflexia
d. instability
d. muscle
d. pressure
d. stability
devascularization
gastric d.
paraesophagogastric d.
devascularized parathyroid remnant
DeVega tricuspid valve annuloplasty
development
discontinuation-emergent symptom d.
pouch d.
sternal d.
developmental
d. coordination disorder
d. landmark
d. line
d. retardation
Deventer pelvis
Devereux-Reichek method
Deverle fixation
deviant articulation
deviated septum
deviation to the right
device therapy
Devine
D. antral exclusion
D. colostomy
D. hypospadias repair
Devine-Devine procedure
devitalization
pulp d.
devitalized
d. bone graft
d. tissue
devolvulization
endoscopic d.
Devonshire
D. colic
D. technique
Dewar
D. posterior cervical fixation procedure
D. posterior cervical fusion
D. posterior cervical fusion technique
Dewar-Barrington
D.-B. arthroplasty
D.-B. clavicular dislocation technique
Dewar-Harris shoulder technique
DeWecker
D. anterior sclerotomy
D. operation
dewy appearance
dexter
Dexter-Grossman classification
dextra
dextrae
dextri
dextrocardia
dextrogyration
dextromethorphan
dextrorotation
dextrotorsion
dextroversion
dextrum
Deyerle femoral fracture technique
DFI
disease-free interval
DFS
disease-free survival
DG-L
deep-gastric longitudinal
DG-L image
DG-T
deep-gastric transverse
DG-T image
DH
deliberate hypotension
DHCA
deep hypothermic circulatory arrest

NOTES

diabetes mellitus
diabetic
d. coma
d. complication
d. gangrene
d. ketoacidosis
d. patient
d. pseudotabes
d. puncture
d. retinal treatment
d. retinopathy
diacele
diacetylcholine
diacondylar fracture
diagnosis, pl. **diagnoses**
anatomic d.
clinical d.
colposcopic d.
cytologic d.
frozen section d.
genetic d.
histologic d.
histopathologic d.
microscopic d.
noninvasive d.
nonoperative d.
operative d.
pathologic d.
postoperative d.
preoperative d.
presumptive d.
surgical d.
diagnostic
d. accuracy
d. anesthesia
d. arthroscopy and débridement
d. arthroscopy, operative arthroscopy, and possible operative arthrotomy
d. articulation test
d. biopsy
d. cardiac catheterization
d. colonoscopy
d. dilemma
d. fiberoptic stomatoscopy
d. finding
d. IGBB
d. imaging evaluation
d. investigation
d. laparoscopy
d. modality
d. and operative arthroscopy
d. peritoneal lavage (DPL)
d. procedure
d. program
d. radiation
d. small bowel series
d. step
d. study
d. surgical therapy
d. technique
d. tube
d. value
d. workup
diagonal section
dial
d. pelvic osteotomy
d. periacetabular osteotomy
dialysate preparation module
dialysis
d. access surgery
arteriovenous d.
d. clinic
continuous ambulatory peritoneal d. (CAPD)
d. disequilibrium syndrome
d. encephalopathy syndrome
extracorporeal d.
d. fistula
inpatient d.
maintenance d.
outpatient d.
peritoneal d.
postoperative d.
d. treatment
dialysis-dependent patient
dialytic ultrafiltration
dialyzer membrane
diameter
biparietal d. (BPD)
corneal d.
end-diastolic d. (EDD)
end-systolic d. (ESD)
maximal rectal d.
rectal d.
diametric pelvic fracture
diamond
D. classification
d. ejection murmur
d. inlay bone graft
Diamond-Gould
D.-G. reduction syndactyly
D.-G. syndactyly operation
diamond-shaped incision
Dianoux operation
diaphragm
bare area d.
central tendon d.
d. eventration
d. injury
d. laceration
laryngeal d.
pelvic d.
d. perforation

sternal part of d.
urogenital d.
diaphragma, pl. **diaphragmata**
diaphragmatic
d. crural repair
d. defect
d. elevation
d. eventration
d. hernia
d. herniation
d. injury
d. laceration
d. node
d. pleura
d. reflection
d. respiration
d. rupture
d. surface
diaphragmatica
diaphragmatic-abdominal respiration
diaphragmatis
diaphysial, diaphyseal
d. fracture
d. osteotomy
diaphysis, pl. **diaphyses**
femoral d.
diarthric
diarthrodial
d. cartilage
d. joint
diarthrosis
diarticular
Dias-Giegerich
D.-G. fracture technique
D.-G. open reduction
Dias-Tachdijian physical injury classification
diastasis
ankle mortise d.
d. fibula
iris d.
palpable rib d.
pubic d.
rectus d.
sutural d.
tibiofibular d.
diastatic skull fracture
diastolic
d. blood pressure (DBP)
d. filling pressure
d. hypertension
d. pressure-time index
d. pressure-volume relation
d. relaxation
d. suction
diathermic
d. fistulotomy
d. loop biopsy
d. resection
d. therapy
diathermocoagulation
diathermy
coagulating d.
d. dissection
electrocoagulation d.
d. hemorrhoidectomy
medical d.
d. operation
d. puncture
short wave d.
surgical d.
diazo staining method
Dibbell cleft lip-nasal reconstruction
DIC
disseminated intravascular coagulation
dichotomization
dichotomous classification
dichotomy
Dickey-Fox operation
Dickey operation
Dickhaut-DeLee
D.-D. classification of discoid meniscus
D.-D. discoid meniscus classification
Dickinson
D. approach
D. calcaneal bursitis technique
Dickinson-Coutts-Woodward-Handler osteotomy
Dick method
Dickson
D. geometric osteotomy
D. transplant technique
Dickson-Diveley procedure
Dickson-Wright operation
dicondylar fracture
Didiee projection
Diebold-Bejjani osteotomy
Dieffenbach
D. method
D. operation
Dieffenbach-Duplay hypospadias technique

NOTES

die punch fracture
dieresis
dieretic
diet
advance to regular d.
clear liquid d.
Dieterle method
Dieulafoy
D. lesion
D. vascular malformation
D. vascular malformation of the stomach
Dieulafoy-like lesion
difference
alveolar-arterial pressure d.
alveolar end-capillary d.
field-echo d.
morphological d.
differential
d. blood pressure
d. force technique
d. nerve block
d. relaxation
d. spinal anesthesia
d. spinal block
d. spinal block anesthetic technique
d. ureteral catheterization test
differentiated thyroid carcinoma
differentiation failure
difficult ventilation
diffuse
d. abdominal pain
d. abdominal tenderness
d. abscess
d. acute inflammation
d. air space disease
d. aneurysm
d. breast involvement
d. carcinomatosis
d. change
d. chronic inflammation
d. colloid goiter
d. esophageal spasm (DES)
d. fatty infiltration
d. fibroma
d. fibromus
d. fusiform dilatation
d. GI hamartoma polyp
d. hemorrhagic pancreatitis
d. idiopathic skeletal hyperostosis (DISH)
d. illumination
d. intravascular coagulation
d. lobular fibrosis
d. lymphatic tissue
d. metastasis
d. microcalcification
d. microvascular thrombosis
d. mucosal polyposis
d. multinodular goiter
d. necrosis
d. papillomatosis
d. peritonitis
d. plane
d. pulmonary alveolar hemorrhage
d. reflection
d. toxic non-nodular goiter
d. transmural ganglioneuromatosis
d. tumor
d. ulceration
d. ulcerative lesion
d. variety
d. vasculitis
diffusely tender abdomen
diffusion
d. anoxia
exchange d.
d. hypoxia
d. respiration
d. root canal filling method
digastric
d. branch
d. fossa
d. groove
d. line
d. muscle
d. muscle flap
d. space
d. triangle
digastrica
digastrici
digastricus
digestive
d. apparatus
d. bleeding
d. continuity
d. glandular cancer
d. manifestation
d. system
d. system vascular disease
d. tract
d. tract malignancy
d. tube
digestorium
digestorius
digit
digital
d. artery protection
d. beam attenuation
d. block anesthesia
d. collateral artery
d. dilation
d. divulsion
d. extensor mechanism
d. extensor tendon
d. flap

d. flexion crease
d. furrow
d. imaging colposcopy
d. mammography
d. manipulation
d. nail
d. pad
d. pressure
d. pulp
d. rectal evacuation
d. rectal examination
d. retinacular ligament
d. subtraction technique
d. vein

digitalization
digitally-guided biopsy
digitatae
digitate impression
digitation
digiti (*pl. of* digitus)
digitization
digitonin method
digitorum
Digit Symbol Substitution Test
digitus, pl. **digiti**
dilacerated canal
dilaceration

sharp d.

dilatable lesion
dilatation

aneurysmal d.
balloon d.
bile duct d.
blind d.
cardiac d.
congenital cystic d.
cricopharyngeal d.
d. and curettage (D&C)
cystic d.
diffuse fusiform d.
ductal d.
endoscopic retrograde balloon d.
esophageal d.
d. and evacuation (D&E)
ex vacuo d.
fusiform d.
gaseous d.
homatropine d.
junctional d.
pancreatic duct d.
percutaneous stricture d. (PSD)
periportal sinusoidal d.
pneumatic d.
poststenotic d.
pouch d.
prestenotic d.
pupillary d.
secondary arrest of d.
segmental d.
transurethral balloon d.
Virchow-Robin space d.

dilatator
dilated loop of bowel
dilating window
dilation

achalasia balloon d.
anal d.
aneurysmal d.
balloon d.
biliary d.
bootstrap d.
bowel d.
Brown-McHardy pneumatic mercury bougie d.
capillary d.
cardiac d.
catheter d.
cervical d.
colonic d.
d. and curettage (D&C)
cystic d.
digital d.
ductal d.
ectatic d.
Eder-Puestow d.
endoscopic papillary balloon d.
episcleral vascular d.
esophageal d.
d. and evacuation (D&E)
extrahepatic biliary cystic d.
finger d.
Frank technique of d.
gastric d.
Grüntzig balloon d.
hepatic web d.
hydrostatic balloon d.
idiopathic d.
inadequate d.
intrahepatic biliary cystic d.
intrahepatic ductal d.
junctional d.
lag d.
d. lag
mechanical ureteral d.

NOTES

dilation *(continued)*
medical d.
mucosal vascular d.
percutaneous balloon d.
periportal sinusoidal d.
peroral esophageal d.
pneumatic bag esophageal d.
pneumatic balloon catheter d.
pneumostatic d.
postoperative ductal d.
poststenotic d.
progressive d.
pupil d.
pyloric d.
reactive d.
rectal d.
serial d.
submucosal vascular d.
d. therapy
through-the-scope balloon d.
tract d.
transurethral balloon d.
TTS balloon d.
urethral d.
Uromat d.
ventricular d.
Wirsung d.

dilator
d. muscle
d. placement
d. placement failure

dilator-and-sheath technique

dilemma
diagnostic d.

Dillwyn-Evans
D.-E. osteotomy
D.-E. resection

dilution
tracer d.

dilution-filtration technique

dimensions

Dimon-Hughston
D.-H. fracture fixation
D.-H. intertrochanteric osteotomy
D.-H. technique

dimorphism
gender d.

dimple
celiac d.
coccygeal d.

dioiodine ablation

dioptric
d. aberration
d. correction

dioxide
arterial carbon d.
carbon d. (CO_2)
end-tidal carbon d.
partial pressure of arterial carbon d. ($PaCO_2$)
partial pressure of carbon d. (PCO_2)
partial pressure of intramuscular carbon d. ($PiCO_2$)
partial pressure of mesenteric venous carbon d. ($PmvCO_2$)

DIP
distal interphalangeal
DIP fusion

diphtheritic membrane

diploë

diploic
d. artery
d. canal
d. vein

diploici

dipole-dipole
d.-d. relaxation
d.-d. relaxation rate

Diprivan technique

direct
d. acrylic restoration
d. brain stimulation
d. cardiac puncture
d. cautery puncture
d. cholecystoenterostomy
d. closure
d. composite resin restoration
d. compression
d. current electrocoagulation
d. cystenterostomy
d. defect
d. electrical nerve stimulation
d. embolectomy
d. flap
d. fluoroscopic visualization
d. Fourier transformation imaging
d. fracture
d. gold restoration
d. histologic investigation
d. illumination
d. inguinal hernia
d. insertion technique
d. intraperitoneal insemination
d. laparoscopic vision
d. laryngoscopy
d. ligation
d. manipulation
d. mechanical ventricular actuation
d. method
d. method for making inlays
d. muscle lysis
d. needle puncture
d. neural stimulation
d. obturator nerve block
d. ophthalmoscopy

d. pressure
d. pyramidal tract
d. resin restoration
d. respiration
d. SSPCS
d. suturing
d. thrombin inhibitor
d. transfusion

direct-current shock ablation
direct/indirect technique
direction
anterograde d.
caudal d.
cephalad d.
clockwise d.
counterclockwise d.
flow d.
line of d.
pelvic d.
phase-encoding d.
principal visual d.
retrograde d.
visual d.
Z d.

directional coronary atherectomy
direct-vision
d.-v. internal urethrotomy
d.-v. liver biopsy

dirty
d. operative wound classification
d. surgery

disarticular amputation
disarticulation
Batch-Spittler-McFaddin knee d.
Boyd hip d.
Burger technique for scapulothoracic d.
elbow d.
hip d.
joint d.
Lisfranc d.
Mazet d.
metatarsophalangeal joint d.
sacroiliac d.
shoulder d.
wrist d.

disassociation
disc (*var. of* disk)
discectomy (*var. of* diskectomy)
discharge
breast d.
pathologic breast d.
physiologic breast d.
same-day d.

disci (*pl. of* discus)
discission
disclosing solution
discoid skin lesion
disconnection syndrome
disconnect wedge
discontinuation-emergent symptom development
discontinuous
d. endothelium
d. neck dissection
d. sterilization

discotomy
discrete
d. bleeding source
d. lesion
d. mass
d. stenosis
d. tumor

discrimination
d. curve
d. loss
d. score

discus, pl. **disci**
disease
abdominal hydatid d.
Abrami d.
acute graft-versus-host d.
adaptation d.
adhesive d.
adult familial hyaline membrane d.
advanced d.
air space d.
amyloid oral cavity d.
aneurysmal d.
antiglomerular basement membrane antibody d.
aortic aneurysmal d.
aortic arch d.
aortic atheromatous d.
aortic occlusive d. (AOD)
aortic valve d.
aortoiliac occlusive d.
Arbuthnot Lane d.
arterial occlusive d.
atherosclerotic heart d.
autosomal dominant polycystic kidney d.
Behçet d.
benign inflammatory d.

NOTES

disease *(continued)*
Berger d.
biliary tract d.
bilobar d.
bone d.
Bright d.
Budd-Chiari syndrome with Behçet d.
Budd-Chiari syndrome without Behçet d.
calcium pyrophosphate deposition d.
carcinoid valve d.
cardiovascular d.
carotid artery d.
cement d.
central core d. (CCD)
central nervous system d.
cerebrovascular d.
choledochal cyst d.
chronic graft-versus-host d.
chronic liver d.
colorectal d.
combined system d.
complex aortic d.
complicated diverticular d.
congestive heart d.
connective tissue d.
coronary artery d.
Crohn d.
Crouzon d.
cutaneous graft-versus-host d.
cystic kidney d.
decompensated liver d.
degenerative discogenic end-plate d.
denervation d.
diffuse air space d.
digestive system vascular d.
distant nodal d.
diverticular d.
early-onset graft-versus-host d.
echinococcal cyst d.
Economo d.
elevator d.
endogenous d.
endomyocardial d.
end-stage renal d. (ESRD)
eosinophilic endomyocardial d.
eventration d.
exanthematous d.
exogenous d.
exophytic joint d.
extensive-stage d.
extraabdominal d.
extracapsular d.
extracranial carotid artery d.
extracranial carotid occlusive d.
extracranial occlusive vascular d.
extrahepatic nodal d.
extramammary Paget d.
extranodal d.
extraorbital d.
extrapyramidal d.
exudative papulosquamous d.
eye d.
familial multigland d.
femoropopliteal occlusive d.
fibrocystic d.
Fournier d.
fracture d.
gallstone d.
gastroesophageal reflux d. (GERD)
glomerular basement membrane d.
graft-versus-host d.
gross cystic d.
hard metal d.
hard pad d.
hepatic venous web d.
heritable connective tissue d.
Hirschsprung d.
humeroperoneal neuromuscular d.
Huntington d.
hyaline membrane d.
hydatid d.
hyperacute graft-versus-host d.
idiopathic eczematous d.
idiopathic peptic ulcer d.
inclusion body d.
inflammatory bowel d.
intraabdominal d.
in-transit d.
intraperitoneal endometrial metastatic d.
intrathoracic d.
irresectable d.
ischemic aortic d.
ischemic heart d.
Jackson and Parker classification of Hodgkin d.
Killip classification of heart d.
Lafora body d.
late-onset d.
late-stage d.
Leri-Weill d.
lichenoid graft-versus-host d.
liver d.
localization of d.
locally advanced d.
lower extremity occlusive d.
lung d.
lupus-associated valve d.
lysosomal storage d.
M_0 d.
malignant pancreatic d.
Marion d.
Ménière d.
mesenteric nodal d.

metastatic d.
microcystic d.
micrometastatic peritoneal d.
microscopic d.
minimal-change d.
mixed connective-tissue d.
Mondor d.
multifocal-extensive d.
multigland d.
multiglandular d.
multilevel atherosclerotic arterial occlusive d.
multiple hydatid d.
neurologic d.
nil d.
nodal d.
node-negative d.
node-positive d.
noncirrhotic metabolic liver d.
nonfamilial multiglandular d.
nonmalignant d.
occlusive carotid artery d.
occlusive coronary artery d.
occult extrahepatic d.
occult hepatic d.
occult irresectable d.
occult systemic d.
omental nodal d.
Ormond d.
osteoarthritis d.
Paget extramammary d.
pancreatic d.
Parkinson d.
pelvic adhesive d.
peptic ulcer d.
periodontal d.
peripheral arterial aneurysmal d.
peripheral vascular d.
peritoneal d.
Peyronie d.
polycystic kidney d. (PKD)
popliteal artery occlusive d. (PAOD)
posttransplant lymphoproliferative d. (PTLD)
preeclamptic liver d.
Preiser d.
progressive d.
pulmonary valve d.
radiation-induced d.
radiation lung d.
Recklinghausen d. type I
d. recurrence rate
recurrent thromboembolic d.
Reiter d.
renal artery occlusive d.
renal artery stenotic d.
renal vascular d.
resectable hepatic d.
residual d.
sclerodermoid graft-versus-host d.
short-segment d.
single hydatid d.
sinonasal d.
sixth venereal d.
small bowel diverticular d.
space-occupying d.
sporadic multigland d.
d. stage
Steinert d.
stenotic d.
surgical pancreatic d.
systemic d.
Takayasu d.
thin basement membrane d.
thoracic aortic d.
thromboembolic d.
thrombotic d.
tricuspid valve d.
unanticipated hepatic d.
undifferentiated connective tissue d.
unilobar d.
unresectable extrahepatic d.
upper tract d.
urinary tract d.
valvular aortic d.
valvular heart d.
van Buren d.
vascular d.
vasculo-Behçet d.
venous stasis d.
venous web d.
vertebral artery d.
vibration d.
von Economo d.
von Hippel-Lindau d.
Winiwarter-Buerger d.

disease-associated mortality

disease-free

d.-f. interval (DFI)
d.-f. patient
d.-f. survival (DFS)

disease-related complication

NOTES

DISH
diffuse idiopathic skeletal hyperostosis
DISH syndrome
dish face
dishpan fracture
disinfecting solution
disinfection
chemical d.
high-level d.
root canal d.
spray-wipe-spray d.
surface d.
thermal d.
disintegration
endoscopic stone d.
d. rate
disinvagination
disjoined pyeloplasty
disk, disc
acromioclavicular d.
articular d.
d. compression
d. diffusion method
d. drusen hemorrhage
d. excision
extruded d.
d. extrusion
d. fragment
free fragment d.
herniated d.
d. herniation
intercalated d.
interpubic d.
intervertebral d.
d. lesion
mandibular d.
d. neovascularization
optic d.
d. oxygenation
d. plication
d. pressure
protruded d.
ruptured d.
sacrococcygeal d.
d. sensitivity method
d. space
d. space infection
d. space narrowing
d. space saline acceptance test
sternoclavicular d.
temporomandibular articular d.
diskectomy, discectomy
anterior d.
automated percutaneous d.
cervical d.
Cloward fusion d.
laminotomy and d.
lumbar d.
microlumbar d.
microsurgical d.
partial d.
percutaneous lumbar d.
Robinson anterior cervical d.
Smith-Robinson anterior cervical d.
thoracic d.
thoracoscopic d.
transthoracic d.
Williams d.
diskography
provocative d.
dislocation
acromioclavicular joint d.
antenatal d.
anterior complete d.
anterior hip d.
anterior-inferior d.
anterior shoulder d.
anterolateral d.
atlantoaxial d.
atlantooccipital joint d.
atypical d.
Bankart shoulder d.
bayonet d.
Bell-Dally cervical d.
Bennett d.
bilateral interfacetal d.
bilateral intrafacetal d.
boutonnière hand d.
bursting d.
carpometacarpal joint d.
central d.
Chopart ankle d.
closed d.
complete anterior d.
complete inferior d.
complete posterior d.
complete superior d.
compound d.
congenital hip d.
congenital lens d.
consecutive d.
d. contour abnormality
dashboard d.
Desault wrist d.
divergent elbow d.
dorsal perilunate d.
dorsal transscaphoid perilunar d.
dysplasia d.
elbow d.
facet d.
d. fracture
fracture d.
frank d.
gamekeeper thumb d.
glenohumeral joint d.
habitual d.

Hill-Sachs shoulder d.
hip d.
incomplete d.
inferior complete closed d.
inferior complete compound d.
interphalangeal joint d.
intraocular lens d.
isolated d.
Kienböck d.
knee d.
lens d.
Lisfranc d.
lumbosacral d.
lunate d.
luxatio erecta shoulder d.
mandibular d.
metatarsophalangeal joint d.
midcarpal d.
milkmaid elbow d.
Monteggia d.
Nélaton ankle d.
occipitoatlantal d.
Otto pelvis d.
Palmer transscaphoid perilunar d.
panclavicular d.
parachute jumper d.
partial d.
patellar intraarticular d.
pathologic d.
perilunar transscaphoid d.
perilunate carpal d.
peroneal d.
phalangeal d.
posterior hip d.
posterior shoulder d.
posteromedial d.
prenatal d.
primitive d.
proximal tibiofibular joint d.
radial head d.
radiocarpal d.
recent d.
recurrent patellar d.
retrosternal d.
rotational d.
sacroiliac d.
scapholunate d.
shoulder d.
Smith d.
spontaneous hyperemic d.
sternoclavicular joint d.
subastragalar d.
subcoracoid shoulder d.
subglenoid shoulder d.
subtalar d.
superior d.
swivel d.
talar d.
tarsal d.
tarsometatarsal d.
temporomandibular joint d.
teratologic d.
tibialis posterior d.
tibiofibular joint d.
transscaphoid perilunate d.
traumatic atlantooccipital d.
triquetrolunate d.
unilateral interfacetal d.
unilateral intrafacetal d.
unreduced d.
volar semilunar wrist d.
wrist d.

dismembered
d. anastomosis
d. pyeloplasty
d. reimplanted appendicocystostomy

disobliteration

disorder
accommodation d.
acquired cornification d.
anorectal d.
arterial d.
articulation d.
autoimmune connective tissue d.
benign esophageal d.
bipolar affective d. (BAD)
blood coagulation d.
cartilaginous growth plate d.
chronic multisystem d.
coagulation d.
coagulopathic d.
colorectal d.
complex adrenal endocrine d.
complex gonadal endocrine d.
complex pituitary endocrine d.
complex thyroid endocrine d.
connective tissue d.
cornification d.
cumulative trauma d.
Curth-Maklin cornification d.
dermatologic d.
developmental coordination d.
ejaculation d.
elimination d.

NOTES

disorder *(continued)*
endocrine d.
endonasal d.
esophageal d.
evacuation d.
experimental d.
gamma loop d.
gonadal endocrine d.
gynecologic d.
hematologic d.
immune-mediated coagulation d.
intestinal ischemic d.
keratitis-deafness cornification d.
lymphoproliferative d.
lysosomal enzyme d.
mastication d.
metabolic d.
mitral valve d.
mixed connective tissue d.
movement d.
multisystem d.
musculoskeletal d.
nail d.
neurologic d.
ocular motility d.
organic articulation d.
pituitary endocrine d.
posttransplant lymphoproliferative d. (PTLD)
posttraumatic stress d.
somatization d.
thrombogenic d.
thyroid endocrine d.
unilateral hemidysplasia cornification d.
urinary tract d.
disparate point
displaced fracture
displacement
d. analysis
anterior d.
d. curve
d. implantation
d. osteotomy
port d.
d. threshold
water d.
disproportion
cephalopelvic d.
disruption
wound d.
dissected tissue arm
dissecting
d. aneurysm
d. intramural hematoma
dissection
acute aortic d.
d. of aorta
aortic d.
arterial wall d.
axillary lymph node d. (ALND)
axillary node d.
balloon d.
bilateral neck d.
blunt and sharp d.
bone d.
bone-ligament d.
bony d.
capsular d.
carotid artery d.
cervical node d.
circumferential mucosal d.
complete axillary d.
complex d.
condyle d.
confirmatory axillary d.
coronary artery d.
cranial nerve d.
D2 d.
DeBakey-type aortic d.
deep iliac d.
diathermy d.
discontinuous neck d.
elective lymph node d. (ELND)
elective neck d.
en bloc d.
endoscopic d.
epiphenomena of d.
esophageal d.
extensive lymph node d.
extracapsular d.
extrahepatic d.
extraperitoneal endoscopic pelvic lymph node d.
field of d.
finger fracture d.
fingertip d.
flank d.
Freer d.
full axillary d.
functional lymph node d.
functional neck d.
gauze d.
groin d.
hard palate d.
hydraulic d.
incisural d.
inguinal canal d.
inguinal-femoral node d.
intracapsular d.
intradural d.
intramural air d.
intraparenchymal digital d.
jugular vein d.
laparoscopic pelvic lymph node d.
lateral cervical node d.

lateroaortic lymph node d.
limited obturator node d.
lymphatic d.
lymph node d.
d. margin
medial d.
mediastinal lymph node d.
mesoesophageal d.
modified radical neck d.
muscle d.
nasal d.
neck d.
nerve-sparing d.
node d.
Pack-Ehrlich deep iliac d.
para-aortic lymph node d.
parenchymal d.
parotid d.
partial zonal d.
pelvic lymph node d. (PLND)
pelvic node d.
periesophageal lymph node d.
perirectal pelvic d.
plane of d.
postradical neck d.
preadventitial d.
precise d.
radical axillary d.
radical lymph node d.
radical mediastinal d.
radical neck d.
retroperitoneal pelvic lymph node d. (RPLND)
scissors d.
selective inguinal node d.
sharp and blunt d.
in situ d.
soft-tissue d.
spiral d.
sponge d.
spontaneous coronary artery d.
Stanford type A, B aortic d.
Stanford-type aortic d.
subligamentous d.
submucosal d.
subperiosteal d.
subtemporal d.
suction d.
suprahyoid neck d.
supraomohyoid neck d.
sylvian d.
symptomatic traumatic d.
systemic d.
Taussig-Morton node d.
therapeutic d.
therapeutic lymph node d. (TLND)
thoracic aortic d.
three-field d.
tissue d.
tongue-jaw-neck d.
transthoracic d.
traumatic internal carotid artery d.
d. tubercle
two-field d.
two-team d.
ultrasonic d.
vertebral d.
water d.

disseminated
d. asymptomatic unilateral neovascularization
d. carcinoma
d. CMV infection
d. gonococcal infection
d. inflammation
d. intravascular coagulation (DIC)

dissemination
hematologic d.
intraperitoneal d.
neoplastic d.
peritoneal d.

Disse space

dissipation
circle d.

dissociable tetrameric hemoglobin

dissociated
d. anesthesia
d. position

dissociation
d., analgesia, immobility, and tension scale
atrial d.
atrioventricular d.
A-V d.
complete atrioventricular d.
complete A-V d.
d. curve
electromechanical d.
electromyocardial d.
hypnotic d.
incomplete atrioventricular d.
incomplete A-V d.
interference d.
intracavitary pressure-electrogram d.

D

NOTES

dissociation *(continued)*
isorhythmic d.
longitudinal d.
lunotriquetral d.
microbic d.
d. movement
radioulnar d.
scapholunate d.
scapulothoracic d.
sleep d.
syringomyelic d.
tabetic d.
dissociative anesthesia
distal
d. anastomosis
d. aortic perfusion
d. biceps brachii tendon rupture
d. bile duct
d. bleeding
d. catheter lengthening
d. cavity
d. centriole
d. clavicular excision
d. clot
d. ectasia
d. esophageal diverticulum
d. esophageal ring
d. esophagectomy
d. extension restoration
d. femoral epiphysial fracture
d. femoropopliteal bypass graft
d. fragment
d. gastrectomy
d. humeral epiphysis
d. humeral fracture
d. interphalangeal (DIP)
d. interphalangeal fusion
d. interphalangeal joint approach
d. laparoscopic pancreatectomy
d. ligation
d. limb
d. metaphysis
d. metastasis
d. nail matrix
d. nerve graft
d. neurolysis
d. pancreas
d. pancreatectomy (DP)
d. pancreaticojejunostomy
d. phalanx
d. portion
d. radial fracture
d. radioulnar joint stabilization
d. remnant
d. shave section
d. splenoadrenal shunting
d. splenorenal shunt (DSRS)
d. stump
d. tibiofibular fusion
d. tumor
d. ureterectomy
d. vein cuff
d. vertebral artery reconstruction
d. visceral perfusion
d. with excision of ulcer gastrectomy
distal-occlusal (DO)
distal-row carpectomy
distance
interincisor d.
skin-to-tumor d.
thyromental d.
tube-carina d.
tube-patient d.
tube-to-film d.
distant
d. flap
d. metastasis
d. nodal disease
d. recurrence
d. recurrence-free survival (DRFS)
distantial aberration
distended
d. abdomen
d. afferent loop
d. colon
d. gallbladder
distention
abdominal d.
bladder d.
cecal d.
colonic d.
gallbladder d.
gaseous d.
gastric d.
liver d.
postprandial d.
progressive abdominal d.
proximal bowel d.
rectal d.
vessel d.
distilled water
distoangular position
distobuccal line angle
distobuccoocclusal point angle
distolabial line angle
distolabioincisal point angle
distolingual line angle
distolinguoincisal point angle
distoocclusal point angle
distortion
d. aberration
corneal d.
pin-cushion d.
distraction
d. arthroplasty

d. of fracture
muscle d.
d. osteogenesis
d. technique

distraction/compression scoliosis treatment

distractive extension

distress
D. Risk Assessment Method (DRAM)
D. Scale for Ventilated Newborn Infants (DSVNI)

distribution
lesion d.
loop d.
pattern of d.
d. pattern
stocking-glove pain d.
ventilation/perfusion d.

disturbance
acid-base d.
chronic motor d.
hemodynamic d.
interdigestive motility d.
microcirculatory d.
motility d.
motor d.
postsurgical d.
sensitive visceral postsurgical d.
upper small bowel motor d.
visceral postsurgical d.

diuresis
balanced salt solution volume d.

diuretic therapy

diurnal
d. enuresis
d. intraocular pressure measurement

divergent
d. elbow dislocation
d. ray projection

diversion
Camey enterocystoplasty urinary d.
Duke pouch cutaneous urinary d.
fecal d.
Gil-Vernet ileocecal cystoplasty urinary d.
ileal conduit urinary d.
ileocolonic pouch urinary d.
Indiana continent reservoir urinary d.
Khafagy modified ileocecal cystoplasty urinary d.
Koch pouch cutaneous urinary d.
Laparostat with fiber d.
Mainz pouch cutaneous urinary d.
orthotopic urinary d.
simple d.
Studer reservoir urinary d.
temporary fecal d.

diversionary ileostomy

diverticula (*pl. of* diverticulum)

diverticular
d. disease
d. hemorrhage
d. hernia

diverticularization

diverticulation abnormality

diverticulectomy
bladder d.
endocavitary bladder d.
Harrington esophageal d.
d. of hypopharynx
Meckel d.
open d.
pharyngoesophageal d.
urethral d.
vesical d.
d. with myotomy

diverticulitis
cecal d.

diverticulopexy

diverticulum, pl. **diverticula**
acquired d.
caliceal d.
cervical d.
congenital d.
distal esophageal d.
esophageal d.
false d.
Meckel d.
midesophageal traction d.
pulsion d.
traction d.
true d.
Zenker d.
Zuckerkandl d.

diverting
d. loop colostomy
d. loop ileostomy
d. proximal colostomy
d. stoma

divided
doubly ligated and d.
d. respiration

NOTES

divided-stoma colostomy
division
anterior primary d.
d. I–IV lesion
intrahepatic vascular d.
maturation d.
posterior primary d.
reduction d.
vascular ring d.
divulse
divulsion
digital d.
Dix-Hallpike maneuver
Dixon
D. fat suppression method
D. method opposed imaging
D. technique
DKS
Damus-Kaye-Stansel
DKS operation
DKS procedure
D-loop transposition of the great artery
DMFC
demand minimum functional capacity
DNA ploidy abnormality
DO
distal-occlusal
DO cavity
dobutamine stress echocardiography (DSE)
Döderlein
D. method
D. roll-flap operation
Dodge area-length method
dog-ear repair
dog-leg fracture
Dohlman operation
DOI
depth of insertion
Dolenc technique
dolichocephalic head
dolichoectatic artery
dolichopellic pelvis
doll's
d. eye maneuver
d. head maneuver
d. head phenomenon
Doll trochanteric reattachment technique
dolorosa
anesthesia d.
domain
abdominal d.
D'ombrain operation
dome
d. excursion
d. fracture
d. osteotomy
dome-shaped osteotomy
dominant
d. component
d. gland
d. mass
domino
d. procedure
d. transplant
DOMS
delayed onset muscle soreness
Donald-Fothergill operation
Donald procedure
donation
autologous blood d.
blood d.
designated blood d.
organ d.
Donders
D. line
D. pressure
D. procedure
space of D.
donor
bacteremic d.
cadaver d. (CAD)
cadaveric d.
CMV-positive d.
cytomegalovirus-positive d.
extended criteria d. (ECD)
d. hepatectomy
d. iliac Y graft
d. kidney
living-related d. (LRD)
living relative d.
non-heart-beating d. (NHBD)
organ d.
d. pancreatectomy
subhuman primate d.
d. tissue
donor-specific bone marrow augmentation
donut mastopexy
Dooley nail
dopamine receptor
dopaminergic
d. medication
d. tract
Doppler
D. auto-correlation technique
D. color flow
D. color flow imaging
D. duplex ultrasonography
endoscopic color D.
D. flow probe examination
D. interrogation
D. method
D. pressure gradient
D. pulse evaluation
D. signal

D. study
D. tissue imaging
transcranial D. (TCD)
D. ultrasound
D. ultrasound segmental blood pressure testing

dopplergram

Doppler-guided artery ligation hemorrhoidectomy

Dor
D. anterior fundoplication
D. fundoplication method
D. fundoplication procedure
D. fundoplication technique

Dorello canal

Dormia noose

Dorrance procedure

dorsa (*pl. of* dorsum)

dorsabdominal

dorsal
d. aspect
d. branch
d. closing wedge osteotomy
d. column stimulation (DCS)
d. column tractotomy
d. cordotomy
d. cord stimulation
d. cross-finger flap
d. digital artery
d. elevated position
d. enteric fistula
d. excision
d. expansion
d. finger approach
d. fissure
d. horn
d. induction
d. inertia position
d. intercalary segmental instability
d. interosseous artery
d. interosseous nerve
d. linear incision
d. lithotomy
d. lithotomy position
d. longitudinal incision
d. lumbotomy incision
d. midline approach
d. pancreatic artery
d. penis
d. perilunate dislocation
d. point
d. proximal metatarsal osteotomy
d. radius tubercle
d. rami nerve
d. recumbent position
d. rhizotomy
d. rigid position
d. root
d. root entry zone (DREZ)
d. root entry zone lesion
d. root entry zone procedure
d. root ganglion
d. root ganglionectomy
d. rotation flap
d. sacrococcygeal muscle
d. scapular artery
d. scapular nerve
d. spine
d. supine position
d. surface
d. synovectomy
d. talonavicular bone
d. tegmental decussation
d. tenosynovectomy
d. thoracic artery
d. thyroid mobilization
d. tissue
d. translation
d. transposition flap
d. transscaphoid perilunar dislocation
d. transverse capsulotomy
d. transverse incision
d. vein patch graft
d. vertebra
d. wire-loop fixation

dorsale

dorsales

dorsalis

dorsal-V osteotomy

dorsalward approach

dorsi

dorsiflexion
d. of ankle

dorsiflexory wedge osteotomy

dorsiscapular

dorsispinal vein

dorsocephalad

dorsolateral
d. approach
d. incision
d. and medial capsulotomy
d. tract

dorsolumbar

NOTES

dorsomedial
d. approach
d. incision
dorsopancreaticus
dorsoplantar
d. approach
d. projection
dorsoradial approach
dorsorostral approach
dorsosacral position
dorsoulnar approach
dorsoventrad
dorsum, pl. **dorsa**
dose
d. escalation
fixed d.
fixed subcutaneous d.
physiologic d.
preoperative d.
priming d.
subcutaneous d.
subparalyzing d.
tissue tolerance d.
dose-effect curve
dose-related effect
dose-response curve
dosing
around-the-clock d.
ATC d.
dot-and-blot hemorrhage
dot-blot
d.-b. procedure
d.-b. technique
dot hemorrhage
Dotter-Judkins technique
Dotter technique
Doubilet sphincterotomy
double
d. adenomas
d. antibody method
d. aortic arch
d. chin
d. decidual sac
d. enterostomy
d. exposure
d. extra stimulus
d. fracture
d. freeze-stalk cryopexy
d. freeze-thaw cryopexy
d. graft
d. incision
d. jaw surgery
d. Maddox rod test
d. osteotomy
d. pedicle TRAM flap
d. pyloroplasty
d. ring
d. simultaneous stimulation
d. stapling technique (DST)
d. unilateral cysts
double-armed suture technique
double-balloon
d.-b. technique
d.-b. valvotomy
d.-b. valvuloplasty
double-barrel
d.-b. colostomy
d.-b. ileostomy
double-burst
d.-b. stimulation
d.-b. transmission
double-button suture technique
double-contrast
d.-c. barium enema examination
d.-c. enema
d.-c. visualization
double-doughnut approach
double-dummy technique
double-exposed rib
double-folded cup-patch technique
double-freeze technique
double-incision fasciotomy
double-inlet ventricle anomaly
double-loop
d.-l. hernia
d.-l. pouch
double-looped semitendinosus technique
double-lumen intubation
double-needle chemonucleolysis
double-point threshold
double-puncture laparoscopy
double-rod
d.-r. technique
double-sealant technique
double-seton modified surgical approach
double-skin mastopexy
double-stapled
d.-s. ileoanal reservoir method
d.-s. ileoanal reservoir procedure
d.-s. ileoanal reservoir technique
double-staple technique
double-stick technique
double-tube technique
double-umbrella closure
double-volume exchange transfusion
double-wire technique
double-wrap graciloplasty
doubly
d. ligated
d. ligated and divided
d. sutured
doughnut ring
doughy
d. abdomen
d. mass

Douglas
D. abscess
D. bag collection method
D. bag technique
cul-de-sac of D.
D. cul-de-sac
D. fold
D. graft
D. line
D. pouch
D. procedure
semicircular line of D.
douglasi
douloureux
tic d.
dowel
d. bone graft
d. spinal fusion
d. technique
doweling spondylolisthesis technique
Dow method
Downey-McGlamery procedure
downregulate
downstream
d. sampling method
d. signaling
d. venous pressure
downward
d. drainage
d. retraction
Doyen vaginal hysterectomy
Doyle operation
DP
distal pancreatectomy
DPL
diagnostic peritoneal lavage
DR-70 tumor marker test
dragon worm infection
drain
d. site evisceration
transcystic d.
d. volume
drainage
abdominal d.
bile tract d.
biliary d.
bladder d.
capillary d.
catheter d.
caval d.
cerebral spinal fluid d.
chest tube d. (CTD)
circle loop biliary d.
closed suction d.
computed tomography-guided selective d.
continuous catheter d.
CT-guided selective d.
dependent d.
downward d.
endoscopic biliary d.
endoscopic nasobiliary catheter d.
endoscopic pancreatic d.
endoscopic transpapillary cyst d.
endosonography-guided d.
enteric d.
external bile d.
external bile tract d.
external biliary d.
external ventricular d.
extrapetrosal d.
fluid d.
d. gastrostomy
hematoma d.
incision and d. (I&D)
internal d.
lymphatic d.
lymphocele d.
Molteno d.
nephrostomy d.
open d.
operative d.
d. pattern
pattern of d.
percutaneous abscess d. (PAD)
percutaneous catheter d.
percutaneous external d. (PED)
percutaneous transhepatic biliary d. (PTBD)
peripancreatic abdominal d.
peritoneal d.
portal d.
postoperative irrigation-suction d.
postural d.
pseudocyst d.
sclerotomy with d.
simple external d.
spinal fluid d.
stereotactic catheter d.
suction d.
thorascopic d.
tidal d.
transcystic d.
T-tube d.

NOTES

drainage *(continued)*
video thoracoscopic d.
Wangensteen d.
wound d.
draining abscess
drain-trap stomach
Drake tandem clipping technique
DRAM
de-epithelialized rectus abdominis muscle
Distress Risk Assessment Method
DRAM flap
draped
prepped and d.
draping
preparation and d.
draw-over vaporizer
dressing therapy
DREZ
dorsal root entry zone
DREZ lesion
DREZ modification of Eriksson technique
DREZ procedure
DREZ surgery
DRFS
distant recurrence-free survival
drilling technique
drip
d. infusion
intravenous d.
d. transfusion
drip-infusion cholangiography
Dripps-American Surgical Association score
Dripps classification
drip-tube feeding
drive
exploratory d.
hypercapnic d.
driven
d. equilibrium Fourier transform (DEFT)
d. equilibrium Fourier transform technique
drop
flow-dependent pressure d.
d. metastasis
droplet infection
drop-lock ring
Drualt
D. bundle
drug
d. administration
gastroprotective d.
d. infusion
nonsteroidal antiinflammatory d. (NSAID)
d. resistance
second-line d.
d. synergy
drum membrane
Drummond
D. spinous wiring technique
D. wire technique
Drummond-Morison operation
drunken sailor effect
drusen
dry
d. abscess
d. amputation
d. colostomy
d. field technique
d. gangrene
d. heat oven sterilization
d. hernia
d. mucous membrane
DSE
dobutamine stress echocardiography
DSRS
distal splenorenal shunt
DST
double stapling technique
DSVNI
Distress Scale for Ventilated Newborn Infants
dual
d. compression scoliosis treatment
d. impression technique
d. onlay cortical bone graft
d. percutaneous endoscopic gastrostomy
d. therapy
Duane
D. anomaly
D. classification
Duane-Hunt relation
Dubin-Amelar varicocele classification
Dubowitz
D. evaluation
D. examination
Duckett procedure
duct
aberrant bile d.
accessory pancreatic d.
anomalous junction of the pancreatobiliary d. (AJPBD)
Arantius d.
Bartholin d.
Bernard d.
bile d.
biliary d.
Blasius d.
bucconeural d.
canalicular d.
d. cannulation
d. carcinoma

d. cell adenocarcinoma
cochlear d.
collecting d.
common bile d. (CBD)
common hepatic d.
craniopharyngeal d.
cystic d.
deferent d.
distal bile d.
d. ectasia
efferent d.
ejaculatory d.
endolymphatic d.
excretory d.
extrahepatic bile d.
frontonasal d.
galactophorous d.
gall d.
Gartner d.
genital d.
hemithoracic d.
Hensen d.
hepatic d.
hepatocystic d.
Hoffmann d.
hypophyseal d.
incisive d.
inferior lacrimal d.
d. injury
intrahepatic bile d.
jugular d.
lactiferous d.
d. of Luschka
lymphatic d.
main pancreatic d. (MPD)
mamillary d.
mammary d.
mesonephric d.
metanephric d.
milk d.
minor sublingual d.
Müller d.
nasofrontal d.
pancreatic d.
papillary d.
paramesonephric d.
paraurethral d.
parotid d.
Pecquet d.
perilymphatic d.
periotic d.
pronephric d.
prostatic d.
reuniens d.
right lymphatic d.
Rivinus d.
salivary d.
Santorini d.
Schüller d.
secretory d.
segmental d.
semicircular d.
seminal d.
spermatic d.
Stensen d.
d. stone
striated d.
subclavian d.
sublingual d.
submandibular d.
submaxillary d.
sudoriferous d.
superior lacrimal d.
sweat d.
d. system
testicular d.
thoracic d.
thymic d.
thyroglossal d.
thyrolingual d.
uniting d.
utriculosaccular d.
d. wall
Walther d.
Wharton d.
Wirsung d.
wolffian d.

ductal

d. adenoma
d. calculus
d. cancer
d. carcinoma
d. carcinoma in situ (DCIS)
d. cystadenoma
d. dilatation
d. dilation
d. ectasia
d. hyperplasia
d. obstruction
d. proliferation
d. system
d. system perforation

NOTES

ductal-dependent
d.-d. lesion
d.-d. pulmonary circulation
ductectasia
ductibus
ductless gland
ductography
ductopenic rejection
duct-to-duct (D-D)
d.-t.-d. anastomosis
duct-to-mucosa
d.-t.-m. anastomosis
d.-t.-m. pancreaticojejunostomy
d.-t.-m. technique
ductule
aberrant d.
biliary d.
efferent d.
inferior aberrant d.
interlobular d.
prostatic d.
superior aberrant d.
transected d.
ductulus, pl. **ductuli**
ductus
Duddell membrane
Duecollement
D. hemicolectomy
D. maneuver
Dufourmentel technique
Duhamel
D. colon operation
D. laparoscopic pull-through
D. procedure
Dührssen
D. incision
D. vaginofixation
Duke
D. bleeding time
D. pouch cutaneous urinary diversion
Duke-Elder operation
Dukes
D. classification
D. classification of carcinoma
D. procedure
D. stage
dull to percussion abdomen
dumbbell
d. mass
d. tumor
dumping
d. stomach
d. syndrome
Duncan-Lovell modification
Duncan position
dunking technique
Dunn
D. biopsy
D. osteotomy
D. technique
Dunn-Brittain foot stabilization technique
Dunnett test
Dunn-Hess trochanteric osteotomy
Dunnington operation
duodenal
d. adenocarcinoma
d. adenoma
d. ampulla
d. bulb
d. bulb deformity
d. cap
d. compression
d. content examination
d. duplication
d. endoscopic polypectomy
d. fistula
d. fluid collection
d. foreign body
d. gland
d. hematoma
d. hernia
d. ileus
d. impression
d. loop
d. mass
d. metastasis
d. migrating activity
d. perforation
d. scarring
d. seromyectomy
d. sphincter
d. stump
d. stump leak
d. tumor
d. ulcer
d. ulceration
d. web
duodenales
duodenalis
duodenectomy
duodeni
duodenobiliary pressure gradient
duodenocaval fistula
duodenocholecystostomy
duodenocholedochotomy
duodenocolic fistula
duodenocystostomy
duodenoduodenostomy
duodenoenterocutaneous fistula
duodenoenterostomy
duodenogastroscopy
retrograde d.

duodenojejunal
d. angle
d. flexure
d. fold
d. fossa
d. hernia
d. junction
d. motor recording
d. recess
d. sphincter
duodenojejunalis
duodenojejunostomy
suprapapillary Roux-en-Y d.
duodenolysis
duodenomesocolica
duodenomesocolic fold
duodenopyloric constriction
duodenorenale
duodenorenal ligament
duodenorrhaphy
duodenoscopy
duodenostomy
Witzel d.
duodenotomy
transverse d.
duodenum
Duplay I, II technique
duplex-guided compression
duplex ultrasonography
duplication
alimentary tract d.
d. anomaly
complete d.
congenital d.
cranial d.
d. cyst
duodenal d.
esophageal d.
fetal d.
gallbladder d.
gastric d.
incomplete d.
partial d.
renal d.
symmetric thumb d.
thumb d.
trunk d.
tubular colonic d.
ureteral d.
Wassel thumb d.
Dupuy-Dutemps
D.-D. dacryocystorhinostomy dye test
D.-D. dacryostomy
D.-D. operation
Dupuytren
D. canal
D. contracture
D. fracture
D. suture technique
dural
d. arteriovenous fistula
d. arteriovenous malformation
d. cavernous sinus fistula
d. ectasia
d. incision
d. nerve root
d. patch reconstruction
d. puncture
d. repair
d. ring
d. shunt syndrome
d. venous sinus
dura mater
Duran approach
duraplasty
duration
d. tetany
d. time
Duret
D. hemorrhage
D. lesion
Durham
D. flatfoot operation
D. plasty
Durkan carpal compression test
Durr
D. nonpenetrating keratoplasty
D. operation
dusky stoma
dust-borne infection
Dutcher body
duToit-Roux
d.-R. arthroplasty
d.-R. staple capsulorrhaphy
Duval
D. pancreaticojejunostomy
D. procedure
Duverger-Velter operation
Duverney
D. fissure
D. fracture

NOTES

D

Duverney *(continued)*
D. gland
D. muscle
DuVries
D. approach
D. deltoid ligament reconstruction technique
D. hammertoe repair
D. incision
D. plantar condylectomy
DuVries-Mann modified bunionectomy
DVT
deep venous thrombosis
concurrent DVT
DVT prevention
DVT prophylaxis
Dwar-Barrington resection
dwarf pelvis
Dwyer
D. clawfoot operation
D. incision
D. osteotomy
D. procedure
Dyban technique
Dyck-Lambert classification
dye
d. dilution technique
d. exclusion test
d. injection
d. reduction spot test
d. scattering method
d. sham intrarenal lesion
d. worker's carcinoma
dye-dilution method
dyed starch method
dynamic
d. bolus tracking technique
d. cardiomyoplasty
d. closure pressure
d. compliance
d. compression
d. compression-plate fixation
d. condylar-screw fixation
d. cystourethroscopy
d. end-tidal forcing
d. fluorescence video endoscopy
d. graciloplasty
d. image
d. lumbar stabilization
d. relation
d. relaxation
d. repair
d. storage allocation
d. traction method
dynamometry
isometric force d.
dysarthric lesion
dysautonomia
familial d.
dyscrasic fracture
dysesthesia
burning d.
dysesthetic pain
dysfunction
bone marrow d.
chronic obstructive pulmonary d.
ejaculatory d.
end organ d.
endothelial cell d.
erectile d.
esophageal body motor d.
extensor mechanism d.
hepatic d.
hepatocellular synthetic d.
late graft d.
multiorgan system d.
multiple organ d. (MOD)
neuromotor d.
obstructive pulmonary d.
organ d.
pancreatitis d.
pelvic floor d.
postanesthetic central nervous system d.
postgastrectomy d.
postoperative renal d.
proximal myofascial d.
pulmonary d.
renal d.
sphincter of Oddi d.
superoxide-mediated endothelial cell d.
vocal d.
dysgenesis
dysgnathic anomaly
dyskinesia
extrapyramidal d.
levodopa-induced d.
retrolisthesis positional d.
dysmenorrheal membrane
dysmotility
esophageal d.
dysmyelination
dysosteogenesis
dysostosis
dyspepsia
postcholecystectomy flatulent d.
dysphagia
benign d.
contractile ring d.
postoperative d.
postvagotomy d.
recurrent d.
dysphasia
expressive d.

dysphoric mood state
dyspigmentation
dysplasia
asphyxiating thoracic d.
bronchopulmonary d. (BPD)
cortical d.
d. dislocation
focal cortical d.
high-grade d.
low-grade d.
oculoauriculovertebral d.
dysplasia-associated
d.-a. lesion
d.-a. mass
dysplastic epithelium
dyspnea
exertional d.
expiratory d.
one-flight exertional d.
d. on exertion
two-flight exertional d.
dysraphic malformation
dysreflexia
autonomic d.
dysregulation
autonomic d.
dysrhythmogenicity
dystonia
muscle d.
posttraumatic cervical d.
dystonic
d. pain
d. tic
dystrophic nail
dystrophy
Becker muscular d.
corneal d.
Emery-Dreifuss muscular d.
facioscapulohumeral muscular d.
myotonic d.
oculopharyngeal muscular d.
reflex sympathetic d.
dysuria
dysuric

NOTES

D

EA
epidural anesthesia
Eagle-Barrett syndrome
Eagle syndrome
Eagleton operation
Eames technique
ear
e. anesthesia
e. bone
e. canal
e. cartilage inflammation
external e.
e. lobe
earlobe adipose tissue
early
e. cancer lesion
e. enteral feeding
e. gastric cancer
e. graft thrombosis
e. infection rate
e. oversewing
e. postoperative period
e. supraclavicular compression
e. thoracoscopic repair
e. thrombectomy
e. unequivocal shock
early-onset graft-versus-host disease
easily reducible hernia
Eastern Cooperative Oncology Group (ECOG)
Eastwood technique
Eaton
E. closed reduction
E. implant arthroplasty
E. volar plate arthroplasty
Eaton-Littler
E.-L. ligament reconstruction
E.-L. technique
Eaton-Malerich
E.-M. fracture-dislocation operation
E.-M. fracture-dislocation technique
E.-M. reduction
Ebbehoj procedure
Eberle contracture release technique
EBM
evidence-based medicine
Ebner
imbrication line of von E.
E. line
E. reticulum
ebonation
ébranlement
Ebstein
E. cardiac anomaly
E. malformation
eburnation
EBV
Epstein-Barr virus
EBV infection
ECA
external carotid artery
ECA-PCA bypass surgery
ECC
endocervical curettage
extracorporeal circulation
ECCE
extracapsular cataract extraction
eccentric
e. exercise
e. fixation
e. hypertrophy
e. interocclusal record
e. jaw position
e. jaw relation
e. ledge
e. maxillomandibular record
e. narrowing
e. occlusion
eccentricity index
ecchondrosis
ecchymosed
ecchymosis, pl. **ecchymoses**
ecchymotic
e. mark
e. mask
eccouchement forcé
eccrine
e. carcinoma
e. sweat gland
ECD
extended criteria donor
ECF-A
eosinophilic chemotactic factor of anaphylaxis
ECFV
extracellular fluid volume
ECG signal-averaging technique
echinococcal
e. cyst disease
e. liver abscess
e. liver cyst
echinococcotomy
echinococcus cyst
echo
e. formation
e. imaging
inconsequential e.
magnitude preparation-rapid acquisition gradient e. (MP-RAGE)

echo *(continued)*
- e. rephasing
- e. reverberation
- e. score
- e. texture
- e. zone

echocardiographic assessment
echocardiography
- dobutamine stress e. (DSE)
- transesophageal e. (TEE)

echodense
- e. mass
- e. structure

echodensity
echoduodenoscopy
echo-free space
echogenic
- e. liver
- e. plaque
- e. tissue

echographic layer
echolucency
echolucent plaque
echopenic liver metastasis
echoplanar magnetic resonance imaging
echo-poor layer
echovirus infection
Ecker fissure
Ecker-Lotke-Glazer
- E.-L.-G. patellar tendon repair
- E.-L.-G. tendon reconstruction technique

Eckert-Davis classification
Eck fistula
Eckhout vertical gastroplasty
eclipse
- e. amblyopia
- e. phase

ECLS
extracorporeal life support
ECMO
extracorporeal membrane oxygenation
ECOG
Eastern Cooperative Oncology Group
ECoG
electrocorticography
- ECoG monitoring
- ECoG performance status scale

Economo disease
ECOR
extracorporeal CO_2 removal
ECPL
endocavitary pelvic lymphadenectomy
ECRB
extensor carpi radialis brevis
ECRL
extensor carpi radialis longus
ECS
elective cosmetic surgery
electrocerebral silence
ECST
European Carotid Surgery Trial
ectal origin
ectasia
- alveolar e.
- aortoannular e.
- artery e.
- corneal e.
- coronary artery e.
- distal e.
- duct e.
- ductal e.
- dural e.
- iris e.
- mammary duct e.
- papillary e.
- scleral e.
- senile e.
- vascular e.

ectasis
ectatic
- e. aneurysm
- e. bronchus
- e. carotid artery
- e. dilation
- e. emphysema
- e. vascular lesion
- e. vessel

ecthyma gangrenosum
ectocolostomy
ectoderm
ectodermal
ectopia
- cerebellar e.
- gallbladder e.
- macular e.
- renal e.
- testicular e.
- ureteral e.

ectopic
- e. ACTH syndrome
- e. anus
- e. atrial tachycardia
- e. bone
- e. craniopharyngioma
- e. cutaneous schistosomiasis
- e. endometrial tissue
- e. eruption
- e. eyelash
- e. focus
- e. gastric mucosa
- e. hyperparathyroidism
- e. impulse
- e. kidney
- e. pancreas

e. parathormone production
e. parathyroid adenoma
e. pregnancy
e. rhythm
e. sebaceous gland
e. spleen
e. ureter
e. ureterocele
e. varix
ectoscopy
ectosteal
ectostosis
ectothrix infection
ECTR
endoscopic carpal tunnel release
ectropion
ECU
extensor carpi ulnaris
eczematoid pruritic plaque
eczematous
e. lesion
e. patch
e. polymorphous light eruption
e. reaction
EDA
end-diastolic cross-sectional area
EDD
end-diastolic diameter
edea
Edebohls
E. incision
E. position
edema
antral e.
brain e.
bullous e.
cerebral e.
corneal e.
endothelial cell e.
ileocecal e.
laryngeal e.
lower extremity e.
lymphatic e.
massive pulmonary hemorrhagic e.
nephrotic e.
neurogenic pulmonary e. (NPE)
pericholecystic e.
peripheral extremity e.
stasis e.
subglottic e.
transient e.
visceral e.
edematous
e. bowel
e. bowel wall
e. mesentery
Eden-Hybbinette
E.-H. arthroplasty
E.-H. procedure
Eden-Lange procedure
Eden-Lawson hysterectomy
edentulous space
Eder-Puestow dilation
edge
anastomotic e.
chondral e.
inferior e.
lateral e.
shelving e.
spectral e.
superior e.
edge-detection method
edge-to-edge suture technique
edgewise technique
Edinburgh 2 Coma Scale
Edinger-Westphal nucleus
Edlan-Mejchar operation
Edmondson grading system for hepatocellular carcinoma
Edmondson-Steiner classification
Edmonton
E. Staging System for Cancer Pain
E. Symptom Assessment Schedule
EDR
extreme drug resistance
EDT
emergency department thoracotomy
education
Accreditation Council for Graduate Medical E. (ACGME)
Edwards
E. procedure
E. septectomy
Edwards-Tapp arterial graft
EEG
electroencephalography
EELV
end-expiratory lung volume
effect
amnestic e.
analgesic e.
antiangiogenic e.
anticoagulant e.
Bernoulli e.

NOTES

effect *(continued)*
biological e.
Bohr e.
cardioprotective e.
cardiotoxic e.
cardiovascular adverse e.
chemoradiotherapy e.
dose-related e.
drunken sailor e.
esophageal e.
Hawthorne e.
hypnotic e.
hypothermic e.
immunomodulating e.
motilin e.
negative e.
oxygen e.
e. parameter
pulmonary e.
second gas e.
sedative e.
stimulating e.
therapeutic e.
effective
e. function
e. renal blood flow
e. renal plasma flow
e. setting expansion
effector
e. operation
e. organ
e. pathway
efferens
efferent
e. duct
e. ductule
e. glomerular arteriole
e. limb
e. loop
e. nerve activity
PGA e.
PJA e.
efficacy
therapeutic e.
Effler-Groves mode of Allison procedure
Effler hiatal hernia repair
effluent
clear e.
effort thrombosis
effusion
chylous e.
exudative pleural e.
pleural e.
subdural e.
Efron jackknife classification
Eftekhar broken femoral stem technique
EG/BUS
external genitalia, Bartholin, urethral, and Skene
EGD
esophagogastroduodenoscopy
EGF
epidermal growth factor
salivary EGF
serum EGF
urinary EGF
egg
e. activation
e. membrane
e. shell nail
Egger line
Eggers
E. neurectomy
E. tendon transfer technique
Eggleston method
Eglis gland
egmentectomy
EHL
electrohydraulic lithotripsy
extensor hallucis longus
EHPO
extrahepatic portal vein obstruction
Ehrenritter ganglion
Ehrlich
E. inner body
Ehrlich-Türck line
EIC
extensive intraductal component
Eicken method
eight-ball hemorrhage
eighth cranial nerve
EIS
endoscopic injection sclerotherapy
Eisenberger technique
ejaculation disorder
ejaculatorius
ejaculatory
e. duct
e. dysfunction
ejection
e. murmur
e. phase
e. phase index
e. rate
e. shell image
e. time
ejection-fraction image
Ejrup maneuver
Ekehorn
E. operation
E. rectopexy
Eklund technique
El-Ahwany humeral supracondylar fracture classification

elastance
airway e.
elastic
e. band fixation
e. band ligation
e. barrier
e. compression
e. lamella
e. recoil
e. recoil pressure
e. tissue
elastica
elastic-fiber fragmentation
elasticus
elastofibroma
elastolysis
generalized e.
Elaut triangle
elbow
e. arthroplasty
e. disarticulation
e. dislocation
e. extensor tendon
e. fracture
elective
e. aneurysmectomy
e. cosmetic surgery (ECS)
e. dilatational tracheostomy
e. hernia repair
e. herniorrhaphy
e. laparotomy
e. lymphadenectomy
e. lymph node dissection (ELND)
e. neck dissection
e. sigmoid resection
e. surgery
e. surgical procedure
electric
e. anesthesia
e. aversion therapy
e. coagulation
e. differential therapy
e. induction
e. stimulation
electrical
e. activation abnormality
e. catheter ablation
e. fulguration
e. heart position
e. nerve stimulation
e. stimulation therapy
e. stimulator waveform
e. surface stimulation
electroanalgesia
electroanesthesia
electrobioscopy
electrocardiogram
electrocardiography
electrocauterization
electrocautery
bipolar e.
bleeding controlled with e.
hook e.
low-current e.
monopolar e.
multipolar e.
needlepoint e.
e. resection
electrocerebral silence (ECS)
electrocholecystectomy
electrocoagulation
bipolar e.
e. diathermy
direct current e.
endoscopic e.
monopolar e.
multipolar e.
e. necrosis
pinpoint e.
snare e.
transendoscopic e.
electroconvulsive therapy
electrocorticography (ECoG)
electrode
e. impedance
e. migration
e. placement
e. potential
e. response time
electrodesiccated bleeding point
electrodesiccation
electrode-skin interface
electrodiaphake
electrodispersive skin patch
electroejaculation
rectal probe e.
electroencephalography (EEG)
electroepilation
electroexcision
electrofulguration
electrogalvanic stimulation
electrogastroenterostomy
electrogenesis

NOTES

E

electrohemostasis
electrohydraulic
e. fragmentation
e. lithotripsy (EHL)
e. shock wave lithotripsy (ESWL)
electrolaryngogram
electrolysis
Faraday law of e.
electrolyte
e. abnormality
e. flush solution
e. imbalance
e. imbalance coma
electrolytic solution
electromagnetic
e. interference (EMI)
e. radiation exposure
e. signal
e. system
e. tracking
electromechanical dissociation
electromyocardial dissociation
electromyographic study
electromyography
laryngeal e.
electronarcosis
electroneurolysis
electronic
e. bone stimulation
e. magnification
electron microscopy
electroparacentesis
electrophoresis
hemoglobin e.
electrophrenic respiration
electrophysiologic
e. function
e. monitoring
electrophysiological stimulation
electrophysiology
flickering blockade e.
patch clamp e.
e. study
electropuncture
electroresection
electroscission
electrosection
electrosterilization
root canal e.
electrosurgery unit (ESU)
electrosurgical
e. desiccation
e. fulguration
e. snare polypectomy
electrotherapeutic sleep therapy
electrotherm
electrotomy
element
glandular e.
elementary
e. fracture
e. lesion
elevated
e. hemidiaphragm
e. lesion
elevation
e. angle
blanched cutaneous e.
chin e.
congenital scapular e.
diaphragmatic e.
e. of extremity
flap e.
e. paresis
periosteal e.
scapular e.
ST segment e.
unilateral diaphragmatic e.
elevator
e. disease
e. esophagus
e. extraction
e. muscle
elevatus deformity
eleventh
e. cranial nerve
e. rib flank incision
e. rib transperitoneal incision
elimination
carbon dioxide e. ($VECO_2$)
e. clearance
CO_2 e.
e. curve
e. disorder
e. half-life
nonpulmonary route of e. (NPE)
e. pocket
e. procedure
e. reaction
Elizabethtown osteotomy
Elliot
E. operation
E. position
ellipsoidal joint
ellipsoidea
ellipsoid method
elliptica
elliptical
e. anastomosis
e. biopsy
e. excision technique
e. recess
e. uterine incision
ellipticus
elliptocytosis

Ellis
E. classification
E. skin traction technique
Ellis-Jones peroneal tendon technique
Ellison
E. lateral knee reconstruction
E. technique
Elmslie procedure
Elmslie-Trillat
E.-T. patellar procedure
E.-T. patellar realignment method
ELND
elective lymph node dissection
Eloesser flap
Elsberg incision
Elschnig
E. blepharorrhaphy
E. body
E. canthorrhaphy
E. canthorrhaphy operation
E. central iridectomy
E. keratoplasty
Ely operation
embedded toenail
embolectomy
arterial e.
balloon e.
catheter e.
direct e.
femoral e.
pulmonary e.
emboli (*pl. of* embolus)
embolic gangrene
emboliform
embolism
air e.
amniotic fluid e.
atheroma e.
catheter e.
gas e.
paradoxical e.
pulmonary e. (PE)
transfusion-related air e.
tumor e.
venous air e. (VAE)
embolization
angiographic e.
arterial e.
hepatic artery e. (HAE)
pulmonary e.
renal arterial e.
selective arterial e.
subselective e.
superselective microcoil e.
venous e.
embolotherapy
embolus, pl. **emboli**
air e.
fatal air e.
hemodynamically significant air e.
e. migration
embouchement
embrasure space
embryectomy
embryo
e. biopsy
e. encapsulation
e. reduction
embryonal
e. cell carcinoma
e. tumor
embryonic
e. fixation syndrome
e. neural tube
e. sac
embryotomy
emedullate
emergence
e. agitation
anesthetic e.
e. delirium
metachronous e.
synchronous e.
emergency
access e.
e. airway management
e. appendectomy
e. colonoscopy
e. department thoracotomy (EDT)
e. indication
e. laparotomy
e. medicine
e. operation
e. procedure
e. room (ER)
e. room thoracotomy
e. SSPCS
e. surgery
surgical e.
e. tracheal intubation
e. tracheostomy
e. ventilation
emergency-department resuscitation

E

NOTES

emergent
e. appendectomy
e. endoscopic sclerotherapy
e. herniorrhaphy
e. intubation
e. operation
e. surgery
Emery-Dreifuss muscular dystrophy
emesis
coffee-grounds e.
EMI
electromagnetic interference
EMI scan
eminence
arcuate e.
cruciate e.
cruciform e.
deltoid e.
frontal e.
genital e.
hypothenar e.
ileocecal e.
iliopectineal e.
iliopubic e.
intercondylar e.
intertubercular e.
orbital e.
parietal e.
pyramidal e.
thenar e.
thyroid e.
eminentia, pl. **eminentiae**
emissaria
emissarium
emissary
e. sphenoidal foramen
e. vein
emission
gas e.
e. line
EMLA
eutectic mixture of local anesthetics
EMLA anesthetic
Emmet
E. operation
E. suture technique
Emmon osteotomy
EMMV
extended mandatory minute ventilation
Emory Pain Estimate Model (EPEM)
emphysema
colonoscopy-related e.
ectatic e.
endoscopy-related e.
nonbullous e.
subcutaneous e.
subgaleal e.
surgical e.
emphysematous
e. cholecystitis
e. gangrene
emprosthotonos position
empty
e. gestational sac
e. sella
emptying
delayed gastric e.
gastric e.
empyema
bilious e.
postpneumonectomy tuberculous e.
empyemic
EMR
endoscopic mucosal resection
en
en bloc
en bloc dissection
en bloc distal pancreatectomy
en bloc excision
en bloc lymphadenopathy
en bloc, no-touch technique
en bloc removal
en bloc resection
en face position
enamel
e. crypt
e. excrescence
e. fracture
e. knot
e. membrane
e. projection
e. rod inclination
e. sac
enameloplasty
enantiomer
enarthrodial joint
enarthrosis
encapsulated
e. brain abscess
e. breast implant
encapsulation
embryo e.
peritoneal e.
tumor e.
encasement
encatarrhaphy
encephalemia
encephali
encephalitis
encephalization
encephalocele
encephaloid gastric carcinoma
encephaloma
encephalomeningocele
encephalomyelitis
experimental allergic e.

encephalomyelocele
encephalopathy
- clinical e.
- degenerative e.
- hepatic e.
- ischemic e.
- portal-systemic e. (PSE)
- refractory e.
- traumatic progressive e.

encephaloscopy
encephalotomy
enchondral
enchondroma of bone
enchondrosarcoma
encircling
- e. cryoablation
- e. endocardial ventriculotomy
- e. explant

encroachment
encrustation
- bile e.

encu method
encysted
- e. calculus
- e. hernia
- e. intraabdominal collection

end
- blind e.
- e. colostomy
- cut e.
- e. exhalation
- e. expiration
- e. expiratory
- e. ileostomy
- e. inspiration
- e. organ dysfunction
- e. point
- proximal e.
- stapled blind e.
- e. stoma
- e. tube
- upper e.

endarterectomy
- blunt eversion carotid e.
- carotid e. (CEA)
- conventional e.
- coronary e.
- eversion e.
- eversion carotid e.
- femoral e.
- gas e.
- open e.
- surgical e.

endaural mastoid incision
end-diastolic
- e.-d. cross-sectional area (EDA)
- e.-d. diameter (EDD)
- e.-d. left ventricular pressure

endemic fungal infection
Ender femoral fracture technique
end-expiratory
- e.-e. intragastric pressure
- e.-e. lung volume (EELV)
- e.-e. phase

endgut
end-inspiratory volume
Endius approach
endless-loop tachycardia
end-loop
- e.-l. colostomy
- e.-l. ileocolostomy
- e.-l. ileostomy
- e.-l. stoma

endoabdominal fascia
endoalveolar crest
endoanal
- e. anastomosis
- e. mucosectomy
- e. ultrasonography

endoaneurysmoplasty
endoaneurysmorrhaphy
- ventricular e.

endoauscultation
endobrachyesophagus
endobronchial
- e. brachytherapy
- e. cancer
- e. fistula
- e. intubation
- e. intubation anesthetic technique
- e. tree
- e. tuberculosis

endocapsular
endocardiac
endocardial
- e. flow
- e. mapping
- e. murmur
- e. resection
- e. stain
- e. thickening

endocarditic

NOTES

endocarditis
prosthetic valve e. (PVE)
endocardium
endocavitary
e. bladder diverticulectomy
e. pelvic lymphadenectomy (ECPL)
e. radiation therapy
endoceliac
endocervical
e. canal
e. curettage (ECC)
e. mucosa
e. polyp
e. sampling
endocervix
endochondral bone
endocolitis
endocolpitis
endocranial
endocranium
endocrinae
endocrine
e. adenomatosis
e. disorder
e. fracture
e. gland
e. imaging
e. pancreas
e. screening
e. surgeon
e. surgery
e. toxicity
e. tumor
endocrinology
endocrinopathy
multiple e.
endocryopexy
endocryoretinopexy
endocyst
endodermal sinus
endodiathermy
endodontia
endodontic
e. armamentarium
e. cavity
e. irrigation
e. surgery
e. technique
endodontics
one-sitting e.
pedodontic e.
surgical e.
endodontist
endodontium
endodontologist
endodontology
endofaradism
endofluoroscopic technique
endofluoroscopy
flexible e.
percutaneous e.
rigid e.
endogalvanism
endogastric
endogenous
e. algogenic agent
e. aneurysm
e. A-V fistula
e. disease
e. event-related potential
e. fiber
e. flora
e. infection
e. lipid pneumonia
e. opiate receptor
e. opioid
e. opioid peptide
e. opioid system
e. protection
e. pyrogen
e. smile
e. steroid
e. uveitis
endoglobar
endoherniotomy
endoillumination
endolacrimal procedure
endolaryngeal
endoleak
proximal e.
endoligature
endolith
endoluminal
e. excision
e. repair
e. stenting
e. technology
e. therapy
endolymph
endolymphatic
e. cavity
e. duct
e. fluid
e. hydrops
e. sac
e. space
endolymphaticus
endolymphic
endometria (*pl. of* endometrium)
endometrial
e. ablation
e. adenocarcinoma
e. atrophy
e. biopsy
e. cancer
e. carcinoma

e. cavity
e. chemical shift imaging
e. curettage
e. cytology
e. island
e. jet washing
e. morphology
e. polyp
e. receptor
e. resection
e. sampling
e. shedding
e. spiral artery
e. thickness
e. tuberculosis
endometric epithelium
endometrioid
endometrioma
endometriosis
endometriotic focus
endometritis
endometrium, pl. **endometria**
endometropic
endomyocardial
e. biopsy
e. disease
endonasal disorder
endoneurolysis
end-on mattress suture technique
endo-osseous
endopelvic fascia
endophlebitis
endophotocoagulation
argon laser e.
endophytic
endoplasmic recticulum
endoprosthesis, pl. **endoprostheses**
endopyelotomy
endopyeloureterotomy
percutaneous e.
endorectal
e. coil magnetic resonance imaging
e. flap
e. ileal pouch
e. ileal pull-through
e. ileoanal pull-through
e. ileoanal pull-through method
e. ileoanal pull-through procedure
e. ileoanal pull-through technique
endoretinal
end-organ
e.-o. damage
e.-o. failure
endoribonuclease
endorrhachis
endoscope-assisted technique
endoscope-body position relationship
endoscope impaction
endoscopic
e. ampullary stenting
e. anterior cruciate ligament reconstruction
e. aspiration lumpectomy
e. band ligation
e. biliary decompression
e. biliary drainage
e. biliary stent placement
e. biopsy site
e. bladder neck suspension
e. breast augmentation
e. brush cytology
e. cardiac surgery
e. carpal tunnel release (ECTR)
e. color Doppler
e. color Doppler assessment
e. control
e. cystenterostomy
e. cystgastrostomy
e. cystoduodenostomy
e. cystogastrostomy
e. devolvulization
e. dissection
e. electrocoagulation
e. electrohydraulic lithotripsy
e. esophagectomy
e. esophagogastric variceal ligation
e. ethmoidectomy
e. examination
e. extirpation cicatricial obliteration
e. extraction
e. extraction pancreatic duct stone
e. finding
e. fine-needle aspiration cytology
e. fine-needle puncture
e. fistulotomy
e. frontal craniotomy
e. fulguration
e. fundoplication
e. gastrostomy
e. healing
e. hemostasis
e. hemostatic therapy

E

NOTES

endoscopic *(continued)*
e. image
e. incision
e. India ink injection
e. injection sclerotherapy (EIS)
e. injection therapy
e. jejunostomy
e. laser therapy
e. light source
e. management
e. mastopexy
e. microwave coagulation
e. mitral valve repair
e. mucosal ablation
e. mucosal resection (EMR)
e. mucosal resection method
e. mucosal resection procedure
e. mucosal resection technique
e. nasobiliary catheter drainage
e. optical urethrotomy
e. pancreatic drainage
e. pancreatic duct sphincterotomy
e. pancreatic stenting
e. pancreatic therapy
e. papillary balloon dilation
e. papillotomy
e. papillotomy and stenting
e. parathyroidectomy
e. photodynamic therapy
e. photography
e. plantar fasciotomy
e. pulsed dye laser lithotripsy
e. reflectance
e. reflectance spectrophotometry
e. removal
e. retroflexion
e. retrograde balloon dilatation
e. retrograde biliary stenting
e. retrograde cannulation
e. retrograde cholangiography
e. retrograde cholangiopancreatography (ERCP)
e. retrograde cholecystoendoprosthesis
e. retrograde sclerotherapy
e. route
e. sessile polypectomy
e. sigmoidopexy
e. sinus surgery
e. small bowel biopsy
e. snare resection
e. sphenoidal biopsy
e. sphincterectomy
e. sphincterotomy (ES)
e. spinal fusion
e. stent exchange
e. stone disintegration
e. stricturotomy
e. strip craniectomy
e. technology
e. transesophageal fine-needle aspiration
e. transpapillary cannulation
e. transpapillary cyst drainage
e. treatment
e. ultrasonographic imaging
e. ultrasonography (EUS)
e. ultrasonography-guided cytology
e. ultrasound evaluation
e. variceal sclerotherapy
e. video-assisted surgery
e. video image
e. visualization

endoscopically
e. normal patient
e. performed longitudinal incision

endoscopic-assisted
e.-a. microsurgical technique
e.-a. technique

endoscopic-controlled lithotripsy

endoscopist

endoscopy
advanced therapeutic e.
American Society for Gastrointestinal E. (ASGE)
anal e.
biliary e.
colorectal cancer e.
e. complication
computerized electronic e.
dynamic fluorescence video e.
fiberoptic intraosseous e.
flexible fiberoptic e.
fluorescent electronic e.
gastrointestinal e.
high-altitude e.
high-magnification e.
intestinal e.
intragastric provocation under e.
intralacrimal e.
intraoperative biliary e.
intraventricular e.
laser-assisted spinal e.
lumbar epidural e.
lung-imaging fluorescent e.
nasal e.
outpatient e.
pancreatic e.
pancreaticobiliary e.
pediatric e.
percutaneous e.
peripartum e.
peroral e.
postsurgical e.
primary diagnostic e.
e. procedure

sinus e.
small intestinal e.
e. suite
surveillance e.
therapeutic upper e.
transesophageal e.
transnasal e.
transoral e.
UGI e.
ultra-high-magnification e.
upper alimentary e.
upper gastrointestinal e.
upper intestinal e.
video e.

endoscopy-related emphysema
endosellar structure
endoskeleton
endosonography
endosonography-guided drainage
endosonoscopy
endosseous
endosteal
e. implant arm
e. surface
e. vessel

endosteum
endostitis
endostoma
endothelia (*pl. of* endothelium)
endothelial
e. barrier
e. bleb
e. cell basement membrane
e. cell dysfunction
e. cell edema
e. damage
e. denudation
e. injury
e. lysis
e. tube

endothelial-dependent relaxation
endothelin
e. A, B receptor
e. plasma level

endotheliochorial placenta
endothelio-endothelial placenta
endothelioma
endotheliosis
endothelium, pl. **endothelia**
capillary e.
continuous e.
corneal e.
discontinuous e.
fenestrated e.
gastrointestinal e.
sinusoidal e.
vascular e.

endothelium-dependent fibrinolysis
endothelium-derived relaxing factor
endothelium-mediated relaxation
endothoracica
endothoracic fascia
endothorax
tension e.

endothrix infection
endothyropexy
endotoxemia
systemic e.

endotoxic
e. exposure
e. shock

endotoxicosis
endotoxin
bacterial e.
e. shock

endotracheal
e. anesthesia
e. aspirate
e. induction
e. insufflation
e. intubation
e. suctioning
e. tube placement

endotrachelitis
endoureterotomy
cold knife e.

endourologic
endourological
e. cold-knife incision
e. therapy

endourology
endovaginal
e. finding
e. imaging

endovascular
e. aneurysm
e. approach
e. balloon occlusion
e. coagulation
e. coiling
e. graft insertion
e. graft treatment
e. intervention
e. repair

NOTES

endovascular *(continued)*
e. stent graft
e. stenting
e. stenting technique
e. surgery
e. technology
e. therapy
endovasculitis
hemorrhagic e.
endovenous septum
endoventricular circular patch plasty
endplate invagination
endpoint
e. measurement
primary e.
resuscitation e.
resuscitative e.
therapeutic e.
end-sigmoid colostomy
end-stage
e.-s. cirrhosis
e.-s. intestinal failure
e.-s. lymphangiomyomatosis
e.-s. renal disease (ESRD)
end-systolic
e.-s. cross-sectional area
e.-s. diameter (ESD)
e.-s. left ventricular pressure
e.-s. pressure-length relationship (ESPLR)
e.-s. pressure-volume relation
e.-s. stress-dimension relation
e.-s. wall thickness (ESWT)
end-tidal
e.-t. carbon dioxide
e.-t. nitrogen concentration
end-to-back bowel anastomosis
end-to-end
e.-t.-e. enterostomy
e.-t.-e. esophagogastrostomy
e.-t.-e. esophagojejunostomy
e.-t.-e. ileo-anal anastomosis without mucosal resection
e.-t.-e. intussuscepted pancreaticojejunostomy
e.-t.-e. invaginating
e.-t.-e. inverting pancreaticojejunostomy
e.-t.-e. jejunoileal bypass
e.-t.-e. reconstruction
e.-t.-e. reconstruction method
e.-t.-e. reconstruction procedure
e.-t.-e. reconstruction technique
e.-t.-e. splenoadrenal anastomosis
e.-t.-e. tendon repair
end-to-side
e.-t.-s. anastomosis
e.-t.-s. arteriotomy
e.-t.-s. choledochojejunostomy
e.-t.-s. esophagogastrostomy
e.-t.-s. esophagojejunostomy
e.-t.-s. jejunoileal bypass
e.-t.-s. nerve coaptation
e.-t.-s. portocaval shunt
e.-t.-s. reimplantation
e.-t.-s. repair
e.-t.-s. splenorenal shunt
e.-t.-s. vasoepididymostomy technique
endurance
cardiorespiratory e. (CRE)
end-viewing sector
end-weave anastomosis
enema
air e.
air-contrast barium e.
antegrade continence e. (ACE)
barium e.
contrast e.
double-contrast e.
small bowel e.
water-soluble contrast e.
energy
e. expenditure
hepatic intracellular e.
enervation
engaged head
engineering
islet cell e.
Englisch sinus
English
E. position
E. rhinoplasty
engorged
engorgement
engraftment
engulf
enhanced external counterpulsation
enhancing
e. brain lesion
e. ring
enlarged
e. parathyroid gland
e. spleen
enlargement
asymmetric parathyroid e.
mediastinal e.
Enna classification
Enneking
E. classification
E. resection-arthrodesis
ensiform
e. appendix
e. cartilage
e. process
ensisternum

ensu method
entangling technique
enteral
e. alimentation
e. feeding
e. nutrition
enterelcosis
enteric
e. cyst
e. drainage
e. fistula
e. infection
e. intussusception
e. nervous system
e. organism
e. plexus
entericus
enteritis
radiation e.
enteroanastomosis
enterocele sac
enterocentesis
enterocholecystostomy
enterocholecystotomy
enterocleisis
omental e.
enterocolic fistula
enterocolitis
necrotizing e. (NEC)
enterocolostomy
enterocutaneous fistula
enterocystoplasty
Camey e.
clam e.
seromuscular e.
sigmoid e.
enteroenteral fistula
enteroenteric fistula
enteroenterostomy
two-layer e.
enterogenital fistula
enterogenous cyst
enterohepatic circulation
enterohepatopexy
enterolith
enterolithiasis
enterolithotomy
enterolysis
enteropathy
radiation e.
enteropeptidase
enteroperitoneal abscess
enteropexy
enteroplasty
enterorenal
enterorrhagia
enterorrhaphy
enteroscopy
intraoperative e.
push e.
push-type e.
Roux-en-Y limb e.
small bowel e.
transgastrostomic e.
video small-bowel e.
enterostomal therapy
enterostomy
double e.
end-to-end e.
percutaneous e.
enterotomy
antimesenteric e.
inadvertent e.
longitudinal e.
occult e.
small bowel e.
enterourethral fistula
enterourethrostomy
enterovaginal fistula
enterovesical fistula
enteroviral infection
entity
pathologic e.
entocranial
entocranium
entomion
entoptoscopy
entrainment
air e.
entrapment
catheter e.
lateral canal e.
peroneal nerve e.
e. syndrome
entrapped
e. gland
e. nerve
entropionize
entropy
approximate e.
entry
air e.
implant e.
e. phenomenon

NOTES

entry *(continued)*
e. point
e. site
e. zone
e. zone lesion
enucleate
enucleation
eye e.
Foix e.
leiomyoma e.
e. method
e. procedure
surgical e.
e. technique
enuresis
diurnal e.
nocturnal e.
envelope
axillary e.
breast skin e.
e. flap
peritoneal e.
soft-tissue e.
enveloping scar tissue
environmental mycobacterial infection
environment modification
enzymatic
e. débridement
e. zonulolysis
enzyme
cyclooxygenase e. (COX-2)
e. induction
pancreatic e.
EORTC
European Organization for Research and Treatment of Cancer
eosin
eosinophilic
e. chemotactic factor of anaphylaxis (ECF-A)
e. endomyocardial disease
e. fibrohistiocytic lesion
epactal bone
eparterial bronchus
epaulet flap
epauxesiectomy
epaxial
EPEM
Emory Pain Estimate Model
ependymal cell
ependymoastrocytoma
ependymoblastoma
ependymoma
anaplastic e.
EPH
episodic paroxysmal hemicrania
ephaptic sprouting
ephippii
epiaortic imaging technique
epicanthal
e. correction
e. fold
epicardial
e. fat pad
e. monitoring
epicondylar avulsion fracture
epicondyle
epicondylectomy
epicondylian
epicondylic
epicondylus, pl. **epicondyli**
epicoracoid
epicranial
e. aponeurosis
e. muscle
epicranialis
epicranium
epicranius
e. muscle
epicystotomy
epidemiologic study
epidermal
e. growth factor (EGF)
e. inclusion cyst
e. necrolysis
e. ridge
epidermalization
epidermatoplasty
epidermic graft
epidermidis
Staphylococcus e.
epidermization
epidermoid
e. carcinoma
e. cyst
e. resection
epidermoidoma
black e.
incisural e.
intradural e.
prepontine white e.
epidermolysis
epididymal
e. sperm
e. sperm aspiration
epididymectomy
epididymidectomy
epididymidis
epididymis, pl. **epididymides**
cauda e.
corpus e.
e. lesion
lobule of e.
epididymisoplasty
epididymitis

epididymoorchitis
epididymoplasty
epididymotomy
epididymovasectomy
epididymovasostomy
epidural
e. abscess
e. abscess evacuation
e. administration
e. anesthesia (EA)
e. anesthetic
e. block
e. blockade
e. blood patch
e. blood patch anesthetic technique
e. cavity
e. delivery
e. electrode array
e. extramedullary lesion
e. hematoma
e. hemorrhage
e. neural blockade
e. neuroplasty
e. opioid
e. opioid infusion
e. pressure waveform (EPWF)
e. space
e. space infection
e. steroid injection
e. top-up
e. tumor evacuation
epidurography
epifascicular epineurotomy
epifluorescent microscopy
epigastric
e. angle
e. artery
e. fold
e. fossa
e. fullness
e. hernia
e. incision
e. pain
e. region
e. vein
epigastrica
epigastrium
epigastrius
epigastrocele
epigastrorrhaphy
epiglottic
e. cartilage
e. reconstruction
epiglottica
epiglottis
epiglottoplasty
epihyal ligament
epihyoid
epi-illumination
epikeratophakic keratoplasty
epikeratoplasty
tectonic e.
epilation
epilepidoma
epilepsy
intractable e.
e. surgery
epilepticus
status e.
epileptogenic process
epimorphic regeneration
epimysiotomy
epinephrine-anesthetic mixture
epinephros
epineural
e. repair
e. suture technique
epineurectomy
interfascicular e.
epineurial neurorrhaphy
epineurolysis
volar e.
epineurotomy
anterior e.
epifascicular e.
interfascicular e.
local e.
epipapillary membrane
epipharynx
epiphenomena of dissection
epiphrenic
epiphyseal (*var. of* epiphysial)
epiphyseolysis
epiphyseos
epiphyses (*pl. of* epiphysis)
epiphysial, epiphyseal
e. bar resection
e. closure
e. growth plate fracture
e. line
e. plate injury
e. ring

E

NOTES

epiphysial *(continued)*
e. slip fracture
e. tibial fracture
epiphysialis
epiphysial-metaphysial osteotomy
epiphysiodesis
open bone graft e.
screw e.
epiphysiolysis
femoral e.
proximal femoral e.
epiphysis, pl. **epiphyses**
atavistic e.
ball-and-socket e.
balloon e.
capital femoral e.
capitular e.
clavicular e.
congenital stippled e.
distal humeral e.
femoral e.
humeral e.
iliac e.
ossifying e.
pressure e.
ring e.
slipped capital femoral e.
stippled e.
tibial e.
traction e.
epiphyte
epiplocele
epiploectomy
epiploic, pl. **epiploicae**
e. appendage
e. appendicitis
e. appendix
e. branch
epiploica
epiploitis
epiplomerocele
epiplomphalocele
epiploon abscess
epiplopexy
epiplosarcomphalocele
epiploscheocele
epipteric bone
epiretinal membrane
episcleral
e. circulation
e. explant
e. ganglion
e. space
e. tissue
e. vascular dilation
episioperineoplasty
episioperineorrhaphy
episioplasty
episiorrhaphy
episiotomy
median e.
mediolateral e.
e. repair
ruptured e.
e. scar
episode
bleeding e.
thrombotic e.
episodic
e. colic
e. paroxysmal hemicrania (EPH)
epispadias
epispadias-exstrophy complex
epispinal
epistasis
epistaxis
episternal bone
episternum
epistropheus
epitarsus
epithelia (*pl. of* epithelium)
epithelial
e. barrier
e. basement membrane
e. breakdown
e. cell
e. cyst
e. hemangioendothelioma
e. inlay
e. invagination
e. migration
epithelialization technique
epithelioserosa
epithelium, pl. **epithelia**
Barrett e.
bile duct e.
colic e.
colon e.
columnar e.
corneal e.
crypt e.
dysplastic e.
endometric e.
esophageal e.
external dental e.
external enamel e.
follicular e.
gastric e.
germinal e.
glandular e.
gut e.
junctional e.
metaplastic e.
pseudostratified e.
pyramidal e.
regenerated esophageal e.

salivary e.
salmon-pink e.
squamous e.
stratified e.
surface e.
transitional e.
villous e.
epithelization
epithesis
epitrochlea
epitrochlear
epituberculous infiltration
epitympanic
e. cell
e. recess
Epley maneuver
épluchage
E point
epoophorectomy
epoöphori
epoophoron
Eppright dial osteotomy
Epstein
E. hip dislocation classification
E. method
Epstein-Barr
E.-B. viral infection
E.-B. virus (EBV)
Epstein-Thomas classification
epulofibroma
EPWF
epidural pressure waveform
equal sagittal flap
equation
alveolar gas e.
Bohr e.
Henderson-Hasselbalch e.
equator
anatomic e.
crystalline lens e.
eyeball e.
geometric e.
lens e.
equatorial plane
equilibrating operation
equilibration
mandibular e.
occlusal e.
equilibrium
acid-base e.
sedimentation e.
equinovalgus deformity
equinovarus deformity
equinus
e. deformity
e. position
equipotent
equipotential line
equivalence
e. point
e. relation
equivalent
human skin e. (HSE)
e. refracting plane
ventilation e.
equivocal
e. finding
e. pancreatic cytology
ER
emergency room
ER thoracotomy
eradication therapy
Erbakan inferior fornix operation
Erb point
ERCP
endoscopic retrograde cholangiopancreatography
ERCP cannulation
postoperative ERCP
preoperative ERCP
ERCP-guided biopsy
ERCP-induced splenic rupture
Erdheim cystic medial necrosis
erectile dysfunction
erect illumination
erection
intraoperative penile e.
penile e.
pharmacologically induced e.
reflex e.
reflexogenic e.
erector
e. spinae muscle
e. spinae tendon
erector-spinal reflex
ergonovine provocation test
Erickson-Leider-Brown technique
erigentes
Eriksson
E. brachial block technique
E. ligament technique
Erlangen pull-type sphincterotomy
Erlenmeyer flask deformity

NOTES

erosion
corneal e.
implant e.
infraspinatus insertion e.
limiting plate e.
recurrent corneal e.
tumor e.
wedge-shaped e.
erosive inflammation
erroneous projection
eruption
ectopic e.
eczematous polymorphous light e.
erythema nodosum-like e.
surgical e.
erysipelas
surgical e.
erysipelas-like skin lesion
erysipeloid
erysiphake
corneal e.
oval cup e.
e. technique
erythema
cold e.
e. nodosum-like eruption
erythroblastoma
erythrocyte
e. mass
e. membrane
erythrocytolysis
erythrodermatous lesion
erythroid colony formation
erythrokeratolysis hiemalis
erythrolysis
erythromelalgia
erythromycin-induced cholecystitis
erythropoietin therapy
ES
endoscopic sphincterotomy
escalation
dose e.
Escapini cataract operation
eschar
escharectomy
escharotomy
ESD
end-systolic diameter
esodic nerve
esophagea
esophageae
esophageal
e. A, B ring
e. achalasia
e. adenocarcinoma
e. artery
e. banding technique
e. band ligation
e. biopsy
e. body motor dysfunction
e. branch
e. cancer
e. carcinoma
e. colic
e. compression
e. constriction
e. contractile ring
e. contraction ring
e. dilatation
e. dilation
e. dilation treatment
e. disorder
e. dissection
e. diverticulum
e. duplication
e. dysmotility
e. ectopic sebaceous gland
e. effect
e. epithelium
e. fistula
e. foreign body
e. fungal infection
e. hernia
e. hiatus
e. impression
e. infection
e. inflammation
e. intubation
e. Lewy body
e. manometry
e. mass
e. measurement
e. mobilization
e. mucosal ring
e. muscular ring
e. myotomy
e. obstruction
e. perforation
e. peristaltic pressure
e. pH
e. pH monitoring
e. photodynamic therapy
e. plexus
e. remnant
e. resection
e. rupture
e. shortening
e. sling procedure
e. spasm
e. sphincter
e. sphincter pressure
e. sphincter relaxation
e. stenosis
e. stricture
e. tear
e. transection

e. tumor
e. ulceration
e. variceal bleeding
e. variceal sclerotherapy
e. varix
e. vein
e. web
esophageales
esophageal-jejunal anastomosis
esophagectasis
esophagectomy
distal e.
endoscopic e.
Ivor Lewis two-stage subtotal e.
laparoscopic-assisted e.
laparoscopic transhiatal e.
mediastinoscopy-assisted transhiatal e.
minimally invasive e.
near-total e.
open e.
subtotal e.
thoracoabdominal e.
thoracoscopic-assisted e.
total endoscopic e.
total laparoscopic e.
total thoracic e.
transhiatal e. (THE)
transhiatal blunt e.
transthoracic e.
video-assisted transsternal radical e.
e. with thoracotomy
esophagei
esophageus
esophagi (*pl. of* esophagus)
esophagitis
pill-induced e.
reflux e.
esophagobronchial fistula
esophagocardiomyotomy
esophagocardioplasty
esophagocolic anastomosis
esophagocutaneous fistula
esophagodiverticulostomy
esophagoduodenostomy
esophagoenterostomy
esophagogastrectomy
Ivor Lewis e.
thoracoabdominal e.
esophagogastric
e. anastomosis
e. cancer
e. fat pad
e. fundoplasty
e. intubation
e. junction
e. orifice
e. resection
e. variceal bleeding
e. vestibule
esophagogastroanastomosis
esophagogastroduodenoscopy (EGD)
pediatric e.
esophagogastromyotomy
esophagogastroplasty
Grondahl-Finney e.
esophagogastroscopy
Abbott e.
intrathoracic e.
Johnson e.
Thal e.
Woodward e.
esophagogastrostomy
Abbott e.
cervical e.
Clagett-Barrett e.
end-to-end e.
end-to-side e.
intrathoracic e.
Johnson e.
Thal e.
thoracic e.
Woodward e.
esophagogram
barium e.
water-soluble contrast e.
esophagojejunostomy
end-to-end e.
end-to-side e.
loop e.
mechanical e.
mediastinal e.
Roux-en-Y e.
stapled e.
transhiatal e.
esophagomediastinal fistula
esophagomyotomy
circumferential e.
Heller e.
laparoscopic e.
modified Heller e.
open e.
thoracic short e.
thoracoscopic e.

NOTES

esophagoplasty
balloon e.
behind-sternum column e.
Belsey e.
cervical e.
colic patch e.
colonic e.
gastric patch e.
gastric tube e.
Grondahl e.
Grondahl-Finney e.
intrathoracic e.
laparoscopic e.
one-stage posterior mediastinal e.
patch e.
pectoralis myocutaneous e.
pediatric e.
reverse gastric tube e.
single-step e.
subtotal e.
transmediastinal posterior e.
esophagoplication
esophagoproximal gastrectomy
esophagopulmonary fistula
esophagorespiratory fistula
esophago-Roux-en-Y-jejunostomy
esophagoscopy
fiberoptic e.
video e.
esophagostomy
cervical e.
palliative e.
esophagotomy
cervical e.
esophagotracheal fistula
esophagus, pl. **esophagi**
anterior e.
Barrett e.
cervical e.
columnar-lined e.
elevator e.
proximal e.
e. temperature
thoracic e.
esotropia
congenital e.
ESPLR
end-systolic pressure-length relationship
ESRD
end-stage renal disease
essential
e. brown induration of lung
e. hypertension
e. tremor
Esser
E. graft
E. inlay operation
Essex-Lopresti
E.-L. axial fixation technique
E.-L. calcaneal fracture classification
E.-L. calcaneal fracture technique
E.-L. joint depression fracture
E.-L. open reduction
established cell line
esterase-metabolized opioid
Estersohn osteotomy
Estes
E. operation
E. procedure
esthetic
e. restoration
e. rhinoplasty
e. septorhinoplasty
e. surgery
esthetics
gingival tissue e.
estimated
e. Fick method
e. time of ovulation (ETO)
Estlander
E. flap
E. operation
Estlander-Abbe flap
estrogen-assisted colposcopy
estrogen receptor localization
ESU
electrosurgery unit
ESWL
electrohydraulic shock wave lithotripsy
ESWT
end-systolic wall thickness
ethanol
e. ablation
e. injection
e. injection therapy
ethanol-induced tumor necrosis
ether
e. convulsion
methyl-*tert*-butyl e. (MTBE)
etherization
ethmocranial
ethmofrontal
ethmoid
e. bone
e. bulla
e. canal
e. cell
e. exenteration
e. fistula
e. registration point
e. sinus carcinoma
ethmoidal
e. artery
e. crest

e. foramen
e. groove
e. infundibulum
e. labyrinth
e. lacrimal fistula
e. nerve
e. notch
e. osteotomy
e. vein
ethmoidale
ethmoidales
ethmoidalia
ethmoidalis
ethmoidectomy
anterior e.
endoscopic e.
external e.
internal e.
intranasal e.
partial e.
total e.
transantral e.
ethmoidolacrimalis
ethmoidolacrimal suture
ethmoidomaxillaris
ethmoidomaxillary suture
ethmolacrimal
ethmomaxillary
ethmonasal
ethmopalatal
ethmosphenoid
ethmoturbinals
ethmovomerine
ethylene
e. oxide (ETO)
e. oxide sterilization
etiology
infectious e.
malignant e.
ETO
estimated time of ovulation
ethylene oxide
ETO sterilization
eucupine
eugnathic anomaly
euplastic
European
E. Carotid Surgery Trial (ECST)
E. Organization for Research and Treatment of Cancer (EORTC)
euryon
EUS
endoscopic ultrasonography
EUS-guided
EUS-g. cytology
EUS-g. fine-needle aspiration
eustachian
e. tube
e. tube orifice
eutectic mixture of local anesthetics (EMLA)
euthyroid sick syndrome
euthyscopy
euvolemia
euvolemic
evacuating clot
evacuation
CT-guided stereotactic e.
digital rectal e.
dilatation and e. (D&E)
dilation and e. (D&E)
e. disorder
epidural abscess e.
epidural tumor e.
fimbrial e.
fluid e.
hematobilia e.
hematoma e.
e. procedure
e. proctography
rectal e.
e. score
stool e.
transsphenoidal e.
evagination
optic e.
evaluation
acute physiologic assessment and chronic health e.
acute physiology and chronic health e. (APACHE)
angiographic e.
anthropometric e.
audiological e.
baseline capacity e.
clinical e.
cosmetic e.
cytologic e.
diagnostic imaging e.
Doppler pulse e.
Dubowitz e.
endoscopic ultrasound e.
followup e.

E

NOTES

evaluation *(continued)*
functional capacity e.
genitourinary e.
hearing aid e.
hormonal e.
infertility e.
job capacity e.
laparoscopic e.
mammographic e.
manometric e.
medical care e.
mental status e.
metabolic e.
neurodiagnostic e.
neurologic e.
neuroradiologic e.
noninvasive e.
pedicle e.
physical capacity e.
postoperative followup e.
preoperative staging e.
presurgical medical e.
pretransplant e.
pretreatment e.
e. protocol
quantitative e.
radiographic e.
radiologic e.
roentgenographic e.
serial radiographic e.
sexual e.
Smith physical capacities e.
static e.
status e.
stent e.
urological e.
uterine e.
videoscopic e.
videourodynamic e.
visual function e.
wake-up e.
Wright-Giemsa e.

Evans
E. ankle reconstruction technique
E. anterior calcaneal osteotomy
E. intertrochanteric fracture classification
E. procedure
E. reconstruction

Evans-Steptoe procedure
Eve method
even-echo rephasing
event
acute cardiac e.
adverse e.
anatomic e.
cardiac e.
catastrophic e.
cerebral e.
cerebrovascular e.
fatal cardiac e.
intraanesthetic e.
neuroelectric e.
precipitating noxious e.
soft e.
thromboembolic e.

eventration
diaphragm e.
diaphragmatic e.
e. disease

Everard Williams procedure
Eversbusch operation
eversion
e. carotid endarterectomy
e. endarterectomy
e. operation
e. orchiopexy
e. osteotomy
e. technique

eversion-external rotation deformity
evert
everting
e. interrupted suture technique

evidement
evidence
biochemical e.
clinical e.
macroscopic e.
radiologic e.
sonographic e.

evidence-based medicine (EBM)
eviration
evisceration
abdominal e.
drain site e.
e. operation
total abdominal e.
upper abdominal e.

evisceroneurotomy
EVM
eye, motor, voice
EVM grading of Glasgow Coma Scale

evoked
e. external urethral sphincter potential monitoring
e. potential technique
e. twitch

evolution
lesion e.
e. time

evolving myocardial infarction
evulsion
Ewald capitellocondylar total elbow arthroplasty

Ewald-Walker kinematic knee arthroplasty

Ewing

extraosseous E.
E. operation

ex

ex amblyopia
ex situ
ex situ bench surgery
ex situ hepatectomy
ex situ-in situ hepatectomy
ex situ-in situ liver resection
ex situ-in situ technique
ex situ in vivo procedure
ex vacuo dilatation
ex vivo
ex vivo cannulation
ex vivo count
ex vivo fertilization
ex vivo gene therapy
ex vivo marrow treatment
ex vivo perfusion
ex vivo technique

exacerbated

exacerbation of pain

exaggerated sniffing position

examination

abdominal e.
arthroscopic e.
Ballard e.
barium e.
bench e.
bile fluid e.
bimanual pelvic e.
bone marrow e.
cardiac e.
chest e.
clinical e.
colonoscopic e.
comparative radiographic e.
cytologic e.
cytology e.
dark-field e.
digital rectal e.
Doppler flow probe e.
double-contrast barium enema e.
Dubowitz e.
duodenal content e.
endoscopic e.
eye e.
fiberoptic e.
flashlight e.
followup e.
full-body cutaneous e.
full-spine radiographic e.
funduscopic e.
gastric residue e.
gray scale e.
hand-held Doppler flow probe e.
histologic e.
histopathologic e.
history and physical e.
immunofluorescent e.
laparoscopic e.
limited e.
LUS e.
mediastinoscopic e.
mental status e.
motor e.
neonate e.
neurologic e.
neurological nerve conduction velocity e.
neuroophthalmologic e.
neurophysiologic e.
neurotologic e.
newborn e.
ophthalmic e.
oral peripheral e.
palpatory e.
parasternal e.
pathologic e.
pathology e.
pelvic e.
pericardial fluid e.
peritoneal fluid e.
physical e.
pleural fluid e.
postmortem e.
proctoscopic e.
radiological e.
rectal e.
rectovaginal e.
reflex e.
retinal e.
self-breast e.
sensory e.
serologic e.
small bowel followthrough e.
soft x-ray e.
speculum e.
sterile vaginal e.
suboptimal e.
supraclavicular e.

E

NOTES

examination *(continued)*
suprasternal e.
synovial fluid e.
systemic e.
tangent screen e.
thermographic e.
transvaginal ultrasonographic e.
ultrasound e.
vaginal e.
Wood light e.
examnialis
exam under anesthesia
exanthema
exanthematous
e. disease
e. fever
e. inflammation
excavated
e. gastric carcinoma
e. lesion
excavatio
excavation
atrophic e.
glaucomatous e.
physiologic e.
retinal e.
excavatum
excementosis, pl. **excementoses**
extension e.
intraepithelial e.
pronglike e.
ultraterminal e.
excess
e. androgen
mandibular e.
marginal e.
maxillary e.
morbidity e.
e. mucus
vertical maxillary e.
excessive
e. bleeding
e. blood loss
e. callus formation
e. fatigue
e. heat production
e. lacrimation
e. lip support
e. spacing
e. straining
e. tearing
e. weight loss
exchange
air e.
air-fluid e.
blood-gas e.
body-fluid e.
catheter e.
cation e.
chemical e.
e. diffusion
endoscopic stent e.
fetal-maternal e.
fluid-gas e.
gas e.
gas-fluid e.
lens e.
multiple inert gas e.
plasma e.
pulmonary-gas e.
respiratory e.
e. technique
e. transfusion
wire-guided balloon-assisted endoscopic biliary stent e.
exchangeable mass
exchanger
countercurrent heat e.
thymocyte NA^+/H^+ e.
excimer
e. laser coronary angioplasty
e. laser photorefractive keratectomy
e. vascular recanalization
excipient
excised specimen
excision
abdominoperineal e.
alar wedge e.
Arlt-Jaesche e.
e. arthroplasty
Bartlett nail-fold e.
e. biopsy
bone cyst e.
Bose nail-fold e.
cervical disk e.
circumferential mesorectal e.
clavicle e.
cold snare e.
complete circumferential mesorectal e.
complete mesh e.
conjunctiva-Müller muscle e.
Curtin plantar fibromatosis e.
Dahlman diverticulum e.
Das Gupta scapular e.
disk e.
distal clavicular e.
dorsal e.
en bloc e.
endoluminal e.
extended mesorectal e.
extratemporal e.
Ferciot e.
Ferciot-Thomson e.
Flatt e.
funicular e.

fusiform e.
goiter e.
hemivertebral e.
incomplete e.
interdental e.
intralesional e.
laser hemorrhoid e.
local e.
marginal e.
mass e.
McKeever-Buck fragment e.
meniscal e.
mesorectal e.
microlumbar disk e.
operative e.
partial mesh e.
pentagonal block e.
radical compartmental e.
rectal e.
retropulsed bone e.
ruptured disk e.
sentinel node e.
sheet mesh e.
Stewart distal clavicular e.
subperichondrial e.
superficial e.
surgical e.
tangential e.
Thompson e.
thymus gland e.
total mesorectal e. (TME)
transanal e.
ulnar head e.
wedge e.
wide local e.
William microlumbar disk e.

excisional
e. arthrodesis
e. biopsy
e. biopsy method
e. biopsy procedure
e. biopsy site
e. biopsy technique
e. cardiac surgery
e. removal

excision-curettage technique
excitability test
excitatory
e. junction potential
e. postsynaptic potential
e. synapse

excited skin syndrome
excitement phase
exciting eye
excitoreflex nerve
excitor nerve
exclave
exclusion
antral e.
e. bypass
Devine antral e.
hepatic vascular e. (HVE)
intermittent vascular e.
partial hepatic vascular e. (PHVE)
subtotal gastric e.
total vascular e.
vascular e.

excoriate
excoriation
neurotic e.

excrement
excrementitious
excrescence
bony e.
enamel e.
Lambl e.
wart-like e.

excrete
excretion
urinary calcium e.

excretorius
excretory duct
excursion
dome e.
insertional e.
lateral e.
protrusive e.
range of e.
respiratory e.
retrusive e.
tendon e.

excystation
execution time
exemia
exencephalia
exencephalic
exencephalocele
exencephalous
exencephaly
exenteration
anterior pelvic e.
ethmoid e.
Iliff e.
orbital e.

E

NOTES

exenteration *(continued)*
pelvic e.
petrous pyramid e.
posterior pelvic e.
supralevator pelvic e.
total pelvic e.
exercise
e. capacity
concentric e.
eccentric e.
e. hyperemia blood flow
e. imaging
e. index
e. ischemia
e. physiology
plyometric e.
e. study
treadmill e.
exercise-associated acute renal failure
exercise-induced
e.-i. arrhythmia
e.-i. asthma
e.-i. bronchospasm
e.-i. incontinence
e.-i. silent myocardial ischemia
e.-i. ventricular tachycardia
exeresis
palliative e.
exergonic reaction
exertion
dyspnea on e.
perceived e.
rated perceived e.
rating of perceived e.
exertional
e. amblyopia
e. anterior compartment syndrome
e. compartment syndrome
e. deep posterior compartment syndrome
e. dyspnea
e. rhabdomyolysis
Exeter bone lavage
exfoliant
exfoliate
exfoliation
lamellar e.
e. syndrome
true e.
exfoliative cytology
exhalation
end e.
exhaustion
e. atrophy
nervous e.
ovarian follicle e.
postactivation e.
e. state
exhilarant
existential pain
exit
e. access
e. block
e. block murmur
e. point
e. pupil
e. site
e. site infection
e. wound
Exner plexus
exocardia
exocardial murmur
exoccipital bone
exocelomic
e. cavity
e. membrane
exocentric construction
exocervix
exocranial orifice
exocrine
e. pancreas
e. pancreatic insufficiency
exocrinopathic process
exodic nerve
exodontia
exodontics
exodontist
exodontology
exogamy
exogenous
e. aneurysm
e. anticoagulant coagulation
e. disease
e. fiber
e. fibrin clot
e. flora
e. hormone
e. IGF-1
e. infection
e. reconstruction
e. smile
e. substance
exognathia
exognathion
exophoria
exophoric
exophthalmic
exophthalmica
exophthalmogenic
exophthalmometric
exophthalmometry
exophthalmos, exophthalmus
recurrent e.
exophthalmos-producing substance
exophytic
e. carcinoma

e. growth
e. gut mass
e. joint disease
exoplant
scleral e.
exopneumopexy
exoserosis
exoskeletal
exoskeleton
exosmosis
exostectomy
exostosectomy
exostosis, pl. **exostoses**
hereditary multiple exostoses
multiple exostoses
exothermic
exotropia
exotropic
expandable
expanded plasma
expanding retroperitoneal hematoma
expansible
expansile
e. abdominal mass
e. unilocular well-demarcated bone lesion
expansion
e. and activator therapy
e. of the arch
clonal e.
controlled e.
delayed e.
dental arch e.
dorsal e.
effective setting e.
field e.
hygroscopic e.
infarct e.
intravascular volume e.
investment e.
lateral extensor e.
linear thermal e.
maxillary e.
mercuroscopic e.
mesangial matrix e.
monoclonal e.
palatal e.
perceptual e.
plasma volume e.
rapid maxillary e.
repeated tissue e.
secondary e.
setting e.
slow maxillary e.
stent e.
thermal coefficient e.
tissue e.
volume e.
wax e.
expansive laminaplasty
expectancy
life e.
expectant management
expectorate
expectoration
prune-juice e.
expenditure
caloric e.
energy e.
resting energy e.
experimental
e. allergic encephalomyelitis
e. disorder
e. method
e. neurasthenia
e. pain
e. pathology
e. threshold
expiration
end e.
expiratory
e. computed tomography
e. dyspnea
end e.
e. flow rate
e. grunt
e. murmur
e. nitrogen
e. positive airway pressure
e. prolongation
e. reserve volume
e. residual volume
e. retard
e. rhonchi
e. valve
e. wheezing
expired
e. air
e. air collection
explant
encircling e.
episcleral e.
Molteno episcleral e.
posterior e.

E

NOTES

explant *(continued)*
segmental e.
sponge e.
explantation
explanted heart
explicit memory
exploding head syndrome
exploration
abdominal e.
bilateral neck e.
bile duct e.
common bile duct e.
complete surgical e.
contralateral groin e.
e. and débridement
formal surgical e.
groin e.
laparoscopically guided transcystic e.
laparoscopic common bile duct e.
laparoscopic transcystic common bile duct e. (LTCBDE)
laparoscopic transcystic duct e.
neck e.
open common bile duct e.
petrous pyramid air cell e.
remedial inguinal e.
routine bilateral neck e.
routine unilateral e.
sclerotomy with e.
standard neck e.
unilateral neck e.
exploratory
e. celiotomy
e. drive
e. laparotomy
e. operation
e. puncture
e. stroke
e. surgery
explosion
colonic e.
e. fracture
e. injury
explosive doubling time
exponential phase
exposed pulp
exposure
Abbott-Gill epiphysial plate e.
accidental pulp e.
aerosolized pollutant e.
allergen e.
anesthetic gas e.
anterior surgical e.
bone e.
bony e.
carious pulp e.
chemical e.
cold e.
cue e.
double e.
electromagnetic radiation e.
endotoxic e.
extradural e.
extrapharyngeal e.
fast film e.
graded e.
heat e.
Henry posterior interosseous nerve e.
imaginal e.
incident e.
industrial e.
e. keratopathy
Kocher-Langenbeck e.
light e.
log relative e.
magnetic radiation e.
maternal mercury e.
mechanical pulp e.
methamphetamine e.
midline e.
noise e.
occupational toxin e.
operative e.
operator e.
prenatal diethylstilbestrol e.
prior drug e.
radiation e.
repeated e.
subclavian vessel e.
subperiosteal e.
sun e.
surgical e.
surgical pulp e.
thoracolumbar junction surgical e.
thoracolumbar spine anterior e.
toxin e.
transperitoneal e.
upper cervical spine anterior e.
in utero e.
vertebral e.
vessel e.
vinyl chloride e.
expressed skull fracture
expression
facial e.
intragraft e.
expressive dysphasia
expressivity
expressor loop
expulsion
graft e.
expulsive
e. coughing

e. hemorrhage
e. pain
exquisitely tender abdomen
exquisite pain
exsanguinate
exsanguinating hemorrhage
exsanguination
fetal e.
e. protocol
e. tourniquet control
e. transfusion
exsanguine
exsanguinotransfusion
exsect
exsection
exsiccant
exsiccate
exsiccation fever
exstrophy closure
exstrophy-epispadias complex
extended
e. criteria donor (ECD)
e. end-to-end anastomosis
e. field irradiation therapy
e. iliofemoral approach
e. jargon paraphasia
e. left hepatectomy
e. left subcostal incision
e. mandatory minute ventilation (EMMV)
e. maxillotomy
e. mesorectal excision
e. pancreatoduodenectomy
e. pelvic lymphadenectomy
e. pyelotomy
e. radical mastectomy
e. resection
e. right hemicolectomy
e. right hepatectomy
e. Ross procedure
e. shoulder flap
e. subfrontal approach
extensibility
penile e.
extensible
extensile approach
extension
atlantooccipital e.
attached gingiva e.
e. base
e. block splinting method
e. bridge
caliceal e.
clot e.
compression e.
cranial e.
e. deformity
distractive e.
e. excementosis
extranodal tumor e.
extrapancreatic e.
extrascleral e.
femoral-trunk e.
e. fiber
finger-like e.
flexion and e.
flexion, abduction, external rotation, e. (fabere)
e. form
full e.
groove e.
hip e.
infarct e.
e. injury
e. injury posterior atlantoaxial arthrodesis
e. instability
internal rotation in e.
intrasellar e.
knee e.
local tumor e.
lumbar e.
e. malposition
orbital e.
e. osteotomy
paraplegia in e.
e. for prevention
radiolucent operating room table e.
e. restriction
ridge e.
subependymal e.
e. teardrop fracture
thrombus e.
extension-type cervical spine injury
extensive
e. bilateral pneumonia
e. intraductal component (EIC)
e. lymph node dissection
e. posterior decompression
extensive-stage disease
extensor
e. carpi radialis brevis (ECRB)
e. carpi radialis brevis muscle
e. carpi radialis brevis tendon

E

NOTES

extensor *(continued)*
e. carpi radialis longus (ECRL)
e. carpi radialis longus flap
e. carpi radialis longus muscle
e. carpi radialis longus tendon
e. carpi ulnaris (ECU)
e. carpi ulnaris muscle
e. carpi ulnaris tendon
e. digiti minimi muscle
e. digiti minimi tendon
e. digiti quinti
e. digiti quinti muscle
e. digiti quinti tendon
e. digitorum brevis
e. digitorum brevis muscle
e. digitorum brevis tendon
e. digitorum communis muscle
e. digitorum communis tendon
e. digitorum longus
e. digitorum longus muscle
e. digitorum longus tendon
e. digitorum tendon
e. hallucis
e. hallucis brevis muscle
e. hallucis longus (EHL)
e. hallucis longus muscle
e. hallucis longus strength
e. hallucis longus tendon
e. hood mechanism
e. indicis proprius muscle
e. indicis proprius musculus
e. indicis proprius tendon
knee e.
e. lengthening
e. mechanism dysfunction
e. pollicis brevis
e. pollicis brevis muscle
e. pollicis brevis tendon
e. pollicis longus
e. pollicis longus muscle
e. pollicis longus tendon
e. quinti tendon
radial wrist e.
e. retinaculum
e. surface
e. tendon injury
e. tendon repair
e. tenodesis
e. tenotomy
e. tetanus
e. thrust reflex
toe e.
wrist e.

extensus
exteriorization colostomy
exteriorize
exteriorized
e. stuttering
e. uterine repair

externa
externae
external
e. absorption
e. acoustic foramen
e. acoustic meatus artery
e. arcuate fiber
e. auditory canal
e. auditory larynx
e. auditory meatus
e. beam irradiation
e. beam radiation therapy
e. bevel incision
e. bile drainage
e. bile tract drainage
e. biliary drainage
e. biliary fistula
e. biliary lavage
e. bleeding
e. bracing
e. branch
e. canthotomy
e. canthus
e. capsule
e. cardiac massage
e. carotid
e. carotid artery (ECA)
e. carotid plexus
e. clot
e. cooling
e. cuneate nucleus
e. dental epithelium
e. direct pressure
e. ear
e. elastic lamina
e. enamel epithelium
e. ethmoidectomy
e. female genital organ
e. fetal monitoring
e. geniculate body
e. genitalia
e. genitalia, Bartholin, urethral, and Skene (EG/BUS)
e. genitalia, Bartholin, urethral, and Skene glands
e. grid
e. hemipelvectomy
e. hemorrhage
e. hemorrhoid
e. hordeolum
e. iliac artery
e. iliac plexus
e. ilium
e. ilium movement
e. inguinal ring

e. ligament
e. male genital organ
e. mammary artery
e. maxillary artery
e. maxillary plexus
e. nasal nerve
e. nose
e. oblique
e. oblique aponeurosis
e. oblique fascia
e. oblique line
e. oblique reflex
e. oblique ridge
e. occipital crest
e. orbital fracture
e. orthovoltage irradiation
e. os
e. pancreatic fistula
e. pin fixation
e. pneumatic calf compression
posteroinferior e.
e. pudendal artery
e. rectal sphincter
e. respiration
e. rotation
e. rotation-abduction stress test
e. rotation-recurvatum test
e. rotator
e. route
e. saphenous nerve
e. scanning
e. shock wave lithotripsy
e. spermatic artery
e. spermatic fascia
e. spermatic nerve
e. sphincterotomy
e. spinal fixation
e. stimulus
e. support
e. surface
e. swelling
e. trauma
e. urethral orifice
e. urethral sphincter
e. urethrotomy
e. vacuum therapy
e. ventricular drainage
e. x-ray therapy

external-coil electrical stimulation
external-internal rotation
externalization
externally
e. releasable knot
e. rotated
externi
externum
externus
extinction
e. phenomenon
sensory e.
visual e.
extinguishing
extirpate
extirpation
Amreich vaginal e.
dental pulp e.
nodal e.
pulp e.
Rubbrecht e.
sac e.
surgical e.
extorsion
extortor
extraabdominal
e. anastomosis
e. anastomotic healing
e. disease
e. infective complication
e. injury
e. operation
e. position
e. site
extraalveolar
extraanatomic
e. bypass
e. bypass method
e. bypass procedure
e. bypass technique
extraanatomical renal revascularization technique
extraarachnoid injection
extraarticular
e. ankylosis
e. arthrodesis
e. augmentation
e. graft
e. hip fusion
e. pain syndrome
e. procedure
e. reconstruction
e. resection
e. structure
e. subtalar fusion

NOTES

extraarticular *(continued)*
- e. subtalar joint
- e. technique
- e. tissue
- e. tuberculosis

extraaxial
- e. compartment
- e. fluid collection

extrabuccal
extrabursal approach
extracaliceal
extracanthic
extracapillary crescent formation
extracapsular
- e. ankylosis
- e. aphakia
- e. arterial ring
- e. cataract extraction (ECCE)
- e. cataract extraction operation
- e. disease
- e. dissection
- e. extraction
- e. fracture
- e. metastasis
- e. tissue

extracardiac
- e. mass
- e. murmur

extracellular
- e. compartment
- e. fluid
- e. fluid volume (ECFV)
- e. granule
- e. ground substance
- e. matrix
- e. matrix remodeling
- e. matrix system
- e. plasma
- e. space
- e. toxin

extracellular-like, calcium-free solution
extracerebral fluid collection
extrachorial placenta
extrachromosomal
extraciliary fiber
extracolonic
extraconal fat reticulum
extracoronal
- e. retention
- e. splinting

extracoronary
extracorporeal
- e. anastomosis
- e. cardiopulmonary circuit
- e. circulation (ECC)
- e. CO_2 removal (ECOR)
- e. dialysis
- e. exchange hypothermia
- e. heart
- e. irradiation
- e. jamming knot
- e. life support (ECLS)
- e. liver perfusion
- e. membrane oxygenation (ECMO)
- e. method
- e. partial nephrectomy
- e. piezoelectric shock wave lithotripsy
- e. procedure
- e. renal preservation
- e. repair
- e. shock wave lithotripsy
- e. surgery
- e. technique
- e. ultrafiltration
- e. venous bypass

extracranial
- e. carotid artery disease
- e. carotid circulation
- e. carotid occlusive disease
- e. cerebral vasculature
- e. mass lesion
- e. occlusive vascular disease
- e. vasculature

extracraniale
extracranial-intracranial
- e.-i. bypass
- e.-i. bypass surgery

extract
- adipose tissue e.
- adrenocortical e.
- aqueous e.
- ceanothus e.
- lyophilized e.
- pancreatic e.
- parathyroid e.
- phenol-preserved e.
- Rauwolfia e.
- venom e.
- whole-body e.

extraction
- allograft e.
- Arroyo cataract e.
- Arruga cataract e.
- bag e.
- Baker pyridine e.
- e. balloon technique
- e. bile duct stone
- breech e.
- Burhenne biliary duct stone e.
- cataract e.
- Chandler-Verhoeff lens e.
- comedo e.
- countercurrent e.
- elevator e.
- endoscopic e.

extracapsular e.
extracapsular cataract e. (ECCE)
first-pass e.
e. flap
forceps e.
foreign body e.
harpoon e.
e. incision
intracapsular cataract e.
intraocular cataract e.
lactate e.
laparoscopic stone e.
liquid e.
magnetic e.
manual e.
Marshall-Taylor vacuum e.
menstrual e.
micro liquid e.
e. pancreatic stone
partial breech e.
planned extracapsular cataract e.
podalic e.
progressive e.
rubber-band e.
serial e.
e. site
solid phase e.
solvent e.
e. space
spontaneous breech e.
stone e.
systemic oxygen e.
tooth e.
total breech e.
vacuum e.

extracystic
extradental projection
extradomain A positive
extradural
e. abscess
e. anesthesia
e. anesthetic technique
e. block
e. clinoidectomy
e. exposure
e. granulation
e. hematoma
e. hematorrhachis
e. hemorrhage
e. phase
e. space
e. vertebral artery

extraembryonic
e. mesoderm
extraepiphysial
extrafascial hysterectomy
extrafective
extragenital
extraglandular conversion
extraglomerular mesangium
extragonadal
extrahepatic
e. abdominal carcinoma
e. access
e. bile duct
e. bile duct cancer
e. bile duct obstruction
e. biliary atresia
e. biliary cystic dilation
e. biliary obstruction
e. biliary tree
e. binary obstruction
e. control
e. dissection
e. lesion
e. metastasis
e. nodal disease
e. portal vein obstruction (EHPO)
e. portal venous hypertension
e. stone
e. tumor
e. tumor site
extraintestinal complication
extrajection
extralaryngeal approach
extraligamentous
extralobar
extraluminal
e. gas
e. hemorrhage
extralymphatic metastasis
extramammary Paget disease
extramaxillary anchorage
extramedullary
e. alignment
e. alignment arch
e. involvement
e. myelopoiesis
e. segment
e. toxicity
extramucosal
e. mass
e. pyloromyotomy
e. stitch

NOTES

extramural
e. lesion
e. upper airway obstruction
extraneous movement
extranodal
e. disease
e. site
e. tumor extension
extraoctave fracture
extraocular
e. movement
e. muscle
e. muscle involvement
e. muscles of Tillaux
extraoral
e. anchorage
e. radiographic examination profile
extraorbital disease
extraosseous Ewing
extraovular
extrapancreatic
e. extension
e. nerve plexus
extrapapillary
extraperineal
extraperiosteal
extraperitoneal
e. approach
e. carbon dioxide insufflation
e. cesarean section
e. CO_2 insufflation
e. endoscopic hernia repair
e. endoscopic pelvic lymph node dissection
e. fascia
e. laparoscopic bladder neck suspension
e. laparoscopic herniorrhaphy
e. laparoscopic nephrectomy
e. location
e. space
e. tissue
totally e. (TEP)
extrapetrosal drainage
extrapharyngeal
e. approach
e. exposure
extraplacental
extrapleural
e. air
e. anastomosis
e. apicolysis
e. pneumothorax
e. space
extrapolate
extrapolated end-tidal carbon dioxide tension ($PETCO_2$)
extrapolation
extraprostatic
extrapsychic
extrapulmonary
e. cough
e. *Pneumocystis carinii* infection
e. site
e. tuberculosis
extrapyramidal
e. disease
e. dyskinesia
e. function assessment
e. nucleus
e. pathway
e. reaction
e. syndrome
e. tract
extrarectus
extrarenal
e. mass
e. renal pelvis
extraretinal
extrasaccular hernia
extrascleral extension
extrasensory
extraskeletal
extrasphincteric anal fistula
extraspinal osteoid osteoma
extrastimulus test
extratemporal excision
extratesticular lesion
extrathoracic
e. metastasis
e. position
e. tuberculosis
extrathyroid
e. invasion
e. spread
extra toe
extratracheal
extrauterine pelvic mass
extravaginal testicular torsion
extravasate
extravasation
e. extremity
e. extrusion
e. feces
fluid e.
e. gas
e. injury
e. irrigation solution
e. phenomenon
extravascular
e. compartment
e. granulomatous feature
e. lung water
e. mass
e. space
extraventricular

extraversion
urinary e.
extravesical
e. anastomosis
e. infrasphincteric ectopic ureter
e. Lich approach
e. ureteral reimplantation technique
e. ureterolysis
extrema
extreme
e. capsule
e. drug resistance (EDR)
e. hearing loss
e. lateral transcondylar approach
e. somatosensory evoked potential
extremis
in e.
extremital
extremitas
extremity
e. abnormality
acromial e.
e. amputation
anterior e.
elevation of e.
extravasation e.
flaccid e.
e. injury
e. ischemia
left lower e.
left upper e.
e. lesion
lower e.
e. malformation
e. melanoma
e. mobilization technique
e. preservation
right lower e.
right upper e.
upper e.
extrinsic
e. allergic alveolitis
e. asthma
e. bladder compression
e. denervation
e. entrapment test
e. environmental staining
e. esophageal impression
e. lesion
e. mass
e. mechanism
e. muscle
e. muscle strength
e. nerve
e. pathway
e. semiconductor
e. sphincter
extrodactyly
extrospection
extroversion
extruded
e. disk
e. disk fragment
e. teeth
extrusion
bone graft e.
disk e.
extravasation e.
implant e.
oocyte e.
placental e.
sealer e.
tube e.
wire e.
extubate
extubation
e. anesthetic technique
postoperative e.
exuberant granulation tissue
exudate
acute inflammatory e.
circinate e.
conjunctival e.
cotton-wool e.
fatty e.
fibrinous e.
fluffy cotton-wool e.
foaming e.
gingival e.
hard e.
inflammatory e.
mucopurulent e.
pharyngeal e.
purulent e.
retinal e.
sanguineous e.
serous e.
soft e.
suppurative e.
waxy e.
exudation
fibrinous e.
gingival e.

NOTES

E

exudation *(continued)*
proteinaceous aqueous e.
purulent e.
exudative
e. ascites
e. eye
e. granulomatous inflammation
e. papulosquamous disease
e. pleural effusion
e. retinal detachment
e. tuberculosis
e. vitreoretinopathy
e. zone
exude
exumbilication
eye
e. disease
e. enucleation
e. examination
exciting e.
exudative e.
e. irrigating solution
e., motor, voice (EVM)
e. muscle surgery
pineal e.
e. point
e. rotation
stony-hard e.
e. tumor
e. tumor localization
web e.
eyeball
e. compression reflex
e. equator
eyebrow
e. fixation
e. laceration
eye-closure reflex
eye-ear plane
eyelash
ectopic e.
e. reflex
eyelid
e. fusion
e. molluscum contagiosum infection
e. surgery
e. tumor
upper e.
eyelid-closure reflex
Eyler flexorplasty

F2 focal point

FA

failure analysis

FA technique

FAB

French-American-British

FAB classification

FAB staging of carcinoma

fabere

flexion, abduction, external rotation, extension

fabere sign

Fabricius ship

FAC

fractional area change

face

cow f.

dish f.

f. form

inferior f.

f. line

f.s rating scale for children

superior f.

face-down position

facelift

facet

f. anomaly

articular f.

clavicular f.

corneal f.

costal f.

f. dislocation

f. excision technique

f. fracture stabilization wiring

f. fusion

inferior costal f.

f. joint

f. joint injection

f. joint preparation

f. plane

f. rhizotomy

f. subluxation stabilization wiring

superior costal f.

transverse costal f.

f. tropism

facetectomy

O'Donoghue f.

partial f.

face-to-face venacavaplasty

face-to-pubes position

facetted corneal scar

facial

F. Action Coding System

f. angiofibroma

f. angle

f. artery

f. axis

f. bone

f. butt joint preparation

f. canal

f. cleft

f. colliculus

f. deformity

f. excursion measurement

f. expression

f. foundation

f. fracture

f. height

f. index

f. muscle

f. nerve

f. nerve-preserving parotidectomy

f. nerve root

f. osteosynthesis

f. plane

f. plexus

f. profile

f. reanimation

f. restoration

f. root

transverse f.

f. triangle

f. vein

faciales

facialis

faciei

facies

acromial articular f.

Potter f.

facilitated angioplasty

facilitating restoration

facilitation

convergence f.

neuromuscular f.

postactivation f.

posttetanic f.

proprioceptive neuromuscular f.

Wedensky f.

facioplasty

facioscapulohumeral muscular dystrophy

faciotelencephalic malformation

F.A.C.S.

Fellow of American College of Surgeons

factor

acidic fibroblast growth f.

atrial natriuretic f. (ANF)

circulating MEN I-specific growth f.

clotting f.

coagulating f.

factor *(continued)*
coagulation f.
endothelium-derived relaxing f.
epidermal growth f. (EGF)
gut proliferative f.
hepatocyte growth f. (HGF)
human epidermal growth f. (hEGF)
inflammatory transcription f.
luminal f.
pathophysiologic f.
patient-dependent f.
patocyte growth f.
perioperative risk f.
polypeptide growth f.
predisposing f.
preoperative f.
prognostic f.
proliferative f.
f. replacement therapy
risk f.
technical f.
thromboembolic risk f.
transforming growth f. (TGF)
tumor necrosis f. (TNF)
vascular endothelial growth f. (VEGF)
f. V Leiden mutation
von Willebrand f.

factor-alpha
tumor necrosis f.-a. (TNF-alpha)

faculty
fusion f.

fade
tetanic f.

Faden
F. operation
F. procedure

Fahey
F. approach
F. technique

Fahey-O'Brien technique

Fahraeus method

failed
f. anesthesia
f. back surgery syndrome
f. femoral osteotomy
f. intubation
f. procedure
f. spinal
f. surgery

failure
acute respiratory f.
f. analysis (FA)
anastomotic f.
f. to awaken
bone marrow f.
bypass f.
chronic intestinal f.
chronic renal f. (CRF)
cocaine-induced respiratory f.
congestive heart f.
differentiation f.
dilator placement f.
end-organ f.
end-stage intestinal f.
exercise-associated acute renal f.
fulminant hepatic f. (FHF)
functional intestinal f.
graft f.
Harrington rod instrumentation f.
heart f.
hepatic f.
hepatorenal f.
implant f.
implantation f.
instrumentation f.
intestinal f.
intubation f.
irradiation f.
late graft f.
late wound f.
liver f.
microcirculatory f.
multiorgan f. (MOF)
multiorgan system f.
multiple organ f. (MOF)
multiple organ system f.
multiple system organ f.
multisystem f.
multisystem organ f. (MSOF)
pacemaker f.
postburn bone marrow f.
postoperative hepatic f.
postoperative liver f.
posttraumatic renal f.
pouch f.
progressive liver f.
progressive respiratory f.
renal f.
respiratory f.
sclerotherapy f.
surgeon-dependent technique f.
surgical f.
suture f.
technical f.
wound f.

Fairbanks-Sever procedure

Fairbanks technique

falcate

falces (*pl. of* falx)

falciform
f. cartilage
f. crest
f. ligament
f. margin

f. process
f. retinal fold
falciforme
falciformis
Falconer lobectomy
Falk-Shukuris operation
Falk vesicovaginal fistula technique
Fallat-Buckholz method
falling hematocrit
fallopian
f. canal
f. hiatus
f. ligament
f. tube
f. tube carcinoma
f. tube mass
f. tube metastasis
fallopiana
Fallot
tetralogy of F.
false
f. aneurysm
f. channel formation
f. cord carcinoma
f. diverticulum
f. knot
f. membrane
f. negative
f. pelvis
f. positive
f. projection
f. rib
f. suture
f. vertebra
f. vocal cord
false-negative
f.-n. cholangiogram
f.-n. result
false-positive
f.-p. interpretation
f.-p. result
falx, pl. **falces**
familial
f. adenomatous polyposis (FAP)
f. aortic ectasia syndrome
f. atypical mole and melanoma (FAM-M)
f. atypical multiple mole melanoma syndrome
f. breast cancer
f. cardiac myxoma syndrome
f. cholestasis syndrome
f. colon cancer (FCC)
f. consequence
f. dysautonomia
f. exudative vitreoretinopathy
f. hemiplegic migraine
f. HPT
f. hypocalciuric hypercalcemia
f. indication
f. Mediterranean fever
f. multigland disease
f. osteochondrodystrophy
f. paroxysmal rhabdomyolysis
f. polyposis syndrome
FAM-M
familial atypical mole and melanoma
FAM-M syndrome
fan beam projection
Fanconi anemia
Fanta cataract operation
FAP
familial adenomatous polyposis
far
f. lateral inferior suboccipital approach
f. point
Farabeuf
F. amputation
F. ischiopubiotomy
F. triangle
Faraday
F. law of electrolysis
F. law of induction
far-and-near suture technique
Farmer
F. operation
F. technique
Farre white line
Fasanella operation
Fasanella-Servat
F.-S. procedure
F.-S. ptosis operation
fascia, pl. **fascias, fasciae**
f. of abdomen
Abernethy f.
alar f.
anal f.
antebrachial f.
anterior rectus f.
axillary f.
brachial f.
broad f.
buccopharyngeal f.

NOTES

fascia *(continued)*
Buck f.
bulbar sheath f.
Camper f.
clavipectoral f.
Cloquet f.
Colles f.
Cooper f.
cremasteric f.
cribriform f.
crural f.
Cruveilhier f.
dartos f.
deep cervical f.
deltopectoral f.
Denonvilliers f.
endoabdominal f.
endopelvic f.
endothoracic f.
external oblique f.
external spermatic f.
extraperitoneal f.
fusion f.
geniohyoid f.
Gerota f.
gluteal f.
Godman f.
Hesselbach f.
iliac f.
iliopectineal f.
incised f.
infundibuliform f.
intercolumnar f.
internal spermatic f.
investing f.
lacrimal f.
f. lata
lumbodorsal f.
masseteric f.
muscular f.
nuchal f.
obturator f.
orbital f.
palpebral f.
pancreatic f.
parietal pelvic f.
parotid f.
parotideomasseteric f.
pectineal f.
pectoral f.
pectoralis f.
pelvic f.
perirenal f.
pharyngobasilar f.
phrenicopleural f.
popliteal f.
Porter f.
prepubic f.
presacral f.
pretracheal f.
prevertebral f.
psoas f.
rectal f.
rectovesical f.
renal f.
retrosacral f.
retrovisceral f.
salpingopharyngeal f.
scalene f.
Scarpa f.
Sibson f.
subcutaneous f.
subperitoneal f.
superficial inguinal f.
superior f.
temporal f.
thoracolumbar f.
Toldt f.
transversalis f.
transverse f.
Treitz f.
triangular f.
Tyrrell f.
umbilical prevesical f.
umbilicovesical f.
visceral pelvic f.
Zuckerkandl f.

fascial
f. arthroplasty
f. bridge
f. closure
f. defect
f. flap
f. graft
f. hernia
f. layer
f. plane
f. shutter mechanism
f. sling approach
f. sling procedure
f. space
f. space infection
f. stranding

fasciaplasty

fascias (*pl. of* fascia)

fascia-splitting incision

fascicular
f. graft
f. repair

fasciculata

fasciculation
benign f.
contraction f.
malignant f.

f. potential
tongue f.
fasciculus, pl. **fasciculi**
wedge-shaped f.
fasciectomy
dermal f.
limited f.
partial f.
radical palmar f.
fasciitis
fasciocutaneous
f. free flap
f. island flap
fasciodesis
fasciola
fascioplasty
fasciorrhaphy
fascioscapulohumeral
fasciotomy
decompression f.
double-incision f.
endoscopic plantar f.
Fronet f.
percutaneous plantar f.
plantar f.
prophylactic f.
Rorabeck f.
single-incision f.
Skoog f.
subcutaneous f.
Yount f.
fashion
concertina-like f.
isolated f.
perpendicular f.
standard f.
Z f.
FAST
fluorescent antibody staining technique
Fourier-acquired steady-state technique
fast
f. exposure technique
f. film exposure
f. neutron radiation therapy
f. spin echo sequence
fast-flush test
fastigiobulbar tract
fasting
preoperative f.
f. recording
fast-pathway radiofrequency ablation
fast-track cardiac anesthesia
fat
abdominal f.
body f.
f. body
f. cell space
creeping f.
f. flap
f. globule
f. graft
herniated preperitoneal f.
f. herniation
f. line
f. necrosis
f. pad
periesophageal f.
f. plane
preperitoneal f.
properitoneal f.
total body f.
fatal
f. air embolus
f. cardiac event
fat-density line
fat-free mass
fatigue
excessive f.
f. fracture
implant f.
postoperative f.
suture f.
fat-patch graft
fat-suppression technique
fatty
f. apron
f. ascites
f. exudate
f. hernia
f. infiltration
f. prostatic tissue
f. renal capsule
fauces
faucial branch
faucium
faulty
f. contact point
f. restoration
Favaloro saphenous vein bypass graft
FBS
fetal bovine serum
FCC
familial colon cancer

F

NOTES

FDPCA
fixed-dose patient-controlled analgesia
Feagin shoulder dislocation test
fear subscale
feather-edged proximal finishing line
featural surgery
feature
clinical manifestations, etiologic factors, anatomic involvement, pathophysiologic f.'s (CEAP)
clinicopathologic f.
cytologic f.
extravascular granulomatous f.
histopathologic f.
immunohistochemical f.
preoperative f.
tumor f.
febrile morbidity
fecal
f. abscess
f. contamination
f. diversion
f. diversion colostomy
f. fistula
f. impaction
f. incontinence
f. load
f. loading
f. soiling
f. stream
fecalith
appendiceal f.
fecaloma
stercoral f.
fecaluria
feces
extravasation f.
Federation of Gynecology and Obstetrics classification
feedback reduction circuit
feeder-frond technique
feeding
f. complication
drip-tube f.
early enteral f.
enteral f.
f. gastrostomy
gastrostomy f.
jejunostomy elemental diet f.
jejunostomy tube f.
oral f.
postoperative regimen for oral early f. (PROEF)
tube f.
f. tube placement
Feiss line
Feist-Mankin position
fellea
fellis
Fellow of American College of Surgeons (F.A.C.S.)
felon infection
Felson
silhouette sign of F.
feltwork
female
f. castration
f. gonad
f. prostate
f. urethra
f. urethral syndrome
femineus
feminina
femininae
femininum
feminization syndrome
feminizing genitoplasty
femoral
f. arch
f. artery
f. artery aneurysm
f. artery approach
f. canal
f. circulation
f. cortical ring allograft
f. diaphyseal fracture
f. diaphysis
f. embolectomy
f. endarterectomy
f. epiphysiolysis
f. epiphysis
f. fossa
f. head
f. head line
f. hernia
f. intertrochanteric fracture
f. metaphysis
f. muscle
f. nailing
f. neck fracture
f. neck fracture reduction
f. nerve
f. nerve block
f. nerve traction test
f. osteotomy
f. plexus
f. prosthesis fixation
f. puncture
f. region
f. resection
f. ring
f. septum
f. shaft
f. shaft fracture
f. sheath
f. supracondylar fracture

f. 3-in-1 technique
f. triangle
f. vein
femorale
femoralis
femoral-popliteal artery bypass
femoral-tibial-peroneal bypass
femoral-trunk extension
femoris
femorodistal
f. bypass
f. reconstructive surgery
femorofemoral (FF)
f. crossover
femoroischial transplantation
femoropopliteal
f. bypass
f. bypass graft
f. occlusive disease
femorotibial
fender fracture
fenestra, pl. **fenestrae**
fenestrated
f. endothelium
f. Fontan operation
f. membrane
f. sheath
fenestration
alveolar plate f.
aortopulmonary f.
apical f.
atrophic f.
baffle f.
catheter-directed f.
cusp f.
cyst f.
dental f.
intercellular f.
laparoscopic f.
Lempert f.
f. operation
tracheal f.
Fenton vaginoplasty
Ferciot excision
Ferciot-Thomson excision
Ferguson
F. hemorrhoidectomy
F. scoliosis measuring method
Fergus operation
Fergusson incision
Ferkel torticollis technique
fermentation
mixed acid f.
Fernandez
F. extensile anterior approach
F. osteotomy
ferning technique
Ferrein
F. canal
F. cord
F. foramen
F. ligament
F. pyramid
ferreini
ferromagnetic microembolization treatment
Ferry line
fertility
fertilization
f. age
ex vivo f.
in vitro f.
in vivo f.
FESS
functional endoscopic sinus surgery
festination
fetal
f. acoustic stimulation test
f. aspiration syndrome
f. body movement
f. bone fracture
f. bovine serum (FBS)
f. cardiac anomaly
f. chest anomaly
f. circulation
f. cystic adenomatoid malformation
f. drug therapy
f. duplication
f. exsanguination
f. gastrointestinal anomaly
f. growth acceleration
f. growth retardation
f. head
f. head:abdominal circumference ratio
f. head circumference
f. head position
f. heart rate acceleration
f. heart rate monitoring
f. hemorrhage
f. infection
f. intracranial anatomy
f. intrahepatic vein

NOTES

fetal *(continued)*
f. liver biopsy
f. liver transplantation
f. lymphoid tissue
f. malpresentation
f. medicine
f. membrane
f. reduction
f. rejection
f. scalp oxygenation
f. skin biopsy
f. surgery
f. thymus transplantation
f. tissue sampling
f. tissue transplant
f. urogenital tract
f. vascular anomaly
fetal-maternal
f.-m. exchange
f.-m. hemorrhage
fetation
fetomaternal
fetoplacental circulation
fetoscopy
fetus growth elevation
FEV_1
forced expiratory volume in 1 second
fever
dehydration f.
exanthematous f.
exsiccation f.
familial Mediterranean f.
fracture f.
inundation f.
Mediterranean exanthematous f.
syphilitic f.
FF
femorofemoral
FF crossover
FGF
fresh gas flow
FHF
fulminant hepatic failure
fiber
accelerator f.
anastomotic f.
association f.
f. bundle
bundle f.
f. bundle volume
endogenous f.
exogenous f.
extension f.
external arcuate f.
extraciliary f.
Gerdy f.
intercolumnar f.
intercrural f.
Nélaton f.
f. optic laryngoscopy
osteogenetic f.
postganglionic parasympathetic f.
postganglionic sympathetic f.
preganglionic parasympathetic f.
preganglionic sympathetic f.
projection f.
pupillodilator f.
rod f.
Rosenthal f.
Sappey f.
Sharpey f.
skinned muscle f.
f. tip modification
zonular f.
fiberglass graft
fiberoptic
f. bronchoscopy
f. bronchoscopy anesthetic technique
f. bundle
f. endoscopy anesthetic technique
f. esophagoscopy
f. examination
f. injection sclerotherapy
f. intraosseous endoscopy
f. intubation method
f. intubation procedure
f. panendoscopy
f. sigmoidoscopy
f. tracheal intubation anesthetic technique
fiberotomy
fiber-splitting incision
fibra, pl. **fibrae**
fibrillary astrocyte
fibrillation
atrial f.
auricular f.
cardiac f.
chronic atrial f.
continuous atrial f.
idiopathic ventricular f.
lone atrial f.
paroxysmal atrial f. (PAF)
f. potential
f. rhythm
synchronized f.
f. threshold
ventricular tachycardia/ventricular f.
fibrillation-flutter
atrial f.-f.
fibrillogranuloma
fibrin
f. calculus
f. degradation product

f. plate method
postvitrectomy f.
fibrinogen
f. degradation product
f. method
fibrinogen-fibrin degradation product
fibrinogenolysis
fibrinoid necrotizing inflammation
fibrinolysin coagulation
fibrinolysis
endothelium-dependent f.
primary f.
fibrinopeptide A
fibrinopurulent inflammation
fibrinoscopy
fibrinous
f. adhesion
f. exudate
f. exudation
f. inflammation
fibroadenolipoma
degenerated f.
fibroadenoma
giant f.
fibroadipose tissue
fibroangioma
fibroblast
f. chemoattraction
f. culture
dermal f.
harvested f.
human lung f. (HLF)
keloid f.
f. migration
f. proliferation
fibroblastic tissue
fibroblastoma
fibrocalcification
fibrocalcific lesion
fibrocarcinoma
fibrocartilage
basilar f.
circumferential f.
interarticular f.
semilunar f.
stratiform f.
fibrocartilaginous
fibrocartilago
fibrocaseous inflammation
fibrocementoma
fibrochondroma
fibrocystic
f. change
f. complex
f. condition
f. disease
fibrocystoma
fibrodentinoma
fibroelastic tissue
fibroelastoma
fibroenchondroma
fibroepithelioma
fibrofascial compartment syndrome
fibrofatty breast tissue
fibrofolliculoma
fibrogliosis
fibrogranuloma
fibrohemangioma
fibrohistiocytic lesion
fibrohistiocytoma
fibroid
f. adenoma
f. inflammation
fibroidectomy
fibrokeratoma
fibroleiomyoma
fibrolipoma
fibroliposarcoma
fibroma
ameloblastic f.
diffuse f.
ungual f.
fibromectomy
fibromus
diffuse f.
fibromuscular
fibromusculoelastic lesion
fibromyalgia trigger point
fibromyectomy
fibromyoma
uterine f.
fibroneuroma
fibroosseous
f. lesion
f. ring of Lacroix
fibroplate
fibroproliferative membrane
fibrosa
fibrosae
fibrosarcoma
fibroscopy
fibrosis
diffuse lobular f.

NOTES

fibrosis *(continued)*
hepatic f.
idiopathic pulmonary f. (IPF)
interstitial pulmonary f. (IPF)
periductal f.
pulmonary f.
fibrosum
fibrotic
f. nub
f. tissue
f. wall
fibrotomy
fibrous
f. adhesion
f. articular capsule
f. bone lesion
f. cap
f. connective tissue
f. ingrowth
f. integration
f. joint
f. loose body
f. obliteration
f. polypoid lesion
f. repair
f. ring
f. scar tissue
f. skeleton
f. tendon sheath
f. union
fibula
diastasis f.
fibulae
fibular
f. flap
f. fracture
f. head
f. metaphysis
f. ostectomy
f. sesamoidectomy
f. strut graft
fibularis
f. brevis muscle
f. longus muscle
f. longus tendon
f. tertius muscle
f. tertius tendon
fibulectomy
partial f.
fibulocalcaneal ligament
Ficat procedure
Fick
F. cardiac output measurement
F. oxygen extraction method
F. position
F. principle
F. technique
Ficoll-Hypaque technique
field
f. block
f. block anesthesia
bloodless f.
f. cancerization
f. of dissection
f. expansion
f. method
operative f.
pulsed electromagnetic f. (PEMF)
surgical f.
field-echo
f.-e. difference
f.-e. image
f.-e. imaging
Fielding
F. femoral fracture classification
F. membrane
F. modification of Gallie technique
Fielding-Magliato subtrochanteric fracture classification
fierce cellular rejection
fifth
f. cranial nerve
f. metatarsal base fracture
fighter fracture
FIGO
International Federation of Gynecology and Obstetrics
FIGO classification staging
figure-eight
f.-e. preparation
f.-e. stitch
figure-four position
figure-of-eight
f.-o.-e. suture technique
fila (*pl. of* filum)
filament
corneal f.
filar mass
Filatov
F. flap
F. keratoplasty
F. operation
Filatov-Gillies
F.-G. flap
F.-G. tubed pedicle
Filatov-Marzinkowsky operation
fill breast implant
filled
decayed, extracted, and f.
filler graft
filleted graft
fillet local flap graft
filling
bead technique f.
brush technique f.
f. canal

f. defect
f. first technique
flow technique f.
f. material condensation
nature root canal f.
postresection f.
pressure technique f.
root canal f.

film
abdominal f.
f. identification
f. oxygenation
plain abdominal f.

filmy adhesion
filopressure
filter
f. placement
f. tilt

filtered-back projection
filtered radioisotope
filtering
f. operation
f. procedure

filtration
f. angle
gel f.
glass-wool f.
glomerular f.
f. method
rate of fluid f.
spontaneous ascites f.
f. surgery

filtration-slit membrane
filtrum
filum, pl. **fila**
fimbria, pl. **fimbriae**
ovarian f.

fimbrial evacuation
fimbriated fold
fimbriectomy
fimbrioplasty
Bruhat laser f.

final
f. cementation
f. cone position
f. consonant position
f. growth
f. outcome

finding
barium enema f.
diagnostic f.
endoscopic f.
endovaginal f.
equivocal f.
histologic liver biopsy f.
intraoperative ultrasound f.
irresectable f.
mammographic f.
manometric f.
operative f.
physical f.
prognostic f.
suspicious f.
ultrasonic endovaginal f.

fine manipulation
fine-needle
f.-n. aspiration (FNA)
f.-n. aspiration biopsy
f.-n. aspiration cytology

finger
f. deformity
f. dilation
f. flap
f. fracture
f. fracture dissection
f. fracture technique
f. indicator
f. joint arthroplasty
F. Oscillation Test
ring f.
f. web

finger-fillet flap
finger-like extension
fingerprint line
fingertip
f. amputation
f. dissection

fingertrap
f. suspension

Finkelstein maneuver
Fink operation
Finney
F. gastroenterostomy
F. operation
F. pyloroplasty
F. strictureplasty
F. stricturoplasty

Finochietto-Billroth I gastrectomy technique
fire
nosocomial f.

Fired-Hendel procedure
firm
f. lesion

NOTES

firm *(continued)*
f. mass
f. texture
first
f. arch syndrome
f. carpometacarpal joint fracture
f. cone position
f. cranial nerve
f. cuneiform bone
f. metacarpal artery
f. parallel pelvic plane
f. ray surgery
f. rib resection via subclavicular approach technique
f. twitch height (T1)
f. web space
first-degree
f.-d. burn
f.-d. hemorrhoid
f.-d. radiation injury
f.-d. tuberculum
first-echelon
first-grade fusion
first-line screening technique
first-pass
f.-p. extraction
f.-p. technique
first-set graft rejection
first-stage repair
first-strand cDNA synthesis
Fischer projection
Fish cuneiform osteotomy technique
Fisher advancement flap
fisherman's knot
Fishgold line
fishmouth
f. amputation
f. anastomosis
f. fracture
f. incision
fishtail deformity
fissura, pl. **fissurae**
fissure
abdominal f.
anal f.
auricular f.
azygos f.
caudal transverse f.
f. cavity
corneal f.
dorsal f.
Duverney f.
Ecker f.
glaserian f.
horizontal f.
inferior accessory f.
inferior orbital f.
major f.
minor f.
oral f.
palpebral f.
petrooccipital f.
petrosquamous f.
petrotympanic f.
portal f.
pterygoid f.
pterygomaxillary f.
rectal f.
right sagittal f.
Rolando f.
sagittal f.
Santorini f.
sphenoidal f.
sphenomaxillary f.
sphenopetrosal f.
squamotympanic f.
superior orbital f.
sylvian f.
tympanomastoid f.
tympanosquamous f.
umbilical f.
vestibular f.
fissured fracture
fistula, pl. **fistulae**
abdominal wall f.
alveolar f.
amphibolic f.
amphibolous f.
anal f.
anastomotic f.
f. in ano
anorectal f.
antecubital arteriovenous f.
aortocaval f.
aortoduodenal f.
aortoenteric f.
aortoesophageal f.
aortogastric f.
aortograft duodenal f.
aortosigmoid f.
arterial-arterial f.
arterial-enteric f.
arterial-portal f.
arteriobiliary f.
arterioportal f.
arterioportobiliary f.
arteriosinusoidal penile f.
arteriovenous f. (AVF)
arteriovenous subclavian f.
aural f.
autocaval f.
A-V f.
benign duodenocolic f.
biliary f.
biliary-bronchial f.
biliary-cutaneous f.

biliary-duodenal f.
biliary-enteric f.
biliocystic f.
biliopleural f.
f. bimucosa
bladder f.
blind f.
Blom-Singer tracheoesophageal f.
bowl f.
BP f.
brachioaxillary bridge graft f.
brachiosubclavian bridge graft f.
branchial f.
Brescia-Cimino A-V f.
bronchobiliary f.
bronchoesophageal f.
bronchopleural f.
bronchopleurocutaneous f. (BPCF)
bronchopulmonary f.
calyceal f.
cameral f.
carotid-cavernous sinus f.
carotid-dural f.
cavernous sinus f.
cerebrospinal fluid f.
cervical f.
cervicovaginal f.
cholecystenteric f.
cholecystocholedochal f.
cholecystocolic f.
cholecystocolonic f.
cholecystoduodenal f.
cholecystoduodenocolic f.
choledochal-colonic f.
choledochocolonic f.
choledochoduodenal f.
choledochoenteric f.
chyle f.
Cimino f.
Cimino-Brescia arteriovenous f.
closure of f.
coccygeal f.
colobronchial f.
colocutaneous f.
cologastrocutaneous f.
coloileal f.
colonic f.
colorectal f.
colovaginal f.
colovesical f.
communicating f.
complete f.
complex anorectal f.
congenital pulmonary
  arteriovenous f.
congenital tracheobiliary f.
congenital urethroperineal f.
controlled f.
corneal f.
coronary artery f. (CAF)
coronary artery-right ventricular f.
craniosinus f.
cutaneobiliary f.
cystogastric f.
dental f.
dialysis f.
dorsal enteric f.
duodenal f.
duodenocaval f.
duodenocolic f.
duodenoenterocutaneous f.
dural arteriovenous f.
dural cavernous sinus f.
Eck f.
endobronchial f.
endogenous A-V f.
enteric f.
enterocolic f.
enterocutaneous f.
enteroenteral f.
enteroenteric f.
enterogenital f.
enterourethral f.
enterovaginal f.
enterovesical f.
esophageal f.
esophagobronchial f.
esophagocutaneous f.
esophagomediastinal f.
esophagopulmonary f.
esophagorespiratory f.
esophagotracheal f.
ethmoid f.
ethmoidal lacrimal f.
external biliary f.
external pancreatic f.
extrasphincteric anal f.
fecal f.
forearm graft arteriovenous f.
gastric f.
gastrocolic f.
gastrocutaneous f.
gastroduodenal f.
gastroenteric f.

NOTES

fistula *(continued)*
gastrointestinal f.
gastrointestinal-cutaneous f.
gastrojejunocolic f.
gastropleural f.
genitourinary f.
gingival f.
graft-enteric f.
Gross tracheoesophageal f.
hepatic artery-portal vein f.
hepatopleural f.
hepatoportal biliary f.
horseshoe f.
H-type tracheoesophageal f.
iatrogenic arteriovenous f.
ileoduodenal f.
ileosigmoid f.
ileovesical f.
incomplete f.
inflammatory f.
internal lacrimal f.
intersphincteric anal f.
intestinal f.
intracranial arteriovenous f.
intrahepatic arterial-portal f.
intrahepatic A-V f.
intrahepatic spontaneous arterioportal f.
intralabyrinthine f.
intraocular f.
jejunocolic f.
labyrinthine f.
lacrimal f.
lacteal f.
mammary f.
Mann-Bollman f.
mesenteric arteriovenous f.
metroperitoneal f.
mucous f.
oroantral f.
orocutaneous f.
orofacial f.
oronasal f.
pancreatic cutaneous f.
pancreaticopleural f.
pararectal f.
parietal f.
perianal f.
perilymph f.
perilymphatic f.
perineal urinary f.
perineovaginal f.
pharyngocutaneous f.
pilonidal f.
pleurobiliary f.
pleuroesophageal f.
postbiopsy renal A-V f.
postoperative pleurobiliary f.
postradiation f.
posttraumatic pancreatic-cutaneous f.
preauricular f.
primary arteriovenous f.
pseudocystobiliary f.
pulmonary arteriovenous f. (PAF)
radiculomedullary f.
rectal f.
rectolabial f.
rectourethral f.
rectourinary f.
rectovaginal f.
rectovesical f.
rectovestibular f.
rectovulvar f.
renal f.
renogastric f.
respiratory-esophageal f.
retroperitoneal f.
reverse Eck f.
salivary f.
scleral f.
sigmoid cutaneous f.
sigmoidovesical f.
solitary pulmonary arteriovenous f.
spermatic f.
spinal dural arteriovenous f.
splanchnic A-V f.
splenic A-V f.
splenobronchial f.
stercoral f.
subclavian arteriovenous f.
submental f.
suprasphincteric f.
sylvian f.
synovial f.
systemic arteriovenous f.
TE f.
f. test
thigh graft arteriovenous f.
Thiry f.
Thiry-Vella f.
thoracic duct f.
thromboembolic f.
thyroglossal f.
tracheobiliary f.
tracheobronchoesophageal f.
tracheocutaneous f.
tracheoesophageal f. (TEF)
transsphincteric anal f.
traumatic f.
ulcerogenic f.
umbilical f.
urachal f.
ureteral f.
ureterocolic f.
ureterocutaneous f.
ureteroperitoneal f.

ureterouterine f.
ureterovaginal f.
urethrocavernous f.
urethrorectal f.
urethrovaginal f.
urinary f.
urinary-umbilical f.
urinary-vaginal f.
urogenital f.
uteroperitoneal f.
vaginal f.
vasocutaneous f.
Vella f.
venobiliary f.
vesical f.
vesicoacetabular f.
vesicocolic f.
vesicocutaneous f.
vesicoenteric f.
vesicointestinal f.
vesicoovarian f.
vesicorectal f.
vesicosalpingovaginal f.
vesicouterine f.
vesicovaginal f.
vesicovaginorectal f.
vitelline f.

fistular formation

fistulation

artificial f.
spreading f.

fistulectomy

fistulization

cholecystobiliary f.

fistulizing surgery

fistuloenterostomy

fistulography

fistulotomy

choledochoduodenal f.
diathermic f.
endoscopic f.
laying-open f.
Parks method of anal f.
Parks staged f.

fistulous tract

Fite method

fitness for general anesthesia

fitting

five-chamber transverse (5C-T)

five-incision procedure

five-one

f.-o. knee ligament repair
f.-o. reconstruction

five-port fan placement

fixation

adjunctive screw f.
alcohol f.
angled blade plate f.
anomalous f.
f. anomaly
anterior internal f.
anterior metallic f.
anterior plate f.
anterior screw f.
anterior spinal f.
AO external f.
AO rigid f.
AO spinal internal f.
APR cement f.
atlantoaxial rotatory f.
autotrophic f.
axial f.
axis f.
bar bolt f.
Barr open reduction and internal f.
Barr tibial fracture f.
f. base
bicortical screw f.
bifocal f.
bifoveal f.
binocular f.
biologic f.
biphase pin f.
blade plate f.
bolt f.
bone-ingrowth f.
bridge plate f.
brow f.
capsular f.
carbon dioxide f.
catheter f.
central f.
cerclage wire f.
cervical spine internal f.
cervical spine screw-plate f.
chest wall f.
circumalveolar f.
circumferential wire-loop f.
circummandibular f.
circumzygomatic f.
closed reduction and percutaneous f. (CRPF)

NOTES

fixation *(continued)*
cloverleaf condylar-plate f.
Cole tendon f.
complement f.
compression plate f.
condylar screw f.
coracoclavicular screw f.
coracoclavicular suture f.
Cotrel-Dubousset f.
craniofacial f.
crossed f.
f. delay
Denham external f.
dens anterior screw f.
Deverle f.
Dimon-Hughston fracture f.
dorsal wire-loop f.
dynamic compression-plate f.
dynamic condylar-screw f.
eccentric f.
elastic band f.
external pin f.
external spinal f.
eyebrow f.
femoral prosthesis f.
formalin f.
four-point f.
fracture f.
Galveston pelvic f.
Gouffon pin f.
graft f.
greenstick f.
Guyton-Noyes f.
Hackethal intramedullary bouquet f.
half-pin f.
hook f.
hook-plate f.
iliac f.
Ilizarov external f.
ingrowth f.
interference fit f.
intermaxillary f.
internal spinal f.
interosseous wire f.
intestinal f.
intramedullary rod f.
intraosseous f.
Kavanaugh-Brower-Mann f.
Kirschner pin f.
Kirschner wire f.
Kronner external f.
Kyle internal f.
lag screw f.
line of f.
loop f.
lumbar pedicle f.
lumbar spine segmental f.
lumbar spine transpedicular f.
Luque-Galveston f.
Luque loop f.
Luque rod f.
Magerl posterior cervical screw f.
mandibular f.
mandibulomaxillary f.
Matta-Saucedo f.
maxillomandibular f.
McKeever medullary clavicle f.
medial malleolus f.
medullary nail f.
metallic rod f.
microwave f.
monocular f.
multiple-point sacral f.
nail-plate f.
nasomandibular f.
near f.
neutralization plate f.
Nichols sacrospinous f.
f. object
occipitocervical f.
odontoid fracture internal f.
odontoid screw f.
open reduction and internal f.
osseous f.
pedicle screw-rod f.
pedicular f.
pelvic f.
percutaneous f.
phalangeal fracture f.
Phemister acromioclavicular pin f.
pin-and-plaster f.
plate f.
plate-screw f.
f. point
porous ingrowth f.
posterior cervical f.
posterior screw f.
posterior segmental f.
prophylactic skeletal f.
provisional f.
pubic f.
f. reflex
restorative f.
rigid internal f.
rigid plate f.
rod sleeve f.
role f.
sacral pedicle screw f.
sacral spine f.
sacroiliac extension f.
sacroiliac flexion f.
sacrospinous ligament vaginal f.
sacrum fusion screw f.
Schneider f.
scoliotic curve f.
screw f.

screw-and-plate f.
screw-and-wire f.
secondary f.
segmental f.
spinal f.
split f.
spring f.
standard formalin f.
staple f.
static f.
Steinmann pin f.
strut plate f.
sublaminar f.
sulcus f.
suture f.
f. suture technique
f. target
f. technique
tension band f.
transarticular wire f.
transcapitellar wire f.
transiliac rod f.
transpedicular screw-rod f.
transverse f.
TSRH rod f.
tunnel and sling f.
visual f.
white f.
wire loop f.

fixator
f. interne
f. muscle

fixed
f. deformity
f. dose
f. drain pipe urethra
f. lung
f. maintainer space
f. point
f. sediment method
f. subcutaneous dose

fixed-dose
f.-d. analysis
f.-d. patient-controlled analgesia (FDPCA)

fixture
implant f.

fixus

flabby abdomen

flaccida

flaccid extremity

flag flap

flail
f. chest
f. knee

FLAIR
fluid-attenuated inversion recovery
FLAIR image
FLAIR sequence

Flajani operation

FLAK
flow artifact killer
FLAK technique

flame hemorrhage

flame-shaped hemorrhage

flammable anesthetic

Flamm technique

flank
f. approach
f. bone
f. dissection
f. gunshot wound
f. incision
f. incisional hernia
f. mass
f. position

flap
Abbe f.
abdominal fasciocutaneous f.
access f.
advancement of rectal f.
anconeus muscle f.
anterior helical rim free f.
aponeurotic f.
apron f.
arm f.
arterial f.
arterialized f.
artery island f.
Atasoy-Kleinert f.
Atasoy palmar f.
Atasoy triangular advancement f.
Atasoy volar V-Y f.
axial flag f.
axial pattern scalp f.
axillary f.
bicoronal scalp f.
bilateral V-Y Kutler f.
bilobed skin f.
bilobed transposition f.
bipedicle dorsal f.
bladder f.
Blaskovics f.
Boari bladder f.

F

NOTES

flap *(continued)*
Boari-Ockerblad f.
bone f.
brachioradialis f.
bridge pedicle f.
buccal mucosal f.
bulbocavernosus fat f.
buried f.
bursal f.
butterfly f.
Byers f.
cartilage f.
caterpillar f.
cellulocutaneous f.
cervical f.
cheek advancement f.
cheek rotation f.
Chinese f.
cocked-half f.
composite f.
compound f.
f. congestion
conjunctival f.
conjunctivo-Tenon f.
corneal f.
cross f.
crossarm f.
cross-finger f.
cross-leg f.
cross-lip f.
cross-lip pedicle f.
C-shaped scalp f.
cutaneous forearm f.
Cutler-Beard bridge f.
Dandy myocutaneous scalp f.
deep circumflex iliac artery-iliac crest f.
de-epithelialized rectus abdominis muscle f.
delayed f.
deltoid f.
deltopectoral f.
deltoscapular f.
dermal fat-free f.
dermal fat pedicle f.
digastric muscle f.
digital f.
direct f.
distant f.
dorsal cross-finger f.
dorsal rotation f.
dorsal transposition f.
double pedicle TRAM f.
DRAM f.
f. elevation
Eloesser f.
endorectal f.
envelope f.
epaulet f.
equal sagittal f.
Estlander f.
Estlander-Abbe f.
extended shoulder f.
extensor carpi radialis longus f.
extraction f.
fascial f.
fasciocutaneous free f.
fasciocutaneous island f.
fat f.
fibular f.
Filatov f.
Filatov-Gillies f.
finger f.
finger-fillet f.
Fisher advancement f.
flag f.
flat f.
foot first-web f.
foramen ovale f.
forearm f.
forehead f.
foreskin f.
fornix-based f.
free bone f.
free fasciocutaneous f.
free fibular harvest f.
free latissimus dorsi f.
free microsurgical f.
free radial forearm f.
free skin f.
free temporal f.
French f.
full-thickness periodontal f.
fusiform f.
galeal f.
gastrocnemius sliding f.
Gilbert scapular f.
gingival f.
glabellar bilobed f.
glabellar rotation f.
gluteus maximus f.
gracilis muscle f.
f. graft
groin f.
Gunderson conjunctival f.
hemipulp f.
hemitongue f.
hinged corneal f.
horizontal f.
horseshoe-shaped f.
Hughes tarsoconjunctival f.
hypogastric f.
ideal f.
iliac crest free f.
iliac crest osseous f.
iliac crest osteocutaneous f.

iliac crest osteomuscular f.
iliac osteocutaneous free f.
iliofemoral pedicle f.
immediate f.
Imre sliding f.
Indian f.
inferior f.
intercostal f.
interdigitating skin f.
internal oblique osteomuscular f.
interpolated f.
interpolation f.
intimal f.
intraoral f.
inverted skin f.
I-shaped scalp f.
island pedicle scalp f.
island skin f.
Italian f.
jejunal free f.
jump f.
Karapandzic f.
Karydakis f.
Koerner f.
Kutler digital f.
Kutler double lateral
advancement f.
Kutler V-Y f.
lateral cartilage f.
latissimus dorsi island f.
latissimus dorsi muscle f.
latissimus dorsi musculocutaneous f.
latissimus dorsi myocutaneous f.
latissimus-scapular muscle f.
latissimus-serratus muscle f.
limbal-based f.
Limberg f.
lined f.
lingual tongue f.
Linton f.
lip switch f.
liver f.
local muscle f.
local skin f.
lower trapezius f.
lumbrical muscle f.
maple leaf f.
Martius bulbocavernosus fat f.
masseter muscle f.
Mathieu island onlay f.
McCraw gracilis myocutaneous f.
McFarlane skin f.
medial f.
melolabial f.
f. meniscal tear
mesiolabial bilobed transposition f.
microsurgical free f.
microvascular free f.
midline forehead f.
Moberg advancement f.
modified dorsalis pedis
myofascial f.
Morrison neurovascular free f.
mucoperichondrial f.
mucoperiosteal periodontal f.
mucoperiosteal sliding f.
mucosal periodontal f.
multistaged carrier f.
muscle f.
muscle-periosteal f.
musculocutaneous free f.
musculotendinous f.
Mustardé rotational cheek f.
myocutaneous f.
myodermal f.
myofascial f.
nasolabial rotation f.
neck f.
f. necrosis
necrotic f.
neurocutaneous island f.
neurovascular free f.
neurovascular island pedicle f.
nutrient f.
oblique f.
Ockerblad-Boari f.
omental f.
omocervical f.
onlay island f.
open f.
opening f.
f. operation
f. operation cataract
Oriental V-Y f.
osteocutaneous f.
osteomusculocutaneous f.
osteomyocutaneous f.
osteoperiosteal f.
osteoplastic bone f.
palatal f.
palmar advancement f.
palmar cross-finger f.
parabiotic f.
paraexstrophy skin f.

NOTES

F

flap *(continued)*
parascapular f.
parasitic f.
partial-thickness f.
pectoralis major myocutaneous f.
pectoralis myofascial f.
pedicled myocutaneous f.
pedicle groin f.
peg f.
penile island f.
pericardial f.
pericoronal f.
pericranial temporalis f.
perineal f.
periodontal f.
periosteal f.
permanent pedicle f.
pharyngeal f.
f. physiology
platysma myocutaneous f.
Pontén fasciocutaneous f.
postangioplasty intimal f.
posterior f.
proneal island f.
pulp f.
racket-shaped f.
radial-based f.
radial forearm f.
random cutaneous f.
random pattern f.
rectus abdominis free f.
rectus abdominis muscle f.
rectus abdominis musculocutaneous f.
rectus abdominis myocutaneous f.
rectus femoris f.
regional f.
remote pedicle f.
retinal f.
retroauricular free f.
reversal pedicle f.
reverse crossfinger f.
reverse forearm island f.
rhomboid transposition f.
rope f.
rotation f.
rotational f.
rotator f.
Rubens breast f.
saphenous f.
scalping f.
scalp sickle f.
scapular f.
Scardino f.
scleral f.
segmented f.
semilunar f.
serratus anterior muscle f.
sickle f.
simple periodontal f.
single pedicle TRAM f.
skew f.
skin f.
sliding f.
soft-tissue f.
split-thickness periodontal f.
Steichen neurovascular free f.
subcutaneous f.
superior f.
supramalleolar f.
supraorbital pericranial f.
supraperiosteal f.
surgical f.
Tait f.
tarsoconjunctival f.
f. technique
temporalis fascia f.
temporalis muscle f.
tensor fascia femoris f.
tensor fascia lata muscle f.
Tenzel rotational cheek f.
thenar f.
thoracoacromial f.
thoracoepigastric f.
three-square f.
tongue f.
f. tracheostomy
TRAM f.
transposition f.
transverse rectus abdominis muscle f.
trapezius f.
triangular advancement f.
triceps f.
Truc f.
tubed groin f.
tubed pedicle f.
tubularized cecal f.
tumbler f.
tummy tuck f.
turned-down tendon f.
turnover f.
tympanomeatal f.
unipedicled f.
unrepositioned f.
upper trapezius f.
Urbaniak neurovascular free f.
Urbaniak scapular f.
U-shaped scalp f.
Van Lint f.
vascularized free f.
ventrum penis f.
vertical f.
f. viability
visor f.

von Langenbeck bipedicle mucoperiosteal f.
von Langenbeck pedicle f.
V-Y advancement f.
V-Y Kutler f.
waltzed f.
Warren f.
web space f.
Widman f.
winged V double f.
wraparound neurovascular free f.
Zimany bilobed f.

flapping valve syndrome
flap-valve mechanism
flashback protocol
flashlight examination
flash photolysis
flash-point temperature
flask closure
flat
f. abdomen
f. back deformity
f. chest
f. condyloma
f. depressed lesion
f. elevated lesion
f. flap
f. pelvis
f. substrate method
flatfoot
peroneal spastic f.
Flatt
F. classification
F. excision
F. technique
flattened duodenal fold
flatulence
flatulent colic
flatus tube insertion
flava
flavum
Flechsig tract
Fleischmann bursa
Fleischner line
Fletcher rule of irradiation tolerance
flexed
f. incision
f. position
flexibility
flexible
f. collodion
f. endofluoroscopy
f. endoscopic surgery
f. fiberoptic bronchoscopy
f. fiberoptic endoscopy
f. fiberoptic myeloscopy
f. hinge suspension
f. laparoscopy
f. nephroscopy
f. sigmoidoscopy
f. ureteropyeloscopy
flexion
f. in abduction and external rotation
f., abduction, external rotation, extension (fabere)
f. in adduction and internal rotation
f. adduction, internal rotation
f. compression spine injury stabilization
f. crease
f. deformity
f. and extension
f. osteotomy
f. teardrop fracture
flexion-extension
f.-e. arc
f.-e. axis
f.-e. injury
f.-e. maneuver
f.-e. plane
f.-e. reflex
flexion-internal rotational deformity
flexion-rotation-drawer knee instability test
flexor
f. carpi radialis tendon
f. digitorum longus tendon
f. digitorum profundus tendon
f. digitorum superficialis tendon
f. hallucis brevis muscle
f. hallucis brevis tendon
f. hallucis longus tendon
f. pollicis longus abductorplasty
f. pollicis longus tendon
f. sheath
f. tendon anastomosis
f. tendon laceration
f. tendon repair
f. tendon rupture
f. tenosynovectomy
flexorplasty
Bunnell modification of Steindler f.

NOTES

flexorplasty *(continued)*
Eyler f.
Steindler f.
flexor-pronator
f.-p. origin
f.-p. origin release
flexura, pl. **flexurae**
flexural
flexure
anorectal f.
colic f.
colon f.
duodenojejunal f.
fluctuant f.
hepatic f.
iliac f.
inferior f.
lumbar f.
perineal f.
sigmoid f.
splenic f.
superior f.
flicker-fusion
f.-f. frequency technique
f.-f. stimulus
f.-f. threshold
flicker fusion
flickering
f. blockade
f. blockade electrophysiology
Flick-Gould technique
flip-flap
Mathieu-Horton-Devine f.-f.
f.-f. procedure
f.-f. technique
floating
f. forehead operation
f. gallbladder
f. kidney
f. organ
f. rib
f. spleen
floccillation
floccular fossa
flocculation
cephalin-cholesterol f.
limit of f.
Ramon f.
thymol f.
flocculonodular arteriovenous malformation
floor
f. fracture
rectal f.
floor-of-mouth
f.-o.-m. closure
f.-o.-m. lesion
floppy
f. Nissen fundoplication
f. Nissen fundoplication method
f. Nissen fundoplication procedure
f. Nissen fundoplication technique
f. valve syndrome
floppy-type Nissen fundoplication
flora
aerobic f.
bacterial f.
endogenous f.
exogenous f.
GI tract f.
intestinal f.
florid
f. duct lesion
f. hyperplasia
flotation rate
flow
anastomotic f.
f. artifact killer (FLAK)
blood f.
carotid arterial blood f.
cerebral blood f. (CBF)
f. convergence method
f. detection technique
f. direction
Doppler color f.
effective renal blood f.
effective renal plasma f.
endocardial f.
exercise hyperemia blood f.
free f.
fresh gas f. (FGF)
hepatofugal f.
hepatopetal f.
f. interruption technique
intraluminal f.
f. mapping technique
f. misregistration
f. pattern
peak expiratory f.
plug f.
regional cerebral blood f. (rCBF)
f. technique filling
tracheal blood f. (TBF)
tricuspid valve f.
flow-dependent
f.-d. oxygen
f.-d. pressure drop
flower
F. bone
F. dental index
flowmetry
fluorescein f.
laser Doppler f. (LDF)
scanning laser Doppler f.
flow-on gradient-echo image

flow-over vaporizer
floxuridine in hepatic metastasis
fluctuans
myotonia f.
fluctuant
f. abscess
f. flexure
f. mass
fluctuantes
fluctuation test
fluence
instantaneous f.
fluffy cotton-wool exudate
fluid
ascitic f.
f. aspiration
bloody peritoneal f.
body f.
f. bolus
carrier f.
cerebrospinal f. (CSF)
chylous ascitic f.
clear f.
cloudy f.
f. collection
cul-de-sac f.
cytospin collection f.
f. drainage
endolymphatic f.
f. evacuation
extracellular f.
f. extravasation
free peritoneal f.
infused f.
f. loading anesthetic technique
loculation of f.
maintenance f.
f. management
motor oil peritoneal f.
oxygen-carrying resuscitative f.
pancreatic f.
perilymphatic f.
peritoneal cavity f.
pleural f.
prostatic f.
prune-juice peritoneal f.
Rees-Ecker f.
f. replacement
respiratory tract f.
f. resuscitation
resuscitative f.
scolicidal f.
seminal f.
serosal f.
f. shift
subphrenic f.
supraphysiologic f.
synovial f.
turbid peritoneal f.
f. warmer
wound f.
fluid-attenuated
f.-a. inversion recovery (FLAIR)
f.-a. inversion recovery image
fluid-filled sac
fluid-gas exchange
fluitantes
fluke
tissue f.
fluorescein
f. angiography
f. flowmetry
f. fundus angioscopy
f. instillation test
f. string test
fluorescence
f. microscopy
f. polarization method
fluorescent
f. antibody staining technique (FAST)
f. electronic endoscopy
f. optode technology
fluorodeoxyglucose-positron
f.-p. emission tomography
f.-p. emission tomography scanning
fluoroscopic
f. control
f. guidance
f. insertion
f. method
f. placement
f. pushing technique
f. visualization
fluoroscopy
f. beam
biplanar f.
biplane f.
C-arm f.
kV f.
lateral f.
portable C-arm image intensifier f.
rapid scan f.

NOTES

F

fluoroscopy *(continued)*
two-plane f.
video f.
flush-and-bathe technique
flushing technique
flush method
fluximetry
laser Doppler f.
Flynn
F. femoral neck fracture reduction
F. technique
fMRI
functional magnetic resonance imaging
FNA
fine-needle aspiration
FNA biopsy
follicular FNA
Hürthle FNA
indeterminate FNA
nondiagnostic FNA
percutaneous FNA
FNA sample
suspicious FNA
FNH
focal nodular hyperplasia
foaming exudate
focal
f. bleeding point
f. calcification
f. cortical dysplasia
f. DCIS
f. fatty infiltration
f. granulomatous inflammation
f. hemorrhage
f. illumination
f. image point
f. infection
f. nodular hyperplasia (FNH)
f. parenchymal brain lesion
f. peritonitis
f. plane
f. segmental glomerulosclerosis (FSGS)
f. splenic lesion
f. tumor
focus, pl. **foci**
ectopic f.
endometriotic f.
hemorrhage f.
image-space f.
necrotic f.
object-space f.
residual f.
septic f.
f. of tumor
focused
f. abdominal sonography
f. radiation therapy

Föerster operation
fogging retinoscopy
Foix enucleation
fold
adipose f.
alar f.
amniotic f.
anterior axillary f.
aryepiglottic f.
axillary f.
Bartlett nail f.
caval f.
cecal f.
cholecystoduodenocolic f.
circular f.
circulator f.
Douglas f.
duodenojejunal f.
duodenomesocolic f.
epicanthal f.
epigastric f.
falciform retinal f.
fimbriated f.
flattened duodenal f.
gastric f.
gastropancreatic f.
glossoepiglottic f.
glossopalatine f.
Guérin f.
Hasner f.
haustral f.
hepatopancreatic f.
Houston f.
ileocecal f.
incudal f.
inferior duodenal f.
inferior rectal f.
inferior transverse rectal f.
inguinal aponeurotic f.
interureteric f.
Kerckring f.
labioscrotal f.
lacrimal f.
f. of laryngeal nerve
lateral glossoepiglottic f.
lateral nail f.
longitudinal f.
malar f.
mallear f.
median glossoepiglottic f.
mucobuccal f.
nail f.
nasojugal f.
Nélaton f.
palatoglossal f.
palatopharyngeal f.
palmate f.
palpebronasal f.

Passavant f.
pharyngoepiglottic f.
pleuroperitoneal f.
presplenic f.
rectal f.
rectouterine f.
rectovesical f.
retinal f.
right umbilical f.
sacrogenital f.
sacrouterine f.
sacrovaginal f.
sacrovesical f.
salpingopalatine f.
salpingopharyngeal f.
sigmoid f.
spiral f.
sublingual f.
superior duodenal f.
superior rectal f.
synovial f.
tarsal f.
tonsillar f.
transverse palatine f.
transverse rectal f.
transverse vesical f.
Treves f.
triangular f.
urachal f.
ureteric f.
uterosacral f.
uterovesical f.
vascular f.
Vater f.
ventricular f.
vestibular f.
vocal f.

folding
f. larynx
skin f.

Foley
F. operation
F. Y-plasty pyeloplasty
F. Y-V plasty

foliate papilla

Folin and Wu method

follicle maturation stimulation

follicular
f. carcinoma
f. cell
f. cholecystitis
f. cyst
f. epithelium
f. FNA
f. hematoma
f. inflammation
f. lesion
f. neoplasm
f. proliferation

folliculoma

folliculus, pl. **folliculi**

followup
clinical f.
f. data
f. evaluation
f. examination
long-term f.
f. time

Fones
F. method
F. technique

Fontan
F. atriopulmonary anastomosis
F. fenestration closure
F. modification of Norwood procedure
F. operation
F. repair

Fontana
F. canal
F. space
space of F.

Fontana-Masson staining method

Fontan-Baudet procedure

fontanelle
anterior f.
anterolateral f.
bregmatic f.
cranial f.
occipital f.
posterior f.

Fontan-Kreutzer procedure

fonticulus, pl. **fonticuli**

foot
f. deformity
f. first-web flap
f. reticulin method
f. rotation

forage
f. core biopsy
f. procedure

foramen, pl. **foramina**
alveolar foramina
anterior condyloid f.

F

NOTES

foramen *(continued)*
aortic f.
f. of Arnold
blind f.
caroticoclinoid f.
carotid f.
cecal f.
f. compression test
conjugate f.
costotransverse f.
emissary sphenoidal f.
ethmoidal f.
external acoustic f.
Ferrein f.
frontal f.
great f.
Huschke f.
Hyrtl f.
incisive f.
inferior dental f.
infraorbital f.
internal auditory f.
internal neurocranial f.
intervertebral f.
jugular f.
lacerated f.
Luschka and Magendie f.
f. magnum
f. magnum line
malar f.
mandibular f.
mastoid f.
mental f.
Monro f.
Morgagni f.
nasal f.
foramina nervosa
nutrient f.
obturator f.
oculomotor f.
optic f.
f. ovale
f. ovale flap
palatine f.
papillary f.
parietal f.
petrosal f.
pleuroperitoneal f.
posterior condyloid f.
round f.
sacral f.
Scarpa f.
solitary f.
sphenoid emissary f.
sphenopalatine f.
sphenotic f.
stylomastoid f.
supraorbital f.
transverse f.
venous f.
vertebral f.
vertebroarterial f.
Vesalius f.
zygomaticofacial f.
zygomaticoorbital f.
zygomaticotemporal f.

foraminal
f. approach
f. compression test
f. herniation
f. node

foraminalis

foraminotomy

Forbes modification of Phemister graft technique

force
f. application
f. feedback system
f. translation (FTR)

forcé
eccouchement f.
redressement f.

force-couple splint reduction

forced
f. alimentation
f. expiratory capacity
f. expiratory spirogram
f. expiratory time
f. expiratory volume
f. expiratory volume in 1 second (FEV_1)
f. generation test
f. mandatory intermittent ventilation
f. respiration

forced-air
f.-a. warming

forced-eye closure

force-frequency relation

force-length relation

forceps
f. extraction
f. maneuver
f. removal
f. rotation

force-velocity-length relation

force-velocity relation

force-velocity-volume relation

forcing
dynamic end-tidal f.

forcipate

forcipressure

Ford triangulation technique

fore-and-aft suture technique

forearm
f. amputation
anterior f.

deep f.
f. flap
f. fracture
f. graft arteriovenous fistula
f. ischemic exercise test
f. plethysmography
superficial f.
f. supination test

forebrain

forefoot arthroplasty

foregut malformation

forehead flap

forehead-nose position

foreign
f. body
f. body aspiration
f. body carcinogenesis
f. body extraction
f. body loop
f. body management
f. body reaction
f. body removal
f. body response
f. body sclerotomy
f. body trauma
f. body tumorigenesis

forekidney

Forel decussation

forequarter amputation

foreskin
f. flap
f. restoration

Forest-Hastings technique

Forest I, II lesion

forestomach

form
extension f.
face f.
QWB-SA f.

formal
f. celiotomy
f. hemipelvectomy
f. hepatic resection
f. laparotomy
f. method
f. surgical exploration

formaldehyde-induced fluorescence method

formalin-ether sedimentation method

formalin fixation

formatio, pl. **formationes**

formation
abscess f.
adhesion f.
anastomotic stricture f.
anterior synechia f.
antiantibody f.
aspergilloma f.
balloon cell f.
blood vessel f.
bone f.
branching tubule f.
bunion f.
Burnet-Talmadge-Lederberg theory of antibody f.
calculous f.
callous f.
cataract f.
chiasma f.
cloacal f.
clot f.
coagulum f.
colloid f.
colony f.
concept f.
crater f.
cyclops f.
echo f.
excessive callus f.
extracapillary crescent f.
false channel f.
fistular f.
gallstone f.
gender identity f.
germinal center f.
Gothic arch f.
hemostatic plug f.
heterotopic bone f.
identity f.
ileostomy f.
image f.
impulse f.
inflammatory pseudotumor f.
intramembranous f.
keloid f.
kerion f.
ketone body f.
lappet f.
localized plaque f.
mesencephalic reticular f.
micelle f.
midbrain reticular f.
neocartilage f.

NOTES

F

formation *(continued)*
- neointima f.
- osteophyte f.
- pannus f.
- paramedian pontine reticular f.
- periosteal new bone f.
- pontine paramedian reticular f.
- posterior synechia f.
- procallus f.
- pseudoaneurysm f.
- pseudopod f.
- reaction f.
- reticular f.
- root f.
- rouleaux f.
- sac f.
- scar f.
- somite f.
- spur f.
- star f.
- stone granuloma f.
- stricture f.
- struvite crystal f.
- symptom f.
- synechia f.
- trellis f.
- twin f.
- web f.

formocresol pulpotomy

fornix, pl. **fornices**
- anterior vaginal f.
- f. approach
- caliceal f.
- cerebral f.
- conjunctival f.
- pharyngeal f.
- posterior vaginal f.
- f. reformation

fornix-based flap

fortification

fortified topical preparation

forward
- f. coarticulation
- f. head posture
- f. traction test
- f. triangle method
- f. triangle technique

Fosnaugh nail biopsy

fossa, pl. **fossae**
- anterior cranial f.
- axillary f.
- Bichat f.
- Biesiadecki f.
- Broesike f.
- canine f.
- Claudius f.
- crural f.
- Cruveilhier f.
- digastric f.
- duodenojejunal f.
- epigastric f.
- femoral f.
- floccular f.
- gallbladder f.
- Gerdy hyoid f.
- glenoid f.
- greater supraclavicular f.
- Gruber-Landzert f.
- hypophysial f.
- iliac f.
- iliacosubfascial f.
- iliopectineal f.
- incisive f.
- inferior duodenal f.
- infraclavicular f.
- infraduodenal f.
- infraspinous f.
- infratemporal f.
- inguinal f.
- intercondylar f.
- intercondyloid f.
- intrabulbar f.
- ischioanal f.
- ischiorectal f.
- Jobert de Lamballe f.
- Jonnesco f.
- jugular f.
- juxta-auricular f.
- lacrimal sac f.
- Landzert f.
- lesser supraclavicular f.
- Malgaigne f.
- mandibular f.
- mastoid f.
- Merkel f.
- mesentericoparietal f.
- Mohrenheim f.
- Morgagni f.
- mylohyoid f.
- omoclavicular f.
- paraduodenal f.
- parajejunal f.
- pararectal f.
- paravesical f.
- petrosal f.
- piriform f.
- pituitary f.
- popliteal f.
- posterior cranial f.
- preauricular f.
- pterygoid f.
- pterygomaxillary f.
- pterygopalatine f.
- retroduodenal f.
- retromandibular f.
- retromolar f.

Rosenmüller f.
scaphoid f.
sigmoid f.
sphenomaxillary f.
splenic f.
subarcuate f.
subcecal f.
subinguinal f.
sublingual f.
submandibular f.
submaxillary f.
subscapular f.
superior duodenal f.
supramastoid f.
supraspinous f.
supratonsillar f.
supravesical f.
temporal f.
Treitz f.
triangular f.
trochlear f.
umbilical f.
Velpeau f.
vermian f.
Waldeyer f.
zygomatic f.

fossula
petrosal f.

fossulate

Fothergill
F. operation
F. stitch

Fothergill-Donald operation

Fothergill-Hunter operation

Foucher epiphysial injury classification

Fould entropion operation

foundation
anhydrous facial f.
denture f.
facial f.
level f.
f. surface

fountain decussation

four-chamber transverse (4C-T)

four-corner midcarpal fusion

four-cuff technique segmental pressure measurement

four-flap Z-plasty

four-gland hyperplasia

Fourier-acquired steady-state technique (FAST)

four-incision procedure

four-limb Z-plasty

four-maximal breath preoxygenation technique

Fournier
F. disease
F. gangrene
syphiloma of F.

four-part fracture

four-place laminectomy

four-point
f.-p. biopsy
f.-p. fixation

four-port
f.-p. diamond placement
f.-p. method
f.-p. procedure
f.-p. technique

four-quadrant hemorrhoidectomy

four-star exercise program

fourth
f. carpometacarpal joint fracture
f. cranial nerve
f. degree radiation injury
f. lumbar nerve
f. parallel pelvic plane

four-wire trochanter reattachment

fovea, pl. **foveae**
Morgagni f.
pterygoid f.
trochlear f.

foveola, pl. **foveolae**
coccygeal f.

foveolar

Fowler-Philip
F.-P. approach
F.-P. incision

Fowler-Stephens
F.-S. maneuver
F.-S. orchiopexy
F.-S. procedure

Fowles
F. dislocation technique
F. open reduction

Fox-Blazina procedure

Fox operation

fraction
alveolar dead-space f.

fractional
f. area change (FAC)
f. dilation and curettage
f. epidural anesthesia

NOTES

F

fractional *(continued)*
- f. spinal anesthesia
- f. sterilization

fractionated
- f. external beam irradiation
- f. radiation therapy

fractionation
- indicator f.
- f. protocol

fracture
- abduction-external rotation f.
- acetabular rim f.
- acute f.
- agenetic f.
- alveolar process f.
- alveolar socket wall f.
- anatomic f.
- Anderson-Hutchins unstable tibial shaft f.
- angulated f.
- angulation f.
- ankle mortise f.
- anterior column f.
- anterolateral compression f.
- apex f.
- apophysial f.
- arch f.
- articular mass separation f.
- articular pillar f.
- Atkin epiphysial f.
- atlantal f.
- atlas-axis combination f.
- atrophic f.
- avulsion stress f.
- axial loading f.
- axis f.
- axis-atlas combination f.
- backfire f.
- banana f.
- f. band
- Bankart f.
- Barton-Smith f.
- basal neck f.
- basal skull f.
- baseball finger f.
- basilar femoral neck f.
- basilar skull f.
- beak f.
- f. bed
- bedroom f.
- Bennett comminuted f.
- bicondylar T-shaped f.
- bicondylar Y-shaped f.
- bicycle spoke f.
- bimalleolar ankle f.
- birth f.
- f. blister
- blow-in f.
- blow-out f.
- boot-top f.
- Bosworth f.
- both-bone f.
- both-column f.
- bowing f.
- boxer f.
- f. bracing
- bronchial f.
- bucket-handle f.
- buckle f.
- bumper f.
- bunk-bed f.
- burst f.
- butterfly f.
- buttonhole f.
- calcaneal avulsion f.
- calcaneal displaced f.
- f. callus
- capillary f.
- capitate f.
- capitellar f.
- carpal bone stress f.
- carpometacarpal joint f.
- cartwheel f.
- cementum f.
- central f.
- cephalomedullary nail f.
- cerebral palsy pathological f.
- cervical spine f.
- cervicotrochanteric displaced f.
- Chance vertebral f.
- Chaput f.
- chauffeur f.
- chip f.
- chiropractic treatment of f.
- chisel f.
- chondral f.
- circumferential f.
- f. classification
- clavicular birth f.
- clay-shoveler f.
- cleavage f.
- closed-break f.
- closed skull f.
- coccyx f.
- Colles f.
- combined flexion-distraction injury and burst f.
- combined radial-ulnar-humeral f.
- comminuted intraarticular f.
- comminuted orbital f.
- comminuted skull f.
- complete f.
- complex f.
- complicated f.
- compound comminuted f.
- compound skull f.

compressed f.
compression f.
condylar femoral f.
condylar process f.
congenital f.
contrecoup f.
coracoid f.
corner f.
coronal split f.
coronoid process f.
cortical f.
Cotton ankle f.
cough f.
cranial f.
crown f.
crown-root f.
crush f.
crushed eggshell f.
Danis-Weber f.
dashboard f.
dens f.
dentate f.
depressed skull f.
depression f.
de Quervain f.
derby hat f.
Descot f.
diacondylar f.
diametric pelvic f.
diaphysial f.
diastatic skull f.
dicondylar f.
die punch f.
direct f.
f. disease
dishpan f.
dislocation f.
f. dislocation
displaced f.
distal femoral epiphysial f.
distal humeral f.
distal radial f.
distraction of f.
dog-leg f.
dome f.
double f.
Dupuytren f.
Duverney f.
dyscrasic f.
elbow f.
elementary f.
enamel f.
f. en coin
endocrine f.
f. en rave
epicondylar avulsion f.
epiphysial growth plate f.
epiphysial slip f.
epiphysial tibial f.
Essex-Lopresti joint depression f.
explosion f.
expressed skull f.
extension teardrop f.
external orbital f.
extracapsular f.
extraoctave f.
facial f.
fatigue f.
femoral diaphyseal f.
femoral intertrochanteric f.
femoral neck f.
femoral shaft f.
femoral supracondylar f.
fender f.
fetal bone f.
f. fever
fibular f.
fifth metatarsal base f.
fighter f.
finger f.
first carpometacarpal joint f.
fishmouth f.
fissured f.
f. fixation
flexion teardrop f.
floor f.
forearm f.
four-part f.
fourth carpometacarpal joint f.
f. fragment
frontal sinus f.
Gaenslen f.
Galeazzi f.
f. gap
Garden femoral neck f.
glenoid rim f.
Gosselin f.
greater trochanteric femoral f.
greater tuberosity f.
greenstick f.
growing f.
Guérin f.
gunshot f.
Gustilo-Anderson open clavicular f.

F

NOTES

fracture *(continued)*
gutter f.
Hahn-Steinthal f.
hairline f.
hamate tail f.
hangman f.
head-splitting humeral f.
healed f.
healing f.
f. healing
hemicondylar f.
Henderson f.
Hermodsson f.
hickory-stick f.
high-energy f.
Hill-Sachs f.
hip f.
hockey-stick f.
Hoffa f.
Holstein-Lewis f.
hoop stress f.
horizontal maxillary f.
humeral head-splitting f.
humeral physial f.
humeral shaft f.
humeral supracondylar f.
Hutchinson f.
hyoid bone f.
ice skater f.
ileofemoral wing f.
impacted f.
implant f.
impression f.
incomplete compound f.
indirect f.
inflammatory f.
infraction f.
insufficiency f.
intercondylar femoral f.
intercondylar humeral f.
intercondylar tibial f.
internal fixation f.
interperiosteal f.
intertrochanteric femoral f.
intertrochanteric four-part f.
intraarticular proximal tibial f.
intracapsular f.
intraoperative f.
intrauterine f.
inverted-Y f.
ipsilateral acetabular f.
ipsilateral femoral neck f.
ipsilateral femoral shaft f.
ipsilateral pelvic f.
ipsilateral tibial f.
irreducible f.
Jefferson f.
joint depression f.
Jones f.
juxtacortical f.
knee f.
Kocher f.
Kocher-Lorenz fracture
laminar f.
lap seatbelt f.
laryngeal cartilage f.
lateral condylar humeral f.
lateral mass f.
Laugier f.
lead-pipe f.
Le Fort I-III f.
Le Fort fibular f.
Le Fort mandibular f.
Le Fort-Wagstaffe f.
lesser trochanter f.
f. line
linear skull f.
Lisfranc f.
long bone f.
longitudinal f.
loose f.
lorry-driver f.
low-energy f.
lower-extremity f.
low lumbar spine f.
lumbar spine burst f.
lumbosacral junction f.
Maisonneuve fibular f.
malar f.
Malgaigne pelvic f.
malleolar f.
mallet f.
malunited calcaneus f.
malunited forearm f.
malunited radial f.
mandibular body f.
mandibular condyle f.
mandibular ramus f.
mandibular symphysis f.
March f.
marginal ridge f.
maternal f.
maxillary f.
maxillofacial f.
mesiodistal f.
metacarpal neck f.
metaphysial tibial f.
metatarsal f.
midface f.
midfoot f.
midshaft f.
milkman f.
minimally displaced f.
missed f.
Moberg-Gedda f.
molar tooth f.

monomalleolar ankle f.
Monteggia forearm f.
Montercaux f.
Moore f.
Mouchet f.
multangular ridge f.
multilevel f.
multiple f.
multiray f.
nasal f.
nasoorbital f.
navicular f.
naviculocapitate f.
neck f.
neoplastic f.
neurogenic f.
neuropathic f.
nightstick f.
nonarticular distal radial f.
noncontiguous f.
nondisplaced f.
nonphysial f.
nonrotational burst f.
nonunion f.
nonunited f.
nutcracker f.
oblique f.
obturator avulsion f.
occipital condyle f.
occult f.
odontoid condyle f.
odontoid neck f.
olecranon f.
one-part f.
open-book f.
open-break f.
open skull f.
orbital blow-out f.
orbital floor f.
orbital rim f.
orbital wall f.
osteochrondral slice f.
osteoporotic f.
outlet strut f.
pacemaker lead f.
Pais f.
paratrooper f.
patellar sleeve f.
pathologic f.
Pauwels f.
pedicle f.
pelvic avulsion f.
pelvic ring f.
pelvic straddle f.
penetrating f.
periarticular f.
periprosthetic f.
peritrochanteric f.
petrous pyramid f.
phalangeal diaphysial f.
physial f.
Piedmont f.
pillion f.
pillow f.
pilon ankle f.
ping-pong f.
pisiform f.
plafond f.
plaque f.
plastic bowing f.
pond f.
porcelain f.
Posada f.
posterior arch f.
posterior column f.
posterior element f.
posterior ring f.
posterior wall f.
postirradiation f.
postoperative f.
Pott ankle f.
profundus artery f.
pronation-abduction f.
pronation-eversion f.
proximal femoral f.
proximal humeral f.
proximal tibial metaphysial f.
pyramidal f.
radial head f.
radial neck f.
radial styloid f.
f. reduction
f. repair
reverse Barton f.
reverse Colles f.
reverse Monteggia f.
rib f.
ring f.
ring-disrupting f.
Rolando f.
roof f.
root f.
rotation f.
rotational burst f.

F

NOTES

fracture *(continued)*
sacral f.
sacroiliac f.
sacrum f.
sagittal slice f.
Salter I-VI f.
scaphoid f.
scotty-dog f.
seatbelt f.
secondary f.
segmental f.
Segond f.
sentinel spinous process f.
SER-IV f.
shaft f.
shear f.
Shepherd f.
short oblique f.
sideswipe elbow f.
simple skull f.
single f.
f. site
skier f.
Skillern f.
skull f.
sleeve f.
slice f.
slot f.
Smith f.
spinal compression f.
spine f.
spinous process f.
spiral oblique f.
splintered f.
split f.
split-heel f.
splitting f.
spontaneous f.
sprain f.
sprinter f.
f. stabilization
stable burst f.
stairstep f.
stellate skull f.
Stieda f.
straddle f.
stress f.
strut f.
subcapital f.
subperiosteal f.
subtrochanteric femoral f.
supination-adduction f.
supination-eversion f.
supination-external rotation IV f.
supracondylar humeral f.
supracondylar Y-shaped f.
surgical neck f.
T f.
talar avulsion f.
talar neck f.
talar osteochondral f.
tarsal bone f.
T-condylar f.
teacup f.
teardrop f.
temporal bone f.
tension f.
testis f.
thoracic spine f.
thoracolumbar burst f.
thoracolumbar spine f.
three-part f.
through-and-through f.
thrower f.
tibial bending f.
tibial condyle f.
tibial diaphysial f.
tibial open f.
tibial plafond f.
tibial plateau f.
tibial shaft f.
tibial triplane f.
tibial tuberosity f.
Tillaux-Chaput f.
Tillaux-Kleiger f.
toddler f.
tongue f.
tooth f.
torsional f.
torus f.
trabecular bone f.
tracheal f.
traction f.
trampoline f.
transcaphoid f.
transcapitate f.
transcervical femoral f.
transchondral f.
transcondylar f.
transepiphyseal f.
transhamate f.
transiliac f.
translational f.
transsacral f.
transscaphoid dislocation f.
transtriquetral f.
transverse comminuted f.
transverse facial f.
transversely oriented endplate compression f.
transverse maxillary f.
transverse process f.
trapezium f.
traumatic f.
trimalleolar ankle f.
triplane tibial f.

tripod f.
triquetral f.
trophic f.
tuft f.
two-part f.
type I, II, III, IIIA, IIIB, IIIC open f.
type C pelvic ring f.
ulnar f.
uncinate process f.
undisplaced f.
unicondylar f.
unimalleolar f.
unstable f.
ununited f.
vertebral body f.
vertebral stable burst f.
vertebral wedge compression f.
vertebra plana f.
vertical shear f.
vertical tooth f.
Volkmann f.
wagon-wheel f.
Wagstaffe f.
Walther f.
wedge compression f.
wedge-shaped uncomminuted tibial plateau f.
western boot in open f.
willow f.
Wilson f.
Y f.
Y-T f.
zygomatic arch f.
zygomatic maxillary complex f.
zygomaticomaxillary f.

fracture-dislocation
atlantoaxial f.-d.
Bennett f.-d.
carpometacarpal f.-d.
Galeazzi f.-d.
Lisfranc f.-d.
pedicolaminar f.-d.
perilunate f.-d.
posterior f.-d.
f.-d. reduction
tarsometatarsal f.-d.
thoracolumbar spine f.-d.
tibial plateau f.-d.
transcapitate f.-d.
transhamate f.-d.
transtriquetral f.-d.
unstable f.-d.
volar plate arthroplasty technique f.-d.

fragilis

fragment
articular f.
avascular f.
avulsed f.
bone f.
bony f.
butterfly fracture f.
capital f.
catheter f.
caudal f.
cephalad f.
chondral f.
cortical f.
disk f.
distal f.
f. E
extruded disk f.
fracture f.
free disk f.
free-floating cartilaginous f.
hinged f.
Hoskins razor blade f.
hypervascular f.
loose f.
metallic f.
osteochondral f.
placental f.
residual f.
retained placental f.
sternal f.
trapdoor f.
tuberosity f.
wedge-shaped uncomminuted f.

fragmentation
elastic-fiber f.
electrohydraulic f.
graft f.
laser-induced f.
stone f.
ultrasonic f.

Fraley syndrome

frame application

frameless
f. stereotactic guidance
f. stereotaxy

framework
implant f.

NOTES

Franceschetti
F. coreoplasty operation
F. corepraxy operation
F. deviation operation
F. keratoplasty operation
F. pupil deviation operation
F. syndrome
frank
f. dislocation
f. hemorrhage
f. intrabiliary rupture
f. necrosis
f. nonsurgical perineal autodilation
f. perforation
f. permanent gastrotomy technique
f. procedure
f. pus
f. rigors
f. technique of dilation
Fränkel
F. neurologic deficit classification
F. white line
Frankenhäuser ganglion
Franke tabes operation
Frankfort
F. horizontal light line
F. horizontal plane
F. mandibular incisor angle
F. mandibular plane angle
Frank-Starling relation
Franz-O'Rahilly classification
frappage therapy
Fraser syndrome
Fraunfelder no-touch technique
Fraunhofer line
Frazier
F. incision
F. suction
Frazier-Spiller
F.-S. operation
F.-S. rhizotomy
FRC
functional residual capacity
freckle
Hutchinson f.
Fredet-Ramstedt
F.-R. operation
F.-R. procedure
F.-R. pyloromyotomy
Fredrickson hyperlipoproteinemia classification
Fredrickson-Levy-Lees classification
free
f. air
f. bone flap
f. disk fragment
f. fasciocutaneous flap
f. fat graft
f. fibular harvest flap
f. flap transfer
f. flow
f. fragment disk
f. fragment herniation
f. gastric margin
f. hepatic venous pressure
f. latissimus dorsi flap
f. ligature suture technique
f. microsurgical flap
f. node
f. peritoneal fluid
f. radial forearm flap
f. skin flap
f. temporal flap
f. tenia
f. tenotomy
f. tissue transfer
free-beam coagulation
Freebody-Bendall-Taylor fusion technique
free-floating
f.-f. canalith
f.-f. cartilaginous fragment
f.-f. particle
freehand
f. method
f. suturing technique
Freeman calcaneal fracture classification
Freer dissection
free-root insertion technique
freeway space
freeze-cleave method
freeze-etch method
freeze-fracture-etch method
freezing
gastric f.
f. point
frena (*pl. of* frenum)
frenal
French
F. flap
F. fracture technique
F. lateral closing wedge osteotomy
F. method
F. plane
F. position
F. scale
F. supracondylar fracture operation
French-American-British (FAB)
F.-A.-B. classification
frenectomy
frenoplasty
frenotomy
frenulectomy
frenuloplasty
frenulum, pl. **frenula**

lingual f.
synovial frenula
frenum, pl. **frena**
Morgagni f.
synovial f.
Frenzel maneuver
frequency
f. modulation
spectral edge f. (SEF)
wavelength f.
frequency-difference interferential current therapy
frequency-duration index
fresh
f. blood clot
f. extrapelvic ovarian transplantation
f. frozen plasma
f. gas flow (FGF)
f. tissue allocation
f. wound
Fresnel membrane
fretum, pl. **freta**
Freund
F. anomaly
F. operation
Frey
F. pancreaticojejunostomy
F. syndrome
friable clot
Friberg microsurgical agglutination test
Fricke operation
friction
intraabdominal f.
f. knot
Friedenwald-Guyton operation
Friedenwald operation
Friede operation
Friedewald approximation
Fried-Green foot procedure
Fried-Hendel tendon technique
fringe
Richard f.
synovial f.
frogleg
f. lateral projection
f. position
Froimson
F. procedure
F. technique
Froimson-Oh repair
frondlike filling defect
Fronet fasciotomy
frons
frontal
f. abscess
f. arteriovenous malformation
f. artery
f. bone
f. border
f. branch
f. cortical approach
f. craniotomy
f. crest
f. eminence
f. foramen
f. gyrectomy
f. lobotomy
f. margin
f. notch
f. plane
f. plane correction
f. projection
f. recess
f. section
f. sinus
f. sinus cavity
f. sinus fracture
f. sinus mucocele
f. sinus septoplasty
f. squama
f. suture
f. triangle
f. tuber
f. vein
f. x-ray
f. x-ray view
frontale
frontales
frontalis
f. muscle
f. sling technique
frontalium
frontoanterior position
frontoethmoidal
f. mucocele
f. suture
frontoethmoidalis
frontoethmoidectomy
frontolacrimalis
frontolateral laryngectomy
frontomalar
frontomaxillaris
frontomaxillary suture

NOTES

F

frontonasal
f. duct
f. suture
frontonasalis
frontonasomaxillary osteotomy
frontooccipital
frontoorbital osteotomy
frontoparietal
f. arteriovenous malformation
f. suture
frontopontine tract
frontoposterior position
frontosphenoidal process
frontosphenoid suture
frontotemporal
f. approach
f. craniotomy
f. tract
frontotemporale
frontotransverse position
frontozygomatica
frontozygomatic suture
Froriep induration
Frost
F. procedure
F. stitch
F. suture technique
frosted liver
Frost-Lang operation
Frouin
quadrangulation of F.
frown incision
frozen
f. section (FS)
f. section analysis
f. section diagnosis
f. section method
Frykman
F. distal radius fracture classification
F. radial fracture classification
FS
frozen section
FSGS
focal segmental glomerulosclerosis
FTR
force translation
Fuchs
F. canthorrhaphy operation
F. iris bombe transfixation operation
F. position
Fukala operation
Fukunaga-Hayes unbiased jackknife classification
fulcrum line
Fulford procedure
fulgurant
fulgurating
fulguration
electrical f.
electrosurgical f.
endoscopic f.
nephroscopic f.
full
f. axillary dissection
f. cast restoration
f. diagnostic laparoscopy
f. extension
f. mastopexy
f. shoulder preparation
full-body cutaneous examination
fullness
epigastric f.
full-spine radiographic examination
full-thickness
f.-t. burn
corneal f.-t.
f.-t. periodontal flap
f.-t. rectal aspiration
fulminans
fulminant
f. hepatic failure (FHF)
f. hepatitis
f. hyperpyrexia
function
atrioventricular nodal f.
autonomous f.
bowel f.
effective f.
electrophysiologic f.
gait f.
graft f.
hemodynamic f.
hepatocellular f.
liver f.
mucociliary f.
neorectal f.
neurologic f.
preoperative liver f.
pulmonary f.
renal f.
sinoatrial nodal f.
functional
f. activation PET scanning
f. capacity classification
f. capacity evaluation
f. castration
f. contracture
f. electrical stimulation
f. endoscopic sinus surgery (FESS)
f. intestinal failure
f. lymph node dissection
f. magnetic resonance imaging (fMRI)
f. neck dissection

f. neuromuscular stimulation
f. orthodontic therapy
f. parenchyma
f. prepubertal castration syndrome
f. problem
f. renal tissue
f. repair
f. residual capacity (FRC)
f. sphincter
f. stereotactic neurosurgery
f. technique
f. veloplasty

functioning allograft
fundal plication
fundament
fundectomy
fundi (*pl. of* fundus)
fundiform ligament
fundoplasty
anterior f.
Belsey IV f.
270-degree laparoscopic posterior f.
esophagogastric f.
Gomez f.
Hill f.
laparoscopic esophagogastric f.
Nissen f.
posterior f.
Thal f.
Thal-Nissen f.
Toupet f.

fundoplication
Belsey Mark II, IV f.
Belsey Mark IV 240-degree f.
Belsey partial f.
Belsey two-thirds wrap f.
Collis-Nissen f.
Dor anterior f.
endoscopic f.
floppy Nissen f.
floppy-type Nissen f.
Guarner wrap f.
Heller myotomy with Dor f.
herniated f.
high-resistance f.
Hill gastropexy f.
Hunter technique for Toupet f.
intrathoracic Nissen f.
laparoscopic anterior partial f.
laparoscopic esophagogastroplasty with Nissen f.
laparoscopic Nissen f. (LNF)
laparoscopic Nissen and Toupet f.
low-resistance f.
microlaparoscopic Nissen f.
modified Belsey f.
Nissen 360-degree wrap f.
Nissen-Rossetti f.
open f.
open Nissen f. (ONF)
redo f.
Rossetti modification of Nissen f.
slipped Nissen f.
Thal f.
total f.
Toupet hemifundoplication f.
transthoracic Nissen f.
twisted f.
uncut Collis-Nissen f.
videoscopic f.

fundus, pl. **fundi**
f. gland
f. microscopy
f. rotation gastroplasty

funduscopic examination
fundusectomy
fungal
f. antibody
f. organism
f. overgrowth
f. pancreatic infection
f. pathogen
f. sinusitis
f. species
f. superinfection

fungating
f. mass
f. sore
f. tumor

fungemia
fungous infection
fungus, pl. **fungi**
pancreatic f.

funic reduction
funicular
f. excision
f. graft
f. inguinal hernia
f. process

funiculopexy
funiculus, pl. **funiculi**
funnel
f. chest deformity
f. stitch

NOTES

F

funnelization of metaphysis
funnel-shaped pelvis
furcalis
furcal nerve
furcation
- f. canal
- denuded f.
- invaded f.
- root f.

Furlow-Fisher modification of Virag 1 operation
Furnas-Haq-Somers technique
Furniss anastomosis
furrier's suture technique
furrow
- corneal marginal f.
- digital f.
- mentolabial f.

furrowing
fusiform
- f. aneurysm
- f. dilatation
- f. excision
- f. flap

fusing point
fusion
- Adkins spinal f.
- Albee spinal f.
- amplitude of f.
- Anderson ankle f.
- ankle f.
- anterior cervical diskectomy and f.
- anterior lumbar vertebral interbody f.
- anterior spinal f.
- f. area
- atlantoaxial f.
- atlantooccipital f.
- autograft f.
- Bailey-Badgley cervical spine f.
- binaural f.
- binocular f.
- Blair f.
- Bosworth spinal f.
- Bradford f.
- Brooks-type f.
- calcaneotibial f.
- central f.
- centric f.
- cervical interbody f.
- cervical spine posterior f.
- Chandler hip f.
- Charnley compression-type knee f.
- Chuinard-Peterson ankle f.
- clothespin H spinal f.
- Cloward anterior spinal f.
- Cloward back f.
- color f.
- Coltart calcaneotibial f.
- commissural f.
- f. complex
- convex f.
- Copeland-Howard scapulothoracic f.
- Davis f.
- Dewar posterior cervical f.
- DIP f.
- distal interphalangeal f.
- distal tibiofibular f.
- dowel spinal f.
- endoscopic spinal f.
- extraarticular hip f.
- extraarticular subtalar f.
- eyelid f.
- facet f.
- f. faculty
- f. fascia
- first-grade f.
- flicker f.
- four-corner midcarpal f.
- Gallie spinal f.
- Gallie subtalar ankle f.
- Glissane ankle f.
- f. grade
- Hall facet f.
- Harris-Smith cervical f.
- Henry-Geist spinal f.
- H-graft f.
- Hibbs-Jones spinal f.
- Horwitz-Adams ankle f.
- f. implantation
- interbody spinal f.
- interfacet wiring and f.
- intertransverse f.
- intraarticular knee f.
- joint f.
- Kellogg-Speed lumbar spinal f.
- King intraarticular hip f.
- knee f.
- labial f.
- Langenskiöld f.
- lateral f.
- long segment spinal f.
- lower cervical spine f.
- lumbar spinal f.
- lumbar spine f.
- lumbar vertebral interbody f.
- lumbosacral f.
- lunotriquetral f.
- motor f.
- müllerian duct f.
- naviculocuneiform f.
- f. nonunion rate
- occipitocervical f.
- pantalar f.
- f. peptide
- peripheral f.

posterior cervical f.
posterior-interbody lumbar spinal f.
posterior-lateral lumbar spinal f.
posterior lumbar interbody f. (PLIF)
posterior spinal f.
posterolateral interbody f.
posterolateral lumbosacral f.
radiolunate f.
radioscaphoid f.
f. reflex
robertsonian f.
Robinson cervical spine f.
root f.
sacral spine f.
scaphocapitate f.
scapulothoracic f.
second-grade f.
selective thoracic spine f.
sensory f.
short segment spinal f.
Simmons cervical spine f.
single-level spinal f.
f. in situ
in situ spinal f.
Smith-Petersen sacroiliac joint f.
Smith-Robinson anterior f.
Smith-Robinson cervical f.
Smith-Robinson interbody f.
Soren ankle f.
spinal f.
splenogonadal f.
Stamm procedure for intraarticular hip f.
f. stiffness
symmetric vertebral f.
talocalcaneal f.
talonavicular f.
f. technique
third-grade f.
thoracic facet f.
thoracic spinal f.
tibiofibular f.
tibiotalar f.
tibiotalocalcaneal f.
tissue f.
trapeziometacarpal f.
triscaphe f.
two-stage hip f.
upper cervical spine f.
urethrohymenal f.
vertebral f.
Watson scaphotrapeziotrapezoidal f.
f. welding
White posterior ankle f.
whole-arm f.
Wilson ankle f.
Wiltberger f.
Wiltse bilateral lateral f.
Winter convex f.

fusion-free position

Futcher line

NOTES

GA
general anesthesia
Gabastou hydraulic method
Gaenslen
G. fracture
G. split-heel incision
G. split-heel technique
Gail
G. model
G. model of breast cancer risk prediction
gait function
galactocele
galactography
galactophori
galactophorous
g. canal
g. duct
Galanti-Giusti colorimetric method
Galbiati bilateral fetal ischiopubiotomy
galea
galeal flap
Galeati gland
galeatomy
Galeazzi
G. fracture
G. fracture-dislocation
G. patellar operation
Galen
G. anastomosis
G. nerve
galenic
g. preparation
g. venous malformation
gallamine triethiodide
gallbladder
body of g.
calcified g.
calculous g.
g. calculus
g. cancer
g. carcinoma
g. colic
distended g.
g. distention
g. duplication
g. ectopia
g. ejection rate
floating g.
g. fossa
g. neck
g. perforation
g. plate
porcelain g.
stasis g.
g. wall abscess
gallbladder-vena cava line
gall duct
galli
Gallie
G. atlantoaxial fusion technique
G. operation
G. procedure
G. spinal fusion
G. subtalar ankle fusion
G. transplant
G. wiring technique
gallinaginis
gallstone
g. colic
g. disease
g. formation
g. ileus
g. migration
g. pancreatitis
silent g.
GALT
gut-associated lymphoid tissue
galvanic stimulation
galvanocautery
galvanosurgery
Galveston
G. pelvic fixation
G. technique
Gambee suture technique
gamekeeper thumb dislocation
gamete
g. intrafallopian tube transfer (GIFT)
g. manipulation
g. micromanipulation
Gamgee tissue
gamma
g. irradiation
g. loop disorder
g. probe localization
g. thalamotomy
gammagraphy
gamma-probe radiolocalization
Gamna-Gandy body
ganglia (*pl. of* ganglion)
ganglial tissue
gangliated
g. cord
g. nerve
gangliectomy
gangliocytic paraganglionoma of the duodenum
gangliocytoma

ganglioformis
ganglioglioma
gangliolysis
percutaneous radiofrequency g.
ganglioma
intracerebral g.
ganglion, pl. **ganglia**
aberrant g.
Acrel g.
Andersch g.
aorticorenal g.
Arnold g.
Auerbach g.
auricular g.
basal g.
g. blockage
g. blocker
Bock g.
carotid g.
celiac g.
cervicothoracic g.
ciliary g.
coccygeal g.
cochlear g.
g. cyst
dorsal root g.
Ehrenritter g.
episcleral g.
Frankenhäuser g.
gasserian g.
geniculate g.
glossopharyngeal g.
hypogastric g.
g. impar block
inferior cervical g.
inferior mesenteric g.
intermediate g.
intervertebral g.
intracranial g.
jugular g.
lacrimal g.
Laumonier g.
Lee g.
Lobstein g.
Ludwig g.
lumbar g.
Meckel g.
nasociliary g.
nodose g.
oculomotor g.
optic g.
otic g.
parasympathetic g.
paravertebral g.
pelvic g.
petrosal g.
phrenic g.
prevertebral g.
pterygopalatine g.
Remak g.
renal g.
Ribes g.
sacral g.
Scarpa g.
Schacher g.
semilunar g.
solar g.
sphenopalatine g.
spinal g.
spiral g.
splanchnic g.
stellate g.
sublingual g.
submandibular g.
submaxillary g.
superior cervical g.
superior mesenteric g.
thoracic g.
trigeminal g.
vertebral g.
vestibular g.
Vieussens g.
Walther g.
ganglionares
ganglionated
ganglionectomy
dorsal root g.
Meckel sphenopalatine g.
sphenopalatine g.
superior cervical g.
ganglioneuroblastoma
ganglioneuroma
ganglioneuromatosis
diffuse transmural g.
ganglionic
g. blockade
g. branch
ganglionostomy
gangrene
appendiceal g.
arteriosclerotic g.
cold g.
cutaneous g.
decubital g.
diabetic g.
dry g.
embolic g.
emphysematous g.
Fournier g.
gas g.
hemorrhagic g.
hot g.
Meleney g.
moist g.
nosocomial g.
Pott g.

pressure g.
primary g.
progressive bacterial synergistic g.
secondary g.
static g.
thrombotic g.
traumatic g.
venous g.
wet g.
white g.

gangrenosum

gangrenous

g. appendicitis
g. cholecystitis
g. granulomatous inflammation
g. hernia

Ganley technique

gantry rotation

Ganzfeld stimulation

gap

Bochdalek g.
fracture g.
interincisor g.

Garceau

G. cheilectomy
G. tendon technique

garden

G. femoral neck fracture
G. femoral neck fracture classification
g. spade deformity

Gardner

G. meningocele repair
G. operation

Garré

sclerosing osteomyelitis of G.

Garrett orientation line

Gartland

G. humeral supracondylar fracture classification
G. procedure
G. Universal radial fracture classification

Gartner

G. canal
G. duct

Gärtner method

gas

g. abscess
anesthetic g.
g. anesthetic
arterial blood g.
g. chromatography
g. chromatography-mass spectrometry
g. clearance method
g. collection
g. contamination
g. density line
g. embolism
g. emission
g. endarterectomy
g. exchange
extraluminal g.
extravasation g.
g. gangrene
g. incontinence
inspired g.
g. insufflation
g. isotope ratio mass spectrometry
laparoscopic g.
nonanesthetic g.
partial pressure of CO_2 g.
serial blood g.
g. sterilization
venous blood g.
xenon g.

gaseous

g. cholecystitis
g. decompression
g. dilatation
g. distention
g. laparoscopy
g. laparoscopy method
g. laparoscopy procedure
g. laparoscopy technique

gas-fluid exchange

gas-forming

g.-f. liver abscess
g.-f. pyogenic liver infection

Gaskell bridge

gasless

g. endoscopic thyroidectomy
g. laparoscopic approach
g. laparoscopic hysterectomy
g. laparoscopy
g. laparoscopy method
g. laparoscopy procedure
g. laparoscopy technique

gas-producing streptococcal infection

gasserectomy

gasserian

g. ganglion

NOTES

G

gasserian *(continued)*
- g. ganglion block
- g. ganglion blockade

gastrectasis

gastrectomy
- Billroth I, II g.
- Billroth I partial g.
- curative radical total g.
- distal g.
- distal with excision of ulcer g.
- esophagoproximal g.
- hand-assisted laparoscopic g.
- high subtotal g.
- Hofmeister g.
- Horsley g.
- Japanese-style g.
- limited g.
- Maki pylorus-preserving g.
- near-total g.
- palliative total g.
- pancreatic-preserving total g.
- partial g. (PG)
- Pólya g.
- proximal g.
- pylorus-preserving g. (PPG)
- radical g.
- radical total g.
- segmental g.
- g. specimen
- standard D1 g.
- standardized curative radical total g.
- subtotal g.
- total g. (TG)
- video-assisted g.

gastric
- g. accommodation test
- g. adenocarcinoma
- g. angioma
- g. antrum
- g. area
- g. arteriovenous malformation
- g. artery
- g. atony
- g. atrophy
- g. balloon implantation
- g. band
- g. bed
- g. bed metastasis
- g. branch
- g. bulge
- g. bypass
- g. bypass procedure (GBP)
- g. bypass surgery
- g. calculus
- g. canal
- g. cancer
- g. carcinoma
- g. cardia
- g. chloric acid
- g. coin removal
- g. compression
- g. cuff
- g. cytology
- g. decompression
- g. devascularization
- g. dilation
- g. distention
- g. duplication
- g. duplication cyst
- g. electrical stimulation
- g. emptying
- g. emptying procedure (GEP)
- g. epithelial cell infiltration
- g. epithelium
- g. fistula
- g. fluid aspiration
- g. fold
- g. foreign body
- g. freezing
- g. fundus wrap
- g. gland
- g. hemorrhage
- g. hernia
- g. impression
- g. infection
- g. insufflation
- g. leiomyoma resection
- g. loop bypass
- g. malignancy
- g. MALT lymphoma
- g. margin
- g. mass
- g. mucosa
- g. mucosal barrier
- g. mucosal hypercarbia
- g. mucosal pattern classification
- g. mucosal pH
- g. non-Hodgkin lymphoma
- g. pacemaker region
- g. patch esophagoplasty
- g. perforation
- g. perforation peritonitis
- g. pit
- g. polypectomy
- g. pouch
- g. pressure
- g. pull-through procedure
- g. pull-up
- g. pull-up procedure
- g. reduction surgery
- g. reflux
- g. remnant
- g. residue examination
- g. rupture
- g. serosa

g. stapling
g. stromal tumor
g. stump carcinoma
g. tonometry
g. tube esophagoplasty
g. ulcer
g. ulceration
g. vagotomy
g. valve tightening
g. valve tightening method
g. valve tightening procedure
g. valve tightening technique
g. variceal bleeding
g. vein
g. vessel
g. volvulus
g. wall
g. wrap (GW)
gastrica
gastricae
gastrici
gastricus
gastrinoma
gastrin secretion
gastris
gastritis
phlegmonous g.
gastroanastomosis
gastrocardiac
gastrocele
gastrocnemii
gastrocnemius sliding flap
gastrocolic
g. fistula
g. ligament
g. omentum
gastrocolicum
gastrocolostomy
gastrocutaneous fistula
gastrocystoplasty
gastrodiaphragmatic ligament
gastroduodenal
g. anastomosis
g. artery
g. complication
g. fistula
g. mucosa
g. mucosal protection
g. orifice
gastroduodenalis
gastroduodenopancreatectomy
gastroduodenoscopy
gastroduodenostomy
Billroth I g.
Jaboulay g.
vagotomy and antrectomy with g.
gastroendoscopy
gastroenteric fistula
gastroenteroanastomosis
gastroenterocolostomy
gastroenterologist
gastroenteropancreatic (GEP)
gastroenteroplasty
gastroenteroptosis
gastroenterostomy
Balfour g.
Billroth I, II g.
Braun-Jaboulay g.
Courvoisier g.
Finney g.
Heineke-Mikulicz g.
Hofmeister g.
g. intussusception
laparoscopic g.
percutaneous g.
Pólya g.
prophylactic g.
Roux g.
Roux-en-Y g.
Schoemaker g.
short-limb Roux-en-Y g.
side-to-side g.
g. stoma
transomental posterior g.
truncal vagotomy and g.
Von Haberer g.
Wölfler g.
gastroenterotomy
gastroepiploic
g. arcade
g. artery
g. vein
gastroesophageal
g. hernia
g. junction
g. reflux disease (GERD)
g. variceal plexus
g. vestibule
gastroesophagostomy
gastrogastrostomy
gastrogavage
gastrohepatic
g. ligament
g. omentum

NOTES

G

gastroileac augmentation
gastroileostomy
gastrointestinal (GI)
g. anastomosis (GIA)
g. bleeding
g. carcinoma
g. complication
g. condition
g. content
g. continuity
g. endoscopy
g. endothelium
g. fistula
g. infection
g. lesion
g. malignancy
g. metastasis
g. problem
G. Quality of Life Index (GIQLI)
g. resection
g. stoma
g. surgery
g. tract
g. ulceration
gastrointestinal-associated lymphoid tissue
gastrointestinal-cutaneous fistula
gastrojejunal
g. anastomosis
g. loop obstruction syndrome
gastrojejunocolic fistula
gastrojejunostomy
antecolic long-loop isoperistaltic g.
Billroth II g.
compression button g.
loop g.
partial inferior retrocolic end-to-side g.
partial superior retrocolic end-to-side g.
percutaneous endoscopic g.
prophylactic g.
retrocolic end-to-side g.
Roux-en-Y g.
total retrocolic end-to-side g.
gastrolavage
gastrolienale
gastrolienal ligament
gastrolith
gastrolithiasis
gastrolysis
gastromelus
gastronesteostomy
gastroomental
g. artery
g. node
gastropancreatic
g. fold
g. vagovagal reflex
gastropancreaticae
gastroparesis
postvagotomy g.
gastropathy
indomethacin-induced g.
gastropexy
anterior g.
Belsey Mark IV g.
belt loop g.
Boerema anterior g.
circumcostal g.
Hill posterior g.
incisional g.
laparoscopic-assisted g.
percutaneous anterior g.
posterior diaphragmatic g.
T-fastener g.
T-tack g.
gastrophrenic
g. anchorage
g. ligament
gastrophrenicum
gastroplasty
adjustable ring g.
Albert-Lembert g.
Collis g.
Collis-Nissen g.
Eckhout vertical g.
fundus rotation g.
Gomez horizontal g.
greater curvature banded g.
hand-assisted laparoscopic vertical-banded g.
horizontal g.
Kuzmak g.
laparoscopic g.
Laws g.
layer-to-layer g.
Mason vertical banded g.
O'Leary lesser curvature g.
open vertical banded g.
silicone elastomer ring vertical g.
Stamm g.
tubular vertical g.
unbanded g.
V-banded g.
vertical banded g. (VBG)
vertical ring g. (VRG)
vertical Silastic ring g.
V-Y g.
gastropleural fistula
gastroplication
gastropneumonic
gastroptosis
gastroptyxis

gastropulmonary
gastropylorectomy
gastropyloric
gastrorrhagia
gastrorrhaphy
gastrorrhexis
gastroschisis
gastroscopic
gastroscopy
high-magnification g.
infrared transillumination g.
gastrosphincteric pressure gradient
gastrosplenic
g. ligament
g. omentum
gastrosplenicum
gastrostaxis
gastrostenosis
gastrostogavage
gastrostolavage
gastrostomy
Beck g.
button one-step g.
Depage-Janeway g.
drainage g.
dual percutaneous endoscopic g.
endoscopic g.
feeding g.
g. feeding
Gauderer-Ponsky-Izant PEG g.
Gauderer-Ponsky PEG g.
Glassman g.
Janeway g.
Kader g.
laparoscopic g.
Olympus g.
palliative g.
Partipilo g.
percutaneous endoscopic g. (PEG)
Russell percutaneous endoscopic g.
g. scarring
Ssabanejew-Frank g.
Stamm g.
tube g.
ultrasound-assisted percutaneous endoscopic g.
venting percutaneous g.
Witzel g.
gastrotomy
anterior g.
Depage-Janeway g.
gastrulation
gate
spinal g.
gate-control
g.-c. hypothesis
g.-c. theory
gated technique
Gatellier-Chastang
G.-C. ankle approach
G.-C. incision
G.-C. posterolateral approach
Gauderer-Ponsky
G.-P. PEG gastrostomy
G.-P. PEG operation
Gauderer-Ponsky-Izant PEG gastrostomy
Gaur balloon distention technique
gaussian line
gauze dissection
gavage
Gavard muscle
gay
g. bowel infection
G. gland
Gayet operation
Gaynor-Hart position
GBP
gastric bypass procedure
GCS
Glasgow Coma Scale
GD2
melanoma-associated antigen GD2
GD3
melanoma-associated antigen GD3
GEA graft
Geenen sphincterotomy
gelatin compression body
gelatinous
g. acute inflammation
g. ascites
g. carcinoma
g. infiltration
gelation
gel filtration
Gelfoam particles transarterial embolization treatment
Gell and Coombs classification
Gelman
G. procedure
G. technique
gelotripsy
Gelpi-Lowry hysterectomy
Gély suture technique
gemination

NOTES

gemistocyte
gemistocytoma
gena
genal
gender
g. dimorphism
g. identity formation
gene
cancer-causing g.
g. induction
mutator g.
g. replacement therapy
susceptibility g.
tumor suppressor g.
general
g. adaptation reaction
g. anesthesia (GA)
g. anesthetic
g. anesthetic technique
g. bloodletting
g. closure
g. endotracheal anesthesia
g. laparoscopic surgical procedure
g. radiation
g. surgeon
g. thoracic surgery
g. thrust manipulation
generales
generalized
g. cortical hyperostosis
g. elastolysis
g. peritonitis
genetic
g. abnormality
g. anomaly
g. approach
g. condition
g. diagnosis
g. lesion
g. marker
g. testing
geneticist
clinical g.
genetics
cancer g.
molecular g.
gene-transfer therapy
genial tubercle
genicula (*pl. of* geniculum)
genicular
g. anastomosis
g. artery
genicularis
geniculate
g. body
g. ganglion
g. neuralgia
geniculi
geniculocalcarine
g. radiation
g. tract
geniculotemporal tract
geniculum, pl. **genicula**
genioglossal muscle
genioglossus
geniohyoglossus
geniohyoid
g. fascia
g. muscle
g. space
geniohyoideus
genion
genioplasty
augmentation g.
genital
g. branch
g. carcinoma
g. condyloma
g. cord
g. duct
g. eminence
g. gland
g. infection
g. organ
g. papulosquamous lesion
g. reconstruction
g. swelling
g. tract
g. tract trauma
g. tract tumor
g. tubercle
g. ulcer
g. ulceration
genitalia
ambiguous external g.
external g.
indifferent g.
genitocrural nerve
genitofemoral
g. causalgia
g. nerve
g. neurectomy
genitofemoralis
genitoinguinale
genitoinguinal ligament
genitoplasty
feminizing g.
masculinizing g.
genitourinary (GU)
g. anomaly
g. apparatus
g. evaluation
g. fistula
g. infection
g. tract

Gennari
line of G.
gentle
g. compression
g. traction
genu
g. valgum deformity
g. varum deformity
genual
genucubital position
genufacial position
genupectoral position
genus
geographic stippling
geometric
g. equator
g. supracondylar extension osteotomy
George
G. Lewis technique
G. line
GEP
gastric emptying procedure
gastroenteropancreatic
Gerbert-Mellilo method
Gerbert osteotomy
Gerbode annuloplasty
GERD
gastroesophageal reflux disease
Gerdy
G. fiber
G. hyoid fossa
G. tubercle
geriatric
g. anesthesia
g. injury
Gerlach
G. tonsil
G. valvula
germ
g. line
g. tube
g. tube test
German method
germinal
g. center formation
g. cord
g. epithelium
g. matrix
g. matrix hemorrhage
g. membrane
germinoma
Gerota
G. capsule
G. fascia
Ger technique
Gesell test with Knobloch modification
gestant anomaly
gestational sac
Getty decompression technique
GFR
glomerular filtration rate
Ghon
G. complex
G. primary lesion
GI
gastrointestinal
GI oncology
GI tract
GI tract flora
GIA
gastrointestinal anastomosis
Giannestras
G. modification of Lapidus technique
G. oblique metatarsal osteotomy
giant
g. cell arteritis
g. cell astrocytoma
g. cell lesion
g. colon
g. condyloma
g. fibroadenoma
g. prosthetic reinforce
g. prosthetic reinforcement of the visceral sac (GPRVS)
Giardia **infection**
Gibbon hernia
gibbous deformity
Gibson
G. approach
G. long vertical relaxing incision
G. suture technique
Gibson-Piggott osteotomy
Gibson-type incision
Giemsa-stained section
Gierke respiratory bundle
Gifford delimiting keratotomy operation
GIFT
gamete intrafallopian tube transfer
gift wrap suture technique
Gigli operation
Gilbert scapular flap
Gilbert-Tamai-Weiland technique

NOTES

Gilchrist procedure
Giliberty bipolar femoral head
Gill
G. laminectomy
G. lesion
G. massive sliding graft
G. procedure
G. sliding graft technique
Gilles operation
Gilliam-Doleris
G.-D. operation
G.-D. uterine suspension
Gilliam operation
Gillies
G. bone graft
G. scar correction operation
Gillies-Millard cocked-hat technique
Gill-Jonas modification of Norwood procedure
Gill-Manning-White spondylolisthesis technique
Gillquist
G. arthroscopy
G. procedure
Gil-Vernet
G.-V. ileocecal cystoplasty
G.-V. ileocecal cystoplasty urinary diversion
G.-V. operation
G.-V. procedure
G.-V. technique
Gimbernat ligament
gingiva, pl. **gingivae**
gingival
g. anatomy
g. artery
g. augmentation
g. cavity
g. cavity wall
g. deformity
g. exudate
g. exudation
g. finishing line
g. fistula
g. flap
g. hemorrhage
g. inflammation
g. point
g. position
g. space
g. stimulation
g. tissue
g. tissue esthetics
g. zone
gingivectomy
chemosurgical g.
Ochsenbein g.
gingivolabial groove
gingivoplasty
ginglymoarthrodial
ginglymoid joint
ginglymus
helicoid g.
lateral g.
Giordano operation
GIQLI
Gastrointestinal Quality of Life Index
GIQLI score
Girard
G. keratoprosthesis operation
G. procedure
girdle
g. anesthesia
pelvic g.
shoulder g.
thoracic g.
Girdlestone
G. hip procedure
G. laminectomy
G. resection
G. resection arthroplasty
Girdlestone-Taylor procedure
Gironcoli hernia
girth
abdominal g.
Gittes
G. operation
G. procedure
G. technique
G. urethropexy
Gittes-Loughlin
G.-L. bladder neck suspension
G.-L. procedure
glabella
glabellad
glabellar
g. bilobed flap
g. exposure osteotomy
g. rotation flap
g. tapping
gladiate
gladiolus
glancing wound
gland
3-1/2 g.
abnormally hyperplastic g.
abnormal parathyroid g.
accessory parotid g.
accessory suprarenal g.
accessory thyroid g.
acid g.
acinous g.
admaxillary g.
adrenal g.
aggregate g.
agminate g.

Albarran g.
anterior lingual g.
apical g.
apocrine g.
g. appearance
areolar g.
arteriococcygeal g.
arytenoid g.
axillary sweat g.
Bartholin g.
Bauhin g.
Blandin g.
Blandin-Nuhn g.
Boerhaave g.
Bowman g.
brachial g.
bronchial g.
Brunner g.
bulbourethral g.
celiac g.
cervical g.
circumanal g.
coccygeal g.
contralateral parathyroid g.
Cowper g.
cutaneous g.
dominant g.
ductless g.
duodenal g.
Duverney g.
eccrine sweat g.
ectopic sebaceous g.
Eglis g.
endocrine g.
enlarged parathyroid g.
entrapped g.
esophageal ectopic sebaceous g.
external genitalia, Bartholin, urethral, and Skene g.'s
fundus g.
Galeati g.
gastric g.
Gay g.
genital g.
Gley g.
greater vestibular g.
Guérin g.
Havers g.
hematopoietic g.
hypercellular g.
hyperplastic g.
inferior g.
inguinal g.
intestinal g.
ipsilateral g.
Knoll g.
labial g.
lactiferous g.
laryngeal g.
lesser vestibular g.
Lieberkühn g.
lingual g.
Littré g.
Luschka g.
lymph g.
mammary g.
master g.
Meibom g.
meibomian g.
Méry g.
mesenteric g.
milk g.
Moll g.
Montgomery g.
mucilaginous g.
muciparous g.
mucous g.
nondominant g.
Nuhn g.
odoriferous g.
oil g.
palatine g.
parathyroid g.
2-1/2 g. parathyroidectomy
paraurethral g.
parotid g.
peptic g.
perspiratory g.
Peyer g.
pharyngeal g.
pineal g.
pituitary g.
Poirier g.
prehyoid g.
preputial g.
prostate g.
pyloric g.
remnant g.
g. removal
retrosternal g.
Rivinus g.
Rosenmüller g.
salivary g.
seminal g.

G

NOTES

gland *(continued)*
seromucous g.
serous g.
sexual g.
g. size
Skene g.
solitary g.
sublingual g.
substernal g.
sudoriferous g.
supernumerary g.
suprahyoid g.
suprarenal g.
sweat g.
synovial g.
target g.
tarsal g.
thymus g.
thyroid g.
tracheal g.
trachoma g.
Tyson g.
urethral g.
uterine g.
vaginal g.
vesical g.
vestibular g.
g. volume
Von Ebner g.
vulvovaginal g.
Waldeyer g.
Wasmann g.
Wepfer g.
Wölfler g.
Zeis g.
glandes (*pl. of* glans)
glandis
glandular
g. branch
g. cancer
g. carcinoma
g. element
g. epithelium
g. substance
g. tissue
glandulares
glandulectomy
glandulopexy
glans, pl. **glandes**
g. penis
glansplasty
meatal advancement and g.
glanuloplasty
glaserian fissure
Glasgow
G. Coma Scale (GCS)
G. Coma Score
G. Outcome Scale
G. Outcome Score (GOS)
glass-bead retention method
Glassman gastrostomy
glass-rod
g.-r. negative phenomenon
g.-r. positive phenomenon
glass-wool filtration
glassy membrane
glaucoma
g. surgery
uncontrollable g.
glaucomatous
g. cul-de-sac
g. excavation
g. ring
Gleason score
Gledhill technique
Gleich osteotomy
Glen
G. Anderson technique
G. Anderson ureteroneocystostomy
Glenn
G. anastomosis
G. operation
G. procedure
glenohumeral
g. adhesive capsulitis
g. articulation
g. dislocation repair
g. joint
g. joint dislocation
glenoid
g. cavity
g. fossa
g. osteotomy
g. point
g. rim fracture
g. surface
glenoplasty
posterior g.
Scott posterior g.
Gley gland
glial
g. ring
g. tumor
gliding-hole-first technique
gliding joint
gliobla
glioblastoma
glioma
low-grade g.
malignant g.
mixed malignant g.
g. sarcomatosum
glioma-polyposis
gliomatous
glioneuroma

gliosarcoma
gliosis
gliotic membrane
Glissane ankle fusion
Glisson
G. capsule
G. sphincter
glissonian
g. capsule
g. pedicle
g. sheath
global hypoperfusion
globi (*pl. of* globus)
globular collection
globule
fat g.
globus, pl. **globi**
glomangioma
glomangiomatous osseous malformation syndrome
glomangiosarcoma
glomangiosis
pulmonary g.
glomectomy
glomerular
g. basement membrane disease
g. capillary pressure
g. capsule
g. crescent
g. extracellular matrix
g. filtration
g. filtration rate (GFR)
g. hyperfiltration
g. macrophage infiltration
g. neutrophil infiltration
g. tip lesion
g. ultrafiltration
glomerulation
glomeruli (*pl. of* glomerulus)
glomerulitis
glomerulonephritis
membranoproliferative g.
glomerulosa
glomerulosclerosis
focal segmental g. (FSGS)
glomerulus, pl. **glomeruli**
glomus
g. arteriovenous malformation
g. body
glossectomy
Commando radical g.
partial g.
subtotal g.
total g.
glossocinesthetic
glossodynia
glossoepiglottic fold
glossopalatine
g. fold
g. muscle
glossopharyngeal
g. ganglion
g. nerve
g. nerve block
g. nerve root
glossopharyngei
glossopharyngeo
glossopharyngeus
glossoplasty
glossorrhaphy
glossoscopy
glossotomy
labiomandibular g.
median labiomandibular g.
glottic
g. carcinoma
g. closure
g. insufficiency
glottidis
glove anesthesia
gloved-fist technique
Glover suture technique
glucagonoma syndrome
Gluck incision
glucose oxidase method
glucuronidation
glue
g. patch
g. patch leak
glutamate toxicity
glutamic
g. oxaloacetic transaminase
g. pyruvic transaminase
glutaraldehyde sterilization
glutathione modification
glutea
gluteal
g. fascia
g. hernia
g. line
g. region
gluteales
gluteofemoral bursa
gluteoinguinal

NOTES

G

gluteorum
gluteus
g. maximus flap
g. maximus muscle
glycerin method
glycerol
g. chemoneurolysis
g. rhizotomy
glycogen infiltration
Glynn-Neibauer technique
GM2
melanoma-associated antigen GM2
gnathic index
gnathoplasty
gnathoschisis
goblet incision
Godman fascia
Goebel-Frangenheim-Stoeckel technique
Goebel procedure
Goebel-Stoeckel-Frangenheim procedure
Goethe bone
Goffe colporrhaphy
Gohil-Cavolo method
goiter
aberrant g.
colloid g.
congenital g.
diffuse colloid g.
diffuse multinodular g.
diffuse toxic non-nodular g.
g. excision
multinodular g.
g. recurrence
goitrous thyroid
gold
g. foil condensation
g. plate technique
g. ring
g. seed implantation technique
g. weight and wire spring operation
Goldberg technique
Goldblatt
G. kidney
G. phenomenon
Golden closing wedge osteotomy
Goldman
G. classification
G. classification operative risk
Goldmann
G. coherent radiation
G. kinetic technique
G. static technique
Goldmann-Larson
G.-L. foreign body
G.-L. foreign body operation
Goldner-Clippinger technique
Goldner-Hayes procedure
Goldner reconstruction
Goldsmith operation
Goldstein spinal fusion technique
Goldthwait-Hauser procedure
golf-hole ureteral orifice
Golgi membrane
Goligher extraperitoneal ileostomy
Gomco
G. suction
G. technique
Gomez
G. fundoplasty
G. horizontal gastroplasty
Gomez-Marquez lacrimal operation
gomphosis
gonad
female g.
male g.
gonadal
g. artery
g. branch
g. complication
g. cord
g. endocrine disorder
g. vein
gonadectomy
gonadoblastoma
gonadopathy
gonadotrophic
gonaduct
gonangiectomy
gonatocele
gonecyst
gonecystolith
Gonin cautery operation
gonioma
goniometry
goniophotocoagulation
gonioplasty
gonioscopy
indentation g.
goniotomy operation
gonocele
gonococcal
g. arthritis
g. infection
g. perihepatitis
Goodall-Power operation
Goodwin
G. cup-patch principle
G. technique
Goodwin-Hohenfellner technique
Goodwin-Scott technique
gooseneck deformity
Gordon
G. approach
G. elementary body
G. joint injection technique

Gordon-Broström technique
Gordon-Taylor
G.-T. hindquarter amputation
G.-T. technique
Gorlin-Chaudhry-Moss syndrome
GOS
Glasgow Outcome Score
Gosselin fracture
Gothic arch formation
Gouffon pin fixation
Gould
G. procedure
G. suture technique
Goulding procedure
Gowers tract
Goyrand hernia
GPRVS
giant prosthetic reinforcement of the visceral sac
GPRVS hernioplasty
Stoppa GPRVS
grabbing technique
gracilis
g. flap technique
g. muscle flap
g. procedure
g. tendon
graciloplasty
double-wrap g.
dynamic g.
gradation
Levine g. 1–6
grade
coma g.
fusion g.
g. I, II oscillation
g. 1–5 mobilization
nuclear g.
tumor g.
graded
g. exposure
g. spinal anesthesia
gradient
alveolar-arterial oxygen g.
alveolocapillary partial pressure g.
aortic pressure g.
aortic valve g.
biliary-duodenal pressure g.
Doppler pressure g.
duodenobiliary pressure g.
gastrosphincteric pressure g.
intracavitary pressure g.
g. method
mitral valve g.
peak systolic g.
peak transaortic valve g.
pressure g.
pullback pressure g.
pulmonary valve g.
temperature g.
transaortic valve g.
transcapillary hydrostatic pressure g.
transmural hydrostatic pressure g.
gradient-echo
2DFT g.-e. imaging
3DFT g.-e. MR imaging
g.-e. method
g.-e. MR image
g.-e. MR imaging
gradient-recalled
g.-r. echo image
multiple planar g.-r. (MPGR)
gradient-reversal fat suppression method
grading
tumor g.
Gradle keratoplasty operation
graduated tenotomy
Graefe operation
graft
accordion g.
acetabular augmentation g.
adipodermal g.
adipose g.
adrenal medulla g.
advancement flap g.
allogenic bone g.
allogenic fetal g.
allogenous bone g.
anastomosed g.
g. anastomosis
aortofemoral bypass g. (AFBG)
araldehyde-tanned bovine carotid artery g.
g. atrophy
augmentation g.
autogeneic g.
autogenous bone g.
axillobifemoral bypass g.
g. bed
Berens g.
bifurcated vascular g.
bifurcation g.
bilateral myocutaneous g.
Björk-Shiley g.

NOTES

G

graft *(continued)*
Blair-Brown skin g.
bone autogenous g.
bone chip g.
bone graft substitute g.
bone marrow g.
bone peg g.
bone-retinaculum-bone autograft g.
bone-tendon-bone g.
bone-to-bone g.
Bonfiglio bone g.
Boplant g.
brachiosubclavian bridge g.
branched vascular g.
Braun-Wangensteen g.
brephoplastic g.
Brescia-Cimino g.
bridge g.
C g.
calvarial free bone g.
Campbell onlay bone g.
cancellous chip bone g.
cancellous and cortical bone g.
cancellous insert g.
cantilevered bone g.
cardiovascular patch g.
carotid-vertebral vein bypass g.
cartilage g.
cephalic vein g.
chessboard g.
chip g.
Clancy patellar tendon g.
clip g.
g. clotting
compilation autogenous vein g.
composite rib g.
composite skin g.
conjunctival patch g.
connective tissue g.
g. contamination
coronary artery bypass g. (CABG)
cortical bone g.
cortical strut g.
corticocancellous bone g.
Cotton cartilage g.
Cragg endoluminal g.
Creech aortoiliac g.
Crescent corneal g.
cross-facial nerve g.
cutis g.
Daniel iliac bone g.
Dardik umbilical g.
Davis muscle-pedicle g.
DeBakey g.
delayed g.
dermal g.
dermal-fat g.
dermis patch g.
devitalized bone g.
diamond inlay bone g.
distal femoropopliteal bypass g.
distal nerve g.
donor iliac Y g.
dorsal vein patch g.
double g.
double-papilla pedicle g.
Douglas g.
dowel bone g.
dual onlay cortical bone g.
Edwards-Tapp arterial g.
endovascular stent g.
epidermic g.
Esser g.
g. expulsion
extraarticular g.
g. failure
fascial g.
fascicular g.
fat g.
Favaloro saphenous vein bypass g.
femoropopliteal bypass g.
fiberglass g.
fibular strut g.
filler g.
filleted g.
fillet local flap g.
g. fixation
flap g.
g. fragmentation
free fat g.
g. function
funicular g.
GEA g.
Gillies bone g.
Gill massive sliding g.
H g.
Haldeman bone g.
Hancock pericardial valve g.
Hancock vascular g.
Harris superior acetabular g.
g. harvest
Henderson onlay bone g.
Henry bone g.
heterodermic g.
heterogeneous g.
heterologous g.
heteroplastic g.
heterospecific g.
heterotopic g.
Hey-Groves-Kirk bone g.
H-graft bone g.
HLA identical kidney g.
Hoaglund bone g.
homogeneous g.
homogenous g.
homologous g.

homoplastic g.
Horton-Devine dermal g.
Huntington bone g.
HUV bypass g.
hyperplastic g.
IEA g.
IMA g.
g. impingement
implantation g.
g. infection
infusion g.
inlay bone g.
insert g.
interbody bone g.
intercalary g.
internal mammary g.
interposition saphenous vein g.
interspecific g.
g. interstice
intracranial-extracranial nerve g.
intracranial-intratemporal nerve g.
intramedullary g.
island g.
isogeneic g.
isologous g.
isoplastic g.
Jeb g.
Judet g.
jump g.
Kebab g.
Keystone g.
Kiel g.
Kimura cartilage g.
Koenig g.
Krause-Wolfe g.
Kutler V-Y flap g.
Langenskiöld bone g.
Lee anterosuperior iliac spine g.
Lee bone g.
ligament g.
load-bearing g.
loop forearm g.
lyophilized bone g.
mandrel g.
Marqez-Gomez conjunctival g.
Massie sliding g.
matchstick g.
Matti-Russe bone g.
McFarland bone g.
McMaster bone g.
medullary bone g.
mesenteric bypass g.
Meyers quadratus muscle-pedicle bone g.
g. migration
Millesi interfascicular g.
Millesi nerve g.
mitral valve homograft g.
morcellized bone g.
mucoperiosteal periodontal g.
mucosal periodontal g.
mucous membrane g.
Mueller patellar tendon g.
Mules g.
multivisceral g.
murine g.
mushroom corneal g.
Mustardé g.
myocutaneous g.
neuromuscular pedicle g.
neurovascular island g.
Nicoll cancellous bone g.
Nicoll cancellous insert g.
nonisometric g.
g. occlusion
Ollier thick split free g.
Ollier-Thiersch g.
orthotopic g.
osteoarticular g.
osteocartilaginous g.
osteochondral g.
osteoperiosteal bone g.
Ostrup vascularized rib g.
Overton dowel g.
papillary pedicle g.
Papineau bone g.
paraffin g.
particulate cancellous bone g.
g. patency
pattern-cut corneal g.
pedicle fat g.
peg bone g.
Phemister onlay bone g.
pie-crusting skin g.
pigskin g.
pinch skin g.
g. placement
portacaval H g.
postage stamp skin g.
powdered bone g.
preclotted g.
g. preparation
prophylactic bone g.
prosthetic arterial g.

NOTES

graft *(continued)*
proud g.
punch g.
Rastelli g.
reduced-size g.
g. rejection
reoperative coronary artery bypass g. (rCABG)
Reverdin epidermal free g.
reversed left saphenous vein bypass g.
rigid g.
roof-patch g.
Ryerson bone g.
sandwiched iliac bone g.
saphenous vein bypass g.
saphenous vein patch g.
scotty-dog g.
seamless g.
Seddon nerve g.
segmental tendon g.
Sheen tip g.
sieve g.
g. site
skip g.
sleeve g.
sliding inlay bone g.
Soto-Hall bone g.
Sparks mandrel g.
g. spatulation
Speed osteotomy g.
split-thickness skin g.
spreader g.
Stark g.
stent g.
g. strength
g. structure
strut g.
g. surveillance
g. survival
syngeneic g.
Taylor-Townsend-Corlett iliac crest bone g.
tendon g.
Thiersch-Duplay tube g.
Thiersch medium split free g.
Thiersch thin split free g.
Thomas extrapolated bar g.
thrombosed g.
g. thrombosis
transplanted stamp g.
g. treatment
tubed free skin g.
tube flap g.
Tudor-Thomas g.
tumbler g.
tunnel g.
vascularized bone g.
g. vasculopathy
vein g.
venous interposition g.
g. versus host
wedge g.
g. weight
Weiland iliac crest bone g.
white g.
Whitecloud-LaRocca fibular strut g.
whole lobar g.
Wilson bone g.
Wilson-Jacobs patellar g.
Windson-Insall-Vince bone g.
Wolfe-Kawamoto bone g.
Wolfe-Krause g.
Wolf full-thickness free g.
xenogeneic g.
xenograft g.
Y g.
zooplastic g.
Z-plasty local flap g.

graftectomy
graft-enteric fistula
graft-host interface
graft-versus-host
g.-v.-h. disease
g.-v.-h. disease reaction
Graham
G. closure
G. plication
grammatic method
gram-negative
g.-n. aerobe
g.-n. aerobic organism
g.-n. microorganism
g.-n. pneumonia
g.-n. sepsis
gram-positive
g.-p. bacterial infection
g.-p. microorganism
g.-p. sepsis
Gram-stain morphology
granddaughter cyst
Granger
G. line
G. method
G. projection
granny knot
Grantham femur fracture classification
Grant-Small-Lehman supracondylar extension osteotomy
Grant-Ward operation
granular
g. appearance
g. kidney
g. pit
g. respiration
granulares

granulation
arachnoid g.
extradural g.
pacchionian g.
g. phase
red g.
g. stenosis
g. tissue
toxic g.
granule
extracellular g.
membrane-coating g.
rod g.
seminal g.
granuloma
infectious g.
inflammatory g.
sterile g.
Teflon g.
granulomatous
g. bacterial infection
g. colitis
g. fungal infection
g. inflammation
g. mastitis
g. tissue
granulosa cell carcinoma
gras
grasping
g. technique
grasp reflex
grass-line ligature
Gratiolet radiation
grattage
Gräupner method
Graves technique
gravidity
gravimetric technique
gravitation abscess
gravitational
g. line
g. particle collection
gravity
g. line
g. method of Stimson
gray
g. hepatization
g. induration
g. infiltration
g. line
g. patch
g. scale examination
gray-line incision
gray-white corneal scar
great
g. anastomotic artery
g. auricular nerve
g. foramen
G. Ormond Street tracheostomy
g. pancreatic artery
g. radicular artery
g. saphenous vein
g. superior pancreatic artery
g. toe
greater
g. cul-de-sac
g. curvature
g. curvature banded gastroplasty
g. curve position
g. multangular bone
g. occipital nerve block
g. omentectomy
g. omentum
g. palatine artery
g. pelvis
g. peritoneal cavity
g. peritoneal sac
g. rhomboid muscle
g. ring
g. saphenous phlebectomy
g. sciatic notch
g. supraclavicular fossa
g. trochanter
g. trochanteric femoral fracture
g. tuberosity fracture
g. vestibular gland
Greaves operation
Green-Banks technique
Greenfield
G. osteotomy
G. spinocerebellar ataxia classification
Greenhow incision
Green procedure
Green-Reverdin osteotomy
greenstick
g. dorsal proximal metatarsal osteotomy
g. fixation
g. fracture
Greenville gastric bypass
Greenwald and Lewman method
Green-Watermann osteotomy
Gregoir-Lich procedure

NOTES

G

grenz ray therapy
Greulich-Pyle technique
Grice-Green technique
Grice incision
grid
external g.
gridiron incision
Griffen Roux-en-Y bypass
Griffith incision
Grimelius
G. argyrophil method
G. technique
Grimsdale operation
griseotomy
circular g.
Gristina-Webb total shoulder arthroplasty
Gritti-Stokes
G.-S. amputation
G.-S. knee amputation technique
gritty tumor
Grocott-Gomori methenamine-silver method
groin
g. dissection
g. exploration
g. flap
g. hernia
g. mass
grommet
Grondahl esophagoplasty
Grondahl-Finney
G.-F. esophagogastroplasty
G.-F. esophagoplasty
G.-F. operation
groove
alar g.
alveololabial g.
anterior auricular g.
arterial g.
auriculoventricular g.
bicipital g.
carotid g.
cavernous g.
chiasmatic g.
corneal lamellar g.
costal g.
deltopectoral g.
digastric g.
ethmoidal g.
g. extension
gingivolabial g.
inferior petrosal g.
infraorbital g.
intermuscular g.
interosseous g.
intertubercular g.
intraorbital g.
lateral bicipital g.
Lucas g.
median g.
meningeal g.
musculospiral g.
mylohyoid g.
nail g.
nasolabial g.
nasopharyngeal g.
obturator g.
occipital g.
palatovaginal g.
paraglenoid g.
pectoral g.
peroneal g.
pharyngotympanic g.
popliteal g.
posterior auricular g.
preauricular g.
pterygopalatine g.
Sibson g.
skin g.
spiral g.
subclavian g.
subcostal g.
supraacetabular g.
g. suture technique
transverse anthelicine g.
uncinate g.
urethral g.
venous g.
vertebral g.
vomerovaginal g.
grooved incision
gross
g. cystic disease
g. deformity
g. fecal contamination
g. lesion
g. manipulation
g. operation
g. tracheoesophageal fistula
Grosse-Kempf tibial technique
Grossmann operation
ground
lateral g. (LG)
ground-glass
g.-g. appearance
g.-g. body of Hadziyannis
g.-g. lesion
group
g. A beta-hemolytic streptococcal infection
g. A streptococcus infection
Children's Cancer Study g. (CCSG)
Eastern Cooperative Oncology G. (ECOG)

g. fascicular repair
Pediatric Oncology G. (POG)
grouping
tumor stage g.
Groves-Goldner technique
growing
g. fracture
g. point
growth
g. acceleration
g. arrest line
exophytic g.
final g.
hamartomatous g.
monoclonal g.
oligoclonal g.
g. plate abscess
g. plate complex
polyclonal g.
g. retardation
tumor g.
Gruber
G. cul-de-sac
G. ligament
G. suture technique
G. test
Gruber-Landzert fossa
Gruca stabilization
grunt
expiratory g.
grunting
g. maneuver
g. respiration
Grüntzig
G. balloon dilation
G. technique
Grynfelt hernia
Grynfeltt triangle
GSW
gunshot wound
single GSW
G syndrome
GU
genitourinary
guaiac-negative stool
guaiac-positive stool
guard
hypoxic g.
guarding
abdominal g.
involuntary g.
voluntary g.
Guarner wrap fundoplication
gubernacular canal
gubernaculum
Hunter g.
Gubler line
Gudas
G. scarf Z-plasty
G. scarf Z-plasty osteotomy
Guéneau de Mussy point
Guérin
G. fold
G. fracture
G. gland
G. sinus
valve of G.
Guhl technique
guidance
computerized image g.
fluoroscopic g.
frameless stereotactic g.
g. image
laparoscopic g.
magnetic imaging g.
g. method
stereotactic g.
ultrasound g.
video-laparoscopic g.
guidance-cooperation model
guide
image g.
g. plane
guided
g. fine-needle aspiration
g. transcutaneous biopsy
guided-needle aspiration cytology
guidewire
g. exchange technique
g. manipulation
g. and mini-snare technique
g. perforation
g. reflection
guiding plane
guillotine
g. amputation
g. needle biopsy
guinea worm infection
gulae
Guleke-Stookey approach
Guller resection
gullet
gullwing incision

G

NOTES

gum
g. line
g. resection
Gunderson conjunctival flap
Gunderson-Sosin modification
gunpowder lesion
gunshot
g. fracture
g. wound (GSW)
Gunston arthroplasty
Gurd
G. procedure
G. resection
Gussenbauer
G. operation
G. suture technique
gustation
gustatory anesthesia
Gustilo-Anderson
G.-A. open clavicular fracture
G.-A. open fracture classification
Gustilo puncture wound classification
gut
blind g.
g. continuity
g. epithelial cell
g. epithelium
g. lumen
g. mucosal homeostasis
g. mucosal weight
g. proliferative factor
gut-associated lymphoid tissue (GALT)
gut-derived gram-negative aerobic organism
Guthrie muscle
gutta-percha point
gutter
abdominal g.
g. fracture
left g.
paracolic g.
paravertebral g.
g. wound
guttering
corneal g.
Guttmann technique
Gutzeit dacryostomy operation
Guyon
G. ankle amputation technique
G. canal
guy suture technique
Guyton-Friedenwald suture technique
Guyton-Noyes fixation
Guyton ptosis operation
GW
gastric wrap
gynandroblastoma
gynecoid pelvis
gynecologic
g. anesthesia
g. disorder
g. laparoscopy
g. malignancy
g. surgeon
g. tumor
gynecological carcinoma
gynecomastia
mastectomy for g.
gynoplasty
gyration
gyrectomy
frontal g.
postcentral g.
precentral g.
gyrose
gyrus, pl. **gyri**
precentral g.

H
H graft
H space
habena, pl. **habenae**
habenula, pl. **habenulae**
habenular trigone
habenulointerpeduncular tract
Haber-Kraft osteotomy
habit
bowel h.'s
habitual
h. dislocation
h. temporomandibular joint luxation
habitus
body h.
Hackethal
H. intramedullary bouquet fixation
H. stacked nailing technique
Haddad metatarsal osteotomy
Hadju-Cheney acroosteolysis syndrome
Hadziyannis
ground-glass body of H.
HAE
hepatic artery embolization
Hagedorn and Jansen method
Haggitt classification
Haglund deformity
Hahn-Steinthal fracture
HAI
hepatic arterial infusion
Haight anastomosis
hair bulb incubation test
hairline fracture
Hajek incision
Håkanson technique
Halban
H. culdoplasty
H. procedure
Haldeman bone graft
half-and-half nail
half-axial projection
half-body irradiation
half-hitch knot
half-life
elimination h.-l.
plasma h.-l.
half-mouth technique
half-pin fixation
half-time
context-sensitive h.-t.
h.-t. method
Hall
H. facet fusion
H. method
H. technique
Hallberg biliointestinal bypass
Halle point
Haller
H. ansa
H. anulus
H. insula
H. membrane
H. plexus
H. rete
H. tripod
Hallermann-Streiff-François syndrome
Hallermann-Streiff syndrome
hallex, pl. **hallices**
hallices (*pl. of* hallex) (*pl. of* hallux)
Hallpike maneuver
hallucal
hallucis
extensor h.
h. longus laceration
hallus
hallux, pl. **hallices**
h. valgus deformity
h. valgus procedure
h. varus correction
halogenated volatile anesthetic
halothane
h. hepatitis
1-MAC h.
Halpin operation
HALS
hand-assisted laparoscopic surgery
Halsted
H. inguinal herniorrhaphy
H. maneuver
H. operation
H. radical mastectomy
H. suture technique
Halsted-Bassini
H.-B. hernia repair
H.-B. herniorrhaphy
Halverson classification
Halverson-McVay hernia classification
hamartoblastoma
hamartoma
cortical h.
plaque-like h.
visceral h.
hamartomatous
h. growth
h. lesion
Hamas technique
hamate
h. bone
h. tail fracture
hamatum

Hamazaki-Wesenberg body
Hambly procedure
Hamilton
H. method
H. Rating Scale for Depression
Hammerschlag method
hammertoe deformity
Hammon procedure
Hamou technique
Hampton
H. line
H. maneuver
H. operation
hamstring
h. ligament augmentation
h. muscle
h. tendon
hamular procedure
hamulus, pl. **hamuli**
pterygoid h.
Hancock
H. pericardial valve graft
H. procedure
H. vascular graft
hand
h. amputation
h. anomaly
h. assist
h. deformity
h. massage
h. ratio
h. reconstruction
h. ventilation
hand-assisted
h.-a. laparoscopic colectomy
h.-a. laparoscopic gastrectomy
h.-a. laparoscopic gastric bypass
h.-a. laparoscopic hemicolectomy
h.-a. laparoscopic live-donor nephrectomy
h.-a. laparoscopic surgery (HALS)
h.-a. laparoscopic vertical-banded gastroplasty
h.-a. laparoscopy
hand-eye coordination
hand-held Doppler flow probe examination
Handley
H. incision
H. lymphangioplasty
H. operation
handling
rough tissue h.
handmade anastomosis
handsewn anastomosis
hand-sutured ileoanal anastomosis
hanger
yoke h.
hanging
h. chain method
h. hip operation
h. toe operation
hangman fracture
hangnail
Hanhart syndrome
Hankin reduction
Hanley-McNeil method
Hanley rectal bladder procedure
Hannover
H. canal
H. classification
Hansen fracture classification
Hantavirus infection
Hapsburg jaw
Hara
H. gallbladder inflammation classification
H. infiltration block
Harada-Ito procedure
hard
h. adhesion
h. calculus
h. callus stage
h. cataract
h. chancre
h. corn
h. exudate
h. mass
h. metal disease
h. pad disease
h. palate
h. palate cancer
h. palate dissection
h. percussion
h. socket
h. and soft tissue
h. sore
h. stool
h. tubercle
Hardcastle tarsometatarsal joint injury classification
hard-copy image
hardening solution
Hardinge
H. lateral approach
H. technique
hardness
indentation h.
hard-soft palate junction
harelip suture technique
Harewood suspension procedure
Hark
H. procedure
H. technique
Harmon
H. cervical approach

H. hip reconstruction
H. incision
H. modified posterolateral approach
H. operation
H. procedure
H. shoulder approach
H. transfer technique
Harmonic hemorrhoidectomy
Harms-Dannheim trabeculotomy operation
Harper-Warren incision
harpoon extraction
Harriluque
H. sublaminar wiring modification
H. technique
Harrington
H. esophageal diverticulectomy
H. hernia repair
H. rod instrumentation failure
H. total hip arthroplasty
Harrington-Allison repair
Harris
H. anterolateral approach
H. femoral component removal
H. four-wire trochanter reattachment
H. growth arrest line
H. lateral approach
H. superior acetabular graft
H. suture technique
Harris-Beath projection
Harrison method
Harris-Smith cervical fusion
harsh respiration
Hartel technique
Harting body
Hartmann
H. closure
H. colostomy
H. operation
H. point
H. pouch
H. procedure
H. reconstruction technique
H. resection
H. stump
harvest
graft h.
organ h.
harvested fibroblast
harvesting
autograft h.
Hasner
H. fold
H. operation
valve of H.
Hassab operation
Hassall body
Hassmann-Brunn-Neer elbow technique
Hasson technique
Hass procedure
Hastings
H. bipolar hemiarthroplasty
H. open reduction
Hatafuku fundus onlay patch esophageal repair
hatchet-head deformity
Hatle method
Haultain operation
Hauri technique
Hauser
H. bunionectomy
H. patellar realignment technique
H. patellar tendon procedure
haustra (*pl. of* haustrum)
haustral
h. fold
h. indentation
h. pouch
haustration
haustrum, pl. **haustra**
Havers gland
haversian canal
Hawkins
H. inside-out nephrostomy technique
H. line
H. method
H. procedure
H. single-stick technique
H. talar fracture classification
Hawthorne effect
Hayes Martin incision
Hay lateral approach
hazardous concentration
HB_s
hepatitis B surface antigen
H_2 blocker
HCC
hepatocellular carcinoma
HCV
hepatitis C virus
HCV antibody

NOTES

H

HD
hemodialysis
HDR intracavitary radiation therapy
head
breech h.
bulldog h.
h. circumference:abdominal circumference ratio
h. compression
h. compression test
condyle h.
countersink screw h.
coupling h.
h. dependent position
h. distraction test
dolichocephalic h.
engaged h.
femoral h.
fetal h.
fibular h.
Giliberty bipolar femoral h.
h. hip arthroplasty
hourglass h.
humeral h.
h. injury
lateral h.
h. line
mandibular h.
Matroc femoral h.
Medusa h.
metatarsal h.
Morse h.
h. movement
oblique h.
optic nerve h.
pancreatic h.
h. paradoxical reflex
h. posture
radial h.
h. ring
series-II humeral h.
short h.
sternocostal h.
superficial h.
terminal h.
h. tetanus
h. titubation
transverse h.
h. trauma
h. turn technique
ulnar h.
h. weaving
h. zone
headache
analgesic abuse h.
brain tumor h.
cervicogenic h.
cluster h.
postdural puncture h. (PDPH)
rebound h.
spinal h.
traction h.
visually triggered h.
head-bobbing doll syndrome
head:body ratio
head-down
h.-d. tilt
h.-d. tilt test
head-dropping test
head-injured patient
head-splitting humeral fracture
head-tilt
h.-t. method
h.-t. test
head-turning reflex
head-up
h.-u. tilt
h.-u. tilt position
h.-u. tilt-table test
h.-u. tilt test
healed
h. fracture
h. yellow atrophy
healing
anastomotic h.
endoscopic h.
extraabdominal anastomotic h.
h. by first intention
fracture h.
h. fracture
impaired h.
intestinal anastomotic h.
intestinal wound h.
primary h.
h. process
h. retardation
h. by second intention
soft-tissue h.
tertiary h.
h. by third intention
wound h.
heal intubation
healthy tissue
Heaney
H. operation
H. technique
hearing aid evaluation
heart
h. anomaly
h. clot
explanted h.
extracorporeal h.
h. failure
h. laser revascularization
h. position
h. rate (HR)

h. rate variability (HRV)
h. sac
h. synchronized ventilation
h. transplant
h. transplantation
transverse section of h.
h. valve leaflet
h. valve replacement

heart-lung
h.-l. preparation
h.-l. resuscitation
h.-l. transplantation

heart-shaped pelvis

heat
h. application
h. balance
h. exposure
h. hyperalgesia
h. production temperature
h. shock

heater-probe coagulation

Heaton operation

heat-seal pouch

heavy
h. condensation
h. metal injection

heavy-ion irradiation

Hedley procedure

hedrocele

heel
h. bone
h. fat pad
h. pad thickening
h. tendon

heel-toe anastomosis

heel-to-ear maneuver

Heerman incision

hEGF
human epidermal growth factor

Heifetz procedure

height
anterior facial h. (AFH)
facial h.
first twitch h. (T1)
nasal h.
orbital h.
twitch h.

height-length index

Heimlich maneuver

Heinecke method

Heineke-Mikulicz
H.-M. gastroenterostomy
H.-M. incision
H.-M. pyloroplasty
H.-M. strictureplasty

Heineke operation

Heine operation

Heinz body

Heinz-Ehrlich body

Heisrath operation

Heister
valve of H.

Helal flap arthroplasty

helcoma

helcoplasty

Held
H. bundle
H. decussation

helical
h. CT
h. suture technique

helices (*pl. of* helix)

helicine artery

helicis

helicoid ginglymus

helicotrema

helium
h. dilution method
h. equilibration time
h. insufflation

helix, pl. **helices**

helix-loop-helix structure

Helle
laparoscopic H.

Heller
H. cardiomyotomy
H. esophagomyotomy
H. myotomy
H. myotomy with Dor fundoplication
H. operation
H. plexus

Heller-Belsey operation

Heller-Dor operation

Heller-Nissen operation

Helmholtz line

helminthic infection

helminthoma

heloma

helotomy

helplessness subscale

Helweg bundle

NOTES

H

hemal
h. arch
h. spine
hemangiectasia
hemangiectasis
hemangiectatic hypertrophy
hemangioameloblastoma
hemangioblastoma
hemangioendothelioblastoma
hemangioendothelioma
epithelial h.
hemangioendotheliosarcoma
hemangioepithelioma
hemangiofibroma
juvenile h.
hemangiolipoma
hemangiolymphangioma
hemangioma
capillary h.
cavernous h.
choroidal h.
port-wine h.
hemangioma-thrombocytopenia syndrome
hemangiomatous tissue
hemangiopericytoma
hemangiosarcoma
hematencephalon
hemathorax
hematobilia evacuation
hematocele
pelvic h.
pudendal h.
scrotal h.
hematocrit
falling h.
h. measurement
hematocystis
hematogenic metastasis
hematogenous
h. mechanism
h. metastasis
h. micrometastasis
hematologic
h. complication
h. disorder
h. dissemination
h. workup
hematolymphangioma
hematolysis
hematoma
acute subdural h.
aneurysmal h.
aortic intramural h.
h. aspiration
axillary h.
basal ganglia h.
bladder flap h.
bowel wall h.
cerebellar h.
chronic subdural h.
communicating h.
corpus luteum h.
dissecting intramural h.
h. drainage
duodenal h.
epidural h.
h. evacuation
expanding retroperitoneal h.
extradural h.
follicular h.
interhemispheric subdural h.
interstitial loculated h.
intracerebral h.
intracranial h.
intrahepatic h.
intramural h.
intraparenchymal h.
isodense subdural h.
mesenteric h.
nasopharyngeal h.
orbital h.
organized h.
para-aortic h.
parenchymal h.
perianal h.
periaortic mediastinal h.
pericardial h.
peridiaphragmatic h.
perigraft h.
perinephric h.
perirenal h.
puerperal h.
pulsatile h.
rectal sheath h.
rectus sheath h.
renal h.
retroperitoneal h.
retropharyngeal h.
retroplacental h.
sciatic nerve palsy h.
septal h.
solid visceral h.
spinal h.
subcapsular renal h.
subchorionic h.
subcutaneous h.
subdural h.
subfascial h.
subgaleal h.
subgluteal h.
sublingual h.
submembranous placental h.
submental h.
subperiosteal h.
subungual h.
sylvian h.

traumatic intracranial h.
umbilical cord h.
wound h.
wrap h.
hematomphalocele
hematomyelia
hematomyelopore
hematopoietic
h. gland
h. metastasis
h. tissue
hematorrhachis
extradural h.
subdural h.
hematospermatocele
hematospermia
hematoxylin body
hemendothelioma
heme-negative stool
heme-positive stool
hemiacidrin irrigation
hemiacrosomia
hemianopsia
homonymous h.
hemiarthroplasty
Bateman h.
Hastings bipolar h.
I-beam hip h.
large-humeral-head h.
McKeever and MacIntosh h.
Neer h.
prosthetic h.
Smith-Petersen h.
hemiazygos
h. vein
hemibody irradiation
hemic calculus
hemicentrum
hemicircular incision
hemicolectomy
Duecollement h.
extended right h.
hand-assisted laparoscopic h.
laparoscopic-assisted h.
laparoscopic left h.
left h.
standard right h.
hemicondylar fracture
hemicorporectomy
hemicorticectomy
cerebral h.
hemicrania
chronic paroxysmal h. (CPH)
episodic paroxysmal h. (EPH)
hemicraniectomy
hemicraniosis
hemicraniotomy
hemidiaphragm
elevated h.
left h.
right h.
h. rupture
hemidouble stapling method
hemielliptica
hemifacial
hemi-Fontan
h.-F. operation
h.-F. procedure
hemifundoplication
laparoscopic posterior h.
Toupet h.
hemigastrectomy
hemiglossal
hemiglossectomy
hemihepatectomy
hemihepatic vascular occlusion
hemihydranencephaly
hemi-Koch procedure
hemilaminectomy
complete lateral h.
lumbar h.
partial h.
unilateral h.
hemilaryngectomy
hemilingual
hemiliver
hemimandible reconstruction
hemimandibulectomy
hemimaxillectomy
hemimyelocele
hemimyelomeningocele
heminephroureterectomy
hemiorchiectomy
hemipancreatectomy
hemipancreaticosplenectomy
hemipelvectomy
complete internal h.
external h.
formal h.
internal h.
partial internal h.
hemipelvis
hemipulp flap

NOTES

hemiresection interposition arthroplasty
hemiscrotectomy
hemisection
tooth h.
triple h.
hemisectomy
hemisphere
cerebellar h.
cerebral h.
hemispherectomy
hemispherica
hemispheric disconnection syndrome
hemispherium
hemistrumectomy
hemithoracic duct
hemithoracicus
hemithorax
hemithyroidectomy
hemitongue flap
hemivertebral excision
hemivulvectomy
hemoaccess
hemobilia
hemocholecyst
hemocholecystitis
hemochromatosis
hemochromogen
hemocryoscopy
hemocytoblastoma
hemocytolysis
hemodialysis (HD)
anemia of h.
continuous venovenous h. (CVVHD)
h. treatment
hemodialysis-dependent patient
hemodilution
acute normovolemic h. (ANH)
hemodynamic
h. change
h. collapse
h. disturbance
h. function
h. instability
h. intolerance
h. maneuver
h. monitoring
h. pertubation
h. push
h. response
h. stability
hemodynamically
h. significant air embolus
h. stable
hemodynamics
hemofiltration
arteriovenous h.
continuous arteriovenous h. (CAVH)
continuous venovenous h.
h. therapy
hemoglobin
dissociable tetrameric h.
h. electrophoresis
hemoglobin-oxygen dissociation curve
hemoglobinuria
paroxysmal nocturnal h.
hemolith
hemolymphangioma
hemolysis
acid h.
chronic h.
hemolytic
h. mechanism
h. uremic syndrome
hemomediastinum
hemonephrosis
hemoperfusion
hepatic venous isolation by direct h. (HVI-DHP)
hemopericardium
hemoperitoneum
Hemophan membrane
hemophilic
h. arthritis
h. arthropathy
hemoplasty
hemopneumopericardium
hemopyelectasis
hemorrhage
abdominal h.
accidental h.
active h.
adrenal h.
alveolar h.
aneurysmal h.
antepartum h.
arachnoid h.
arterial h.
bilateral adrenal h.
bladder h.
blot h.
brainstem h.
catheter-induced pulmonary artery h.
cerebellar h.
cerebral h.
choroidal h.
colonic diverticular h.
colorectal h.
concealed h.
conjunctival h.
h. control
diffuse pulmonary alveolar h.
disk drusen h.

diverticular h.
dot h.
dot-and-blot h.
Duret h.
eight-ball h.
epidural h.
expulsive h.
exsanguinating h.
external h.
extradural h.
extraluminal h.
fetal h.
fetal-maternal h.
flame h.
flame-shaped h.
focal h.
h. focus
frank h.
gastric h.
germinal matrix h.
gingival h.
hepatic h.
Icelandic form of intracranial h.
intermediate h.
internal h.
intestinal h.
intraabdominal arterial h.
intraalveolar h.
intracapsular h.
intracerebral h.
intracranial h. (ICH)
intraluminal h.
intramural intestinal h.
intraocular h.
intraoperative h.
intraparenchymal h.
intrapartum h.
intraperitoneal h.
intraplaque h.
intraventricular h.
laryngeal h.
lobar h.
lower gastrointestinal h.
massive h.
mediastinal h.
mesencephalic h.
nasal h.
nasopharyngeal h.
neonatal intracranial h.
neonatal intraventricular h.
nonaneurysmal perimesencephalic subarachnoid h.
ochre h.
oropharyngeal h.
pancreatitis-related h.
parenchymatous intracerebral h.
perianeurysmal h.
perinephric space h.
periventricular-intraventricular h.
h. per rhexis
petechial h.
placental h.
pontine h.
postextraction h.
postgastrectomy h.
postoperative h.
postpartum h.
postpolypectomy h.
posttraumatic h.
posttreatment h.
preplacental h.
preretinal h.
primary h.
punctate h.
refractory variceal h.
renal cyst h.
reperfusion-induced h.
retinal h.
retinopathy h.
retrobulbar h.
retroperitoneal h.
retropharyngeal h.
round h.
salmon-patch h.
scleral h.
secondary h.
signal h.
slit h.
splinter h.
spontaneous renal h.
sternocleidomastoid h.
stigmata of recent h.
stress ulcer h.
subarachnoid h.
subcapsular h.
subchorial h.
subchorionic h.
subconjunctival h.
subcortical h.
subdural h.
subependymal h.
subepithelial h.
subgaleal h.
subhyaloid h.

NOTES

H

hemorrhage *(continued)*
subintimal h.
submucosal gastric h.
subperiosteal h.
subretinal h.
suprachoroidal h.
syringomyelic h.
thalamic-subthalamic h.
torrential h.
transplacental h.
unavoidable h.
upper GI h.
variceal h.
venous h.
vitreal h.
vitreous breakthrough h.
white-centered h.
yellow-ochre h.

hemorrhagic
h. angiomyolipoma
h. ascites
h. complication
h. endovasculitis
h. gangrene
h. infarction
h. inflammation
h. lesion
h. metastasis
h. radiation injury
h. shock
h. stroke
h. transformation

hemorrhoid
cutaneous h.
external h.
first-degree h.
internal h.
ligation of h.
Lord dilation of h.
mixed h.
mucocutaneous h.
necrotic h.
prolapsed h.
rubber-band ligation of h.
second-degree h.
strangulated h.
third-degree h.
thrombosed internal and external h.

hemorrhoidal
h. nerve
h. plexus
h. vein
h. zone

hemorrhoidalis

hemorrhoidectomy
ambulatory h.
anoderm-preserving h.
closed h.
diathermy h.
Doppler-guided artery ligation h.
Ferguson h.
four-quadrant h.
Harmonic h.
laser h.
ligation h.
limited h.
Longo h.
Lord h.
Milligan-Morgan h.
modified Whitehead h.
Morinaga h.
nonmucosal h.
open h.
Parks h.
radical h.
rubber band h.
scissors-excision h.
semiopen h.
stapled h.
three-quadrant h.
two-quadrant h.

hemospermia

hemostasia

hemostasis
chemical h.
complete h.
endoscopic h.
immaculate h.
meticulous h.
proactive h.

hemostatic
h. agent
h. collodion
h. plug formation
h. staple line
h. suture technique

hemostat technique

hemostyptic

hemotherapy

hemothorax, pl. **hemothoraces**

Henderson
H. classification
H. fracture
H. onlay bone graft
H. posterolateral approach
H. posteromedial approach
H. skin incision

Henderson-Hasselbalch equation

Hendler unitunnel technique

Henke
H. space
H. triangle

Henle
H. body
H. elastic membrane
H. fenestrated membrane

H. loop
H. tubule
Henning inside-to-outside technique
Henry
H. acromioclavicular technique
H. anterior strap approach
H. anterolateral approach
H. bone graft
H. extensile approach
H. incision
H. operation
H. posterior interosseous nerve approach
H. posterior interosseous nerve exposure
H. radial approach
H. resection
H. splenectomy
Henry-Geist spinal fusion
Hensen
H. body
H. canal
H. cell
H. duct
H. plane
Hensing ligament
hepaplastin test
heparin
h. cofactor II plasma level
h. irrigation
h. neutralized thrombin time (HnTT)
heparinase correction
heparin-binding protein
heparin-induced
h.-i. lipolysis
h.-i. thrombocytopenia (HIT)
heparinization procedure
hepatectomize
hepatectomy
cadaveric donor h.
central h.
concomitant h.
donor h.
ex situ h.
ex situ-in situ h.
extended left h.
extended right h.
laparoscopic h.
laparoscopic-assisted h. (LAH)
LCVP-aided h.
LCVP-assisted h.
left h.
limited h.
living donor partial h.
local h.
partial h.
recipient h.
regional h.
right lobe h.
segmental h.
simultaneous segmental h.
standardized h.
subsegmental h.
subtotal h.
total left h.
triple lobe h.
wedge h.
hepatic
h. abscess
h. adenoma
h. allograft
h. arterial buffer response
h. arterial infusion (HAI)
h. arterial therapy
h. artery
h. artery embolization (HAE)
h. artery-portal vein fistula
h. branch
h. candidal infection
h. capsule
h. cell carcinoma
h. circulation
h. colic
h. colorectal metastasis
h. coma
h. complication
h. congestion
h. dearterialization
h. decompensation
h. duct
h. duct calculus
h. dysfunction
h. encephalopathy
h. failure
h. fibrosis
h. flexure
h. function reserve
h. fungal infection
h. gunshot wound
h. hemorrhage
h. hilum
h. injury
h. intracellular energy

NOTES

H

hepatic *(continued)*
h. intracellular energy status
h. ischemia
h. ischemic time
h. lobectomy
h. lobule
h. malignancy
h. margin
h. mass lesion
h. necrosis
h. neoplasm
h. outflow block
h. outflow tract
h. parasitic cyst
h. parenchyma
h. parenchymal transection
h. pedicle
h. perfusion
h. plexus
h. portal vein
primary h.
h. regeneration
h. resection
h. resectional surgery
h. rupture
h. scintigraphy
h. segment
h. sinusoid
h. subsegmentectomy
h. surface
h. territory
h. transplant
h. transplantation
h. trauma
h. triad
h. tumor
h. vascular exclusion (HVE)
h. vascular isolation (HVI)
h. vascular isolation technique
h. venous confluence
h. venous isolation by direct hemoperfusion (HVI-DHP)
h. venous outflow obstruction
h. venous trunk
h. venous web disease
h. web
h. web dilation
hepatica
hepaticae
hepatici
hepaticocholangiojejunostomy
hepaticocutaneous jejunostomy
hepaticocystojejunostomy
hepaticodochotomy
hepaticoduodenostomy
hepaticoenterostomy
hepaticogastrostomy
hepaticojejunostomy
Hepp-Couinaud h.
mucosa-to-mucosa Roux-en-Y h.
Roux-en-Y h.
wide mucosa-to-mucosa Roux-en-Y h.
hepaticolithotomy
hepaticolithotripsy
hepaticoportoenterostomy
hepaticopulmonary
hepaticostomy
hepaticotomy
hepatic-renal angle
hepaticus
hepatis
hepatitis
H. Activity Index Classification
h. A-E infection
anesthetic h.
autoimmune h.
h. B surface antigen (HB_s)
h. C virus (HCV)
fulminant h.
halothane h.
peliosis h.
radiation h.
short incubation h.
hepatization
gray h.
red h.
yellow h.
hepatobiliary
h. imaging
h. manifestation
h. surgery
hepatoblastoma
unresectable h.
hepatocarcinoma
hepatocele
hepatocellular
h. acidosis
h. cancer
h. carcinoma (HCC)
h. function
h. synthetic dysfunction
hepatocholangioenterostomy
hepatocholangiojejunostomy
hepatocholangiostomy
hepatocolic ligament
hepatocolicum
hepatocystic duct
hepatocyte
h. growth factor (HGF)
h. transplantation
hepatoduodenal
h. ligament
h. reflection
hepatoduodenale

hepatoduodenal-peritoneal reflection
hepatoduodenostomy
hepatoenteric
hepatoesophageal ligament
hepatoesophageum
hepatofugal flow
hepatogastric ligament
hepatogastricum
hepatojejunal anastomosis
hepatojejunostomy
complex h.
high h.
hilar h.
intracystic h.
laparoscopic h.
palliative h.
pediatric h.
peripheral h.
Roux-en-Y h.
side-to-side h.
simple h.
hepatolith
hepatolithectomy
hepatolithiasis
intrahepatic h.
hepatoma
hepatomegaly
congestive h.
hepatomphalocele
hepatomphalos
hepatonephric
hepatonephromegaly
hepatopanc
hepatopancreatic
h. ampulla
h. fold
h. sphincter
hepatopancreatica
hepatopancreaticae
hepatopathy
radiation h.
hepatoperitonitis
hepatopetal flow
hepatopexy
hepatopleural fistula
hepatopneumonic
hepatoportal biliary fistula
hepatoportoenterostomy
Kasai-type h.
hepatoptosis
hepatopulmonary
hepatorenal
h. angle
h. bypass
h. failure
h. ligament
h. pouch
h. recess
h. syndrome
hepatorenale
hepatorenalis
hepatorrhagia
hepatorrhaphy
hepatorrhexis
hepatoscopy
hepatostomy
hepatotomy
hepatotoxemia
hepatotoxicity
anesthetic h.
hepatotrophic nutrient
Hepp-Couinaud
H.-C. biliary tract procedure
H.-C. hepaticojejunostomy
herald patch
herbal
h. medicine
h. therapy
Herbert operation
hereditary
h. breast cancer
h. cancer syndrome
h. coproporphyria
h. flat adenoma syndrome
h. malignancy
h. multiple exostoses
h. nonpolyposis colon cancer (HNPCC)
h. nonpolyposis colon carcinoma (HNPCC)
h. predisposition
Hering
canal of H.
H. nerve
Hering-Breuer reflex
heritable connective tissue disease
Herman-Gartland osteotomy
Hermodsson
H. fracture
H. internal rotation technique
H. tangential projection
hernia
abdominal incisional h.

NOTES

H

hernia *(continued)*
abdominal wall h.
acquired h.
amniotic h.
antevesical h.
axial hiatal h.
Barth h.
Béclard h.
bilateral inguinal h. (BIH)
bilocular femoral h.
Birkett h.
bladder h.
Bochdalek h.
broad ligament h.
cecal h.
cerebral h.
Cheatle-Henry h.
Cloquet h.
combined hiatal h.
complete h.
concealed h.
concentric h.
congenital diaphragmatic h. (CDH)
Cooper h.
crural h.
h. defect
diaphragmatic h.
direct inguinal h.
diverticular h.
double-loop h.
dry h.
duodenal h.
duodenojejunal h.
easily reducible h.
h. en bissac
encysted h.
epigastric h.
esophageal h.
extrasaccular h.
fascial h.
fatty h.
femoral h.
flank incisional h.
funicular inguinal h.
gangrenous h.
gastric h.
gastroesophageal h.
Gibbon h.
Gironcoli h.
gluteal h.
Goyrand h.
groin h.
Grynfelt h.
Hesselbach h.
Hey h.
hiatal h.
Holthouse h.
iliacosubfascial h.
incarcerated h.
h. incarceration
h. incision
incisional h.
incomplete h.
indirect inguinal h.
infantile h.
inguinal h.
inguinocrural h.
inguinofemoral h.
inguinolabial h.
inguinoproperitoneal h.
inguinoscrotal h.
inguinosuperficial h.
intermuscular h.
internal h.
interparietal h.
intersigmoid h.
interstitial h.
intraepiploic h.
intrailiac h.
intrapelvic h.
irreducible h.
ischiatic h.
Krönlein h.
labial h.
laparoscopic repair of paraesophageal h. (LRPH)
Larrey h.
Laugier h.
left inguinal h. (LIH)
Lesgaft h.
lesser sac h.
levator h.
Littré h.
Littré-Richter h.
lower quadrant abdominal incisional h.
lumbar h.
Madden repair of incisional h.
Malgaigne h.
Maydl h.
meningeal h.
mesenteric h.
mesocolic h.
h. metastasis
midline incisional h.
Morgagni h.
Morgagni-Larrey type h.
mucosal h.
multiorgan h.
muscle h.
nontraumatic h.
oblique h.
obturator h.
omental h.
orbital h.
ovarian h.

pannicular h.
pantaloon h.
paraduodenal h.
paraesophageal diaphragmatic h.
paraesophageal hiatal h.
parahiatal h.
paraileostomal h.
h. paralysis
paraperitoneal h.
parapubic h.
parasaccular h.
parastomal h.
paraumbilical h.
parietal h.
pectineal h.
pediatric h.
pericolostomy h.
perineal h.
peritoneal h.
peritoneopericardial diaphragmatic h.
periumbilical h.
Petit h.
pleuroperitoneal h.
port site h.
posterior vaginal h.
postoperative h.
h. pouch
primary indirect inguinal h.
properitoneal inguinal h.
pudendal h.
pulsion h.
rectal h.
h. in recto
recurrent incisional h.
reducible h.
retrocecal h.
retrocolic h.
retrograde h.
retroperitoneal h.
retropubic h.
retrosternal h.
Richter h.
Rieux h.
right inguinal h. (RIH)
Rokitansky h.
rolling hiatal h.
h. rupture
h. sac
sciatic h.
scrotal h.
secondary h.
Serafini h.
short esophagus type hiatal h.
sliding abdominal h.
sliding esophageal hiatal h.
slipped h.
spigelian h.
Spigelius h.
spontaneous lateral ventricle h.
spontaneous ventrolateral h.
stoma h.
strangulated incisional h.
strangulated paraesophageal h.
subpubic h.
suprapubic h.
synovial h.
thyroidal h.
tonsillar h.
transient hiatal h.
transmesenteric h.
traumatic diaphragmatic h.
Treitz h.
trocar site h.
true h.
tunicary h.
umbilical h.
unilateral h.
uterine h.
vaginal h.
vaginolabial h.
Velpeau h.
ventral h.
ventrolateral h.
vesicle h.
vitreous h.
Von Bergman h.
W h.
wound h.

hernial aneurysm

herniated

h. disk
h. fundoplication
h. preperitoneal fat
h. presacral fat pad
h. viscus

herniation

brain h.
cardiac h.
caudal transtentorial h.
central h.
cerebral h.
cervical midline disk h.
cingulate h.
cisternal h.

NOTES

H

herniation *(continued)*
diaphragmatic h.
disk h.
fat h.
foraminal h.
free fragment h.
intercervical disk h.
intervertebral disk h.
lumbar disk h.
midline disk h.
nucleus pulposus h.
h. pit
posterolateral h.
rostral transtentorial h.
sphenoidal h.
subfalcial h.
synovial h.
tentorial h.
thoracic disk h.
tonsillar h.
transtentorial h.
traumatic cervical disk h.
uncal h.
ureteroneocystostomy h.
visceral h.
vitreous h.
hernioappendectomy
hernioenterotomy
hernioid
herniolaparotomy
hernioplasty
abdominal midline incisional h.
classical Judd-Mayo overlap midline incisional h.
GPRVS h.
incisional h.
Judd-Mayo overlap midline incisional h.
laparoscopic h.
Lichtenstein tension-free h.
massive incisional h.
mesh plug h.
midline incisional h.
modified Shouldice h.
modified TAPP h.
overlap midline incisional h.
prosthetic incisional h.
Shouldice h.
tension-free h.
transabdominal preperitoneal h.
herniopuncture
herniorrhaphy
Adden h.
anterior inguinal h.
Bassini inguinal h.
h. chronic inguinodynia
elective h.
emergent h.
extraperitoneal laparoscopic h.
Halsted-Bassini h.
Halsted inguinal h.
Hill-type hiatus h.
inguinal h.
laparoscopic total extraperitoneal h.
Lichtenstein h.
Macewen h.
Madden incisional h.
McVay h.
mesh h.
modified Bassini h.
modified McVay h.
open h.
pants-over-vest h.
Ponka h.
primary inguinal h.
Shouldice h.
sutureless laparoscopic extraperitoneal inguinal h.
totally extraperitoneal inguinal h.
transabdominal laparoscopic h.
umbilical h.
ventral h.
vest-over-pants h.
herniotomy
Petit h.
herpes
h. epithelial tropic ulceration
h. simplex virus infection
h. zoster infection
h. zoster pain
herpetic infection
herpetoid lesion
Herring lateral pillar classification
hersage
hesitation phenomenon
Hess
H. eyelid operation
H. ptosis operation
Hesselbach
H. fascia
H. hernia
H. ligament
H. triangle
heteroautoplasty
heterocheiral
heterodermic graft
heterogeneity characteristic
heterogeneous
h. attenuation
h. gland size
h. graft
h. keratoplasty
heterograft
autogenous fascial h.
heterokeratoplasty
heterolateral

heterologous
h. graft
h. insemination
heterolysis
heterophoric position
heteroplastic graft
heteroplastid
heteroplasty
heteroscopy
heterospecific graft
heterotopic
h. bone formation
h. graft
h. ossification prevention
h. transplantation
heterotransplantation
heterozygosity
Hetzel forward triangle method
heuristic method
Heuser membrane
hexametazime
hexokinase method
hex procedure
hexylcaine
Hey-Groves
H.-G. fascia lata technique
H.-G. ligament reconstruction technique
Hey-Groves-Kirk
H.-G.-K. bone graft
H.-G.-K. technique
Hey hernia
Heyman-Herndon clubfoot procedure
Heyman-Herndon-Strong technique
HFJV
high-frequency jet ventilation
H-flap incision
HFOV
high-frequency oscillatory ventilation
HFPPV
high-frequency positive-pressure ventilation
HFV
high-frequency ventilation
HGF
hepatocyte growth factor
H-graft
H-g. bone graft
H-g. fusion
mesocaval H-g.
HHCA
hypothermic hypokalemic cardioplegic arrest

hiatal hernia
hiatopexy
hiatoplasty
tension-free h.
hiatotomy
hiatus
adductor h.
aortic h.
Breschet h.
esophageal h.
fallopian h.
maxillary h.
pleuroperitoneal h.
sacral h.
saphenous h.
scalene h.
Scarpa h.
semilunar h.
Hibbs-Jones spinal fusion
Hibbs procedure
hibernal epidemic viral infection
hibernation
myocardial h.
hibernoma
Hickman line
hickory-stick fracture
hidden
h. layer
h. nail skin
hidradenitis
h. suppurativa
hidradenoma
clear cell h.
cystic h.
nodular h.
papillary h.
poroid h.
solid h.
hidrocystoma
hiemalis
Hiff operation
Higgins
H. incision
H. technique
high
h. attenuation
h. blood pressure
h. cellularity
h. endothelial venule
h. hepatojejunostomy
h. intraluminal pressure
h. intrauterine insemination

NOTES

H

high *(continued)*
h. ligation
h. lip line
h. lithotomy
h. neurological lesion
h. output ileostomy
h. predictive value
h. pressure zone (HPZ)
h. smile line
h. spinal anesthesia
h. subtotal gastrectomy
h. threshold receptor
h. tibial osteotomy
high-affinity progestin receptor
high-altitude
h.-a. endoscopy
h.-a. simulation test
high-amplitude sucking technique
high-capacity fluid warmer
high-dose
h.-d. radioiodine therapy
h.-d. scan
h.-d. thrombin time (HiTT)
high-energy fracture
high-flux dialysis membrane
high-frequency
h.-f. jet
h.-f. jet ventilation (HFJV)
h.-f. jet ventilator
h.-f. oscillation
h.-f. oscillation ventilation
h.-f. oscillatory ventilation (HFOV)
h.-f. percussive ventilation
h.-f. positive pressure
h.-f. positive-pressure ventilation (HFPPV)
h.-f. positive-pressure ventilator
h.-f. ventilation (HFV)
high-grade
h.-g. astrocytoma
h.-g. dysplasia
h.-g. MALT lymphoma
h.-g. squamous intraepithelial lesion
high-heat casting technique
high-intensity lesion
high-kV technique
high-level disinfection
high-loop cutaneous ureterostomy
highly selective vagotomy
high-magnification
h.-m. colonoscopy
h.-m. endoscopy
h.-m. gastroscopy
Highmore
H. abscess
antrum of H.
H. body
highmori
high-resistance fundoplication
high-resolution
h.-r. image
h.-r. ultrasonography
high-risk
h.-r. angioplasty
h.-r. papillary cancer
h.-r. patient
high-speed rotational atherectomy
high-tension suturing technique
high-voltage
h.-v. pulsed galvanic stimulation
h.-v. therapy
hila (*pl. of* hilum)
hilar
h. biopsy
h. carcinoma
h. cholangiocarcinoma
h. cylinder
h. hepatojejunostomy
h. mass
h. plate
h. region
h. structure scar tissue
Hilgenreiner horizontal Y line
Hilgenreiner-Perkins line
Hill
H. antireflux operation
H. fundoplasty
H. gastropexy fundoplication
H. hiatus hernia repair
H. median arcuate repair
H. posterior gastropexy
H. procedure
Hillis-Müller maneuver
Hill-Nahai-Vasconez-Mathes technique
hillock
seminal h.
Hill-Sachs
H.-S. deformity
H.-S. fracture
H.-S. shoulder dislocation
H.-S. shoulder lesion
Hill-type hiatus herniorrhaphy
HILP
hyperthermic isolated limb perfusion
Hilton
H. method
H. white line
hilum, pl. **hila**
hepatic h.
splenic h.
h. stimulation
hilus
Hinchey diverticulitis grade classification
hindbrain deformity

hindfoot
h. amputation
h. deformity
hindgut
hindquarter amputation
hinge
h. joint
h. osteotomy
h. position
soft-tissue h.
hinge-axis point
hinged
h. corneal flap
h. fragment
Hinman
H. procedure
H. syndrome
Hinsberg operation
hip
h. arthroplasty
h. bone
h. deformity
h. disarticulation
h. dislocation
h. extension
h. fracture
h. pinning
h. reduction
h. replacement surgery
h. rotation
transient osteoporosis of h.
Hippel operation
hippocampectomy
Hippocrates manipulation
hippocratica
Hippocratic maneuver
Hirano body
Hirayma osteotomy
Hirschberg method
Hirschfeld
H. canal
H. method
Hirschsprung disease
Hirst operation
hirudin
hirudinization
His
angle of H.
H. bundle
H. bundle ablation
H. bundle heart block
H. canal
H. line
H. perivascular space
H. plane
His-Purkinje tissue
histangic
histiocyte
histiocytic tissue
histiocytoma
histiocytosis
histioma
histoangic
histochemical method
histocompatibility
histologic
h. assessment
h. characteristic
h. diagnosis
h. examination
h. investigation
h. lesion
h. liver biopsy finding
h. marker
h. pattern
h. result
h. study
h. tolerance
h. tooth repair
h. type
histological assessment
histology
histolysis
histonectomy
histopathologic
h. analysis
h. confirmation
h. data
h. diagnosis
h. examination
h. feature
h. information
h. validation
***Histoplasma* infection**
histotoxic anoxia
HIT
heparin-induced thrombocytopenia
immune-mediated HIT
Hitchcock tendon technique
HiTT
high-dose thrombin time
HIV
human immunodeficiency virus
HIV classification

NOTES

H

HIV-1, -2 infection
HLA identical kidney graft
HLF
human lung fibroblast
HNPCC
hereditary nonpolyposis colon cancer
hereditary nonpolyposis colon carcinoma
HNPCC syndrome
HnTT
heparin neutralized thrombin time
Hoaglund bone graft
Hoaglund-States classification
hobnailed appearance
hobnail liver
Hoche
H. bundle
H. tract
Hochenegg operation
hockey-stick
h.-s. deformity
h.-s. fracture
h.-s. incision
Hodge
H. maneuver
H. plane
Hodgson technique
Hodor-Dobbs procedure
Hoechst dye method
Hoffa
H. fat pad
H. fracture
Hoffman jejunoplasty
Hoffmann
H. approach
H. duct
H. panmetatarsal head resection
Hoffmann-Clayton procedure
Hofmeister
H. anastomosis
H. gastrectomy
H. gastroenterostomy
H. operation
H. procedure
H. technique
Hofmeister-Pólya anastomosis
Hogan operation
Hoguet
H. maneuver
H. operation
H. pantaloon hernia repair
Hohl-Luck tibial plateau fracture classification
Hohl-Moore
H.-M. classification
H.-M. technique
Hohl tibial condylar fracture classification
Hohmann procedure
Hoke-Kite technique
Hoke-Miller procedure
Hoke procedure
Holdaway line
Holden line
hold-relax
h.-r. method
h.-r. technique
Holdsworth spinal fracture classification
hole
bur h.
lag screw thread h.
h. preparation method
hole-in-one technique
Hollander test
Holl ligament
hollow
h. bone
Sebileau h.
h. visceral injury
h. viscus
h. viscus injury
Holmes method
Holmgren method
holoacrania
holocord
hologastroschisis
holoprosencephaly
holorachischisis
Holstein fracture of humerus
Holstein-Lewis fracture
Holth
H. iridencleisis
H. operation
H. sclerectomy
Holthouse hernia
Holzer method
Holzknecht space
homatropine dilatation
homeostasis
gut mucosal h.
mucosal h.
operational h.
homocladic
homogeneity
tissue h.
homogeneous
h. ablation
h. graft
homogenous
h. graft
h. keratoplasty
h. radiation
h. tooth transplantation
homograft
h. aortic valve replacement
cryopreserved aortic h.
homovital h.

pulmonary h.
h. reaction
h. rejection
homokeratoplasty
homolateral
homologous
h. artificial insemination
h. blood transfusion
h. graft
homolysis
homomorphic
homonomous
homonomy
homonymous hemianopsia
homoplastic graft
homoplasty
homotopic transplantation
homotransplantation
homotype
homotypic
homovital homograft
homozygous achondroplasia
honeycombed appearance
honeycomb lesion
Hood
H. and Kirklin incision
H. procedure
H. technique
hood
laminar flow h.
hook
h. cautery
h. electrocautery
h. fixation
hooked
h. bone
h. bundle of Russell
h. intramedullary nail
h. wire localization
hook-lying position
hook-nail deformity
hook-plate fixation
hook-to-screw L4-S1 compression construct
hoop stress fracture
Hopkins operation
Hoppenfeld-Deboer
H.-D. approach
H.-D. technique
Horay operation
hordeolum
external h.
Hori technique
horizontal
h. angulation
h. canal
h. external rotation
h. fissure
h. flap
h. gastroplasty
h. incision
h. mattress suture technique
h. maxillary fracture
h. osteotomy
h. plane
h. position
h. projection
h. section
hormonal evaluation
hormone
circulating h.
exogenous h.
intact parathyroid h. (iPTH)
parathyroid h. (PTH)
steroid h.
horn
coccygeal h.
dorsal h.
lesser h.
nail h.
sacral h.
superior h.
Horner
H. muscle
H. syndrome
hornification
hornpipe position
horripilation
horseshoe
h. abscess
h. fistula
h. incision
horseshoe-shaped
h.-s. flap
h.-s. incision
Horsley
H. anastomosis
H. gastrectomy
Horton-Devine dermal graft
Horvath operation
Horwitz-Adams ankle fusion
Hoskins razor blade fragment
hospital
H. Anxiety and Depression Scale

NOTES

H

hospital *(continued)*
Imperial College London H.
h. monitoring
h. mortality
h. pneumoperitoneum
h. stay
Texas Scottish Rite H. (TSRH)
hospital-acquired infection
host
graft versus h.
reservoir h.
hostile abdomen
hot
h. abscess
h. axilla
h. axillary bed
h. biopsy
h. biopsy technique
h. defect
h. gangrene
h. lesion
h. line
h. nodule
h. sentinel node
Hotchkiss-McManus PAS technique
hot-dog technique
hot-knife conization
hottest spot
Hotz-Anagnostakis operation
Hotz entropion operation
Houghton-Akroyd
H.-A. fracture technique
H.-A. open reduction
Hounsfield unit (HU)
hour
postoperative h.
postprandial h.
hourglass
h. deformity
h. head
h. membrane
h. stomach
House
H. advancement anoplasty
H. flap anoplasty
H. reconstruction
H. stapedectomy
H. technique
House-Brackmann classification
Houston
H. fold
H. muscle
valve of H.
Hovanian
H. procedure
H. transfer technique
Hovius
H. canal
H. membrane
Howard
H. method
H. technique
H. test
Howell-Jolly body
Howe silver precipitation method
Howland lock
Howorth
H. approach
H. procedure
Howorth-Keillor procedure
Ho:YAG laser angioplasty
Hoyer
H. anastomosis
H. canal
HPT
hyperparathyroidism
familial HPT
nonfamilial untreated HPT
primary untreated HPT
secondary HPT
sporadic primary HPT
symptomatic primary HPT
untreated HPT
HPV
hypoxic pulmonary vasoconstriction
H.P. Wright method
HPZ
high pressure zone
anal HPZ
HR
heart rate
HRV
heart rate variability
HS
hypertrophic scar
HSE
human skin equivalent
H-shaped
H.-s. capsular incision
H.-s. ileal pouch-anal anastomosis
H-type tracheoesophageal fistula
HU
Hounsfield unit
hub contamination
Huber adductor digiti quinti opponensplasty
Hubscher maneuver
Hudson line
Hudson-Stähli line
hue
salmon-patch h.
Huebner recurrent artery
Hueck ligament

Hueter
- H. incision
- H. line
- H. maneuver

Hugenholtz method
Huggins operation
Hughes
- H. modification of Burch technique
- H. operation
- H. tarsoconjunctival flap

Hughston
- H. classification
- H. external rotation recurvatum test
- H. procedure

Hughston-Degenhardt reconstruction
Hughston-Hauser procedure
Hughston-Jacobson
- H.-J. lateral compartment reconstruction
- H.-J. technique

Huguier
- H. canal
- H. circle
- H. sinus

Hui-Linscheid procedure
human
- h. AML cell line
- h. bite infection
- h. epidermal growth factor (hEGF)
- h. immunodeficiency virus (HIV)
- h. immunodeficiency virus classification
- h. leukocyte class II DR antigen
- h. lung
- h. lung fibroblast (HLF)
- h. lyophilized dura cystoplasty
- h. monoclonal antibody
- h. ovum fertilization test
- h. papillomavirus infection
- h. skin equivalent (HSE)
- h. subject
- h. thrombin
- h. umbilical vein (HUV)

humeral
- h. approach
- h. artery
- h. articulation
- h. canal
- h. epiphysis
- h. fracture malunion
- h. head
- h. head-splitting fracture
- h. line
- h. physial fracture
- h. shaft fracture
- h. supracondylar fracture

humerale
humeri (*pl. of* humerus)
humeroperoneal neuromuscular disease
humeroradial articulation
humeroradialis
humeroscapular
humeroulnar
- h. articulation

humeroulnaris
humerus, pl. **humeri**
humidity
- absolute h.
- relative h.

Hummelsheim
- H. operation
- H. procedure

humor
- aqueous h.
- vitreous h.

humpback deformity
hump removal
hunger
- bone h.

Hungerford-Krackow-Kenna knee arthroplasty
Hungerford technique
Hunt
- H. and Kosnik classification
- H. operation

Hunt-Early technique
Hunter
- H. canal
- H. gubernaculum
- H. line
- H. operation
- H. technique for Toupet fundoplication

hunterian ligation
Hunter-Schreger line
Huntington
- H. bone graft
- H. disease
- H. tibial technique

Hunt-Transley operation
Hürthle
- H. cell change
- H. FNA

Huschke foramen

NOTES

H

Hutchinson
H. fracture
H. freckle
H. patch
Hutchison syndrome
Hutch ureteral reflux operation
HUV
human umbilical vein
HUV bypass graft
HVE
hepatic vascular exclusion
HVI
hepatic vascular isolation
HVI-DHP
hepatic venous isolation by direct hemoperfusion
hyaline
h. basement membrane
h. body
h. mass
h. membrane disease
h. membrane syndrome
hyalinization
hyalitis anterior membrane
hyalocapsular ligament
hyaloid
h. artery
h. body
h. canal
h. posterior membrane
hyaloideo-capsulario
hyaloidotomy
Hyam conization
hybridization-subtraction technique
hybridoma technique
hydatic liver cyst
hydatid
h. cyst
h. cyst intrahepatic rupture
h. disease
h. material
hydatidocele
hydatidoma
hydatidostomy
hydradenoma
hydranencephaly
hydrate microcrystal theory of anesthesia
hydration
adequate h.
intravenous h.
h. layer water
maternal h.
h. status
h. therapy
vigorous h.
hydraulic dissection
hydrencephalocele
hydrencephalomeningocele
hydrencephalus
hydroappendix
hydrocalycosis
hydrocele
postoperative h.
h. sac
hydrocelectomy
hydrocephalic
hydrocephalocele
hydrocephaloid
hydrocephalus
normal-pressure h.
obstructive h.
post-subarachnoid hemorrhage h.
hydrocephaly
hydrocholecystis
hydrocirsocele
hydrocolpocele
hydrocystoma
hydrodelamination
hydrodelineation
hydrodissection
hydroencephalocele
hydroflotation
hydroflow technique
hydrogen
h. inhalation technique
h. washout method
hydrogenation
hydrogenolysis
hydrolysis
ATP h.
intragastric h.
h. of solution
h. of surfactant
urea h.
hydroma
hydromeningocele
hydromeningoencephalocele
hydromyelia
hydromyelocele
hydromyelomeningocele
hydromyoma
hydronephrosis
hydronephrotic
hydroperitoneum
hydropertubation
hydropneumoperitoneum
hydrops
endolymphatic h.
hydropyonephrosis
hydrorchis
hydrosarca
hydrosarcocele
hydrostatic
h. balloon dilation
h. pressure

Hypafix tape

hydrosyringomyelia
hydrotherapy
chylous h.
hydrotomy
hydrotubation
hydroureter
hydroxyapatite arthropathy
hyfrecation
hygroma
subdural h.
hygroscopic
h. expansion
h. technique
hyla
hyloma
hymenal
h. caruncula
h. membrane
h. ring
h. syndrome
hymenalis
hymenectomy
hymenoplasty
hymenorrhaphy
hymenotomy
Hynes pharyngoplasty
hyoepiglottic ligament
hyoepiglotticum
hyoepiglottidean
hyoglossal
h. membrane
h. muscle
Hyoglossus muscle
hyoid
h. apparatus
h. bone
h. bone fracture
h. bone resection
h. muscle
h. syndrome
hyoidei
hyoideum
hyoideus
hyopharyngeus
hyothyroid
hyothyroidea
Hypaque enema
hyparterial
hypaxial
hypencephalon
hyperacute
h. graft-versus-host disease
h. rejection
hyperaeration
hyperaldosteronism
hyperalgesia
barbiturate-related h.
heat h.
visceral h.
hyperalimentation
central h.
intravenous h.
parenteral h.
peripheral h.
hyperbaric
h. local anesthetic
h. oxygen
h. oxygenation
h. oxygen therapy
h. pressure
h. spinal anesthesia
h. tetracaine
hyperbilirubinemia
hypercalcemia
familial hypocalciuric h.
persistent h.
recurrent h.
hypercapnia
permissive h. (PHC)
hypercapnic
h. drive
h. ventilatory response
hypercarbia
central venous h.
gastric mucosal h.
venous h.
hypercellular gland
hypercoagulable state
hypercoagulation
hypercontractile external sphincter response
hyperdense brain lesion
hyperdeviation
hyperdistended abdomen
hyperdynamic
h. circulation
h. shock
hyperemia
hyperemic
hyperesthesia
hypereuryprosopic
hyperexplexia

NOTES

H

hyperextension deformity
hyperextension-hyperflexion injury
hyperfibrinolysis
hyperfiltration
    capillary h.
    glomerular h.
    h. injury
    renal h.
hyperfractionated total body irradiation
hyperfractionation
hyperfunctioning nodule
hyperglycemia
hyperhydration
hyperhydropexy
hyperinfection
hyperinflation
hyperinsulinemia
    peripheral h.
hyperintense brain lesion
hyperkeratotic lesion
hyperlactation
hyperlactemia
hypermetabolic response
hypermetropia
hypernephroid carcinoma
hypernephroma
hyperorchidism
hyperosmolar
    h. diabetic coma
    h. hyperglycemic nonketotic coma
hyperostosis
    diffuse idiopathic skeletal h. (DISH)
    generalized cortical h.
hyperparathyroidism (HPT)
    ectopic h.
    neonatal severe h.
    primary h.
    sporadic primary h.
    untreated h.
hyperpathia
hyperpigmented lesion
hyperplasia
    adenomatous h.
    asymmetric h.
    atypical h. (AH)
    basal cell h.
    benign prostatic h. (BPH)
    congenital adrenal h.
    ductal h.
    florid h.
    focal nodular h. (FNH)
    four-gland h.
    intimal h.
    intraductal h.
    lobular h.
    moderate h.
    multigland h.
    multiglandular parathyroid h.
    multiple gland h.
    papillary h.
    parathyroid h.
    polyclonal h.
    solid h.
    sporadic multigland h.
    sporadic multiple gland parathyroid h.
    squamous h.
    stent-induced intimal h.
    thyroid h.
hyperplastic
    h. cyst
    h. cystadenoma
    h. gland
    h. graft
    h. inflammation
    h. polyp
    h. tissue
    h. tumor
hyperpronation
hyperpyrexia
    fulminant h.
    malignant h.
hyperreflexic bladder
hyperresonant abdomen
hypersalivation
hypersensitive xiphoid syndrome
hypersensitivity
    h. angiitis
    denervation h.
hypersensitization
hypersplenism
hypertelorism
hypertension
    arterial h.
    diastolic h.
    essential h.
    extrahepatic portal venous h.
    idiopathic intracranial h.
    intraabdominal h.
    intrahepatic h.
    lithotripsy-induced h.
    malignant h.
    neurogenic h.
    pediatric portal h.
    portal h.
    primary pulmonary h. (PPH)
    pulmonary artery h. (PAH)
    renal h.
    renovascular h.
    surgically corrected h.
    unshuntable portal h.
hyperthermia
    malignant h. (MH)
    h. therapy
    whole-body h.

hyperthermic
h. isolated limb perfusion (HILP)
h. temperature
hyperthymization
hypertonic
h. bladder
h. lactated saline
h. saline-epinephrine
hypertonic-hyperoncotic fluid resuscitation
hypertrophic
h. granulation tissue
h. scar (HS)
h. scarring
hypertrophy
benign prostatic h.
eccentric h.
hemangiectatic h.
hypervalvular phonation
hypervascular fragment
hypervascularity
hyperventilation
alveolar h.
isocapnic h.
h. maneuver
h. syndrome
h. test
h. tetany
hypervolemia
hyphema
hypnosis anesthesia
hypnotic
h. dissociation
h. effect
intravenous h.
h. response
hypoactive bowel sounds
hypoaeration
hypoalgesia
somatic h.
hypobaria
hypobaric spinal anesthesia
hypocalcemia
postoperative h.
transient h.
hypocapnia
hypocarbia
hypocellular fibrous tissue
hypochondriaca
hypochondriac region
hypochondrium
hypochordal
hypocystotomy
hypodense brain lesion
hypoderm
hypodermatomy
hypodermic implantation
hypodermoclysis
hypoeccrisis
hypoechoic lesion
hypoesthesia
hypogastric
h. artery
h. artery ligation
h. flap
h. ganglion
h. nerve
h. plexus block anesthetic technique
h. region
h. vein
hypogastrica
hypogastricus
hypogastrium
hypogastrocele
hypogastroschisis
hypogenitalism
hypoglossal
h. artery
h. canal
h. canal venous plexus
h. facial nerve anastomosis
h. facial transfer procedure
hypoglossi
hypoglossus, hypoglossis
hypoglottis
hypoglycemia
hypognathous
hypogonadism
hypohyloma
hypoinflation
hypolobulation
hypomelanotic macule
hyponychium
hypooncotic plasma substitute
hypoparathyroidism
permanent h.
hypoperfusion
global h.
regional h.
splanchnic h.
spreading h.
systemic h.
hypopharyngeus

NOTES

H

hypopharynx
diverticulectomy of h.
hypophysectomize
hypophysectomy
partial central h.
total h.
transsphenoidal h.
unilateral h.
hypophyseoportal vein
hypophyseos
hypophyses
hypophysial
h. artery
h. duct
h. portal circulation
hypophysialis
hypophysis
hypopigmentation
postinflammatory h.
hypopituitarism
hypoplasia
aortic h.
pulmonary h.
hypoplastic
h. left heart repair
h. left heart syndrome
hyposalivation
hyposcheotomy
hypospadiac
hypospadias
hyposplenism
hypostasis
postmortem h.
pulmonary h.
hypostatic abscess
hypostomia
hypotension
catecholamine-resistant h.
deliberate h. (DH)
induced h.
spontaneous intracranial h. (SIH)
systemic h.
hypotensive
h. anesthesia
h. resuscitation
h. surgery
hypothalamic activation
hypothalamic-hypophysial-ovarian-endometrial axis
hypothalamic-hypophysial portal circulation
hypothalamohypophysial tract
hypothalamotomy
hypothenaprimeris
hypothenar
h. eminence
h. muscle
h. prominence
hypothermia
accidental h.
h. anesthetic technique
core h.
deep h.
extracorporeal exchange h.
intraoperative core h.
moderate resuscitative h.
pediatric h.
profound h.
redistribution h.
regional h.
total body h.
hypothermia-induced coagulopathy
hypothermia-related coagulopathy
hypothermic
h. anesthesia
h. circulatory arrest
h. effect
h. hepatic perfusion
h. hypokalemic cardioplegic arrest (HHCA)
hypothesis, pl. **hypotheses**
gate-control h.
hypotonia
skeletal muscle h.
hypotonic
h. solution
hypotympanic cell
hypotympanum
hypouresis
hypoventilation
alveolar h.
benzodiazepine-induced h.
sedation-induced h.
hypovolemia
hypovolemic shock
hypoxia
diffusion h.
hypoxic h.
ischemic h.
local h.
stagnant h.
tissue h.
tumor h.
hypoxia-induced rhabdomyolysis
hypoxic
h. guard
h. hypoxia
h. pulmonary vasoconstriction (HPV)
h. ventilatory decrease
h. ventilatory response
hypsibrachycephalic
hypsiconchous
hypsiloid
h. angle
h. cartilage

hypsistaphylia
hypsistenocephalic
Hyrtl
H. anastomosis
H. foramen
H. loop
H. sphincter
hysterectomy
abdominal h.
abdominovaginal h.
Bonney abdominal h.
cesarean h.
classic abdominal Semm h.
Dellepiane h.
Doyen vaginal h.
Eden-Lawson h.
extrafascial h.
gasless laparoscopic h.
Gelpi-Lowry h.
laparoscopically assisted vaginal h. (LAVH)
laparoscopic-assisted vaginal h.
laparoscopic Döderlein h.
laparoscopic radical h.
Latzko radical abdominal h.
Mayo h.
Meigs-Werthein h.
modified radical h.
obstetrical h.
paravaginal h.
pelviscopic intrafascial h.
radical abdominal h.
radical vaginal h.
Reis-Wertheim vaginal h.
supracervical h.
total abdominal h.
vaginal h.
Ward-Mayo vaginal h.
hysterical
h. anesthesia
h. colic
hystericus
hysterocele
hysterocleisis
hysterocystopexy
hysterolysis
hysteromyoma
hysteromyomectomy
hysteromyotomy
hystero-oophorectomy
hysteropexy
abdominal h.
Alexander-Adams h.
hysteroplasty
hysterorrhaphy
hysterosacropexy
hysterosalpingectomy
laparoscopic h.
hysterosalpingo-oophorectomy
hysterosalpingostomy
hysteroscopic surgery
hysteroscopy
laparoscopic-assisted vaginal h.
hysterotomy
abdominal h.
vaginal h.
hysterotrachelectomy
hysterotracheloplasty
hysterotrachelorrhaphy
hysterotrachelotomy

NOTES

H

IA
inferior apical
IA segment
IAC
intraarterial chemotherapy
IAP
intraabdominal pressure
IAR
immediate asthmatic reaction
IAS
internal anal sphincter
IASP
International Association for the Study of Pain
IASP Classification of Chronic Pain
iatrogenic
i. arteriovenous fistula
i. bowel injury
i. hernia defect
i. infection
i. tension pneumothorax
i. transmission
iatrotechnique
IB
inferior basal
IB segment
I-beam
I-b. hip hemiarthroplasty
I-b. hip operation
IC
Isaacson classification
ICA
internal carotid artery
ICDA
International Classification of Diseases, Adapted for Use in the United States
ice
i. application
i. point
i. skater fracture
i. slush
ice-cold saline
Icelandic form of intracranial hemorrhage
ICH
intracranial hemorrhage
icing liver
ICISS
International Classification of Diseases-9 Version of Injury Severity Score
ICLH double-cup arthroplasty
ICP
intracranial pressure
ICSI
intracytoplasmic sperm injection
ictal abnormality
ICU
intensive care unit
ICU care priority
ICU sedation
I&D
incision and drainage
ideal
i. body weight
i. flap
i. solution
Ideberg glenoid fracture classification
identical point
identification
colonic lesion i.
film i.
lesion i.
nasal mucosal i.
i. phenomenon
identifying canal
identity formation
IDET
intradiscal electrothermal therapy
idiographic approach
idiopathic
i. adult intussusception
i. bone cavity
i. brachial plexopathy
i. brown induration
i. cause
i. constipation
i. dilation
i. eczematous disease
i. hypertrophic subaortic stenosis
i. ileocecal intussusception
i. intracranial hypertension
i. paroxysmal rhabdomyolysis
i. peptic ulcer disease
i. preretinal membrane
i. pulmonary fibrosis (IPF)
i. ventricular fibrillation
IGBB
image-guided breast biopsy
diagnostic IGBB
IG bundle
IGF-1
insulin-like growth factor I
exogenous IGF-1
ignition point
IGPA
infragenicular popliteal artery
IGS
image-guided surgery

I

IINB
ilioinguinal-iliohypogastric nerve block
ileac
ileal
i. artery
i. biopsy
i. bladder
i. conduit
i. conduit urinary diversion
i. crypt
i. inflammation
i. inflow tract
i. J-pouch
i. loop
i. neobladder urinary pouch
i. outflow tract
i. patch ureteroplasty
i. perforation
i. pouch-anal anastomosis (IPAA)
i. pouch-distal rectal anastomosis
i. pouch surgery
i. resection
i. reservoir construction
i. sphincter
i. vein
i. W-pouch
ileales
ilealis
ileal-sigmoid anastomosis
ileectomy
ilei
ileitis
pouch i.
ileoanal
i. anastomosis
i. endorectal pull-through
i. pouch
i. pouch procedure
i. pull-through procedure
ileoascending colostomy
ileocecal
i. cystoplasty
i. edema
i. eminence
i. fat pad
i. fold
i. junction
i. opening
i. orifice
i. pouch
i. region
i. ureterosigmoidostomy
i. valve
ileocecale
ileocecalis
ileocecocolic sphincter
ileocecocystoplasty bladder augmentation
ileocecostomy
ileocecum
ileocolectomy
ileocolic
i. artery
i. conduit
i. intussusception
i. resection
i. vein
ileocolica
ileocolici
ileocolonic
i. pouch
i. pouch urinary diversion
i. resection
ileocolonoscopy
ileocolostomy
end-loop i.
LeDuc-Camey i.
ileocystoplasty
Camey i.
clam i.
LeDuc-Camey i.
ileocystostomy
cutaneous i.
ileoduodenal fistula
ileoentectropy
ileofemoral wing fracture
ileogastrostomy
ileoileostomy
ileojejunal bypass
ileopexy
ileoproctostomy
ileorectal anastomosis (IRA)
ileorectostomy
ileorrhaphy
ileoscopy
ileosigmoid
i. anastomosis
i. colostomy
i. fistula
i. knot
ileosigmoidostomy
ileostomy
Bishop-Koop i.
blowhole i.
Brooke i.
i. closure
i. construction
continent i.
defunctioning loop i.
Dennis-Brooke i.
diversionary i.
diverting loop i.
double-barrel i.
end i.
end-loop i.
i. formation
Goligher extraperitoneal i.

high output i.
incontinent i.
J-loop i.
Koch continent i.
Koch reservoir i.
loop i.
loop-end i.
permanent loop i.
pouched i.
i. reversal
split i.
i. spout
i. stenosis
i. stoma
temporary loop i.
terminal i.
Turnbull end-loop i.

ileotomy

ileotransverse
i. colon anastomosis
i. colostomy

ileotransversostomy

ileovesical
i. anastomosis
i. fistula

ileovesicostomy
incontinent i.

ileum
terminal i.

ileus
adhesive i.
duodenal i.
gallstone i.
occlusive i.
paralytic i.
postoperative i.

iliac
i. apophysis
i. arterial tree
i. artery
i. artery aneurysm
i. artery angioplasty
i. bone
i. branch
i. bursa
i. buttressing procedure
i. colon
i. compression test
i. crest
i. crest biopsy
i. crest bone aspiration
i. crest bone graft stabilization
i. crest free flap
i. crest osseous flap
i. crest osteocutaneous flap
i. crest osteomuscular flap
i. crest resection
i. epiphysis
i. fascia
i. fixation
i. flexure
i. fossa
i. muscle
i. osteocutaneous free flap
i. osteotomy
i. plexus
i. region
i. roll
i. spine
i. steal
i. tubercle
i. vein
i. wing resection

iliaca

iliacae

iliaci

iliacosubfascial
i. fossa
i. hernia

iliacosubfascialis

iliacum

iliacus

Iliff
I. approach
I. exenteration
I. operation

ilii

iliocapsularis

iliococcygeal muscle

iliococcygeus

iliocolotomy

iliocostalis

iliocostal muscle

iliofemoral
i. approach
i. flap artery
i. pedicle flap

iliohypogastric
i. muscle
i. nerve
i. nerve block
i. neurectomy

iliohypogastrici

iliohypogastricus

NOTES

ilioinguinal
i. acetabular approach
i. incision
i. nerve
i. nerve block
i. neurectomy
i. ring
ilioinguinal-iliohypogastric nerve block (IINB)
ilioinguinalis
iliolumbale
iliolumbalis
iliolumbar
i. artery
i. ligament
ilioneoureterocystotomy
iliopectinate line
iliopectinea
iliopectineal
i. arch
i. bursa
i. eminence
i. fascia
i. fossa
i. line
iliopelvic sphincter
iliopsoas
i. muscle
i. ring
i. tendon
iliopubic
i. eminence
i. tract
iliopubica
iliosacral and iliac fixation construct
iliosciatic
iliospinal
iliotibial
i. band
i. band graft augmentation
i. tract
iliotibialis
iliotrochanteric
ilium
external i.
internal-external i.
Ilizarov
I. external fixation
I. limb-lengthening technique
I. method
ill-defined mass
illness
catastrophic i.
life-threatening i.
medical i.
illumination
axial i.
background i.
central i.
coaxial i.
contact i.
critical i.
dark-field i.
dark-ground i.
diffuse i.
direct i.
erect i.
focal i.
Köhler i.
lateral i.
narrow-slit i.
oblique i.
slit i.
vertical i.
ILP
isolated limb perfusion
IM
intramuscular
IMA
inferior mesenteric artery
internal mammary artery
IMA graft
ima
imae
image
i. acquisition
i. analysis
AP-T i.
axial spin-echo i.
body i.
2C-L i.
i. compression
4C-T i.
5C-T i.
DG-L i.
DG-T i.
dynamic i.
ejection-fraction i.
ejection shell i.
endoscopic i.
endoscopic video i.
field-echo i.
FLAIR i.
flow-on gradient-echo i.
fluid-attenuated inversion recovery i.
i. formation
i. formation principle
gradient-echo MR i.
gradient-recalled echo i.
guidance i.
i. guide
i. guide bundle
hard-copy i.
high-resolution i.
i. intensification

i. interpretation
MP-L i.
MP-T i.
multiplanar i.
MV-T i.
i. point
point-counting i.
radiographic i.
real-time echo-planar i.
real-time multiplanar i.
i. registration
sagittal spin-echo i.
second-echo i.
short-pulse repetition time/echo time i.
single-slice gradient-echo i.
spin-echo i.
static i.
i. subtraction
surface-projection rendering i.
thin-section axial i.
transmission i.
T1-weighted spin-echo i.
T2-weighted spin-echo i.
ultrasound i.
video i.

image-guided
i.-g. breast biopsy (IGBB)
i.-g. fine-needle aspiration biopsy
i.-g. interactive neurosurgery
i.-g. pancreatic core aspiration
i.-g. stereotactic brain biopsy
i.-g. surgery (IGS)

image-integrated surgery treatment planning

image-related screening technique

image-selected in vivo spectroscopy

image-space focus

imaginal exposure

imaging
abdominal i.
anatomic i.
B-mode i.
color i.
2DFT gradient-echo i.
3DFT gradient-echo MR i.
direct Fourier transformation i.
Dixon method opposed i.
Doppler color flow i.
Doppler tissue i.
echo i.
echoplanar magnetic resonance i.
endocrine i.
endometrial chemical shift i.
endorectal coil magnetic resonance i.
endoscopic ultrasonographic i.
endovaginal i.
exercise i.
field-echo i.
functional magnetic resonance i. (fMRI)
gradient-echo MR i.
hepatobiliary i.
intraoperative i.
intravenous digital subtraction i.
krypton-8lm ventilation i.
magnetic resonance i. (MRI)
magnetic source i. (MSI)
i. method
i. modality
multiple-echo i.
multiple line scan i.
multiple-plane i.
multiple spin-echo i.
oblique sagittal gradient-echo MR i.
pancreatic i.
paramagnetic enhancement accentuation by chemical shift i.
phase-sensitive gradient-echo MR i.
point i.
power Doppler i.
preoperative i.
projection-reconstruction i.
projection tract i.
rapid acquisition radiofrequency-echo-steady state i.
rapid bedside i.
rotating frame i.
sagittal-plane i.
selective excitation projection reconstruction i.
sensitive plane projection reconstruction i.
sequential line i.
sequential plane i.
sequential point i.
serial i.
short-inversion recovery i.
single-echo diffusion i.
spin-echo magnetic resonance i.
spoiled gradient-echo i.
steady-state gradient-echo i.

NOTES

imaging *(continued)*
i. strategy
stress-redistribution-reinjection thallium-201 i.
i. study
i. technique
three-dimensional Fourier transform gradient-echo i.
three-dimensional projection reconstruction i.
tissue Doppler i.
transverse section i.
tumor i.
two-dimensional Fourier transformation i.
two-dimensional Fourier transform gradient-echo i.
ventilation/perfusion i.
xenon lung ventilation i.
Imanaga method
imbalance
electrolyte i.
imbricate
imbricated suture technique
imbrication
capsular i.
i. line of Pickerill
i. line of von Ebner
MacNab line for facet i.
medial capsular i.
medialis obliquus i.
retinal i.
IML
internal mammary lymphoscintigraphy
immaculate hemostasis
immediate
i. amputation
i. asthmatic reaction (IAR)
i. breast reconstruction
i. extension technique
i. flap
i. postoperative period
i. transfusion
immersion
i. method
i. microscopy
i. technique
imminens
imminent cardiac arrest
immobilization
cast i.
cervical i.
i. method
postoperative i.
rigid cervical i.
Rowe-Zarins shoulder i.
sling i.
spica cast i.
sternal-occipital-mandibular i.
tooth i.
Treponema pallidum i.
Webril i.
immotile cilia syndrome
immovable joint
ImmTher therapy
immune
i. electron microscopy
i. inflammation
i. mechanism
i. modulation
i. response
i. system anatomy
immune-mediated
i.-m. coagulation disorder
i.-m. HIT
i.-m. unfractionated heparin-induced thrombocytopenia
immunity
cellular i.
CTL i.
immunocompetent tissue therapy
immunocytochemical approach
immunocytoma
immunodeficient
immunodepression
immunodiagnostic method
immunofluorescence
i. method
i. microscopy
immunofluorescent examination
immunohistochemical
i. analysis
i. feature
i. marker
i. method
i. stain
i. staining
i. technique
immunohistochemistry
immunoincompetent
immunologic
i. classification
i. complication
i. impairment
i. method of purging
immunometric sandwich method
immunomodulating
i. effect
i. infection
immunomodulation
immunonutrition
immunoperoxidase method
immunoproliferative lesion
immunoreactive parathyroid hormone assay
immunoreactivity

immunoscintigraphy
immunostain
cytokeratin i.
immunostaining
immunostimulation
immunosuppression
pharmacologic i.
short-term i.
tacrolimus-based i.
immunosympathectomy
immunotherapy
active specific i. (ASI)
systemic i.
impacted
i. calculus
i. fracture
impaction
basket i.
endoscope i.
fecal i.
i. lesion
i. point
stool i.
impaired
i. healing
i. mobility
i. oxygen utilization
i. regeneration syndrome
impairment
immunologic i.
impalement
abdominal i.
anorectal i.
impar
impatent
impedance
electrode i.
i. method
pacemaker i.
i. plethysmography
i. pneumography
imperfecta
lethal osteogenesis i.
osteogenesis i.
severe deforming osteogenesis i.
Sillence type II-IV osteogenesis i.
imperforate anus
imperforation
Imperial College London Hospital
impetiginization
impingement
graft i.
implant
i. abutment
i. alloy aluminum
i. arthroplasty
i. biocompatibility
i. cervix
encapsulated breast i.
i. entry
i. erosion
i. extrusion
i. failure
i. fatigue
fill breast i.
i. fixture
i. fracture
i. framework
i. gingival sulcus
i. infrastructure
i. mesostructure
i. migration
i. model
i. neck
neoplastic port site i.
i. placement
i. reaction
i. removal
i. restoration
i. stage
i. structure
i. substructure interspace
i. superstructure neck
i. survival rate
implantable
i. cardioverter-defibrillator/atrial tachycardia pacing
i. infusion port
i. pain modality
implantation
i. bleeding
circumferential i.
cortical i.
displacement i.
i. failure
fusion i.
gastric balloon i.
i. graft
hypodermic i.
interstitial i.
in-the-bag i.
intracavitary i.
intraocular lens i.
intrusive i.

NOTES

implantation *(continued)*
mesh i.
i. metastasis
metastatic i.
needle tract i.
nerve i.
periosteal i.
i. phase
placental i.
radioactive seed i.
radon seed i.
real-time 3-D biplanar transperineal prostate i.
i. response
screw i.
i. site
stent i.
subcutaneous i.
subdural grid i.
submuscular i.
subpectoral i.
superficial i.
tension-free mesh i.
i. test
tubouterine i.
ureter i.
implant-bearing surface
implant-cement interface
implanted suture technique
implication
clinical i.
psychologic i.
implicit memory
implosive therapy
impotence
impregnation
impressio, pl. **impressiones**
impression
cardiac i.
colic i.
digitate i.
duodenal i.
esophageal i.
extrinsic esophageal i.
i. fracture
gastric i.
i. preparation
prepared cavity i.
renal i.
suprarenal i.
surgical bone i.
i. technique
trigeminal i.
imprint
tissue i.
improvement
clinical i.
impulse
ectopic i.
i. formation
mobilization with i.
point of maximum i.
Imre
I. keratoplasty
I. lateral canthoplasty
I. lateral canthoplasty operation
I. sliding flap
Imrie prognostic scoring index
imus
IMV
intermittent mandatory ventilation
IMZ type restoration
in
in extremis
opting in
in situ
in situ bypass
in situ dissection
in situ hypothermic perfusion
in situ photocoagulation
in situ procedure
in situ reconstruction
in situ spinal fusion
in situ split-liver procurement
in situ uterine repair
in utero exposure
in utero repair
in vitro contracture test
in vitro fertilization
in vitro fertilization-embryo transfer
in vivo
in vivo fertilization
in vivo optical spectroscopy
inactivation
trigger-point i.
inadequate
i. dilation
i. surgery
i. visualization
inadvertent
i. enterotomy
i. laceration
i. serosal tear
i. trauma
i. venous injury
in-and-out catheterization
inapparent infection
in-between size
incae
incarcerated hernia
incarceration
colon i.
colonoscopy-related i.
hernia i.
iris i.

penile i.
retrograde i.

incarial bone

incarnant

incarnative

incarnatus

incidence

incident
i. exposure
i. point

incidental
i. appendectomy
i. parathyroidectomy
i. rupture
i. splenectomy

incidentaloma
adrenal i.

incineration

incisal
i. canal
i. cavity
i. mandibular plane angle
i. point
i. preparation

incised
i. fascia
i. wound

incision
abdominal wall i.
abdominoinguinal i.
abdominothoracic i.
ab externo i.
ab interno i.
Agnew-Verhoeff i.
alar i.
Alexander i.
Amussat i.
angular i.
anterior i.
anterolateral thoracotomy i.
anteromedial i.
appendectomy i.
apron skin i.
arcuate i.
areolar i.
Auvray i.
axillary i.
backcut i.
Banks-Laufman i.
Battle i.
battledore i.
Battle-Jalaguier-Kammerer i.
bayonet-type i.
Bergmann i.
Bergmann-Israel i.
Bevan abdominal i.
bicoronal i.
bifrontal i.
bikini skin i.
bilateral subcostal i.
bilateral transabdominal i.
bisubcostal i.
Blair i.
boutonnière i.
Brackin i.
breast i.
Brock i.
Brockman i.
Brunner modified i.
Brunner palmar i.
Bruser skin i.
bucket-handle i.
Burns-Haney i.
buttonhole skin i.
Caldwell-Luc i.
capsular i.
cautery i.
celiotomy i.
cervical i.
cesarean section i.
Chang-Miltner i.
Charnley i.
Cherney lower transverse abdominal i.
Chernez i.
chevron i.
chevron-shaped i.
Chiene i.
choledochotomy i.
chord i.
Cincinnati i.
circular i.
circumareolar i.
circumferential i.
circumlimbal i.
circumlinear i.
circumscribing i.
circumumbilical i.
clamshell i.
classical transverse i.
clavicular i.
i. closure
Codman i.
Coffey i.

NOTES

incision *(continued)*
collar i.
Colonna-Ralston i.
colpotomy i.
confirmatory i.
conjunctival i.
Connell i.
corneal i.
corneoscleral i.
corridor i.
cortical i.
Courvoisier i.
Couvelaire i.
Crawford i.
crisscrossing abdominal wall i.'s
crosshatch i.
cross-tunneling i.
crucial i.
cruciate i.
Cubbins i.
Curtin i.
curved i.
curvilinear i.
cutdown i.
darting i.
Deaver i.
decompression i.
deltoid-splitting i.
deltopectoral i.
Depage i.
diamond-shaped i.
dorsal linear i.
dorsal longitudinal i.
dorsal lumbotomy i.
dorsal transverse i.
dorsolateral i.
dorsomedial i.
double i.
i. and drainage (I&D)
Dührssen i.
dural i.
DuVries i.
Dwyer i.
Edebohls i.
eleventh rib flank i.
eleventh rib transperitoneal i.
elliptical uterine i.
Elsberg i.
endaural mastoid i.
endoscopic i.
endoscopically performed longitudinal i.
endourological cold-knife i.
epigastric i.
extended left subcostal i.
external bevel i.
extraction i.
fascia-splitting i.
Fergusson i.
fiber-splitting i.
fishmouth i.
flank i.
flexed i.
Fowler-Philip i.
Frazier i.
frown i.
Gaenslen split-heel i.
Gatellier-Chastang i.
Gibson long vertical relaxing i.
Gibson-type i.
Gluck i.
goblet i.
gray-line i.
Greenhow i.
Grice i.
gridiron i.
Griffith i.
grooved i.
gullwing i.
Hajek i.
Handley i.
Harmon i.
Harper-Warren i.
Hayes Martin i.
Heerman i.
Heineke-Mikulicz i.
hemicircular i.
Henderson skin i.
Henry i.
hernia i.
H-flap i.
Higgins i.
hockey-stick i.
Hood and Kirklin i.
horizontal i.
horseshoe i.
horseshoe-shaped i.
H-shaped capsular i.
Hueter i.
ilioinguinal i.
infraclavicular i.
inframammary i.
infraumbilical i.
inguinal i.
inner bevel i.
intercartilaginous i.
internal bevel i.
intracapsular i.
intraoral i.
intraperitoneal i.
inverse bevel i.
inverted bevel i.
inverted-U abdominal i.
inverted-Y i.
Jackson i.
Jergesen i.

J-shaped skin i.
Kammerer-Battle i.
Kehr i.
keyhole i.
Killian i.
Koenig-Schaefer i.
Küstner i.
Lanz i.
laparotomy i.
LaRoque herniorrhaphy i.
lateral utility i.
lazy-C i.
lazy-H i.
lazy-S i.
lazy-Z i.
L-curved i.
Lempert i.
Lilienthal i.
limbal i.
i. line
linear i.
Linton i.
lip-splitting i.
Loeffler-Ballard i.
longitudinal i.
low-collar i.
lower uterine segment i.
low-segment transverse i.
low transverse i.
L-shaped capsular i.
Ludloff i.
Lynch i.
MacFee i.
Mackenrodt i.
Mallard i.
marginal i.
Martin i.
Mason i.
mastectomy i.
mastoid i.
Mayfield i.
Maylard i.
Mayo-Robson i.
McArthur i.
McBurney appendectomy i.
McLaughlin-Ryder i.
McVay i.
medial parapatellar i.
median sternotomy i.
Meyer i.
midabdominal transverse i.
midaxillary line i.
midline lower abdominal i.
midline oblique i.
midline upper abdominal i.
Mikulicz i.
minilaparotomy i.
modified Gibson i.
Morison i.
multiple-port i.
muscle-splitting i.
Nagamatsu i.
Nicola i.
non-rib-spreading thoracotomy i.
Ober i.
Ollier i.
omega-shaped i.
Orr i.
ovarian i.
overlapping i.
palmar i.
parainguinal i.
paramedial i.
paramedian i.
paramuscular i.
parapatellar i.
pararectus i.
parasagittal i.
parascapular i.
paraumbilical i.
paravaginal i.
Parker i.
Péan i.
Penduloff i.
perianal i.
periareolar i.
perilimbal i.
perineal i.
periscapular i.
peritoneal i.
periumbilical i.
Perthes i.
Pfannenstiel i.
Phemister i.
Picot i.
plantar longitudinal i.
plaque i.
popliteal i.
port i.
postauricular i.
posterior hemicircular i.
posterior transthoracic i.
posterolateral costotransversectomy i.
preauricular i.

NOTES

incision *(continued)*
precut i.
Pridie i.
proximal i.
Pulvertaft fishmouth i.
puncture i.
racquet i.
racquet-shaped i.
radial skin i.
recently healed surgical i.
rectus muscle-splitting i.
rectus sheath i.
recumbent i.
relaxing i.
relief i.
relieving i.
Rethi i.
retroauricular i.
reverse bevel i.
reverse-Y i.
right-sided submandibular transverse i.
rim i.
Robertson i.
Rodman i.
Rollet i.
Rosen i.
Roux-en-Y jejunal loop i.
Ruddy i.
S i.
saber-cut i.
salmon backcut i.
Sanders i.
Sanger i.
scalp i.
Schobinger i.
Schuchardt relaxing i.
scoring i.
scratch-type i.
Sellheim i.
semiflexed i.
semilunar i.
serpentine i.
S-flap i.
Shambaugh i.
shelving i.
shoulder-strap i.
Simon i.
single midline extraperitoneal i.
Singleton i.
skin i.
skin-crease i.
skin-knife i.
skived i.
Sloan i.
smiling i.
spindle-shaped i.
spiral i.
split i.
split-heel i.
S-shaped i.
stab wound i.
standard clavicular i.
standard Kocher i.
standard retroperitoneal flank i.
stellate i.
steri-stripped i.
sternal-splitting i.
sternotomy i.
Stewart i.
stocking-seam i.
straight i.
subciliary i.
subcostal flank i.
subcostal transperitoneal i.
subinguinal i.
sublabial i.
submammary i.
subtrochanteric i.
subumbilical i.
supracervical i.
suprapubic Pfannenstiel i.
supraumbilical i.
surgical i.
Sutherland-Rowe i.
Swan i.
T i.
tangential i.
temporal i.
Thomas-Warren i.
thoracoabdominal i.
thoracotomy i.
transection i.
transmeatal tympanoplasty i.
transpubic i.
transrectus i.
transurethral laser i.
transverse mastectomy i.
transverse skin i.
trap i.
trapezoidal i.
T-shaped i.
umbilical skin-knife i.
unilateral subcostal i.
upper midline i.
upright-Y i.
U-shaped i.
uterine i.
vertical midline i.
vertical uterine i.
volar midline oblique i.
volar zig-zag finger i.
von Noorden i.
V-shaped i.
Wagner skin i.
Warren i.

Watson-Jones i.
Weber-Fergusson i.
web space i.
wedge i.
Weir i.
Westin-Hall i.
Whipple i.
Wigby-Taylor i.
Wilde i.
Willy Meyer mastectomy i.
W-shaped i.
xiphoid-to-pubis midline abdominal i.
xiphoid-to-umbilicus i.
Y i.
Yorke-Mason i.
Y-shaped i.
Y-V-plasty i.
Z-flap i.
zig-zag finger i.
Z-plasty i.
Z-shaped i.

incisional
i. biopsy
i. corporoplasty
i. gastropexy
i. hernia
i. hernioplasty
i. infiltration
i. metastasis
i. pain
i. scar

incisiva

incisive
i. canal
i. duct
i. foramen
i. fossa

incisor
i. point

incisura

incisurae

incisural
i. dissection
i. epidermoidoma
i. space

inciting pathology

inclination
axial i.
condylar guidance i.
crown i.
enamel rod i.
lateral condylar i.
lingual i.
pelvic i.

inclinatio pelvis

inclusion body disease

incompetent sphincter

incomplete
i. amputation
i. atrioventricular dissociation
i. A-V dissociation
i. colonoscopy
i. compound fracture
i. dislocation
i. duplication
i. excision
i. fistula
i. hernia
i. polypectomy
i. reduction
i. regeneration
i. relaxation
i. right bundle-branch block
i. tumor resection

inconsequential echo

incontinence
anal i.
Blaivas classification of urinary i.
exercise-induced i.
fecal i.
gas i.
neurogenic i.
overflow i.
paradoxical i.
passive i.
postprostatectomy i.
reflex i.
stress urinary i.
urge i.
urinary exertional i.

incontinent
i. ileostomy
i. ileovesicostomy

incorporation
bone graft i.

increased
i. lateral joint space
i. pressure
i. systemic vascular resistance

incremental
i. blood sampling
i. therapy

NOTES

incrustation
  stent i.
incudal fold
incudis
incudomallearis
incudomalleolar
  i. articulation
  i. joint
incudostapedial
incus
indenization
indentation
  i. gonioscopy
  i. hardness
  haustral i.
  i. operation
  prominent i.
  i. tonometer
  i. tonometry
independent exercise program
indeterminate FNA
index, pl. **indices**
  Abdominal Trauma I. (ATI)
  accute physiology prognostic scoring i.
  Addiction Severity I.
  alveolar i.
  American Rheumatism Association i.
  American Urological Association symptom i.
  analgesic i.
  anesthetic i.
  ankle-brachial i.
  ankle-brachial pressure i. (ABPI)
  Arthritis Helplessness I. (AHI)
  articulation i.
  atherectomy i.
  atrial stasis i.
  auricular i.
  basilar i.
  biliary saturation i.
  bispectral i.
  body mass i. (BMI)
  cardiac i. (CI)
  cephalic i.
  cephalorrhachidian i.
  cerebral i.
  cerebrospinal i.
  chest i.
  cholesterol saturation i.
  compliance, rate, oxygenation, and pressure i.
  computed tomography severity i. (CTSI)
  cranial i.
  dental i.
  diastolic pressure-time i.
  eccentricity i.
  ejection phase i.
  exercise i.
  facial i.
  Flower dental i.
  frequency-duration i.
  Gastrointestinal Quality of Life I. (GIQLI)
  gnathic i.
  height-length i.
  Imrie prognostic scoring i.
  irritation i.
  juxtaglomerular granulation i.
  length-breadth i.
  length-height i.
  limb salvage i.
  maturation i.
  mean shunt i.
  i. metacarpophalangeal joint reconstruction
  mitral valve closure i.
  nasal i.
  Neck Disability I.
  orbital i.
  orbitonasal i.
  oxygenation i. (OI)
  oxygen saturation i.
  palatal i.
  palatomaxillary i.
  pectus i.
  penetrating abdominal trauma i. (PATI)
  penile-brachial pressure i.
  phosphate excretion i.
  physical therapy i.
  i. pollicization
  portal shunt i.
  pressure-volume i.
  PSE i.
  pulmonary vascular resistance i. (PVRI)
  Ranson prognostic scoring i.
  i. ray amputation
  relaxation time i.
  Right Ventricular Stroke Work I. (RVSWI)
  Röhrer i.
  sacral i.
  saturation i.
  sedimentation i.
  segmental pressure i.
  Shoulder Pain and Disability I.
  shunt i.
  Singh osteoporosis i.
  systolic pressure time i.
  thoracic i.
  transversovertical i.
  i. of variability

ventilation i. (VI)
vertical i.
zygomaticoauricular i.

Indian
I. flap
I. method
I. operation
I. rhinoplasty

Indiana continent reservoir urinary diversion

indication
clinical i.
emergency i.
familial i.
surgical i.

indicator
i. dilution technique
finger i.
i. fractionation
prognostic i.
redox i.

indicator-dilution curve

indices (*pl. of* index)

indicis

indifferent genitalia

indirect
i. defect
i. fracture
i. hernial sac
i. inguinal hernia
i. laryngoscopy
i. manipulation
i. memory
i. obturator nerve block
i. ophthalmoscopy
i. portography
i. pulpal therapy
i. reduction
i. restorative method
i. technique
i. transfusion
i. triangulation

indiscriminate lesion

indocyanine
i. green clearance result
i. green indicator dilution technique
i. green method
i. green retention test

Indoklon therapy

indomethacin-induced gastropathy

indophenol method

induced
i. apnea
i. bronchospasm
i. hypotension
i. hypotension anesthetic technique
i. tension pneumothorax

induction
i. of anesthesia
anesthetic i.
i. anesthetic technique
i. chemotherapy
dorsal i.
electric i.
endotracheal i.
enzyme i.
Faraday law of i.
gene i.
labor augmentation i.
lysogenic i.
magnetic i.
menstrual cycle i.
negative control enzyme i.
neuromuscular system electric i.
ovulation i.
pain i.
positive control enzyme i.
rapid-sequence i. (RSI)
remission i.
Spemann i.
sputum i.
superovulation i.

induration
brawny i.
cyanotic i.
Froriep i.
gray i.
idiopathic brown i.
plastic i.
red i.

industrial exposure

indwelling

inequality
ventilation/perfusion i.

inertia
colonic i.

inextensible

infant
Distress Scale for Ventilated Newborn I.'s (DSVNI)

infantile
i. articulation
i. choriocarcinoma syndrome

infantile *(continued)*
i. colic
i. embryonal carcinoma
i. hernia
i. perseveration
infantilism
celiac i.
infarct
i. expansion
i. extension
infarction
evolving myocardial i.
hemorrhagic i.
myocardial i. (MI)
renal i.
Thrombolysis in Myocardial I. (TIMI)
infarctive lesion
infected
i. collection
i. necrosis
i. tract
infection
abortive i.
Absidia i.
active systemic bacterial i.
adenoviral i.
adenovirus i.
adnexal i.
aerobic i.
airborne i.
amebic i.
anaerobic ocular i.
antifungal esophageal i.
antifungal-resistant opportunistic i.
apical i.
aspergillosis i.
Aspergillus i.
asymptomatic i.
atypical mycobacterial i.
bacterial i.
benign papillomavirus i.
beta hemolytic streptococci i.
biliary tract i.
blood-borne i.
bloodstream i.
blood stream i.
brain i.
buccal space i.
Bunyavirus i.
i. calculus
Campylobacter i.
Candida i.
candidal i.
catheter tunnel i.
central line i.
cervical i.
cervicovaginal i.
chlamydial i.
Chlamydia trachomatis i.
chorioamnionic i.
chronic Epstein-Barr virus i.
closed-space i.
clostridial i.
CMV i.
Coccidioides i.
coliform urinary i.
colonization i.
community-acquired i.
congenital HIV i.
cross i.
cryptococcal i.
Cryptococcus i.
cryptogenic i.
cryptosporidial i.
cutaneous bacterial i.
cutaneous viral i.
cysticercal i.
cytomegalovirus i.
deep delayed i.
deep-seated fungal i.
deep wound i.
dengue hemorrhagic fever i.
dental i.
dermatophyte fungal i.
disk space i.
disseminated CMV i.
disseminated gonococcal i.
dragon worm i.
droplet i.
dust-borne i.
EBV i.
echovirus i.
ectothrix i.
endemic fungal i.
endogenous i.
endothrix i.
enteric i.
enteroviral i.
environmental mycobacterial i.
epidural space i.
Epstein-Barr viral i.
esophageal i.
esophageal fungal i.
exit site i.
exogenous i.
extrapulmonary *Pneumocystis carinii* i.
eyelid molluscum contagiosum i.
fascial space i.
felon i.
fetal i.
focal i.
fungal pancreatic i.
fungous i.
gas-forming pyogenic liver i.

gas-producing streptococcal i.
gastric i.
gastrointestinal i.
gay bowel i.
genital i.
genitourinary i.
Giardia i.
gonococcal i.
graft i.
gram-positive bacterial i.
granulomatous bacterial i.
granulomatous fungal i.
group A beta-hemolytic streptococcal i.
group A streptococcus i.
guinea worm i.
Hantavirus i.
helminthic i.
hepatic candidal i.
hepatic fungal i.
hepatitis A-E i.
herpes simplex virus i.
herpes zoster i.
herpetic i.
hibernal epidemic viral i.
Histoplasma i.
HIV-1, -2 i.
hospital-acquired i.
human bite i.
human papillomavirus i.
iatrogenic i.
immunomodulating i.
inapparent i.
intestinal i.
intraabdominal i.
intraamniotic i.
intrauterine i.
IUD-related i.
kala-azar i.
laryngeal i.
latent herpes simplex virus i.
line i.
liver cyst i.
local i.
lower genital tract i.
lower respiratory tract i.
MAC i.
MAI i.
mass i.
masticator space i.
maternal i.
Medina i.
Meleney i.
metasynchronous bacterial urinary tract i.
middle ear i.
mixed fungal/bacterial i.
mixed nail i.
monilial i.
mucor i.
multiple hepatitis virus i.
musculoskeletal i.
mycobacterial i.
Mycobacterium avium complex i.
Mycobacterium avium-intracellulare i.
Mycoplasma i.
mycotic i.
necrotizing i.
neisserial i.
nematode i.
neonatal i.
neutropenia-related bacterial i.
nondermatophyte fungal i.
nonopportunistic i.
nontuberculous mycobacterial i.
nosocomial fungal i.
odontogenic i.
opportunistic systemic fungal i.
oral i.
overwhelming postsplenectomy i.
pancreatic bacterial i.
papillomavirus i.
parainfluenza virus i.
parasitic i.
parastomal i.
paravaccinia virus i.
paronychial i.
pelvic i.
percutaneous bone marrow i.
perianal i.
periapical i.
perinatal i.
perineal i.
periorbital i.
peripancreatic i.
peristomal i.
peritoneal fungal i.
persistent tolerant i.
pharyngeal gonococcal i.
pin tract i.
pneumococcal i.
polymicrobial i.
postoperative i.

NOTES

infection *(continued)*
postpartum i.
postsplenectomy i.
i. prevention
primary fungal i.
primary herpes simplex i.
protozoal i.
Pseudomonas i.
puerperal i.
pulmonary bacterial i.
pulmonary fungal i.
pulmonary parenchymal i.
pure fungal i.
pyodermatous i.
pyogenic spinal i.
recurrent upper respiratory tract i.
renal cyst i.
renal fungal i.
repeated respiratory i.
reservoir of i.
respiratory syncytial virus i.
respiratory tract i.
retroperitoneal i.
retrovirus i.
rhinocerebral i.
Rhizopus i.
rickettsial i.
rotavirus i.
Salinem i.
salivary gland i.
scalp i.
secondary fungal i.
serpent i.
Shigella i.
shunt i.
skin i.
spinal i.
spirochetal i.
spirochete i.
staphylococcal i.
streptococcal i.
Streptococcus i.
subclinical i.
subcutaneous fungal i.
subcutaneous necrotizing i.
subperiosteal i.
subumbilical i.
superficial subumbilical i.
suppurative i.
surgical i.
surgical-site i. (SSI)
sycosiform fungous i.
symptomatic i.
synchronous urinary tract i.
systemic fungal i.
tarsal joint i.
temporal space i.
terminal i.
torulopsis i.
trematode i.
Trichomonas i.
tunnel i.
ultralow anterior resection parastomal i.
unusual opportunistic i.
upper genital tract i.
upper respiratory tract i.
urinary tract i.
uterine i.
vaccinia i.
vaginal i.
varicella i.
varicella-zoster virus i.
vertically acquired i.
vesicular viral i.
Vibrio fetus i.
Vincent i.
viral respiratory i.
vulvar i.
vulvovaginal premenarchal i.
web space i.
Western blot i.
whipworm i.
wound i.
xenogenic i.
yeast i.
zoonotic i.

infectious
i. complication
i. etiology
i. granuloma

infective extraabdominal complication

inferior
i. aberrant ductule
i. accessory fissure
i. alveolar artery
i. alveolar nerve
i. alveolar vein
i. apical (IA)
i. arcuate bundle
i. articular pit
i. articular process
i. basal (IB)
i. boundary
i. carotid artery
i. carotid triangle
i. cerebral artery
i. cervical ganglion
i. complete closed dislocation
i. complete compound dislocation
i. costal facet
i. costal pit
i. dental foramen
i. duodenal fold
i. duodenal fossa
i. duodenal recess

i. edge
i. epigastric artery
i. extradural approach
i. face
i. flap
i. flexure
i. fornix reformation
i. gland
i. glenohumeral ligament
i. gluteal artery
i. hemorrhoidal artery
i. hemorrhoidal nerve
i. hemorrhoidal plexus
i. hypogastric plexus
i. hypophysial artery
i. ileocecal recess
i. internal parietal artery
i. interosseous vein
i. labial artery
i. lacrimal duct
i. lacrimal papilla
i. lacrimal punctum
i. laryngeal artery
i. laryngeal cavity
i. laryngotomy
i. lateral genicular artery
i. lateral genicular vein
i. lingular segment
i. longitudinal sinus
i. meatal antrostomy
i. meatus
i. medial genicular artery
i. medial genicular vein
i. mediastinum
i. mesenteric artery (IMA)
i. mesenteric ganglion
i. mesenteric plexus
i. occipital triangle
i. omental recess
i. orbital fissure
i. palpebral nerve
i. pancreatic artery
i. pancreaticoduodenal artery
i. parietal lobe
i. pelvic aperture
i. petrosal groove
i. petrosal sinus
i. petrosal sulcus
i. phrenic artery
i. pole
i. pubic ligament
i. rectal artery
i. rectal fold
i. rectal nerve
i. rectal plexus
i. sagittal sinus
i. suprarenal artery
i. surface
i. tarsus
i. temporal branch
i. thoracic aperture
i. thoracic artery
i. thyroid artery
i. thyroid notch
i. thyroid plexus
i. thyroid tubercle
i. transvermian approach
i. transverse rectal fold
i. transverse scapular ligament
i. ulnar collateral artery
i. vena cava (IVC)
i. vena cava ligation
i. vena cava pressure (IVCP)
i. vena cava reconstruction
i. vertebral notch
i. vesical artery
i. vesical nerve
i. vesical plexus

inferiores
inferioris
inferior-lateral endonasal transsphenoidal approach
inferius
InFerno moist heat therapy
inferolateral
inferomedial aspect
infertility evaluation
infestation
noninvasive i.
infiltrate
infiltrating
i. duct adenocarcinoma
i. ductal carcinoma
i. lobular carcinoma
infiltration
adipose i.
i. anesthesia
i. anesthetic technique
bacterial mucosal i.
i. block
bone marrow i.
brachial plexus i.
calcareous i.
cellular i.

infiltration *(continued)*
choroidal i.
colonic i.
diffuse fatty i.
epituberculous i.
fatty i.
focal fatty i.
gastric epithelial cell i.
gelatinous i.
glomerular macrophage i.
glomerular neutrophil i.
glycogen i.
gray i.
incisional i.
leukemic i.
leukocyte i.
leukocytic i.
lipomatous i.
local i.
local tissue i.
lymphocytic i.
lymphoid i.
massive malignant i.
mononuclear cell i.
neutrophilic i.
panmucosal inflammatory cell i.
paraneural i.
patchy i.
peribronchiolar lymphocyte i.
pericapsular fat i.
perineural i.
plasma cell portal i.
root i.
sanguineous i.
tuberculous i.
tumor i.
infiltrative carcinoma
inflamed synovial pouch
inflammable
inflammation
active chronic i.
acute and chronic i.
acute hemorrhagic i.
adhesive i.
allergic i.
alterative i.
atrophic i.
blenorrhagic i.
bronchial i.
bullous granulomatous i.
calcified granulomatous i.
cartilage i.
caseating granulomatous i.
caseous i.
catarrhal i.
cavitating i.
i. cell
central zone i.
cervical i.
chronic jejunal i.
circumscribed i.
confluent i.
croupous i.
cystic acute i.
cystic chronic i.
cystic granulomatous i.
degenerative i.
diffuse acute i.
diffuse chronic i.
disseminated i.
ear cartilage i.
erosive i.
esophageal i.
exanthematous i.
exudative granulomatous i.
fibrinoid necrotizing i.
fibrinopurulent i.
fibrinous i.
fibrocaseous i.
fibroid i.
focal granulomatous i.
follicular i.
gangrenous granulomatous i.
gelatinous acute i.
gingival i.
granulomatous i.
hemorrhagic i.
hyperplastic i.
ileal i.
immune i.
interstitial i.
intralobular i.
ischemic ocular i.
localized i.
membranous acute i.
microbiliary i.
miliary granulomatous i.
mucosal i.
multifocal i.
myocardial i.
necrotic i.
necrotizing granulomatous i.
neutrophilic i.
nonnecrotizing granulomatous i.
obliterative i.
ocular i.
organizing i.
ossifying i.
pelvic i.
periodontal i.
perirectal i.
portal eosinophilic i.
portal tract i.
prepatellar bursa i.
productive i.
proliferative i.

pseudomembranous acute i.
purulent i.
pustular i.
i. reaction
recurrent i.
retrodiskal temporomandibular joint pad i.
sanguineous i.
sclerosing i.
serofibrinous i.
serous acute i.
spinal i.
subacute i.
suppurative acute i.
suppurative chronic i.
suppurative granulomatous i.
transmural i.
transudative i.
traumatic i.
ulcerative i.
urate-associated i.
uremic i.
vaginal i.
vesicular acute i.
vesicular granulomatous i.

inflammatory
i. arteritis
i. bowel disease
i. breast carcinoma
i. cavity
i. cell
i. cytokine
i. exudate
i. fistula
i. fracture
i. granuloma
i. lesion
i. membrane
i. pain
i. perforation
i. problem
i. pseudotumor formation
i. response
i. rupture
i. sinus tract
i. transcription factor

inflated lung

inflation
balloon i.
i. reflex

inflection, inflexion
point of i.

inflow
arterial i.
i. control
i. occlusion
portal i.
i. tract
i. vessel

infold

informal method

information
anatomic imaging i.
histopathologic i.
prognostic i.

informed consent

infraauricular
i. mass

infra-auriculares

infraclavicular
i. fossa
i. incision
i. part of brachial plexus
i. triangle

infraclavicularis

infraclinoid aneurysm

infracostalis

infracostal line

infracotyloid

infraction fracture

infradentale

infradiaphragmatic

infraduodenal fossa

infragastric pancreoscopy

infragenicular popliteal artery (IGPA)

infraglenoid
i. tubercle

infraglottic
i. cavity
i. space

infraglotticum

infrahepatic
i. cavotomy
i. inferior vena cava

infrahyoid
i. bursa
i. muscle

infrahyoidea

infrahyoidei

infrainguinal bypass

infralabyrinthine approach

inframammaria

inframammary
i. approach

NOTES

inframammary *(continued)*
i. crease
i. incision
i. region
inframandibular
inframarginal
inframaxillary
inframesocolic space
infraorbital
i. anesthesia
i. artery
i. canal
i. foramen
i. groove
i. injection
i. nerve
i. nerve block
i. notch
i. region
i. space
i. space abscess
i. suture
i. vein
infraorbitalis
infrapatellar
i. fat body
i. fat pad
i. tendon rupture
infrapatellare
infrapatellaris
infrapopliteal
i. bypass
i. transluminal angioplasty
i. vessel
infrared
i. coagulation
i. photocoagulation
i. spectroscopy
i. therapy
i. transillumination gastroscopy
infrarenal
i. aorta
i. aortic cross-clamping
i. aortic reconstruction
i. cava
i. endograft placement
i. template procedure
infrascapular
i. artery
i. region
infrascapularis
infraspinata
infraspinati
infraspinatus
i. bursa
i. insertion erosion
infraspinous fossa
infrasplenic
infrasternal angle
infrasternalis
infrastructure
implant i.
infratemporal
i. crest
i. fossa
i. fossa approach
i. space
infratemporalis
infratentorial
i. arteriovenous malformation
i. structure
i. supracerebellar approach
i. tumor
infrathoracic
infratrochlearis
infratrochlear nerve
infraumbilical
i. incision
i. omphalocele
i. position
infraversion
infundibula (*pl. of* infundibulum)
infundibular wedge resection
infundibulectomy
Brock i.
infundibuliform
i. fascia
i. sheath
infundibuliformis
infundibuloma
infundibuloovarian ligament
infundibulopelvic ligament
infundibulotomy
infundibulum, pl. **infundibula**
caliceal i.
ethmoidal i.
infused fluid
infusion
analgesic i.
i. cholangiography
chronic subcutaneous i.
computer-assisted controlled i. (CACI)
drip i.
drug i.
epidural opioid i.
i. graft
hepatic arterial i. (HAI)
intravariceal i.
lipid i.
mesenteric vasodilator i.
nerve block i.
i. port
portal i.
propofol i.
i. rate

target-controlled i. (TCI)
triple-lumen i.
vasodilator i.
infusional chemotherapy
Ingelman-Sundberg gracilis muscle procedure
ingested foreign body
Inglis-Cooper technique
Inglis-Ranawat-Straub
I.-R.-S. elbow synovectomy
I.-R.-S. technique
Inglis triaxial total elbow arthroplasty
Ingram-Bachynski hip fracture classification
Ingram bony bridge resection
Ingram-Canle-Beaty epiphysial-metaphysial osteotomy
Ingram-Withers-Speltz motor test
ingrowing toenail
ingrown nail
ingrowth
fibrous i.
i. fixation
local i.
inguen
inguinal
i. aponeurotic fold
i. approach
i. branch
i. canal
i. canal dissection
i. crest
i. field block
i. fossa
i. gland
i. hernia
i. herniorrhaphy
i. incision
i. ligament
i. lymphadenectomy
i. lymph node metastasis
i. neuralgia
i. perivascular block
i. plexus
i. region
i. ring
i. triangle
i. trigone
inguinale
inguinal-femoral node dissection
inguinalis
inguinocrural hernia
inguinodynia
herniorrhaphy chronic i.
mesh i.
post herniorrhaphy i.
inguinofemoral hernia
inguinolabial hernia
inguinoperitoneal
inguinoproperitoneal hernia
inguinoscrotal hernia
inguinosuperficial hernia
inhalant anesthesia
inhalation
i. aerosol
i. agent
i. analgesia
i. anesthetic technique
i. mask anesthesia
i. method
i. pneumonia
i. therapy
i. tuberculosis
inhalational anesthesia
inhaled anesthetic
inherent risk
inherited cancer syndrome
inhibition
pyruvate dehydrogenase i.
inhibitor
angiotensin-converting enzyme i. (ACE)
COX-2 i.
cytokine receptor i.
direct thrombin i.
proton pump i. (PPI)
selective serotonin reuptake i. (SSRI)
inhibitory
i. nerve
i. role
inhibitory-excitatory mechanism
in-hospital mortality rate
initial
i. colostomy
i. consonant position
i. manifestation
i. necrosectomy
i. operation
i. preparation
i. primary pathogen
i. resection
i. screening procedure

NOTES

initial *(continued)*
i. syphilitic lesion
i. systemic chemotherapy
initialization
initiation
tumor i.
injected
injection
air i.
block i.
blood patch i.
bolus i.
cervical nerve root i.
ciliary i.
circumcorneal i.
collagen i.
conjunctival i.
continuous subcutaneous insulin i.
contrast i.
corticoid i.
dermal i.
dermal route of i.
dye i.
endoscopic India ink i.
epidural steroid i.
ethanol i.
extraarachnoid i.
facet joint i.
heavy metal i.
infraorbital i.
i. injury
intraarticular i.
intracavernosal i.
intracavernous i.
intracordal silicone i.
intracytoplasmic sperm i. (ICSI)
intradermal i.
intralesional i.
intramuscular i.
intraosseous i.
intrapulpal i.
intratendinous i.
intrathecal i.
intratumoral i.
intravariceal i.
intravascular i.
intravenous i.
intraventricular i.
intravitreal i.
ipsilateral i.
isotope i.
local i.
i. of local anesthetic
lumbar facet i.
lumbar nerve root i.
i. mass
mental block i.
i. method
i. molding
nasopalatine i.
nerve root i.
nerve root sleeve i.
paracervical i.
paramagnetic contrast i.
paravariceal i.
parenchymal route of i.
percutaneous alcohol i.
percutaneous ethanol i.
peribulbar i.
periocular i.
peroneal tendon sheath i.
retrobulbar i.
root i.
route of i.
saline i.
i. sclerotherapy
selective i.
sensitizing i.
sham i.
i. site
steroid i.
i. study
subarachnoid i.
subconjunctival i.
subcutaneous i.
tangential colonic submucosal i.
i. technique
test i.
i. therapy
trigger point i.
ultrasonographically-guided i.
Van Lint i.
vocal cord i.
i. volume
injection-molded method
injury
acceleration i.
acceleration/deceleration i.
Ajmalin liver i.
anal sphincter i.
anterior abdominal i.
arterial i.
associated i.
axial compression i.
axillary vascular i.
axonal i.
bile duct i.
blast i.
blunt carotid i.
blunt liver i.
blunt torso i.
bowel i.
brachial plexus traction i.
brain i.
burn i.
Callahan extension of cervical i.

carotid i.
cerebral i.
closed head i.
closed soft tissue i.
combined i.'s
complement-induced lung i.
compression i.
concomitant spinal cord i.
crush i.
cutaneous burn i.
decompensation i.
diaphragm i.
diaphragmatic i.
duct i.
endothelial i.
epiphysial plate i.
explosion i.
extension i.
extension-type cervical spine i.
extensor tendon i.
extraabdominal i.
extravasation i.
extremity i.
first-degree radiation i.
flexion-extension i.
fourth degree radiation i.
geriatric i.
head i.
hemorrhagic radiation i.
hepatic i.
hollow visceral i.
hollow viscus i.
hyperextension-hyperflexion i.
hyperfiltration i.
iatrogenic bowel i.
inadvertent venous i.
injection i.
innominate vascular i.
intestinal radiation i.
intraabdominal i.
intraoperative inadvertent venous i.
intrathoracic i.
I/R i.
irradiation i.
ischemia and reperfusion i.
ischemia-reperfusion i.
ischemic liver i.
isolated arterial i.
isolated liver i.
isolated venous i.
kneecapping i.
lateral compression i.
left-sided i.
levator i.
liver i.
major vascular i.
medication-induced i.
microwave radiation i.
mild traumatic brain i. (mTBI)
minor i.
minor splenic i.
missile i.
needlestick i.
nerve i.
neurologic i.
nonsevered i.
obstetrical traction i.
obturator nerve i.
occult diaphragmatic i.
open head i.
organ-specific pattern of i.
osteochondral i.
pediatric i.
penetrating liver i.
penetrating thoracoabdominal i.
percutaneous i. (PI)
perigenicular vascular i.
peripheral nerve i.
peroneal nerve i.
i. prevention
pronation i.
pronation-abduction i.
pronation-eversion i.
pronation-eversion-external rotation i.
proximal subclavian i.
radiation i.
recurrent nerve i.
reperfusion i.
retroclavicular i.
right-sided i.
second degree radiation i.
severe traumatic brain i.
I. Severity Score (ISS)
soft-tissue extremity i.
sphincter i.
spinal cord i.
splenic i.
stretch i.
subclavian i.
suction i.
supination i.
supination-eversion i.
supination-external rotation i.

NOTES

injury *(continued)*
supination-inversion rotation i.
supination-plantar flexion i.
thermal i.
third-degree radiation i.
thoracic inlet vascular i.
thoracoabdominal i.
torso i.
transfusion-related acute lung i. (TRALD)
transfusion-related lung i. (TRLI)
translation i.
traumatic brain i. (TBI)
trifurcation i.
trocar i.
trocar-related i.
ureteral i.
urinary tract i.
valgus-external rotation i.
vascular i.
venous i.
ventilator-induced lung i. (VILI)
visceral i.
viscus i.
whiplash i.
injury-prevention strategy
inlay
i. bone graft
corneal i.
direct method for making i.'s
epithelial i.
i. restoration
inlet
i. allotransplantation
i. patch mucosa
i. port
thoracic i.
in-line
i.-l. grafting
i.-l. perfusion
inner
i. bevel incision
i. cell mass
i. ear tack procedure
i. limiting membrane
i. table
innervation
cutaneous i.
i. of head and neck
i. problem
striated muscle i.
innominata
innominatal
innominate
i. artery
i. artery compression syndrome
i. artery reconstruction
i. bone
i. bone resection
i. cardiac vein
i. line
i. osteotomy
i. vascular injury
i. vessel
innominatus
innovative therapy
inoperable
i. canal
i. patient
inoscopy
inotrope
i. resuscitation
i. resuscitation technique
inotropic state
inotropism
inotropy
negative i.
Inoue balloon mitral valvotomy
inpatient
i. dialysis
i. dialysis unit
input layer
inquiry
cognitive-attitudinal factor i.
INR
international normalized ratio
Insall
I. anterior cruciate ligament reconstruction
I. ligament reconstruction technique
I. patella alta method
I. patellar injury classification
I. procedure
Insall-Burstein-Freeman knee arthroplasty
inscription
tendinous i.
insemination
artificial intravaginal i.
cervical i.
cup i.
direct intraperitoneal i.
heterologous i.
high intrauterine i.
homologous artificial i.
intrafollicular i.
intratubal i.
intrauterine i.
Makler i.
subzonal i.
i. swim-up technique
therapeutic i.
washed intrauterine i.
insertion
anatomic i.
anomalous i.

axillary i.
biliary endoprosthesis i.
blind i.
buttonhole puncture technique for hemodialysis needle i.
catheter i.
caval i.
depth of i. (DOI)
endovascular graft i.
flatus tube i.
fluoroscopic i.
jejunal tube i.
J-tube i.
i. loss
marginal i.
path of i.
PEG i.
percutaneous catheter i.
percutaneous endoscopic gastrostomy i.
percutaneous pin i.
Pierrot-Murphy advancement i.
i. point
rerouting i.
retrograde catheter i.
route of i.
screw i.
subclavian central venous catheter i.
i. technique
tendinous i.
tensor i.
transjugular i.
velamentous i.
wire i.

insertional excursion

inside-out technique

inside-to-outside technique

insolation

inspiration

crowing i.
degree of i.
end i.
shallow i.
suspended i.
i. time

inspiratory

i. bulbospinal neuron
i. intercostal activity
i. occlusion pressure
i. positive airway pressure
i. pressure support
i. rib cage depression
i. time (Ti)
i. vapor concentration

inspiratory/expiratory

inspiratory-to-expiratory ratio

inspired

i. air
i. gas
i. ventilation (VI)

inspissate

inspissation

instability

atlantoaxial i.
catheter i.
cervical i.
congenital i.
congenital cervical i.
detrusor i.
dorsal intercalary segmental i.
extension i.
hemodynamic i.
membrane i.
one-plane i.
sagittal plane i.
spinal i.

installation procedure

install method

instantaneous

i. fluence

instillation

i. of anesthetic
contrast material i.
lavage i.
i. therapy

institute

Cardiopulmonary Research I. (CAPRI)
Dana-Farber Cancer I.
National Cancer I. (NCI)

instrument

i. migration
i. recirculation

instrumental perforation

instrumentarium

instrumentation failure

instrument-tract seeding

insufficiency

aortic valve i.
atrioventricular valve i.
degenerative mitral valve i.
exocrine pancreatic i.
i. fracture

NOTES

insufficiency *(continued)*
glottic i.
mesenteric i.
mitral valve i.
pulmonary valve i.
renal i.
respiratory i.
transverse plane motion i.
venous i.
insufficient airway maintenance
insufflate
insufflation
air i.
i. anesthesia
i. anesthetic technique
constant flow i.
cranial i.
endotracheal i.
extraperitoneal carbon dioxide i.
extraperitoneal CO_2 i.
gas i.
gastric i.
helium i.
intraperitoneal carbon dioxide i.
intraperitoneal CO_2 i.
perirenal i.
peritoneal i.
presacral i.
i. pressure
retroperitoneal gas i.
Rubin tubal i.
i. of stomach
talc i.
i. test set
thoracoscopic talc i.
tubal i.
insula, pl. **insulae**
Haller i.
insular
i. artery
i. carcinoma
insulares
insulated cautery
insulin
i. coma
i. coma therapy
i. coma treatment
i. preparation
i. resistance
i. secretion
i. shock therapy
insulin-like growth factor I (IGF-1)
insulinoma
insult
macrotraumatic i.
microtraumatic i.
intact
i. gastric serosa
i. membrane
i. parathyroid hormone (iPTH)
i. parathyroid hormone assay
integration
binaural i.
body side i.
competing messages i.
complete i.
fibrous i.
large-scale i.
medium-scale i.
very large scale i.
integrity
anatomic i.
soft-tissue i.
integument
integumentary barrier
integumentum commune
intensification
image i.
intensity
Descriptor Differential Scale of Pain I.
intensity-encoded receptor
intensive care unit (ICU)
intent
curative i.
palliative i.
intention
healing by first i.
healing by second i.
healing by third i.
second i.
secondary i.
intentional
i. rebreathing
i. replantation
i. rotation
i. saccade
i. tooth reimplantation
interaction
additive i.
synergistic i.
interalveolar space
interarticular
i. fibrocartilage
i. joint
interarticularis
interarytenoid notch
interatriale
interatrial septum
interaural attenuation
interbody
i. bone graft
i. spinal fusion
intercalary
i. allograft procedure

i. graft
i. resection
intercalated disk
intercapillary
intercapitales
intercapitular vein
intercarotic
intercarotid nerve
intercarpal articulation
intercarpeae
intercartilaginous incision
intercavernosi
intercavernosus septum
intercavernous venous sinus
intercellular
i. fenestration
i. space
intercentral
interceptive conditioning
intercervical disk herniation
interchangeability
interchondral
i. articulation
i. ligament
interchondrales
interclavicular
i. ligament
i. notch
interclaviculare
interclinoid ligament
intercoccygeal
intercolonoscopy
intercolumnar
i. fascia
i. fiber
intercondylar
i. eminence
i. femoral fracture
i. fossa
i. humeral fracture
i. line
i. space
i. tibial fracture
intercondylare
intercondylaris
intercondyloid
i. fossa
i. notch
intercondyloidea
intercoronary anastomosis
intercostal
i. anesthesia
i. artery
i. bundle
i. flap
i. fossa block
i. membrane
i. nerve
i. nerve block
i. nerve block anesthetic technique
i. neuralgia
i. space
i. vein
i. vessel
intercostale
intercostales
intercostalia
intercostalium
intercostohumeralis
intercostohumeral nerve
intercricothyrotomy
intercristal space
intercrural
i. fiber
intercrurales
intercuspal position
intercuspation
intercutaneomucous
interdeferential
interdental
i. canal
i. denudation
i. excision
i. ligation
i. papilla
i. resection
i. space
i. tissue
interdigestive
i. motility disturbance
i. period
interdigit
interdigital
interdigitating skin flap
interdigitation
interendognathic suture
interface
bone-cement i.
bone-implant i.
cement i.
cement-bone i.
cup-cement i.
electrode-skin i.
graft-host i.

NOTES

interface *(continued)*
implant-cement i.
long-term bone-instrumentation i.
pin-bone i.
prosthesis i.
prosthesis-cement i.
soft-tissue i.
interfacet wiring and fusion
interfacial canal
interfascial
i. approach
i. space
interfasciale
interfascicular
i. epineurectomy
i. epineurotomy
i. fibrous tissue
interfemoral
interference
i. dissociation
electromagnetic i. (EMI)
i. fit fixation
i. modification
i. screw technique
interferential therapy
interforniceal approach
interfoveolare
interfoveolar ligament
interfragmentary compression
interfrontal
interganglionares
interganglionic rami
interglobular space of Owen
intergluteal
intergonial
interhemispheric
i. approach
i. propagation time
i. subdural hematoma
interiliaci
interilioabdominal amputation
interincisor
i. distance
i. gap
interinnominoabdominal amputation
interischiadic
interlamellar space
interlesional therapy
interlobar
interlobular
i. artery
i. artery of kidney
i. ductule
interlobulares
interlocking suture technique
intermaxilla
intermaxillaris
intermaxillary
i. fixation
i. relation
i. suture
intermedia
intermediae
intermediary nerve
intermediate
i. amputation
i. anterior wall
i. bronchus
i. bundle
i. cuneiform bone
i. digastric tendon
i. ganglion
i. hemorrhage
i. laryngeal cavity
i. line
i. mesoderm
i. omohyoid tendon
i. phalangectomy
i. restoration
i. sacral crest
i. temporal artery
intermedii
intermediolateral
intermedium
intermedius
intermesenteric
i. abscess
i. arterial anastomosis
i. plexus
intermesenterica
intermesentericus
intermetacarpal articulation
intermetacarpeae
intermetameric
intermetatarseae
intermittent
i. acute porphyria
i. catheterization
i. demand ventilation
i. inflow occlusion
i. mandatory ventilation (IMV)
i. mechanical ventilation
i. pneumatic compression
i. positive pressure (IPP)
i. positive pressure breathing (IPPB)
i. positive pressure ventilation (IPPV)
i. self-obturation
i. sterilization
i. subclavian vein obstruction
i. vascular exclusion
intermodulation
intermuscular
i. gluteal bursa

i. groove
i. hernia
i. membrane
i. septum
intermusculare
interna
internae
internal
i. abdominal ring
i. anal sphincter (IAS)
i. auditory artery
i. auditory canal
i. auditory foramen
i. auditory vein
i. bevel incision
i. branch
i. canthus
i. carotid artery (ICA)
i. carotid venous plexus
i. clot
i. decompression
i. drainage
i. ethmoidectomy
i. female genital organ
i. fixation, closed reduction
i. fixation fracture
i. hemipelvectomy
i. hemorrhage
i. hemorrhoid
i. hemorrhoidal complex
i. hernia
i. iliac artery
i. inguinal ring
i. jugular vein
i. jugular vein cannulation anesthetic technique
i. jugular vein catheterization anesthetic technique
i. jugular vein puncture anesthetic technique
i. lacrimal fistula
i. male genital organ
i. mammary artery (IMA)
i. mammary graft
i. mammary lymphoscintigraphy (IML)
i. mammary node
i. mammary node biopsy
i. mammary plexus
i. maxillary artery
i. maxillary plexus
i. maxillary vein
i. neurocranial foramen
i. neurolysis
i. oblique aponeurosis
i. oblique line
i. oblique osteomuscular flap
i. occipital crest
i. pudendal artery
i. pudendal vein
i. radiation therapy
i. rectal artery
i. rectal nerve
i. respiration
i. rotation
i. rotation deformity
i. rotation in extension
i. rotator
i. spermatic artery
i. spermatic fascia
i. sphincterotomy
i. spinal fixation
i. spiral sulcus
i. surface
i. thoracic artery
i. thoracic lymphatic plexus
i. thoracic vein
i. urethral orifice
i. urethral sphincter
i. urethrotomy
internal-external
i.-e. ilium
i.-e. rotation
internarial
internasalis
internasal suture
international
I. Association for the Study of Pain (IASP)
i. cancer of cervix classification
I. Classification of Diseases, Adapted for Use in the United States (ICDA)
I. Classification of Diseases-9 Version of Injury Severity Score (ICISS)
I. Federation of Gynecology and Obstetrics (FIGO)
I. Federation of Gynecology and Obstetrics classification
i. normalized ratio (INR)
i. stage classification
interne
fixator i.

NOTES

internervous plane
interni
internist
internodal tract of Bachmann
internum
internus
interocclusal rest space
interorbital
interossea
interosseal
interossei (*pl. of* interosseus)
interosseous
i. border
i. cartilage
i. crest
i. groove
i. margin
i. muscle
i. sacroiliac ligament
i. wire fixation
interosseum
interosseus, pl. **interossei**
interpalpebral
interparietal
i. bone
i. hernia
i. suture
interparietale
interparietalis
interpectorales
interpediculate
interpeduncular
i. cistern
i. fossa lesion
interpeduncularis
interpelviabdominal amputation
interperiosteal fracture
interphalangeal
i. amputation
i. articulation
i. collateral ligament
distal i. (DIP)
i. joint dislocation
interpleural
i. administration
i. analgesia
i. anesthesia
i. anesthetic technique
i. application
i. block
interpolated flap
interpolation flap
interposing
interposition
i. membrane
i. mesocaval shunt
i. saphenous vein graft
soft-tissue i.
tissue i.
interpositional
i. elbow arthroplasty
i. shoulder arthroplasty
interpretation
cholangiographic i.
false-positive i.
image i.
intraoperative i.
mirror-image i.
i. variability
interprismatic space
interproximal
i. reduction
i. space
interpubica
interpubic disk
interpubicus
interpulmonary septum
interradicular
i. alveoloplasty
i. lesion
i. septum
i. space
interradicularia
interrenal
interrogation
deep Doppler velocity i.
Doppler i.
stereoscopic i.
interrupted
i. aortic arch
i. respiration
i. suture technique
interruption
sympathetic i.
interscalene
i. approach
i. blockade
i. block anesthetic technique
i. brachial plexus block
i. triangle
interscapulum
intersection syndrome
intersegmental rotation
intersheath space
intersigmoid
i. hernia
i. recess
intersigmoideus
interspace
implant substructure i.
interspecific graft
intersphincteric
i. abscess
i. anal fistula

i. anorectal space
i. proctectomy

interspinal
i. line
i. muscle
i. plane

interspinale

interspinales

interspinalis

interspinous
i. ligament
i. segmental spinal instrumentation technique
i. wiring

interstice, pl. **interstices**
graft i.

interstimulus interval (ISI)

interstitial
i. brachytherapy
i. cystitis
i. hernia
i. implantation
i. inflammation
i. irradiation
i. loculated hematoma
i. neovascularization
i. nephritis
i. photodynamic therapy
i. pressure
i. pulmonary fibrosis (IPF)
i. radiation therapy
i. rejection
i. space
i. tissue

intertarseae

intertendineus

intertragicus

intertransversalis

intertransversarii

intertransversarium

intertransverse
i. fusion
i. ligament
i. muscle

intertrigo with ulceration

intertrochanteric
i. crest
i. femoral fracture
i. four-part fracture
i. line
i. varus osteotomy

intertrochanterica

intertubercular
i. eminence
i. groove
i. line
i. plane
i. sheath
i. sulcus

intertuberculare

intertubercularis

interureteral

interureterica

interureteric fold

intervaginal
i. space

interval
i. appendectomy
disease-free i. (DFI)
interstimulus i. (ISI)
i. operation
pacemaker escape i.
rupture-delivery i.

interval-strength relation

intervascular

intervening connective tissue

intervention
angiographic i.
endovascular i.
medical i.
neurosurgical i.
operative i.
prophylactic angiographic i.
surgical i.

interventional
i. cardiac catheterization
i. cardiologist
i. option
i. procedure
i. radiologist
i. radiology
i. technique
i. therapy

interventricular
i. septal rupture
i. septum

interventriculare

intervertebral
i. cartilage
i. disk
i. disk herniation
i. foramen
i. ganglion
i. notch

NOTES

intervertebral *(continued)*
i. symphysis
i. vein
intervertebralis
interview
structured pain i. (SPI)
intervolar plate ligament
intestina (*pl. of* intestinum)
intestinal
i. allograft
i. anastomosis
i. anastomotic healing
i. anastomotic leakage
i. arterial arcade
i. artery
i. biopsy
i. bypass procedure
i. calculus
i. colic
i. conduit
i. content
i. endoscopy
i. failure
i. fistula
i. fixation
i. flora
i. gland
i. hemorrhage
i. infection
i. ischemic disorder
i. loop
i. malrotation
i. obstruction
i. perforation
i. radiation injury
i. resection
i. rotation
i. surgery
i. tract
i. transplantation
i. trunk
i. ulceration
i. vein
i. villous atrophy
i. villus
i. web
i. wound healing
intestinales
intestinalis
intestine
absorptive i.
large i.
small i.
intestinum, pl. **intestina**
in-the-bag implantation
intima
intimal
i. flap
i. hyperplasia
i. thrombosis
intimus
intolerance
hemodynamic i.
intonation contour
intortor
intoxication
i. amaurosis
citrate i.
intraabdominal
i. abscess
i. adhesion
i. arterial hemorrhage
i. bleeding
i. catastrophe
i. disease
i. friction
i. hypertension
i. infection
i. injury
i. lesion
i. mass
i. organ
i. pressure (IAP)
i. sepsis
i. spillage
i. surgery
i. tip
intraadenoidal
intraalveolar hemorrhage
intraamniotic infection
intraanal pressure
intraanesthetic event
intraaortic balloon counterpulsation
intraarterial
i. chemoembolization
i. chemotherapy (IAC)
i. counterpulsation
i. therapy
intraarticular
i. anesthetic technique
i. cartilage
i. injection
i. knee fusion
i. loose body
i. osteotomy
i. procedure
i. proximal tibial fracture
i. reconstruction
i. sternocostal ligament
intra-articulare
intraaxial parenchymal brain neoplasm
intrabuccal
intrabulbar fossa
intracanalicular irradiation
intracapsular
i. cataract extraction

i. cataract extraction operation
i. dissection
i. fracture
i. hemorrhage
i. incision
i. ligament
i. metastasis
i. osteotomy
i. temporomandibular joint arthroplasty

intracapsularia

intracardiac
i. mass
i. pressure
i. pressure curve

intracatheter

intracavernosal
i. injection
i. injection treatment

intracavernous
i. injection
i. injection therapy
i. plexus

intracavitary
i. anesthesia
i. implantation
i. pressure-electrogram dissociation
i. pressure gradient
i. radiation boost therapy

intracellular-like, calcium-bearing crystalloid solution

intracellular protein degradation

intracerebral
i. arteriovenous malformation
i. ganglioma
i. hematoma
i. hemorrhage
i. leukostasis
i. vascular malformation

intracerebroventricular

intracholedochal pressure

intracisternal

intracolic

intraconal lesion

intracordal silicone injection

intracorneal

intracoronal-extracoronal retention

intracoronary thrombolysis balloon valvuloplasty

intracorporeal
i. anastomosis
i. injection therapy
i. knot
i. knotting technique
i. laser lithotripsy
i. shock wave lithotripsy
i. suturing

intracostal

intracranial
i. anatomy
i. aneurysm
i. arteriovenous fistula
i. arteriovenous malformation
i. bleeding
i. cavity
i. circulation
i. dural vascular anomaly
i. ganglion
i. hematoma
i. hemorrhage (ICH)
i. mass
i. mass lesion
i. pathology
i. pressure (ICP)
i. pressure monitoring
i. pressure value
i. rhizotomy
i. stimulation
i. tumor
i. vascular malformation
i. venous system

intracranial-extracranial nerve graft

intracranial-intratemporal nerve graft

intracristal space

intractable
i. epilepsy
i. pain

intracutaneous segment

intracuticular
i. stitch

intracystic hepatojejunostomy

intracytoplasmic sperm injection (ICSI)

intradermal
i. anesthetic
i. injection
i. mattress suture technique
i. tattooing technique

intradiscal
i. electrothermal therapy (IDET)
i. pressure

intraductal
i. cancer
i. carcinoma
i. cholangioscopy

NOTES

intraductal *(continued)*
- i. component
- i. hyperplasia
- i. pressure

intradural
- i. abscess
- i. approach
- i. dissection
- i. dorsal spinal root rhizotomy
- i. epidermoidoma
- i. extramedullary lesion
- i. extramedullary mass
- i. tumor surgery

intraepidermal carcinoma

intraepiphysial osteotomy

intraepiploic hernia

intraepithelial
- i. excementosis
- i. nonkeratizing carcinoma

intraesophageal
- i. peristaltic pressure
- i. variceal pressure

intrafaradization

intrafascial space

intrafollicular insemination

intragalvanization

intragastric
- i. anastomosis
- i. hydrolysis
- i. pressure
- i. prosthesis migration
- i. provocation under endoscopy

intraglandular
- i. fluid collection

intraglandulares

intraglomerular pressure

intragraft expression

intrahepatic
- i. abscess
- i. anatomy
- i. arterial-portal fistula
- i. A-V fistula
- i. bile duct
- i. biliary cystic dilation
- i. biliary tree
- i. control
- i. course
- i. ductal dilation
- i. hematoma
- i. hepatolithiasis
- i. hypertension
- i. lesion
- i. metastasis
- i. pathology
- i. portosystemic shunt
- i. spontaneous arterioportal fistula
- i. vascular division

intrahyoid

intrailiac hernia

intrajugularis

intrajugular process

intralabyrinthine fistula

intralacrimal
- i. endoscopy
- i. surgery

intralesional
- i. excision
- i. injection
- i. therapy

intraligamentary anesthesia

intralobular
- i. connective tissue
- i. inflammation

intraluminal
- i. cyst
- i. esophageal pressure
- i. flow
- i. foreign body
- i. hemorrhage
- i. intubation
- i. pH-pressure relationship
- i. pouch
- i. seeding
- i. tumor
- i. urethral pressure

intramammary sentinel node

intramedullary
- i. anesthesia
- i. arteriovenous malformation
- i. canal
- i. demyelination
- i. graft
- i. lesion
- i. nailing
- i. rod fixation
- i. tractotomy
- i. tumor
- i. tumor biopsy

intramembranous
- i. formation
- i. space

intramucosal metastasis

intramural
- i. abscess
- i. air dissection
- i. artery
- i. blood perfusion
- i. colonic air
- i. esophageal rupture
- i. extramucosal lesion
- i. fistulous tract
- i. hematoma
- i. intestinal hemorrhage
- i. involvement
- i. pH

intramuscular (IM)

i. anesthetic
i. injection
i. preanesthetic medication anesthetic technique
i. venous malformation

intramusculature abscess

intramyocardial
i. air
i. pressure
i. tumor

intranasal
i. analgesic
i. anesthesia
i. approach
i. ethmoidectomy
i. polypectomy
i. sinus surgery

intraneural pressure

in-transit
i.-t. disease
i.-t. metastasis

intraocular
i. administration
i. cataract extraction
i. fistula
i. foreign body
i. hemorrhage
i. lens
i. lens dislocation
i. lens implantation
i. pressure

intraoperative
i. assessment
i. bile sample
i. biliary endoscopy
i. biopsy
i. bleeding
i. blood loss
i. bowel lavage
i. bowel preparation
i. cavernous nerve stimulation
i. cholangiogram (IOC)
i. colonic lavage
i. complication
i. computer-assisted spinal orientation technique
i. confirmation
i. contamination
i. core body temperature
i. core hypothermia
i. CVP
i. death
i. dynamic cholangiography
i. enteroscopy
i. fluid management
i. fracture
i. frozen section
i. hemorrhage
i. imaging
i. imaging method
i. inadvertent venous injury
i. interpretation
i. iPTH assay
i. lymphatic mapping
i. monitor
i. morbidity
i. MRI
i. neurophysiologic monitoring (IOM)
i. normothermia
i. parathyroid hormone monitoring
i. penile erection
i. plateletpheresis
i. procedure
i. radiation
i. rupture
i. stress relaxation
i. touch prep cytology
i. transcranial Doppler monitoring
i. ultrasonography (IOUS)
i. ultrasound (IOUS)
i. ultrasound finding
i. urine output
i. vascular accident
i. verification

intraoperatively donated autologous blood

intraoral
i. anesthesia
i. antrostomy
i. cone irradiation
i. flap
i. incision
i. pressure
i. trauma

intraorbital
i. anesthesia
i. foreign body
i. groove
i. surgery

intraosseous
i. abscess
i. anesthesia
i. bone lesion

NOTES

intraosseous *(continued)*
i. fixation
i. injection
i. membrane
intrapancreatic portion
intraparavariceal procedure
intraparenchymal
i. digital dissection
i. hematoma
i. hemorrhage
intraparotideus
intraparotid plexus
intrapartum
i. asphyxiation
i. hemorrhage
intrapatellar bursa
intrapelvic hernia
intrapericardial pressure
intraperitoneal
i. abscess
i. adhesion
i. air
i. anesthesia
i. anesthetic
i. blood transfusion
i. carbon dioxide insufflation
i. cavity
i. CO_2 insufflation
i. dissemination
i. drug administration
i. endometrial metastatic disease
i. fetal transfusion
i. hemorrhage
i. hyperthermic chemotherapy (IPHC)
i. hyperthermic perfusion
i. incision
i. method
i. mobilization
i. perforation
i. position
i. pressure
i. procedure
i. radiation therapy
i. recurrence
i. seeding
i. spillage
i. technique
i. viscus
i. viscus rupture
i. volume
intraperitoneally
intrapharyngeal space
intrapial
intraplaque hemorrhage
intrapleural
i. block
i. catheter placement
i. pressure
i. rupture
intraportal vein
intraprostatic
intrapulmonary
i. metastasis (IPM)
i. shunt ratio
intrapulpal
i. anesthesia
i. injection
i. pressure
intrapyretic amputation
intrarenal chemolysis
intrarrhachidian
intrascrotal
intrasellar
i. extension
i. lesion
i. mass
intraseptal alveoloplasty
intrasheath tenotomy
intraspinal
i. administration
i. anesthesia
i. therapy
intrasplenic
intrasynovial
intratendinous injection
intratentorial supracerebellar approach
intrathecal
i. administration
i. analgesic
i. anesthesia
i. anesthetic
i. antinociception
i. cannulation anesthetic technique
i. injection
i. morphine anesthetic technique
i. neurolysis
i. opioid labor analgesia
i. therapy
intrathoracic
i. anastomosis
i. bleeding
i. disease
i. esophagogastroscopy
i. esophagogastrostomy
i. esophagoplasty
i. injury
i. mass
i. Nissen fundoplication
i. position
i. pressure
i. stomach
intrathyroidal pathology
intrathyroid cartilage

intratracheal
i. anesthesia
i. intubation
intratubal insemination
intratumoral
i. calcification
i. injection
intraultrasonography
intraurethral pressure
intrauterine
i. amputation
i. foreign body
i. fracture
i. growth retardation
i. infection
i. insemination
i. intraperitoneal fetal transfusion
i. pressure measurement
i. respiration
i. resuscitation
intravagale
intravaginal
i. electrical stimulation
i. pouch
i. space
i. torsion
intravariceal
i. infusion
i. injection
i. pressure
i. sclerotherapy
intravasation
venous i.
intravascular
i. coagulation screen
i. endothelial proliferative lesion
i. fluid therapy
i. foreign body
i. foreign body retrieval
i. injection
i. lipolysis
i. mass
i. pressure
i. volume
i. volume expansion
intravenous (IV)
i. administration
i. alimentation
i. analgesic
i. anesthetic
i. antibiotic therapy
i. block anesthesia
i. blood
i. cannulation
i. cannulation anesthetic technique
i. contrast
i. digital subtraction imaging
i. drip
i. hydration
i. hydration therapy
i. hyperalimentation
i. hypnotic
i. injection
i. medication
i. oxygen-15 water bolus technique
i. ozone therapy
i. regional anesthesia (IVRA)
i. saline
i. sedation
i. sedation anesthesia
i. sheath
i. vasopressin
intraventricular
i. aberration
i. endoscopy
i. hemorrhage
i. injection
i. mass
i. therapy
intravesical
i. alum irrigation
i. anastomosis
i. chemotherapeutic treatment
i. chemotherapy
i. migration
i. pressure
i. ureterolysis
intravital microscopy
intravitreal injection
intrinsic
i. brainstem lesion
i. circuitry
i. compression
i. end-expiratory pressure
i. minus deformity
i. minus position
i. muscle
i. plus deformity
i. positive end-expiratory pressure (PEEPi)
i. restoration
i. sphincter
introduction site
introflexion

NOTES

introgastric
introitus
introjection
intromittent organ
introspective method
introvert
intrusive implantation
intubate
intubated ureterotomy
intubation
altercursive i.
i. anesthetic technique
aqueductal i.
blind nasotracheal i.
bronchoscope-guided i.
catheter-guided endoscopic i.
double-lumen i.
emergency tracheal i.
emergent i.
endobronchial i.
endotracheal i.
esophageal i.
esophagogastric i.
failed i.
i. failure
heal i.
intraluminal i.
intratracheal i.
lighted stylet-guided oral i.
mainstem i.
nasal i.
nasogastric i.
nasotracheal i. (NTI)
O'Dwyer i.
oral endotracheal i.
oral lighted-stylet i.
orotracheal i.
pyloric i.
rapid sequence induction i.
RSI orotracheal i.
silicone i.
terminal ileum i.
total time to i. (TTI)
tracheal i.
translaryngeal tracheal i.
intumescence
intumescent
intumescentia
intussuscepted mass
intussuscepting
intussusception
adult i.
appendiceal i.
cecal i.
colocolic i.
colonic i.
enteric i.
gastroenterostomy i.
idiopathic adult i.
idiopathic ileocecal i.
ileocolic i.
pediatric i.
sigmoid-rectal i.
small bowel idiopathic i.
stomal i.
inundation fever
invaded furcation
invaginate
invaginated membrane
invaginating
i. anastomosis
end-to-end i.
i. suture technique
invagination
basilar i.
epithelial i.
stomal i.
stump i.
i. technique
invasion
advanced local i.
blood vessel i. (BVI)
cancer i.
capsular i.
chest wall i.
extrathyroid i.
local i.
lymphatic i.
lymphovascular i.
lymph vessel i. (LVI)
margin i.
microscopic i.
mucosal i.
perineural i.
serosa i.
submucosal i.
tumor i.
vascular i.
venous i.
wall i.
invasive
i. adenocarcinoma
i. breast cancer
i. breast carcinoma
i. ductal cancer
i. ductal carcinoma
i. hemodynamic monitoring
i. lobular carcinoma
i. localization
i. pressure measurement
i. procedure
i. recurrence
i. technique
i. therapy
i. tumor

I

inventory
Brief Pain I. (BPI)
Multidimensional Pain I. (MPI)
Neonatal Facial Pain I. (NFCS)
Pain Appraisal I. (PAI)
State-Trait Anxiety I. (STAI)
inverse bevel incision
inverse-ratio ventilation
inversion appendectomy
inversion-eversion rotation
inversion-ligation appendectomy
inversus
inverted
i. bevel incision
i. L-form osteotomy
i. pelvis
i. skin flap
inverted-U
i.-U abdominal incision
i.-U pouch
inverted-V peritoneotomy
inverted-Y
i.-Y. fracture
i.-Y. incision
inverting knot technique
invertor
investigation
diagnostic i.
direct histologic i.
histologic i.
preoperative i.
soft x-ray i.
investing
i. cartilage
i. fascia
investment expansion
involuntary
i. guarding
i. sterilization
involution cyst
involved-field radiation
involvement
bifurcation i.
border i.
celiac nodal i.
diffuse breast i.
extramedullary i.
extraocular muscle i.
intramural i.
lymph node i.
macroscopic i.
margin resection i.
mesocolic i.
metastatic i.
nervous system i.
nodal i.
node i.
portal nodal i.
pulmonary i.
retinal i.
segmental i.
serosal i.
trifurcation i.
inward-going rectification
inward rotation
IOC
intraoperative cholangiogram
iodide-containing medication
iodine-131 whole-body scan
iodine treatment
iodized oil
IOM
intraoperative neurophysiologic monitoring
ionization
i. chamber pocket
root canal i.
specific i.
ionizing irradiation
iontophoresis
IOUS
intraoperative ultrasonography
intraoperative ultrasound
IPAA
ileal pouch-anal anastomosis
IPC
ischemic preconditioning
IPF
idiopathic pulmonary fibrosis
interstitial pulmonary fibrosis
IPHC
intraperitoneal hyperthermic chemotherapy
IPM
intrapulmonary metastasis
macroscopic IPM
microscopic IPM
IPP
intermittent positive pressure
IPPB
intermittent positive pressure breathing
IPPV
intermittent positive pressure ventilation

NOTES

ipsilateral
i. acetabular fracture
i. adrenalectomy
i. femoral neck fracture
i. femoral shaft fracture
i. gland
i. hemispheric symptom
i. injection
i. nerve root lesion
i. pelvic fracture
i. portal vein obstruction
i. shoulder
i. side
i. thyroid lobectomy
i. tibial fracture
iPTH
intact parathyroid hormone
iPTH assay
iPTH level
I/R
ischemia and reperfusion
I/R injury
IRA
ileorectal anastomosis
iridectomy
argon laser i.
basal i.
Bethke i.
buttonhole i.
Castroviejo i.
central i.
Chandler i.
complete i.
Elschnig central i.
laser i.
i. operation
optic i.
optical i.
patent i.
peripheral i.
preliminary i.
preparatory i.
pupil-to-root i.
i. scar
sector i.
stenopeic i.
superior sector i.
therapeutic i.
iridencleisis
Holth i.
i. operation
iridis
iridization
iridocapsulotomy
iridocele
iridocoloboma
iridocorneal
i. angle
i. endothelial syndrome
i. epithelial syndrome
iridocornealis
iridocorneosclerectomy
iridocyclectomy
iridocyclochoroidectomy
Peyman i.
iridocystectomy
iridodialysis operation
iridodiastasis
iridogoniocyclectomy
iridoplasty
iridosclerotomy
iridotasis operation
iridotomy
Abraham i.
Castroviejo radial i.
laser i.
i. operation
radial i.
iris
i. diastasis
i. ectasia
i. incarceration
i. neovascularization
i. ring
iritoectomy
iritomy
iron-Hudson-Stähli line
iron line
iron-stocker line
irotomy
irradiated melanoma cell
irradiation
abdominal i.
abdominopelvic i.
adjuvant i.
breast i.
cardiac i.
cataract i.
i. cataract
cesium i.
charged-particle i.
childhood thyroid i.
convergent beam i.
cranial i.
craniospinal i.
i. damage
external beam i.
external orthovoltage i.
extracorporeal i.
i. failure
fractionated external beam i.
gamma i.
half-body i.
heavy-ion i.
hemibody i.
hyperfractionated total body i.

i. injury
interstitial i.
intracanalicular i.
intraoral cone i.
ionizing i.
linearly polarized near-infrared i.
local i.
low-dose i.
mantle i.
mediastinal i.
Nd:YAG laser i.
para-aortic node i.
partial-breast i.
pelvic i.
postoperative i.
prophylactic i.
selective i.
single-fraction total body i.
surface i.
therapeutic i.
total axial node i.
total body i.
total lymphoid i.
total nodal i.
ultraviolet blood i.
UV i.
whole-abdomen i.
whole abdominopelvic i.
whole-body i.
whole-pelvis i.

irreducible
i. fracture
i. hernia

irregular bone

irregularly widened lumen

irresectability

irresectable
carcinoma stage i.
i. disease
i. finding

irrespirable

irresuscitable

irreversible
i. coma
i. shock

irrigating solution

irrigation
acetohydroxamic acid i.
antral i.
i. and aspiration
i. burn
caloric i.
canal i.
closed i.
continuous bladder i.
copious i.
endodontic i.
hemiacidrin i.
heparin i.
intravesical alum i.
on-table i.
oral i.
pulsed i.
pulse lavage i.
rectal pulsed i.
rectum i.
sinus i.
i. solution
whole-gut i.
wound i.

irrigation-suction
postoperative i.-s.

irritability
soft-tissue i.

irritable lesion

irritant
i. patch-test reaction
i. patch-test response

irritation
i. callus
i. index
parastomal i.
peritoneal i.

irritative lesion

irruption

irruptive

Irvine operation

Irving tubal ligation

Irwin osteotomy

Isaacson classification (IC)

ischemia, ischaemia
contralateral i.
exercise i.
exercise-induced silent myocardial i.
extremity i.
hepatic i.
limb i.
lower limb i.
mesenteric i. (MI)
myocardial i.
nonocclusive mesenteric i. (NOMI)
normothermic i.
radiation-induced i.
i. and reperfusion (I/R)

NOTES

ischemia *(continued)*
i. and reperfusion injury
tourniquet i.
warm i.
ischemia-guided medical therapy
ischemia-reperfusion injury
ischemic
i. aortic disease
i. cardiomyopathy
i. colitis
i. compression
i. encephalopathy
i. heart disease
i. hypoxia
i. infected ulceration
i. liver injury
i. mesenteric change
i. ocular inflammation
i. preconditioning (IPC)
i. stroke
i. ulcer
ischemic-tourniquet technique
ischia (*pl. of* ischium)
ischiadic
i. plexus
i. spine
ischiadica
ischiadici
ischiadicum
ischial
i. bone
i. bursa
i. ramus
i. spine
i. weightbearing ring
ischiatic hernia
ischii
ischioanal fossa
ischiobulbar
ischiocavernosus
ischiocavernous muscle
ischiocele
ischiococcygeal
ischiococcygeus
ischiofemoral
ischioperineal
ischiopubic ramus
ischiopubiotomy
Farabeuf i.
Galbiati bilateral fetal i.
ischiorectal
i. abscess
i. anorectal space
i. fat pad
i. fossa
i. fossa plane
ischiorectalis
ischiovertebral
ischium, pl. **ischia**
ischuretic
I-shaped scalp flap
Isherwood projection
ISI
interstimulus interval
island
endometrial i.
i. graft
i. pedicle scalp flap
i. skin flap
island-flap procedure
islet
i. cell
i. cell cancer
i. cell engineering
i. cell tumor
i.'s of Langerhans
pancreatic i.
isobaric spinal anesthesia
isobologram analysis
isobolographic analysis
isobolography
isocapnia
isocapnic hyperventilation
isodense subdural hematoma
isodose line
isoelectric
i. line
i. point
isoenzyme
pancrease-specific amylase i.
isoflurane-induced vasoconstriction
isogeneic graft
isogenic graft
isograft
isoinertial
isokinetic collection
isolated
i. annuloplasty
i. arterial injury
i. dislocation
i. fashion
i. hepatic perfusion
i. iliac artery aneurysm
i. limb perfusion (ILP)
i. liver injury
i. metastatic tumor
i. NCRLM
i. procedure
i. venous injury
isolation
hepatic vascular i. (HVI)
i. perfusion therapy
i. technique
total vascular i. (TVI)
isologous graft

I

isolysis
isometric
i. cervical extension strength
i. force dynamometry
i. point
i. technique
i. tubular vacuolization
i. venous tension
isoperistaltic anastomosis
isoplastic graft
isoproterenol
isoquinoline
isorhythmic dissociation
isosbestic point
isosulfan blue-dye mapping
isotope
i. dilution-mass spectrometry
i. injection
i. localization
isotransplantation
isotropic tissue
isovolumetric relaxation
isovolumic
i. relaxation
i. relaxation time
Israel method
ISS
Injury Severity Score
isthmectomy
isthmorrhaphy
isthmus
isthmusectomy
Italian
I. flap
I. method
I. operation
I. rhinoplasty
itchy soft palate
iterative reconstruction
Itis
bundle of I.
Ito
I. method
I. procedure
IUD-related infection
IV
intravenous
IV contrast
IV fluid therapy
IV sedation
Ivalon
I. sponge-wrap operation
I. suture technique
IVC
inferior vena cavum
inferior vena cava
IVC ligation
IVC occlusion
IVC pressure
IVC reconstruction
retrohepatic IVC
suprahepatic IVC
thrombosis of IVC
IVCP
inferior vena cava pressure
Ivor
I. Lewis esophagogastrectomy
I. Lewis two-stage subtotal esophagectomy
Ivor-Lewis resection
ivory membrane
IVRA
intravenous regional anesthesia
Ivy
I. loop wiring
I. method of bleeding time

NOTES

J
J loop technique
J point
J versus S versus W pelvic ileal pouch
Jaboulay
J. amputation
J. gastroduodenostomy
J. pyloroplasty
Jaboulay-Doyen-Winkleman
J.-D.-W. operation
J.-D.-W. technique
jackknife position
Jackson
J. incision
J. membrane
J. and Parker classification of Hodgkin disease
Jackson-Babcock operation
Jacobaeus procedure
Jacob membrane
Jacobs locking-hook spinal rod technique
Jacobson
J. cartilage
J. nerve
Jacoby
border tissue of J.
Jacod syndrome
Jacquart facial angle
Jacquemet recess
Jacques plexus
Jaeger-Hamby procedure
Jaesche-Arlt operation
Jaesche operation
Jaffe procedure
Jahss
J. maneuver
J. ninety-ninety method
J. procedure
Jaime lacrimal operation
James
J. bundle
J. position
Jameson operation
jamming knot
Janecki-Nelson shoulder girdle resection
Janeway
J. gastrostomy
J. lesion
Jannetta microvascular decompression procedure
Jansey
J. procedure
J. technique
Jansky classification
Japanese
J. approach
J. cancer classification
J. Classification for Gastric Carcinoma (JCGC)
J. standard operation
Japanese-style
J.-s. gastrectomy
J.-s. lymphadenectomy
J.-s. operation
Japas
J. osteotomy
J. V-osteotomy
Jarjavay ligament
Jatene arterial switch procedure
jaundice
breast-milk j.
cholestatic j.
obstructive j.
preoperative j.
regurgitation j.
jaw
j. bone
Hapsburg j.
j. joint
j. relation
j. relation record
j. thrust maneuver
upper j.
Jaworski body
jaw-to-jaw
j.-t.-j. position
j.-t.-j. relation
JCGC
Japanese Classification for Gastric Carcinoma
Jefferson fracture
Jeffery
J. radial fracture classification
J. technique
jejunal
j. artery
j. biopsy
j. fasting motor activity
j. free flap
j. interposition of Henle loop
j. lumen
j. manometry
j. motility
j. pouch
j. puncture
j. puncture area
j. Roux-en-Y limb
j. Roux-en-Y loop

J

jejunal *(continued)*
j. serosa
j. submucosa
j. tube insertion
jejunales
jejunectomy
jejunization
jejunocolic fistula
jejunocolostomy
jejunoileal
j. anastomosis
j. bypass (JIB)
j. bypass reversal method
j. bypass reversal procedure
j. bypass reversal technique
j. bypass surgery
jejunoileostomy
Roux-en-Y distal j.
jejunojejunal anastomosis
jejunojejunostomy
jejunoplasty
Hoffman j.
jejunostomy
afferent j.
decompression j.
j. elemental diet feeding
endoscopic j.
hepaticocutaneous j.
laparoscopic j.
loop j.
needle catheter j. (NCJ)
percutaneous endoscopic j. (PEJ)
j. tract choledochoscopy
j. tube feeding
Witzel j.
jejunotomy
jejunum
j. loop
proximal j.
upper j.
Jena method
Jenckel
J. cholecystoduodenostomy
J. method
Jendrassik-Grof method
Jendrassik maneuver
jennerization
Jensen
J. classification
J. operation
J. transposition procedure
Jergesen incision
jerky respiration
Jerne technique
jet
high-frequency j.
j. lesion
j. pilot position
transtracheal j.
j. ventilation
j. ventilation anesthetic technique
Jeune syndrome
Jewett
J. and Strong staging
J. and Whitmore classification
JIB
jejunoileal bypass
JIB reversal
J-loop ileostomy
job capacity evaluation
Jobe-Glousman capsular shift procedure
Jobert
J. de Lamballe fossa
J. suture technique
Johner-Wruhs tibial fracture classification
Johnson
J. chevron osteotomy
J. esophagogastroscopy
J. esophagogastrostomy
J. operation
J. pelvic fracture technique
J. procedure
J. pronator advancement
J. root canal filling method
J. staple technique
Johnson-Spiegl
J.-S. hallux varus correction
J.-S. procedure
Johnston
J. buttonhole procedure
J. method
J. pursestring suture technique
joint
anterior intraoccipital j.
arthrodial j.
j. aspiration
atlantoaxial j.
atlantooccipital j.
axial rotation j.
ball-and-socket j.
biaxial j.
bicondylar j.
bilocular j.
j. branch
capitular j.
j. capsule
j. cavity
coccygeal j.
composite j.
compound j.
costochondral j.
costotransverse j.
costovertebral j.
cotyloid j.
cricothyroid j.

j. deformity
dentoalveolar j.
j. depression fracture
diarthrodial j.
j. disarticulation
ellipsoidal j.
enarthrodial j.
extraarticular subtalar j.
facet j.
fibrous j.
j. fusion
ginglymoid j.
glenohumeral j.
gliding j.
hinge j.
immovable j.
incudomalleolar j.
interarticular j.
jaw j.
lateral atlantoaxial j.
j. line
j. line pain
lumbosacral j.
Luschka j.
mandibular j.
j. manipulation
manubriosternal j.
j. mobilization
j. mouse
movable j.
multiaxial j.
neurocentral j.
j. oil
peg-and-socket j.
petrooccipital j.
pivot j.
plane j.
polyaxial j.
posterior intraoccipital j.
j. protection training
j. reconstruction
rotary j.
rotation j.
sacrococcygeal j.
screw j.
SI j.
simple j.
socket j.
j. space
j. space narrowing
sphenooccipital j.
spheroid j.
spiral j.
sternal j.
sternoclavicular j.
sternocostal j.
suture j.
synarthrodial j.
synchondrodial j.
syndesmodial j.
synovial j.
talocrural j.
temporomandibular j.
thigh j.
trochoid j.
uncovertebral j.
uniaxial j.
unilocular j.
wedge-and-groove j.
xiphisternal j.
zygapophyseal j.

Jonas modification of Norwood procedure

Jones
J. first-toe repair
J. fracture
J. and Jones wedge technique
J. position
J. resection arthroplasty
J. tube procedure

Jones-Barnes-Lloyd-Roberts classification

Jones-Brackett technique

Jones-Politano technique

Jonnesco fossa

Jonnson maneuver

Joplin bunionectomy

Jorgensen technique

Joseph rhinoplasty

J-pexy
omental J-p.

J-pouch
colonic J-p.
ileal J-p.

J. R. Moore procedure

J-sella deformity

J-shaped
J-s. ileal pouch
J-s. ileal pouch-anal anastomosis
J-s. skin incision

J-sign

J-tube insertion

J-type maneuver

Judd-Mayo overlap midline incisional hernioplasty

NOTES

Judd pyloroplasty technique
Judet
J. graft
J. quadricepsplasty
Judkins-Sones
J.-S. technique
J.-S. technique of cardiac catheterization
Judkins technique
juga (*pl. of* jugum)
jugal
j. bone
j. point
jugomaxillary point
jugular
j. bulb anomaly
j. bulb catheter placement assessment
j. bulb oxyhemoglobin desaturation
j. bulb venous oxygen saturation
j. compression maneuver
j. duct
j. foramen
j. foramen syndrome
j. fossa
j. ganglion
j. lymphatic trunk
j. nerve
j. plexus
j. process
j. sinus
j. technique
j. tubercle
j. vein
j. vein dissection
j. venous arch
j. venous bulb
j. venous oxygen saturation ($SjVO_2$)
j. venous pressure
jugulare
jugularis
jugulodigastric
jugulodigastricus
juguloomohyoid
j. node
juguloomohyoideus
jugulum
jugum, pl. **juga**
juice
cancer j.
jumbo biopsy
jump
j. flap
j. graft
jumper-knee position
junction
anorectal j.
atypical j.
cavohepatic j.
choledochoduodenal j.
choledochopancreatic ductal j.
costochondral j.
cystic duct-infundibulum j.
duodenojejunal j.
esophagogastric j.
gastroesophageal j.
hard-soft palate j.
ileocecal j.
manubriosternal j.
mucocutaneous j.
neuroeffector j.
rectosigmoid j.
sacrococcygeal j.
sclerocorneal j.
scotoma j.
squamocolumnar j.
sternoclavicular j.
sternomanubrial j.
ureteropelvic j. (UPJ)
junctional
j. dilatation
j. dilation
j. ectopic tachycardia
j. epithelium
junctura, pl. **juncturae**
Jung muscle
Junod procedure
Jurkat T-cell line
justo
Juvara procedure
juvenile
j. ankylosing spondylitis
j. embryonal carcinoma
j. hemangiofibroma
j. nevoxanthoendothelioma
j. pelvis
j. polyp
j. rheumatoid arthritis
juxta-anal colostomy
juxta-articulation
juxta-auricular fossa
juxtacardiac pleural pressure
juxtacortical fracture
juxtacrine stimulation
juxtacubital reconstruction
juxtaepiphysial
juxtaglomerular
j. body
j. complex
j. granulation index
juxtahepatic vein
juxta-intestinales
juxtaposition
juxtarestiform body

k

k space

k space segmentation

K562 erythroid line

KACT

kaolin-activated clotting time

Kader gastrostomy

Kader-Senn

K.-S. gastrotomy technique

K.-S. operation

Kaes

line of K.

Kajava classification

kala-azar infection

Kalamchi classification

Kaliscinski ureteral procedure

Kalish osteotomy

Kalt suture technique

Kammerer-Battle incision

kangaroo

k. pouch

k. tendon suture technique

kaolin-activated clotting time (KACT)

Kapandji technique

Kapel elbow dislocation technique

Kaplan

K. oblique line

K. open reduction

K. osteotomy

K. technique

Kaplan-Meier method

Karakousis-Vezeridis

K.-V. procedure

K.-V. resection

Karapandzic flap

Karhunen-Loeve procedure

Karlsson procedure

Karnofsky

K. rating scale classification

K. scale

Karr method

Karydakis flap

Kasabach-Merritt syndrome

Kasai

K. operation

K. portoenterostomy

K. procedure

Kasai-type hepatoportoenterostomy

Kashiwagi technique

Kasser-Kennedy method

Kasugai classification

Kates-Kessel-Kay technique

Kato thick smear technique

Katzin operation

Kaufer tendon technique

Kauffman-White classification

Kaufmann technique

Kausch-Whipple pancreatoduodenectomy

Kavanaugh-Brower-Mann fixation

Kawaii-Yamamoto procedure

Kawamura

K. dome osteotomy

K. pelvic osteotomy

Kazanjian operation

Keasbey lesion

Keating-Hart method

Kebab graft

Keen

K. operation

K. point

Kehr

K. incision

K. technique

Keil tumor cell classification

Keith bundle

Keith-Wagener-Barker classification

Keith-Wagener classification

Kelami classification

Kelikian-Clayton-Loseff

K.-C.-L. surgical syndactyly

K.-C.-L. technique

Kelikian-McFarland procedure

Kelikian procedure

Kelikian-Riashi-Gleason

K.-R.-G. patellar tendon repair

K.-R.-G. technique

Kellam-Waddel classification

Keller

K. bunionectomy

K. procedure

K. resection arthroplasty

Keller-Madlener operation

Kelling-Madlener procedure

Kellogg-Speed

K.-S. fusion technique

K.-S. lumbar spinal fusion

Kelly

K. plication

K. plication procedure

K. suture technique

Kelly-Keck osteotomy

Kelly-Kennedy modification

Kelman operation

keloid

k. fibroblast

k. formation

keloplasty

kelotomy

Kelsey unloading exercise therapy

Kelvin body

K

Kempf-Grosse-Abalo Z-step osteotomy
Kendrick
K. method
K. method below-knee amputation
K. procedure
K. technique
Kendrick-Sharma-Hassler-Herndon technique
Kennedy
K. area-length method
K. classification
K. ligament technique
K. procedure
Kennedy-Pacey operation
Kent
K. bundle
K. bundle ablation
bundle of Stanley K.
Kent-His bundle
keratectomy
Castroviejo k.
excimer laser photorefractive k.
k. operation
photorefractive k. (PRK)
phototherapeutic k.
superficial k.
keratinized tissue
keratin scale
keratitis-deafness cornification disorder
keratitis lesion
keratoacanthoma
keratoangioma
keratocele
keratocentesis operation
keratoconjunctivitis
keratocricoid
keratodermatocele
keratoepithelioplasty
keratoglossus
keratohyal
keratoleukoma
keratolysis
pitted k.
keratoma
keratometry
surgical k.
keratomileusis
laser-assisted in situ k. (LASIK)
laser in situ k. (LASIK)
k. operation
keratomy
keratopathy
band k.
exposure k.
keratophakic keratoplasty
keratopharyngeus
keratoplasty
allopathic k.
Arroyo k.
Arruga k.
autogenous k.
Durr nonpenetrating k.
Elschnig k.
epikeratophakic k.
Filatov k.
heterogeneous k.
homogenous k.
Imre k.
keratophakic k.
lamellar refractive k.
layered k.
Morax k.
nonpenetrating k.
k. operation
optic k.
optical k.
partial k.
Paufique k.
penetrating k.
perforating k.
photorefractive k.
punctate epithelial k.
refractive k.
Sourdille k.
superficial lamellar k.
tectonic k.
thermal k.
total k.
keratoscopy
keratostomy
keratotomy
arcuate transverse k.
astigmatic k.
delimiting k.
laser k.
k. operation
radial k. (RK)
refractive k.
Ruiz trapezoidal k.
trapezoidal k.
Kerckring fold
kerectomy
kerion formation
Kerley
K. A, B, C lines
Kernohan
K. notch
K. system of glioma classification
Kern technique
Kerr cesarean section
KESS constipation scoring system classification
Kessel-Bonney
K.-B. extension osteotomy
K.-B. procedure

Kessler
K. repair
K. suture technique
Kestenbaum procedure
ketoacidosis
diabetic k.
ketone body formation
ketoprofen analgesic therapy
Kety-Schmidt
K.-S. inert gas saturation technique
K.-S. method
Kevorkian punch biopsy
Key-Conwell pelvic fracture classification
Keyes punch biopsy
keyhole
k. approach
k. coronary bypass procedure
k. deformity
k. incision
k. mastopexy
k. method
k. surgery
k. tenodesis technique
keyhole-shaped craniectomy
key-in-lock maneuver
Key operation
Keystone
K. graft
K. mastopexy
K. technique
Khafagy modified ileocecal cystoplasty urinary diversion
KHC
knot holding capacity
Khodadoust line
Kidde cannula technique
Kidner
K. foot procedure
K. lesion
kidney
abdominal k.
k. abscess
k. adenocarcinoma
k. adenoma
amyloid k.
k. anomaly
arciform vein of k.
arteriosclerotic k.
artificial k.
Ask-Upmark k.
atrophic k.
k. biopsy
k. carbuncle
cicatricial k.
k. colic
contracted k.
cortical arch of k.
cystic k.
donor k.
ectopic k.
floating k.
Goldblatt k.
granular k.
interlobular artery of k.
k. internal splint/stent (KISS)
medullary sponge k.
mortar k.
movable k.
pelvic k.
k. position
putty k.
pyelonephritic k.
sclerotic k.
sigmoid k.
simultaneous pancreas and k. (SPK)
thoracic k.
k. transplantation
tumor-bearing k.
unicaliceal k.
wandering k.
waxy k.
kidney-sparing operation
Kiehn-Earle-DesPrez procedure
Kiel
K. classification
K. graft
K. Pediatric Tumor Registry
Kienböck dislocation
Kiernan space
Kiesselbach area
Kikuchi-MacNap-Moreau approach
Kilfoyle humeral medial condylar fracture classification
Kilian line
killer
flow artifact k. (FLAK)
Killian
K. bundle
K. frontal sinusotomy
K. frontoethmoidectomy procedure
K. incision
Killian-Jamieson area

NOTES

Killip classification of heart disease
Killip-Kimball heart failure classification
kilogram per meter squared
kilovolt
Kilsyn-Evans principle of frontal plane correction
Kimerle anomaly
Kimmelstiel-Wilson lesion
Kimura cartilage graft
Kinast indirect reduction
kinesthetic method
King
K. ASD umbrella closure
K. biopsy method
K. intraarticular hip fusion
K. open reduction
K. operation
K. technique
K. type IV curve posterior correction
King-Richards dislocation technique
King-Steelquist
K.-S. hindquarter amputation
K.-S. technique
kinking
catheter k.
Kinsey
K. atherectomy
K. rotation atherectomy extrusion angioplasty
Kinzie method
Kirby-Bauer disk diffusion method
Kirby operation
Kirchner cell
Kirk thigh amputation technique
Kirner deformity
Kirschner
K. pin fixation
K. suture technique
K. wire fixation
K. wire placement
Kirstein method
KISS
kidney internal splint/stent
kissing
k. balloon angioplasty
k. balloon technique
Kitano knot
Kitaoka-Leventen medial displacement metatarsal osteotomy
Kitzinger method of childbirth
Kjeldahl method
Kjolbe technique
kleeblatschädel deformity
Klein
K. muscle
K. technique
Kleinert
K. modification
K. repair
Klippel-Feil
K.-F. anomaly
K.-F. deformity
Klippel-Trenaunay syndrome
Klippel-Trenaunay-Weber syndrome
Klisic-Jankovic technique
Kluge method
Knapp
K. operation
K. procedure
Knapp-Wheeler-Reese operation
knee
k. anatomy
k. arthroplasty
descending artery of k.
k. dislocation
k. extension
k. extensor
flail k.
k. fracture
k. fusion
lateral k.
posterior k.
k. replacement surgery
k. rotation
kneecap
kneecapping injury
knee-chest position
knee-elbow position
kneeling position
kneeling-squatting position
knife-edged finishing line
knob
aortic k.
lateral deflection control k.
Knobby-Clark procedure
knock-knee deformity
Knoll
K. gland
K. refraction technique
Knoop hardness indenter point
knot
Aberdeen k.
Ahern k.
bow-tie k.
capstan k.
clinch k.
curved-needle surgeon k.
Dangel slip k.
enamel k.
externally releasable k.
extracorporeal jamming k.
false k.
fisherman's k.
friction k.

granny k.
half-hitch k.
k. holding capacity (KHC)
ileosigmoid k.
intracorporeal k.
jamming k.
Kitano k.
laparoscopic extracorporeal k.
one-handed k.
partial-throw surgeon k.
primitive k.
Roeder loop k.
secure intracorporeal k.
self-tightening slip k.
surgeon's k.
syncytial k.
Tim k.
Topel k.
Tripier operation throw square k.
true k.
vital k.
wire k.

knotting
catheter k.

Knott technique

Knowles pinning

knuckle
k. of tube

Ko-Airan
K.-A. bleeding control procedure
K.-A. maneuver

Koch
K. conduit
K. continent ileostomy
K. pouch cutaneous urinary diversion
K. pouch modified procedure
K. reservoir ileostomy
K. technique

Kocher
K. anastomosis
K. classification
K. curved L approach
K. fracture
K. lateral J approach
K. maneuver
K. method
K. point
K. pylorectomy
K. pyloromyotomy
K. ureterosigmoidostomy procedure

Kocher-Gibson posterolateral approach

Kocher-Langenbeck
K.-L. approach
K.-L. exposure

Kocher-Lorenz fracture

Kocher-McFarland hip arthroplasty

Koch pouch

Kochs operation

Koenig graft

Koenig-Schaefer
K.-S. incision
K.-S. medial approach

Koerner flap

Koffler operation

Köhler
K. illumination
K. line

Kohlrausch muscle

Kolmogorov-Smirnov procedure

Kolobow membrane lung

Kondoleon operation

Kondoleon-Sistrunk elephantiasis procedure

Konno
K. biopsy method
K. operation
K. procedure
K. repair

koronion

koroscopy

Korotkoff test

Kotz-Salzer rotationplasty

Koutsogiannis
K. calcaneal displacement osteotomy
K. procedure

Koutsogiannis-Fowler-Anderson osteotomy

Kovalevsky canal

Krackow
K. maneuver
K. point

Kramer-Craig-Noel basilar femoral neck osteotomy

Kraske
K. operation
K. parasacral approach
K. position
K. procedure
K. transsacral proctectomy

Kraupa operation

Krause
K. bone

NOTES

Krause *(continued)*
K. denervation
K. ligament
K. method
K. muscle
K. respiratory bundle
transverse suture of K.
Krause-Wolfe graft
Krawkow-Cohn technique
Krawkow-Thomas-Jones technique
Kreiker operation
Krempen-Craig-Sotelo tibial nonunion technique
Krempen-Silver-Sotelo nonunion operation
Kreuscher bunionectomy
Krimsky method
Kristeller
K. maneuver
K. method
Kroner tubal ligation
Krönig technique
Krönlein
K. hernia
K. operation
K. orbitotomy
K. procedure
Krönlein-Berke operation
Kronner external fixation
Kropp
K. cystourethroplasty
K. operation
K. procedure
Krukenberg
K. corneal spindle
K. hand reconstruction
K. procedure
Kruskal-Wallis
K.-W. nonparametric analysis
K.-W. test
krypton-8lm ventilation imaging
Kugel
K. anastomosis
K. approach
K. hernia repair
Kugelberg reconstruction
Kuhnt
K. dacryostomy
K. eyelid operation
K. tarsectomy
Kuhnt-Helmbold operation
Kuhnt-Junius repair
Kuhnt-Szymanowski procedure
Kuhnt-Thorpe operation
Kulchitsky cell carcinoma
Kumar
K. application
K. spica cast technique
Kumar-Cowell-Ramsey technique
Küntscher technique
Kussmaul
K. coma
K. respiration
Kussmaul-Kien respiration
Küstner
K. incision
K. uterine inversion correction
Kutes arthroplasty
Kutler
K. digital flap
K. double lateral advancement flap
K. finger amputation technique
K. V-Y flap
K. V-Y flap graft
Kuzmak
K. gastric banding
K. gastroplasty
kV fluoroscopy
KWB classification
K-wire placement
Kwitko operation
Kyle-Gustilo classification
Kyle-Gustilo-Premer classification
Kyle internal fixation
kyphectomy
Sharrard-type k.
kyphosis
k. correction
k. creation
postlaminectomy k.
postradiation k.
kyphos resection
kyphotic
k. angulation
k. deformity
k. deformity pathomechanics

LA
  laparoscopic appendectomy
  lateral apical
    LA segment
Labbé
  L. gastrotomy technique
  L. triangle
  L. vein
labia (*pl. of* labium)
labial
  l. cavity
  l. fusion
  l. gland
  l. hernia
  l. line
  l. pad
  l. tubercle
  l. ulceration
  l. vein
  l. vestibule
labiales
labialization
labii
labile blood pressure
labioglossolaryngeal
labioglossomandibular approach
labioglossopharyngeal
labioincisal line angle
labiolingual
  l. plane
  l. technique
labiomandibular
  l. approach
  l. glossotomy
labiomental
labionasal
labiopalatine
labioperineal pouch
labioplasty
labioscrotal fold
labium, pl. **labia**
  ungual labia
labor
  l. augmentation induction
  l. pain
laboratory
  l. monitoring
  l. parameter
LaBorde method
labored respiration
labral lesion
labrum
labyrinth
  bony l.
  ethmoidal l.
  Ludwig l.
  osseous l.
  renal l.
  Santorini l.
  vestibular l.
labyrinthectomy
labyrinthine
  l. artery
  l. fistula
  l. fistula test
  l. surgery
  l. vein
labyrinthotomy
labyrinthus
lacerable
lacerated foramen
laceration
  aortic l.
  birth canal l.
  bladder l.
  brain l.
  burst-type l.
  canalicular l.
  central stellate l.
  cervical l.
  chevron l.
  concurrent hepatic l.
  conjunctival l.
  corneal l.
  corneoscleral l.
  diaphragm l.
  diaphragmatic l.
  eyebrow l.
  flexor tendon l.
  hallucis longus l.
  inadvertent l.
  lid margin l.
  liver l.
  longitudinal l.
  lower pole l.
  parenchymal l.
  perineal l.
  peripheral l.
  rectal l.
  scalp l.
  splenic l.
  stellate l.
  tarsal l.
  tentorial l.
  through-and-through l.
  vaginal l.
  vascular l.
lacertus
lacerum
lace suture technique

L

Lachman maneuver
lacmoid staining solution
lacrimal, lachrymal
l. angle duct anomaly
l. apparatus
l. artery
l. bone
l. canal
l. canaliculus
l. crest
l. fascia
l. fistula
l. fold
l. ganglion
l. gland repair
l. gland tumor
l. irrigation test
l. lake
l. margin
l. mass
l. nerve
l. notch
l. papilla
l. point
l. punctum
l. sac
l. sac fossa
l. surgery
l. system
l. vein
lacrimale
lacrimalis
lacrimation
excessive l.
l. reflex
lacrimoconchalis
lacrimoconchal suture
lacrimomaxillaris
lacrimomaxillary suture
lacrimotomy
Lacroix
fibroosseous ring of L.
osseous ring of L.
lactate
blood l. (BL)
l. clearance
l. extraction
l. level
normalizing l.
normal serum l.
lactation letdown response
lacteal
l. fistula
l. vessel
lactic
l. acidosis
l. acidosis and stroke-like syndrome
lactiferi
lactiferous
l. duct
l. gland
l. sinus
lactoperoxidase radioiodination
lacuna, pl. **lacunae**
Morgagni l.
osteocytic l.
urethral l.
lacunae
lacunar
l. abscess
l. ligament
lacunare
Ladd
L. band
L. operation
L. procedure
laesa
Lafora body disease
lag
l. dilation
dilation l.
l. screw fixation
l. screw thread hole
l. time
Lagleyze-Trantas operation
Lagrange
L. humeral supracondylar fracture classification
L. operation
LAH
laparoscopic-assisted hepatectomy
Lahey operation
Laimer area
Laird-McMahon anorectoplasty
laissez-faire lid operation
lake
lacrimal l.
lateral l.
Lallemand body
Lallemand-Trousseau body
Lallouette pyramid
LAMA
laser-assisted microanastomosis
Lamaze
L. method
L. technique
lambda suture line
lambdoid
l. margin
l. suture
lambdoidea
Lambert canal
Lambl excrescence
Lamb-Marks-Bayne technique

Lambrinudi
L. osteotomy
L. technique
lamella, pl. **lamellae**
corneal l.
elastic l.
lamellar
l. corneal transplant
l. exfoliation
l. refractive keratoplasty
lamellation
lamina, pl. **laminae**
alar l.
basal l.
basilar l.
cribrous l.
deep l.
external elastic l.
fusca l.
pterygoid l.
suprachoroid l.
thyroid l.
laminaplasty
expansive l.
Tsuji l.
laminar
l. cortex posterior aspect
l. flow hood
l. fracture
laminated
l. acellular mass
l. clot
lamination
laminectomy
cervical spine l.
decompression l.
decompressive l.
four-place l.
Gill l.
Girdlestone l.
multilevel l.
radial l.
laminoforaminotomy
laminoplasty
laminotomy and diskectomy
Lancaster operation
Lancefield classification
lanceolate deformity
Lanchner operation
landmark
anatomic l.
anatomical l.
bony l.
cephalometric l.
developmental l.
pedicle l.
surface l.
Winnie l.
Landolt
L. body
L. operation
Landzert fossa
Lane
L. band
L. operation
L. procedure
Langenbeck
L. operation
L. triangle
Langendorff
L. heart preparation
L. method
L. perfusion
Langenskiöld
L. bone graft
L. bony bridge resection
L. fusion
L. procedure
Langer
L. arch
L. line
Langerhans
islets of L.
Lange tendon lengthening and repair
Langevin updating procedure
Langhans line
Lannelongue ligament
Lanz
L. incision
L. line
L. point
Lanza scale for drug-induced mucosal damage classification
LAO
left anterior oblique
left anterior occipital
LAO position
LAP
left atrial pressure
laparectomy
laparocele
laparocystidotomy
laparoenterotomy
laparogastroscopy

NOTES

L

laparogastrostomy
laparogastrotomy
laparohepatotomy
laparohysterectomy
laparohystero-oophorectomy
laparohysteropexy
laparohysterosalpingo-oophorectomy
laparohysterotomy
laparoileotomy
laparomyomectomy
laparomyositis
laparorrhaphy
laparosalpingectomy
laparosalpingo-oophorectomy
laparosalpingotomy
laparoscopic
l. adjustable silicone gastric banding
l. adrenalectomy
l. anterior partial fundoplication
l. appendectomy (LA)
l. approach
l. artery ligation
l. assistance
l. autopsy
l. bariatric surgery
l. bilioenteric anastomosis
l. bladder neck suture suspension procedure
l. bowel resection
l. Burch procedure
l. bypass procedure
l. cardiomyotomy
l. celiac plexus pain block
l. cholecystectomy (LC)
l. cholecystotomy
l. clip application
l. colectomy
l. colorectal cancer surgery
l. colposuspension technique
l. common bile duct exploration
l. cyst decortication
270-degree l. posterior fundoplasty
l. dismembered pyeloplasty
l. dissection and manipulation
l. distal pancreatectomy
l. Döderlein hysterectomy
l. donor nephrectomy (LDN)
l. Dorr antireflux surgery
l. esophageal myomectomy
l. esophagogastric fundoplasty
l. esophagogastroplasty with Nissen fundoplication
l. esophagomyotomy
l. esophagoplasty
l. evaluation
l. examination
l. extracorporeal knot
l. feeding tube replacement
l. fenestration
l. gallbladder removal
l. gas
l. gastric banding
l. gastric bypass
l. gastroenterostomy
l. gastroplasty
l. gastrostomy
l. guidance
l. Hassab operation
l. Helle
l. Heller myotomy
l. hepatectomy
l. hepatojejunostomy
l. hernioplasty
l. hysterosalpingectomy
l. intracorporeal ultrasonography (LICU)
l. IPOM repair
l. jejunostomy
l. laser cholecystectomy (LLC)
l. left hemicolectomy
l. liver biopsy
l. lymph node dissection method
l. lymph node dissection procedure
l. lymph node dissection technique
l. lymphocelectomy
l. lysis of adhesion
l. management
l. needle colposuspension
l. nephrectomy
l. Nissen fundoplication (LNF)
l. Nissen fundoplication method
l. Nissen fundoplication procedure
l. Nissen fundoplication technique
l. Nissen fundoplication with esophageal lengthening
l. Nissen and Toupet fundoplication
l. orchiopexy
l. paraaortic lymph node sampling
l. paraaortic lymph node sampling method
l. paraaortic lymph node sampling procedure
l. paraaortic lymph node sampling technique
l. paraesophageal hernia repair (LPHR)
l. pelvic lymphadenectomy
l. pelvic lymph node dissection
l. photography
l. pneumodissection
l. port site metastasis
l. posterior hemifundoplication
l. proctectomy
l. PROST
l. prosthetic mesh repair

l. pyloromyotomy
l. radical hysterectomy
l. radical prostatectomy
l. repair of paraesophageal hernia (LRPH)
l. retropubic colposuspension
l. seromyotomy
l. splenectomy
l. staging
l. stone extraction
l. stripping technique
l. surgical procedure
l. technology
l. total extraperitoneal herniorrhaphy
l. total occlusion (LTO)
l. total proctocolectomy
l. Toupet anti-reflux surgery
l. transcystic common bile duct exploration (LTCBDE)
l. transcystic duct exploration
l. transcystic lithotripsy (LTCL)
l. transcystic papillotomy
l. transcystic sphincter of Oddi manometry
l. transhiatal esophagectomy
l. transhiatal view
l. treatment
l. trocar wound
l. tubal banding procedure
l. ultrasonography (LUS)
l. ultrasound
l. ureteral reanastomosis
l. ureterolithotomy
l. uterine nerve ablation
l. uterolysis
l. vagotomy
l. varicocelectomy
l. varicocele repair
l. varix ligation
l. ventral hernia repair
l. vision

laparoscopically
l. assisted endorectal pull-through procedure
l. assisted surgery
l. assisted vaginal hysterectomy (LAVH)
l. guided cryoablation
l. guided transcystic exploration

laparoscopic-assisted
l.-a. aneurysmectomy
l.-a. aortic reconstructive surgery
l.-a. esophagectomy
l.-a. gastropexy
l.-a. hemicolectomy
l.-a. hepatectomy (LAH)
l.-a. living donor nephrectomy
l.-a. procedure
l.-a. small bowel resection
l.-a. vaginal hysterectomy
l.-a. vaginal hysteroscopy

laparoscopic-induced neuralgia

laparoscopist

laparoscopy
ambulatory gynecologic l.
bedside l.
closed l.
diagnostic l.
double-puncture l.
flexible l.
full diagnostic l.
gaseous l.
gasless l.
gynecologic l.
hand-assisted l.
laser l.
mandatory l.
needle l.
open l.
pelvic l.
revision l.
second-look l.
single-port l.
single-puncture l.
therapeutic l.

laparoscopy-assisted colectomy

laparoscopy-guided subhepatic cholecystostomy

Laparostat with fiber diversion

laparotomy
elective l.
emergency l.
exploratory l.
formal l.
l. incision
negative l.
open l.
routine l.
second-look l.
staging l.
standard midline l.

laparotrachelotomy

laparotyphlotomy

laparouterotomy

NOTES

Lapides-Ball urethropexy
Lapides technique
Lapidus
L. bunionectomy
L. hammertoe technique
lappet formation
lap seatbelt fracture
LAR
low anterior resection
lardaceous liver
large
l. canal
l. cell carcinoma
l. intestine
l. mask airway
l. pelvis
l. restoration
large-core
l.-c. needle aspiration biopsy
l.-c. technique
large-humeral-head hemiarthroplasty
large-particle biopsy
large-scale integration
Larmon
L. forefoot arthroplasty
L. forefoot procedure
LaRoque herniorrhaphy incision
Laroyenne operation
Larrey
L. cleft
L. hernia
Larsen syndrome
Larson
L. ligament reconstruction
L. technique
Lartat-Jacob hepatic resection
laryngea
laryngeae
laryngeal
l. anesthesia
l. anomaly
l. aperture
l. bursa
l. carcinoma
l. cartilage fracture
l. cyst
l. diaphragm
l. edema
l. electromyography
l. framework surgery
l. gland
l. hemorrhage
l. infection
l. keel operation
l. mask airway (LMA)
l. mask insertion anesthetic technique
l. muscle
l. nerve paralysis
l. oscillation
l. pharynx
l. pouch
l. prominence
l. repair
l. respiration
l. sinus
l. skeleton
l. vein
l. ventricle
l. web
laryngectomy
anterior partial l.
frontolateral l.
narrow-field l.
near-total l.
partial l.
subtotal supraglottic l.
supracricoid partial l.
supraglottic l.
total l.
vertical partial l.
wide-field total l.
laryngei
larynges (*pl. of* larynx)
laryngeus
laryngis
laryngocele
laryngology
laryngopharyngectomy
partial l.
total l.
laryngopharyngeus
laryngopharynx
laryngoplasty
sternothyroid muscle flap l.
laryngopyocele
laryngoscopy
l. anesthetic technique
direct l.
fiber optic l.
indirect l.
laser l.
mirror-image l.
suspension l.
laryngospasm
postextubation l.
laryngotomy
inferior l.
laryngotracheoplasty (LTP)
larynx, pl. **larynges**
external auditory l.
folding l.
posterior l.
superficial anterior l.
superior l.

laser
l. arthroscopy
l. biliary lithotripsy
l. cavity
l. cervical conization
l. coagulation
l. coagulation vaporization procedure (LCVP)
l. Doppler flowmetry (LDF)
l. Doppler fluximetry
l. hemorrhoidectomy
l. hemorrhoid excision
l. iridectomy
l. iridotomy
l. keratotomy
l. laparoscopic cholecystectomy (LLC)
l. laparoscopic vagotomy
l. laparoscopy
l. laryngoscopy
l. manipulation
l. method
l. partial nephrectomy
l. photoablation
l. photocoagulation
l. photovaporization
l. plume
l. recanalization
l. in situ keratomileusis (LASIK)
l. surgery
l. therapy
l. tissue weld
l. tissue welding
l. trabeculoplasty
l. uterosacral nerve ablation
l. vaporization
l. welding technique
laser-assisted
l.-a. appendectomy
l.-a. balloon angioplasty
l.-a. microanastomosis (LAMA)
l.-a. in situ keratomileusis (LASIK)
l.-a. spinal endoscopy
l.-a. uvulopalatoplasty (LAUP)
laser-evoked potential
laser-filtering surgery
laser-induced
l.-i. fragmentation
l.-i. intracorporeal shock wave lithotripsy
lasering
lasertripsy
Lash
L. operation
L. procedure
LASIK
laser-assisted in situ keratomileusis
laser in situ keratomileusis
LAST
limited anterior small thoracotomy
LAST coronary bypass procedure
lata
fascia l.
latae
Latarget
L. procedure
Latarget nerve
late
l. complication
l. graft dysfunction
l. graft failure
l. infection rate
l. wound failure
latency
postdrug l.
latent herpes simplex virus infection
late-onset disease
latera (*pl. of* latus)
lateral
l. aberration
l. adenoidectomy
l. apex
l. apical (LA)
l. aspiration
l. atlantoaxial joint
l. band mobilization
l. bending technique
l. bicipital groove
l. calcaneal branch
l. canal
l. canal entrapment
l. canthotomy
l. canthus
l. cartilage flap
l. central palmar space
l. cerebral aperture
l. cervical node dissection
l. chest x-ray
l. closing wedge osteotomy
l. column
l. compartment reconstruction
l. compression
l. compression injury
l. condensation

NOTES

lateral *(continued)*
- l. condylar humeral fracture
- l. condylar inclination
- l. condyle
- l. cord
- l. corticospinal tract
- l. crus
- l. decubitus position
- l. deflection control knob
- l. deltoid splitting approach
- l. edge
- l. excursion
- l. extensor expansion
- l. extensor release
- l. extracavitary approach
- l. fluoroscopy
- l. fusion
- l. Gatellier-Chastung approach
- l. geniculate body
- l. ginglymus
- l. glossoepiglottic fold
- l. ground (LG)
- l. ground bundle
- l. head
- l. illumination
- l. J approach
- l. jaw projection
- l. joint of ankle
- l. joint line
- l. joint space
- l. knee
- l. Kocher approach
- l. lake
- l. listhesis
- l. lithotomy
- l. mass
- l. mass fracture
- l. meniscectomy
- l. muscle
- l. nail fold
- l. nasal branch
- l. orbit
- l. perforation
- l. pole
- l. portion
- l. process
- l. prone position
- l. rectus recession
- l. rectus resection
- l. rectus tendon
- l. recumbent position
- l. retraction
- l. rhachotomy
- l. root
- l. sac
- l. sector
- l. sinus
- l. utility incision
- l. ventricle
- l. wall
- l. window technique
- l. wound
- l. x-ray view

laterale

laterales

lateralis

laterality

lateralization
- cortical l.

lateral-lateral pouch

lateral-sector pedicle

lateriflexion

lateroabdominal

lateroaortic
- l. lymph node dissection
- l. metastasis

laterodeviation

lateroflexion

lateropharyngeum

lateroposition

later postoperative period

late-stage disease

latex closure

lathing procedure

latissimus
- l. dorsi island flap
- l. dorsi muscle flap
- l. dorsi musculocutaneous flap
- l. dorsi myocutaneous flap
- l. dorsi procedure
- l. dorsi tendon

latissimus-scapular muscle flap

latissimus-serratus muscle flap

lattice
- l. space

latus, pl. **latera**

Latzko
- L. cesarean section
- L. partial colpocleisis
- L. radical abdominal hysterectomy
- L. vesicovaginal fistula repair

laudable

Lauenstein procedure

Lauge-Hansen ankle fracture classification

Laugier
- L. fracture
- L. hernia

Laumonier ganglion

LAUP
- laser-assisted uvulopalatoplasty

Laurell
- L. method
- L. technique

Lauren gastric carcinoma classification

Lauth
L. canal
L. ligament
lavage
abdominal l.
bowel l.
l. bowel preparation
colonic l.
continuous postoperative closed l.
copious peritoneal l.
diagnostic peritoneal l. (DPL)
Exeter bone l.
external biliary l.
l. instillation
intraoperative bowel l.
intraoperative colonic l.
peritoneal l.
pulsatile pressure l.
saline l.
l. solution
l. and suction
LAVH
laparoscopically assisted vaginal hysterectomy
Lavine reduction
law
l. of association
l. of denervation
Le Chatelier l.
Laws
L. gastroplasty
Lawson operation
layer
aponeurotic l.
barrier l.
echographic l.
echo-poor l.
fascial l.
hidden l.
input l.
meningeal l.
mesothelial cell l.
molecular external l.
nerve fiber bundle l.
nuclear external l.
orbital l.
output l.
parietal l.
plexiform external l.
posterior l.
pretracheal l.
prevertebral l.
seromuscular l.
serous l.
superficial l.
suprachoroid l.
l. technique
visceral l.
layered
l. closure
l. keratoplasty
layer-to-layer gastroplasty
laying-open fistulotomy
Lazaro da Silva technique colostomy
Lazarus-Nelson technique
Lazepen-Gamidov anteromedial approach
lazy-C incision
lazy-H incision
lazy-S incision
lazy-Z incision
LB
LB segment
LC
laparoscopic cholecystectomy
LCAT
lecithin-cholesterol acyltransferase
L-curved incision
LCVP
laser coagulation vaporization procedure
LCVP-aided
LCVP-a. hepatectomy
LCVP-a. hepatic resection
LCVP-a. technique
LCVP-assisted
LCVP-a. hepatectomy
LCVP-a. major liver resection
LDF
laser Doppler flowmetry
LDN
laparoscopic donor nephrectomy
LDN technique
LDR
low dose rate
LDR intracavitary radiation therapy
Le
Le Chatelier law
Le Chatelier principle
Le Dentu suture technique
Le Dran suture technique
Le Fort classification
Le Fort fibular fracture
Le Fort I-III fracture
Le Fort mandibular fracture
Le Fort-Neugebauer operation

NOTES

Le *(continued)*
Le Fort operation
Le Fort osteotomy
Le Fort partial colpocleisis
Le Fort procedure
Le Fort suture technique
Le Fort-Wagstaffe fracture
Le Fort-Wehrbein-Duplay hypospadias repair
Leach-Igou step-cut medial osteotomy
Leach-Schepsis-Paul augmentation
Leach technique
lead
l. appearance
l. colic
l. line
Leadbetter
L. cystourethroplasty
L. hip manipulation
L. maneuver
L. modification technique
L. procedure
Leadbetter-Politano
L.-P. procedure
L.-P. ureterovesicoplasty
lead-pipe
l.-p. colon
l.-p. fracture
leaf
superior l.
leaflet
aortic valve l.
heart valve l.
mitral valve l.
posterior mitral valve l.
valve l.
Leahey operation
leak
anastomotic stump l.
bile l.
chylous l.
cystic duct stump l.
duodenal stump l.
glue patch l.
mask l.
pancreatic stump l.
periprosthetic l.
l. point pressure
postoperative anastomotic l.
Roux limb stump l.
stump l.
trocar gas l.
leakage
anastomotic l.
bile l.
biliary l.
cervical l.
chylous l.
corneal l.
intestinal anastomotic l.
local l.
l. rate
silicone implant l.
tube l.
lean
l. body mass
l. body weight
Leao
spreading depression of L.
leapfrog position
leather-bottle stomach
Leboyer
L. method
L. technique
lecithin-cholesterol acyltransferase (LCAT)
Lecompte maneuver
ledge
eccentric l.
LeDuc
L. anastomosis
L. technique
LeDuc-Camey
L.-C. ileocolostomy
L.-C. ileocystoplasty
Lee
L. anterosuperior iliac spine graft
L. bone graft
L. ganglion
L. procedure
L. reconstruction
L. technique
leech
mechanical l.
LEEP
loop electrocautery excision procedure
loop electrosurgical excision procedure
LEEP conization
leeway space
Lee-White
L.-W. clotting time
L.-W. clotting time method
Lefèvre gastrectomy technique
LeFort III facial advancement
left
l. anterior oblique (LAO)
l. anterior oblique position
l. anterior oblique projection
l. anterior occipital (LAO)
l. atrial isolation procedure
l. atrial pressure (LAP)
l. atrium-to-femoral artery circulatory bypass
l. brachiocephalic vein
l. bundle-branch block
l. colectomy

l. coronary artery
l. coronary valve
l. decubitus position
l. dominant coronary circulation
l. frontal craniotomy (LFC)
l. gutter
l. heart catheterization
l. hemicolectomy
l. hemidiaphragm
l. hepatectomy
l. hypochondriac region
l. inguinal hernia (LIH)
l. lateral decubitus position
l. lateral projection
l. lateral region
l. lower extremity
l. rotation
l. subclavian vein (LSV)
l. thorax
l. upper extremity
l. upper quadrant
l. upper quadrant peritonectomy
l. ventricle
l. ventricular end-diastolic area (LVEDa)
l. ventricular end-diastolic pressure
l. ventricular end-systolic area (LVESa)
l. ventricular outflow tract (LVOT)
l. ventricular puncture
l. ventricular systolic pressure
l. vertebral artery

left-sided
l.-s. colorectal obstruction
l.-s. injury
l.-s. nail
l.-s. thoracotomy

left-side-down position
left-to-right subtotal pancreatectomy
Legat point
Lehman technique
Leibolt technique
leiomyoblastoma
leiomyofibroma
leiomyoma enucleation
leiomyomectomy
leiomyosarcoma
recurrent l.

Leishman classification
LeJour mastopexy
Lejour-type breast reduction
Leksell technique
Lelièvre osteotomy
Lembert suture technique
Lempert
L. fenestration
L. incision

Lenart-Kullman technique
length
bowel l.
pedicle screw path l.
peripheral capillary filtration slit l.
restriction fragment l.
l. of stay (LOS)

length-breadth index
lengthening
distal catheter l.
extensor l.
laparoscopic Nissen fundoplication with esophageal l.
surgical crown l.

length-height index
length-resting tension relation
length-tension relation
lengthwise slit
Lennert
L. classification
L. lesion

lens
l. aberration
C-loop intraocular l.
corneal l.
l. dislocation
l. equator
l. exchange
intraocular l.
l. plane
l. removal
suture of l.
l. suture technique

lensectomy
Charles l.
coal-mining l.

lentectomy
lenticular
l. loop
l. papilla
l. process
l. ring

lenticulostriate artery
lentiform bone
lentigo melanoma
Lepird procedure
L'Episcopo hip reconstruction

NOTES

L'Episcopo-Zachary procedure
leprosy
anesthetic l.
leptomeningeal
l. anastomosis
l. carcinoma
l. metastasis
l. space
leptomeninges
leptomyelolipoma
Leriche
L. operation
L. sympathectomy
Leri-Weill disease
LES
lower esophageal sphincter
LES pressure
Lesgaft
L. hernia
L. space
lesion
accessible l.
acetowhite l.
acneform l.
acute gastric mucosal l.
acute traumatic l.
admixture l.
aggressive l.
anal squamous intraepithelial l.
angiocentric immunoproliferative l.
angiocentric lymphoproliferative l.
angiodysplastic l.
angioinvasive l.
angioproliferative l.
angulated l.
annular constricting l.
anterior labrum periosteum shoulder arthroscopic l.
aphthous-type l.
apple-core l.
l. architecture
l. arrangement
articular cartilage l.
atherosclerotic carotid artery l.
atlantoaxial l.
axial l.
axillary skin l.
Baehr-Lohlein l.
Bankart shoulder l.
barrel-shaped l.
basal ganglionic l.
benign bone l.
benign lymphoepithelial l.
benign lymphoproliferative l.
benign vascular l.
Bennett l.
biceps interval l.
bifurcation l.
bilobed polypoid l.
bird's nest l.
blanchable red l.
blastic l.
bleeding l.
blue-gray l.
Blumenthal l.
bone marrow l.
bony l.
boomerang-shaped l.
Bracht-Wachter l.
braid-like l.
brainstem l.
branch l.
bridge-like l.
brown-black l.
bubbly bone l.
bullous skin l.
bull's eye macular l.
Bywaters l.
calcified l.
cancer l.
carpet l.
cavitary lung l.
cavitary small-bowel l.
cemental l.
central l.
centrilobular l.
cerebral l.
cervical l.
chest l.
chiasmal l.
choroidal l.
circular cherry-red l.
cleavage l.
cochlear l.
coin l.
cold l.
colonic vascular l.
complete common peroneal nerve l.
concentric l.
congenital l.
conjunctival melanotic l.
constricting l.
cornea guttate l.
corneal punctate l.
cortical l.
Councilman l.
culprit l.
cutaneous l.
cylindromatous l.
cystic bone l.
cystic lymphoepithelial AIDS-related l.
demyelinating l.
dendritic l.
de novo l.
depigmented l.

depressed l.
dermal l.
desmoid l.
destructive bone l.
Dieulafoy l.
Dieulafoy-like l.
diffuse ulcerative l.
dilatable l.
discoid skin l.
discrete l.
disk l.
l. distribution
division I–IV l.
dorsal root entry zone l.
DREZ l.
ductal-dependent l.
Duret l.
dye sham intrarenal l.
dysarthric l.
dysplasia-associated l.
early cancer l.
ectatic vascular l.
eczematous l.
elementary l.
elevated l.
enhancing brain l.
entry zone l.
eosinophilic fibrohistiocytic l.
epididymis l.
epidural extramedullary l.
erysipelas-like skin l.
erythrodermatous l.
l. evolution
excavated l.
expansile unilocular well-demarcated bone l.
extracranial mass l.
extrahepatic l.
extramural l.
extratesticular l.
extremity l.
extrinsic l.
fibrocalcific l.
fibrohistiocytic l.
fibromusculoelastic l.
fibroosseous l.
fibrous bone l.
fibrous polypoid l.
firm l.
flat depressed l.
flat elevated l.
floor-of-mouth l.
florid duct l.
focal parenchymal brain l.
focal splenic l.
follicular l.
Forest I, II l.
gastrointestinal l.
genetic l.
genital papulosquamous l.
Ghon primary l.
giant cell l.
Gill l.
glomerular tip l.
gross l.
ground-glass l.
gunpowder l.
hamartomatous l.
hemorrhagic l.
hepatic mass l.
herpetoid l.
high-grade squamous intraepithelial l.
high-intensity l.
high neurological l.
Hill-Sachs shoulder l.
histologic l.
honeycomb l.
hot l.
hyperdense brain l.
hyperintense brain l.
hyperkeratotic l.
hyperpigmented l.
hypodense brain l.
hypoechoic l.
l. identification
immunoproliferative l.
impaction l.
indiscriminate l.
infarctive l.
inflammatory l.
initial syphilitic l.
interpeduncular fossa l.
interradicular l.
intraabdominal l.
intraconal l.
intracranial mass l.
intradural extramedullary l.
intrahepatic l.
intramedullary l.
intramural extramucosal l.
intraosseous bone l.
intrasellar l.

NOTES

lesion *(continued)*
intravascular endothelial proliferative l.
intrinsic brainstem l.
ipsilateral nerve root l.
irritable l.
irritative l.
Janeway l.
jet l.
Keasbey l.
keratitis l.
Kidner l.
Kimmelstiel-Wilson l.
labral l.
Lennert l.
Libman-Sacks l.
lichenified l.
linear l.
lipocytic l.
localized l.
Löhlein-Baehr l.
long l.
low-attenuation l.
lower motor neuron l.
low-grade squamous intraepithelial l.
lucent lung l.
lumbar spinal cord l.
lumbar spine l.
lumbosacral plexus l.
lumbosacral root l.
lymphoepithelial l.
lymphoproliferative l.
lytic bone l.
macrofollicular l.
macroscopic l.
macrovascular coronary l.
malignant l.
malignant pituitary l.
Mallory-Weiss l.
mammographic l.
l. margination
mass l.
medium l.
melanocytic conjunctival l.
melanotic l.
mesencephalic low-density l.
mesenchymal l.
mesenteric vascular l.
metastatic l.
minute polypoid l.
mixed fat-water density l.
mixed sclerotic and lytic bone l.
molecular l.
monotypic l.
Monteggia equivalent l.
Morel-Lavele l.
morphea-like l.
l. morphology
mucocutaneous l.
mucosal l.
mucous membrane l.
mulberry l.
multifocal enhancing l.
multilocular cystic l.
napkin-ring annular l.
neoplastic l.
neural l.
neurovascular l.
nickel-and-dime l.
nodular l.
nodule-in-nodule l.
nonbacterial thrombotic endocardial l.
nonblanchable, abnormally colored l.
nonerosive gastric mucosal l.
nonmeningiomatous malignant l.
nonneoplastic tumor-like l.
nonperforative l.
nucleus ambiguus l.
nummular l.
occult talar l.
ocular adnexal l.
oil drop l.
onion scale l.
orbital l.
organic l.
Osgood-Schlatter l.
osseous l.
osteoblastic l.
osteochondral l.
osteolytic bone l.
osteopathic l.
osteosclerotic l.
ostial l.
papillary l.
papulopustular l.
papulosquamous l.
papulovesicular l.
paraorbital l.
parasagittal l.
patch l.
pathologic l.
perforative l.
periodontal l.
peripheral nerve l.
perisellar vascular l.
periventricular hyperintense l.
periventricular white matter l.
Perthes l.
photon-deficient bone l.
pigmented l.
pigment epithelial l.
plaque-like l.
plexiform l.

polypoid l.
postfracture l.
potentially resectable l.
precancerous l.
prechiasmal optic nerve l.
precipitating l.
precursor l.
preexisting l.
premalignant l.
preoperative l.
presacral cystic l.
primary l.
proliferative l.
pruritic l.
pseudocancerous l.
pseudomedial longitudinal fasciculus l.
pulpoperiapical l.
punched-out l.
purpuric l.
pustular l.
pyodermatous skin l.
radial sclerosing l.
radiodense l.
radiofrequency l.
radiofrequency-generated thermal l.
radiolucent l.
radiopaque l.
reactive lymphoid l.
recurrent nerve l.
regurgitant l.
residual l.
restenosis l.
reticular l.
retroacetabular l.
retrochiasmal l.
retrogeniculate l.
reverse Hill-Sachs l.
right-sided l.
rim-enhancing l.
ring l.
ring-wall l.
rolled shoulder l.
rotationally induced shear-strain l.
rotator cuff l.
ruptured peliotic l.
saddle l.
satellite l.
scaling skin-colored l.
scirrhous l.
sclerosing l.
sclerotic bone l.
secondary l.
semipedunculated l.
sessile l.
shagreen l.
short-segment l.
SIL/ASCUS l.
Sinding-Larsen-Johansson l.
sinonasal l.
sinusoidal l.
l. size
skeletal l.
skin-colored l.
skip l.
SLAP l.
slope-shouldered l.
small bowel l.
smooth skin-colored l.
soft l.
soft-tissue l.
space-occupying brain l.
special l.
spiculated l.
spinal l.
splenic l.
spontaneous l.
squamous intraepithelial l.
square-shouldered l.
stellate border breast l.
Stener l.
stenotic l.
stereotactic l.
stress l.
structural l.
subtentorial l.
supranuclear l.
suprasellar low-density l.
supratentorial l.
suspicious l.
synchronous l.
systemic l.
tandem l.
target l.
thoracic l.
trabeculated bone l.
transient l.
traumatic l.
trophic l.
truncal l.
tuberculous l.
tubulovillar l.
type B-1, -2 l.
typical skin l.

L

NOTES

lesion *(continued)*
uncommitted metaphysial l.
undifferentiated l.
unifocal optic nerve l.
unilocular cystic l.
unresectable l.
uremic gastrointestinal l.
varicelliform l.
vasculitic l.
vegetative l.
venular l.
verrucous l.
vesicobullous l.
violaceous l.
visceral l.
vulvar pigmented l.
vulvovaginal l.
Waldeyer ring l.
weeping l.
well-circumscribed l.
white l.
white-spot l.
wire-loop l.
wraparound periapical l.
Wrisberg l.
yellow l.

lesioning
stereotactic radiofrequency l.

Leslie-Ryan anterior axillary approach

lesser
l. cul-de-sac
l. curvature
l. horn
l. omentectomy
l. omentum
l. palatine artery
l. pancreas
l. pelvis
l. peritoneal cavity
l. peritoneal sac
l. resection
l. ring
l. sac approach
l. sac hernia
l. sac technique
l. sciatic notch
l. supraclavicular fossa
L. triangle
l. trochanter
l. trochanter fracture
l. vestibular gland

Lesshaft triangle

Lester-Jones operation

Lester Martin modification of Duhamel operation

lethal
l. concentration
l. osteogenesis imperfecta

Letournel-Judet
L.-J. acetabular fracture classification
L.-J. approach

letterbox technique

leukemia

leukemic infiltration

leukochloroma

leukocyte infiltration

leukocytic
l. infiltration
l. margination

leukocytoclastic vasculitis

leukocytoma

leukodepletion

leukoencephalopathy
radiation-induced l.

leukolymphosarcoma

leukolysis

leukoma
adherent l.

leukosarcoma

leukostasis
intracerebral l.

leukotomy
prefrontal l.
transorbital l.

Leung thumb loss classification

Levaditi method

levator
l. ani syndrome
l. aponeurosis repair
l. hernia
l. injury
l. palpebrae
l. resection
l. scapulae syndrome
l. span
l. swelling

levatorplasty

level
anterior midpapillary l.
antithrombin III plasma l.
arterial lactate l.
attenuation l.
bilirubin l.
CEA l.
Clark l.
collagenase l.
endothelin plasma l.
l. foundation
heparin cofactor II plasma l.
iPTH l.
lactate l.
motilin l.
multiple shunt l.'s
overall sound l.
pain tolerance l.

parathyroid hormone l.
pentane excretion l.
plasma l.
plasminogen plasma l.
post-injury l.
pretreatment l.
protein C, S plasma l.
PTH l.
saturation sound pressure l.
sensation l.
serum lidocaine l. (SLL)
serum total bilirubin l.
sound pressure l.
total bilirubin l.
uterine lysosome l.
level-dependent
blood oxygenation l.-d.
leverage
Levine
L. dislocation operation
L. gradation 1–6
Levine-Harvey classification
levitation
levodopa dopaminergic medication
levodopa-induced dyskinesia
levo-transposed position
Levret maneuver
Levy, Rowntree, and Marriott method
Lewis
L. and Benedict method
L. intercalary resection
L. operation
L. thoracotomy
Lewis-Chekofsky resection
Lewissohn method
Lewis-Tanner
L.-T. procedure
L.-T. subtotal esophagectomy and reconstruction
Lewit stretch technique
Lexer operation
LFC
left frontal craniotomy
LG
lateral ground
LG bundle
Liang and Pardee method
libera
liberation
liberi
Libman-Sacks lesion
Lich
L. extravesical technique
L. procedure
lichenification
lichenified lesion
lichenoid graft-versus-host disease
Lich-Gregoir
L.-G. anastomosis
L.-G. kidney transplant surgery
L.-G. repair
L.-G. technique
L.-G. ureterolysis
Lichtblau osteotomy
Lichtenstein
L. hernial repair
L. herniorrhaphy
L. mesh repair
L. operation
L. tension-free hernioplasty
Lichtman technique
LICU
laparoscopic intracorporeal ultrasonography
lid
l. closure reaction
l. margin laceration
upper l.
lid-loading technique
Lieberkühn
L. crypt
L. gland
Liebolt radioulnar technique
lien
lienal artery
lienales
lienalis
lienculus
lienectomy
lienis
lienopancreatic
lienophrenic ligament
lienorenale
lienorenal ligament
lienunculus
Lieutaud
L. body
L. triangle
L. trigone
L. uvula
life
l. expectancy
no signs of l.

NOTES

L

life *(continued)*
perceived quality of l. (PQOL)
quality of l. (QOL)
l. space
l. table method
life-saving form of therapy
life-sustaining hepatic reserve
life-threatening
l.-t. cancer
l.-t. complication
l.-t. illness
lift-and-cut biopsy
lifting
abdominal wall l.
sternal l.
ligament
accessory plantar l.
accessory volar l.
acromioclavicular l.
alar l.
anococcygeal l.
anterior costotransverse l.
anterior cruciate l. (ACL)
anterior sternoclavicular l.
anterior tibiotalar l.
Arantius l.
arcuate pubic l.
atlantooccipital l.
auricular l.
Berry l.
broad uterine l.
Camper l.
capsular l.
cardinal l.
caroticoclinoid l.
caudal l.
ceratocricoid l.
cervical l.
cholecystoduodenal l.
chondroxiphoid l.
ciliary l.
Civinini l.
Clado l.
Cloquet l.
collateral l.
Colles l.
Cooper l.
coracoacromial l.
coracoclavicular l.
coracohumeral l.
costoclavicular l.
costocolic l.
costotransverse l.
costoxiphoid l.
cotyloid l.
Cowper l.
cricoarytenoid l.
cricothyroid l.
cricotracheal l.
cruciform l.
cystoduodenal l.
Denonvilliers l.
denticulate l.
digital retinacular l.
duodenorenal l.
epihyal l.
external l.
falciform l.
fallopian l.
Ferrein l.
fibulocalcaneal l.
fundiform l.
gastrocolic l.
gastrodiaphragmatic l.
gastrohepatic l.
gastrolienal l.
gastrophrenic l.
gastrosplenic l.
genitoinguinal l.
Gimbernat l.
l. graft
Gruber l.
Hensing l.
hepatocolic l.
hepatoduodenal l.
hepatoesophageal l.
hepatogastric l.
hepatorenal l.
Hesselbach l.
Holl l.
Hueck l.
hyalocapsular l.
hyoepiglottic l.
iliolumbar l.
inferior glenohumeral l.
inferior pubic l.
inferior transverse scapular l.
infundibuloovarian l.
infundibulopelvic l.
inguinal l.
interchondral l.
interclavicular l.
interclinoid l.
interfoveolar l.
interosseous sacroiliac l.
interphalangeal collateral l.
interspinous l.
intertransverse l.
intervolar plate l.
intraarticular sternocostal l.
intracapsular l.
Jarjavay l.
Krause l.
lacunar l.
Lannelongue l.
Lauth l.

lienophrenic l.
lienorenal l.
Lockwood l.
longitudinal l.
lumbocostal l.
Luschka l.
Mackenrodt l.
mallear l.
Mauchart l.
Meckel l.
nuchal l.
palpebral l.
pancreaticosplenic l.
pectineal l.
peridental l.
periodontal l.
Petit l.
petroclinoid l.
petrosphenoid l.
phrenicocolic l.
phrenicolienal l.
phrenicosplenic l.
phrenoesophageal l.
phrenogastric l.
phrenosplenic l.
pterygomandibular l.
pterygospinal l.
pterygospinous l.
pubic arcuate l.
puboprostatic l.
pulmonary l.
radiate sternocostal l.
radiocapitate l.
radiotriquetral l.
radioulnar l.
l. reconstruction
reflected inguinal l.
reflex l.
rhomboid l.
right prostatic l.
right triangular l.
round uterine l.
sacrodural l.
sacrospinous l.
sacrotuberous l.
serous l.
sphenomandibular l.
spiral l.
splenocolic l.
splenorenal l.
stellate l.
sternoclavicular l.
sternopericardial l.
stylohyoid l.
stylomandibular l.
stylomaxillary l.
suprascapular l.
supraspinous l.
suspensory l.
sutural l.
synovial l.
tarsal l.
temporomandibular l.
Teutleben l.
Thompson l.
thyroepiglottic l.
thyrohyoid l.
Treitz l.
triangular l. of liver
urachal l.
uterosacral l.
uterovesical l.
venous l.
ventral sacrococcygeal l.
ventricular l.
vertebropelvic l.
vesicoumbilical l.
vesicouterine l.
vestibular l.
vocal l.
Whitnall l.
yellow l.
Zaglas l.
Zinn l.

ligamenta (*pl. of* ligamentum)
ligamental anesthesia
ligamentopexy
ligamentoplasty
ligamentous support tissue
ligamentum, pl. **ligamenta**
ligand
tissue l.
ligated
circumferentially l.
doubly l.
staple l.
suture l.
ligate-divide-staple technique
ligation
aneurysm clip l.
artery l.
band l.
Barron l.
bidirectional l.

NOTES

ligation *(continued)*
bile duct l.
Blalock-Taussig shunt l.
bleeding site l.
common bile duct l.
direct l.
distal l.
elastic band l.
endoscopic band l.
endoscopic esophagogastric variceal l.
esophageal band l.
l. of hemorrhoid
l. hemorrhoidectomy
high l.
hunterian l.
hypogastric artery l.
inferior vena cava l.
interdental l.
Irving tubal l.
IVC l.
Kroner tubal l.
laparoscopic artery l.
laparoscopic varix l.
modified Irving-type tubal l.
open retroperitoneal high l.
parotid duct l.
pedicle l.
pole l.
Pomeroy tubal l.
postureteral l.
rubber-band l.
sigmoid sinus l.
sling l.
spermatic vein l.
stump l.
surgical l.
suture l.
l. suture technique
teeth l.
tracheal l.
transesophageal varix l.
transgastric l.
tubal l.
variceal band l.
varicose vein stripping and l.
varix l.
vessel l.
ligature
light
l. coagulation
l. exposure
l. guide bundle
l. microscopy
l. projection
l. wire torque
light-around-wire technique
lighted stylet-guided oral intubation
light-reflecting wedge
LIH
left inguinal hernia
Lilienthal incision
Liliequist
membrane of L.
Lillie allochrome method
limb
afferent l.
l. deformity
distal l.
efferent l.
l. ischemia
l. ischemia pain
jejunal Roux-en-Y l.
l. length angulation
pelvic l.
phantom l.
proximal l.
l. reduction
l. reduction abnormality
l. reduction anomaly
l. replantation
Roux l.
Roux-en-Y l.
l. salvage
l. salvage index
thoracic l.
vertebral, anal, cardiac, tracheal, esophageal, renal, l. (VACTERL)
limbal
l. approach
l. compression
l. incision
l. parallel orientation
limbal-based flap
limb-body wall complex
Limberg
L. flap
L. technique
limbi (*pl. of* limbus)
limbic center
limb-lengthening procedure
limb-salvage
l.-s. procedure
l.-s. surgery
limb-saving
l.-s. method
l.-s. procedure
l.-s. technique
limb-sparing
l.-s. operation
l.-s. procedure
l.-s. surgery
limbus, pl. **limbi**
conjunctival l.
corneal l.

l. mass
Vieussens l.

limited
l. anterior small thoracotomy (LAST)
l. examination
l. fasciectomy
l. gastrectomy
l. hemorrhoidectomy
l. hepatectomy
l. obturator node dissection
l. pancreatectomy
l. resection
l. thoracotomy

limit of flocculation

limiting
l. membrane
l. plate erosion

Limoge current

LINAC
linear accelerator

LINAC-based radiosurgery

Lincoff operation

Lindell classification

Lindeman procedure

Lindesmith operation

Linde Walker Oxygen Program

Lindholm
L. technique
L. tendo calcaneus repair

Lindner
L. operation
L. sclerotomy

Lindsay operation

Lindseth osteotomy

Lindsjö method

line
accretion l.
AC-PC l.
action l.
air-fluid l.
alveolar point-nasal point l.
alveolar point-nasion l.
alveolobasilar l.
alveolonasal l.
Amberg lateral sinus l.
aneuploid cell l.
l. angle
angular l.
anocutaneous l.
anorectal l.
anterior axillary l.
anterior commissure-posterior commissure l.
antitension l.
arcuate l.
Arlt l.
arterial mean l.
atopic l.
axillary l.
azygoesophageal l.
basal l.
base l.
basinasal l.
B cell l.
Beau l.
l. of Bechterew
BeWo choriocarcinoma cell l.
bimastoid l.
bisector l.
bismuth l.
black l.
Blaschko l.
blue l.
Blumensaat l.
Bolton-nasion l.
Brödel bloodless l.
Burton l.
calcification l.
calciotraumatic l.
Camper l.
canthomeatal l.
Cantlie l.
CaSki cell l.
cell l.
cement l.
cemental l.
cementing l.
cervical l.
Chaussier l.
Clapton l.
cleavage l.
clivus canal l.
colonic mucosal l.
Conradi l.
contour l.
corneal iron l.
coronoid l.
Correra l.
costoclavicular l.
costophrenic septal l.
Crampton l.
craze l.
cross-arch fulcrum l.

NOTES

line *(continued)*
curved radiolucent l.
CVP l.
cyma l.
D l.
Daubenton l.
delay l.
Dennie l.
Dennie-Morgan l.
dentate l.
developmental l.
digastric l.
l. of direction
Donders l.
Douglas l.
Ebner l.
Egger l.
Ehrlich-Türck l.
emission l.
epiphysial l.
equipotential l.
established cell l.
external oblique l.
face l.
Farre white l.
fat l.
fat-density l.
feather-edged proximal finishing l.
Feiss l.
femoral head l.
Ferry l.
fingerprint l.
Fishgold l.
l. of fixation
Fleischner l.
l. focus principle
foramen magnum l.
fracture l.
Fränkel white l.
Frankfort horizontal light l.
Fraunhofer l.
fulcrum l.
Futcher l.
gallbladder-vena cava l.
Garrett orientation l.
gas density l.
gaussian l.
l. of Gennari
George l.
germ l.
gingival finishing l.
gluteal l.
Granger l.
gravitational l.
gravity l.
gray l.
growth arrest l.
Gubler l.
gum l.
Hampton l.
Harris growth arrest l.
Hawkins l.
Head l.
Helmholtz l.
hemostatic staple l.
Hickman l.
high lip l.
high smile l.
Hilgenreiner horizontal Y l.
Hilgenreiner-Perkins l.
Hilton white l.
His l.
Holdaway l.
Holden l.
hot l.
Hudson l.
Hudson-Stähli l.
Hueter l.
human AML cell l.
humeral l.
Hunter l.
Hunter-Schreger l.
iliopectinate l.
iliopectineal l.
incision l.
l. infection
infracostal l.
innominate l.
intercondylar l.
intermediate l.
internal oblique l.
interspinal l.
intertrochanteric l.
intertubercular l.
iron l.
iron-Hudson-Stähli l.
iron-stocker l.
isodose l.
isoelectric l.
joint l.
Jurkat T-cell l.
l. of Kaes
Kaplan oblique l.
Kerley A, B, C l.'s
K562 erythroid l.
Khodadoust l.
Kilian l.
knife-edged finishing l.
Köhler l.
labial l.
lambda suture l.
Langer l.
Langhans l.
Lanz l.
lateral joint l.
lead l.

Linton l.
lip l.
load l.
long l.
lorentzian l.
lower midclavicular l.
low lip l.
lumbar gravitational l.
lymphoblastoid cell l.
M l.
Mach l.
MacNab l.
mamillary l.
mammary l.
mare's tail l.
McGregor basal l.
McKee l.
McRae foramen magnum l.
median l.
Mees l.
mercurial l.
Meyer l.
Meyerding spondylolisthesis classification l.
midaxillary l.
midclavicular l.
midheel l.
midhumeral l.
midmalleolar l.
midpoint to meatal l.
midscapular l.
midsternal l.
Moloney l.
Monro l.
Monro-Richter l.
Morgan l.
Morris hepatoma cell l.
mucogingival l.
mucosal l.
Muehrcke l.
murine mesangial cell l.
myelomonocytic cell l.
mylohyoid l.
nasion-alveolar point l.
nasobasilar l.
nasolabial l.
Nélaton l.
neonatal l.
neuronal cell l.
nipple l.
nuchal l.
Obersteiner-Redlich l.
obturator l.
odontoid perpendicular l.
Ohngren l.
orbital l.
orbitomeatal l.
Owen l.
oxygen supply l.
palatooccipital l.
pararectal l.
paraspinal l.
parasternal l.
paravertebral l.
Pastia l.
pectinate l.
percutaneous l.
peripheral arterial l.
Perkins vertical l.
physial l.
Pickerill imbrication l.
pigmentary demarcation l.
pleural l.
pleuroesophageal l.
plumb l.
Poirier l.
Poupart l.
preaxillary l.
principal l.
properitoneal fat l.
protrusive l.
psoas l.
pubic hair l.
pubococcygeal l.
pupillary l.
radiocapitellar l.
radiolucent crescent l.
radio signal l.
recessional l.
rectal floor l.
Reid base l.
rejection l.
resonance l.
resting l.
retentive fulcrum l.
l. of Retzius
reversal l.
Rex-Cantli-Serege l.
Richter-Monro l.
right midinguinal l.
rolandic l.
Roser-Nélaton l.
sacral arcuate l.
sacral horizontal plane l.

NOTES

line *(continued)*
sagittal suture l.
Salter incremental l.
Sampoelesi l.
scapular l.
Schreger l.
Schwalbe l.
sclerotic l.
scurvy l.
semicircular l. of Douglas
semilunar l.
septal l.
Sergent white l.
Shenton l.
simian l.
sinus l.
Snellen l.
soleal l.
spectral l.
Spieghel l.
Spigelius l.
spinolamellar l.
spinolaminar l.
spinous interlaminar l.
spiral l.
stabilizing fulcrum l.
Stähli pigment l.
sternal l.
Stocker l.
stromal l.
subclavian l.
subcostal l.
supracondylar l.
supracrestal l.
survey l.
suture l.
Sydney l.
sylvian l.
T-cell l.
teardrop l.
temporal l.
tender l.
terminal l.
l. test
Thompson l.
tibiofibular l.
l. of Toldt
tram l.
trapezoid l.
triradiate l.
trough l.
Turk l.
Twining l.
Tycos pressure infusion l.
Ullmann l.
V l.
venous l.
Vesling l.
vibrating l.
visual l.
Voigt l.
von Ebner l.
Wackenheim clivus canal l.
water density l.
Wegner l.
white l. of Toldt
l. width
Winberger l.
Z l.
Zahn l.
zero l.
Zöllner l.
Z-shaped suture l.

linea
l. alba

linear
l. l. (LINAC)
l. accelerator-based radiosurgery
l. calcification
l. craniectomy
l. incision
l. lesion
l. osteotomy
l. salpingostomy
l. skull fracture
l. thermal expansion
l. ulceration

linearly polarized near-infrared irradiation
lined flap
Linell-Ljungberg classification
linguae
lingual
l. approach
l. artery
l. bone
l. branch
l. cavity
l. frenulum
l. gland
l. inclination
l. mucosa
l. nerve
l. plexus
l. split-bone technique
l. tongue flap
l. vein

linguales
lingualis
lingualplasty
lingula, pl. **lingulae**
lingular branch
lingularis
linguofacialis
linguofacial trunk
linguoincisal line angle

linguoocclusal line angle
lining
cavity l.
linnaean system of nomenclature
Linton
L. flap
L. incision
L. line
L. operation
L. procedure
lip
acetabular l.
l. adhesion operation
anterior l.
cleft l.
l. line
l. switch flap
upper l.
lipectomy
abdominal l.
lipid
l. infusion
l. peroxidation
l. peroxidation product
lipiodol transarterial embolization treatment
lipoatrophy
postinfection l.
lipoblastoma
lipocele
lipocytic lesion
lipofibroadenoma
lipofibroma
lipogranuloma
lipoid theory of narcosis
lipoleiomyoma
lipolysis
heparin-induced l.
intravascular l.
lipoma
lipoma-like tissue
lipomatous
l. infiltration
l. tissue
lipomeningocele
lipomyelocele
lipomyelocystocele
lipomyelomeningocele
lipomyxoma
liponecrosis
lipophilic opioid
lipoprotein
very low density l. (VLDL)
liposarcoma
liposomal preparation
liposome-encapsulated tetracaine
liposuction
ultrasonic-assisted l. (UAL)
liposuctioning
Lipscomb
L. procedure
L. technique
Lipscomb-Anderson procedure
lip-splitting incision
liquefaction necrosis
liquid
l. extraction
l. scintillation spectrometer
liquor
Scarpa l.
Lisfranc
L. amputation
L. articulation
L. disarticulation
L. dislocation
L. fracture
L. fracture-dislocation
L. tubercle
Lison-Dunn method
Lissauer
L. bundle
L. tract
lissosphincter
Lister
L. method
L. technique
L. tubercle
listerism
listhesis
Listing plane
lithagogue
lithectomy
lithiasis
biliary l.
pancreatic l.
lithium
lithocystotomy
litholapaxy
Bigelow l.
litholysis
chemical l.
litholyte
litholytic

NOTES

lithotomist
lithotomy
bilateral l.
dorsal l.
high l.
lateral l.
marian l.
median l.
percutaneous cholangioscopic l.
percutaneous transhepatic cholangioscopic l. (PTCSL)
perineal l.
l. position
prerectal l.
suprapubic l.
vaginal l.
vesical l.
lithotresis
ultrasonic l.
lithotripsy
biliary l.
blind l.
candela l.
cystoscopic electrohydraulic l.
electrohydraulic l. (EHL)
electrohydraulic shock wave l. (ESWL)
endoscopic-controlled l.
endoscopic electrohydraulic l.
endoscopic pulsed dye laser l.
external shock wave l.
extracorporeal piezoelectric shock wave l.
extracorporeal shock wave l.
intracorporeal laser l.
intracorporeal shock wave l.
laparoscopic transcystic l. (LTCL)
laser biliary l.
laser-induced intracorporeal shock wave l.
mechanical l.
piezoelectric l.
pressure regulated electrohydraulic l.
l. retreatment
rotational contact l.
shock wave l. (SWL)
tunable dye laser l.
ultrasonic l.
lithotripsy-induced hypertension
lithotriptic
lithotriptoscopy
lithotrity
lithuresis
litigation reaction
Little
L. area
L. technique
Littler
L. technique
Littler-Cooley technique
Littré
L. gland
L. hernia
Littré-Richter hernia
Litwak aortic bypass
Livadatis circular myotomy
live donor nephrectomy
liver
l. abscess
alcoholic l.
l. allograft
l. allotransplantation
l. bed
l. biopsy
l. capsule
cirrhotic l.
l. cyst infection
l. damage
l. disease
l. distention
echogenic l.
l. failure
l. flap
frosted l.
l. function
l. function test
l. hanging maneuver
hobnail l.
icing l.
l. injury
l. laceration
lardaceous l.
l. lobe
l. lobule
l. mass
l. metastasis
native l.
nutmeg l.
obstructed l.
l. operation
l. parenchyma
polycystic l.
l. regeneration
l. resection
split l.
stasis l.
steatotic l.
sugar-icing l.
l. tissue
l. tract
l. transplant
l. transplantation
triangular ligament of l.
l. tumor
l. volume

wandering l.
waxy l.
l. wire TC ablation
living
l. donor nephrectomy
l. donor partial hepatectomy
l. relative donor
living-related
l.-r. donor (LRD)
l.-r. donor transplantation
l.-r. liver transplantation (LRLT)
l.-r. small bowel transplant
Livingstone therapy
Livingston peribulbar wedge
LLC
laparoscopic laser cholecystectomy
laser laparoscopic cholecystectomy
Lloyd Davis modified lithotomy position
Lloyd-Roberts-Catteral-Salamon classification
Lloyd-Roberts fracture technique
LMA
laryngeal mask airway
LNF
laparoscopic Nissen fundoplication
load
fecal l.
l. line
load-bearing graft
load-deflection
l.-d. curve
l.-d. rate
load-deformation curve
load-displacement
l.-d. curve
l.-d. plot
loading
fecal l.
lobar
l. bronchus
l. hemorrhage
l. nephronia
l. resection
lobares
lobate
lobatum
hepar l.
lobe
caudate l.
ear l.
inferior parietal l.
liver l.
native caudate l.
paracentral l.
renal l.
l. resection
Riedel l.
right caudate l.
Spiegel l.
spigelian l.
Spigelius l.
superior parietal l.
thyroid l.
lobectomy
Falconer l.
hepatic l.
ipsilateral thyroid l.
pulmonary l.
sleeve l.
temporal l.
thyroid l.
total l.
unilateral l.
lobi (*pl. of* lobus)
lobose
lobotomy
frontal l.
prefrontal l.
radical prefrontal l.
transorbital l.
Lobstein ganglion
lobster-claw deformity
lobular
l. acinus
l. carcinoma
l. hyperplasia
lobulate
lobulated
l. contour
l. mass
lobule
l. of epididymis
hepatic l.
liver l.
posterior l.
posterior-lateral l.
renal cortical l.
secondary pulmonary l.
l. of Zuckerkandl
lobulet
lobulus, pl. **lobuli**
lobus, pl. **lobi**
local
l. abscess

NOTES

local *(continued)*
l. anesthesia
l. anesthetic
l. anesthetic reaction
l. bloodletting
l. epineurotomy
l. excision
l. excitatory state
l. exhaust ventilation
l. hepatectomy
l. hypoxia
l. infection
l. infiltration
l. ingrowth
l. injection
l. invasion
l. irradiation
l. leakage
l. lymphatic uptake
l. muscle flap
l. radical resection
l. recurrence
l. skin flap
l. standby anesthesia technique
l. surgery
l. therapy
l. tissue infiltration
l. treatment
l. tumor extension
l. twitch response (LTR)
Localio-Francis-Rossano resection
Localio procedure
localization
anatomic l.
bleeding site l.
l. of disease
estrogen receptor l.
eye tumor l.
gamma probe l.
hooked wire l.
invasive l.
isotope l.
methylene blue dye l.
needle l.
pancreatic tumor l.
pedicle l.
percutaneous l.
placental l.
preoperative l.
radioisotope l.
sentinel node l.
l. signal
SLN l.
l. study
l. technique
l. test
wire l.
localized
l. abdominal sign
l. abscess
l. inflammation
l. lesion
l. leukocyte mobilization
l. plaque formation
l. prostate cancer
locally advanced disease
locating canal
location
extraperitoneal l.
nonaxillary l.
tumor l.
lock
Howland l.
locking suture technique
lock-stitch suture technique
Lockwood ligament
locoregional
l. management
l. recurrence
l. recurrence-free survival (LRRFS)
l. relapse
l. treatment
loculation
l. of fluid
l. syndrome
Loeffler-Ballard incision
Loesche classification
Loewenthal
L. bundle
L. tract
Löffler suture technique
logadectomy
logical
l. method
l. operation
log relative exposure
logrolling maneuver
Löhlein-Baehr lesion
Löhlein operation
lollipop mastopexy
Londermann operation
lone atrial fibrillation
long
l. axis
l. bone
l. bone fracture
l. cone technique
l. lesion
l. line
l. segment spinal fusion
l. thoracic artery
l. thoracic vein
longa
longer-segment obstruction
longi

longissimus
longitudinal
l. aberration
l. canal
l. choledochotomy
deep-gastric l. (DG-L)
l. dissociation
l. enterotomy
l. fold
l. fracture
l. incision
l. laceration
l. ligament
l. ligament rupture
l. method
midpapillary l. (MP-L)
l. myotomy
l. nephrotomy of Boyce
l. oval pelvis
l. pancreaticojejunostomy
l. relaxation
l. scanning
l. section
l. side-to-side anastomosis
two-chamber l. (2C-L)
l. vertebral venous sinus
longitudinale
longitudinales
longitudinalis
long-limb gastric artery bypass
Longmire
L. operation
L. valvotomy
Longmire-Gutgeman gastric reconstruction
Longo hemorrhoidectomy
long- and short-lever rotational manipulation
long-term
l.-t. bone-instrumentation interface
l.-t. central venous access catheter placement
l.-t. epidural catheterization
l.-t. followup
l.-t. morbidity
l.-t. outcome
l.-t. oxygen therapy
l.-t. paralysis
l.-t. survival
longum
longus
l. capitis muscle
l. colli muscle
extensor carpi radialis l. (ECRL)
extensor digitorum l.
extensor hallucis l. (EHL)
extensor pollicis l.
loop
air-filled l.
Biebl l.
bowel l.
central chemoreflex l.
cerebral-sacral l.
cervical l.
l. choledochojejunostomy
colonic l.
contiguous l.
l. diathermy cervical conization
distended afferent l.
l. distribution
duodenal l.
efferent l.
l. electrocautery excision procedure (LEEP)
l. electrosurgical excision procedure (LEEP)
l. electrosurgical excision procedure conization
l. esophagojejunostomy
expressor l.
l. fixation
l. forearm graft
foreign body l.
l. gastric bypass
l. gastric bypass method
l. gastric bypass procedure
l. gastric bypass technique
l. gastrojejunostomy
Henle l.
Hyrtl l.
ileal l.
l. ileostomy
l. ileostomy construction
intestinal l.
jejunal interposition of Henle l.
jejunal Roux-en-Y l.
l. jejunostomy
jejunum l.
lenticular l.
nephronic l.
N-shaped sigmoid l.
open l.
ostomy l.
l. ostomy bridge

L

NOTES

loop *(continued)*
peduncular l.
peripheral chemoreflex l.
puborectalis l.
Roux-en-Y l.
l. stoma
subclavian l.
l. transverse colostomy
vascular l.
venous l.
looped cautery
loop-end ileostomy
loop-on mucosa suture technique
loose
l. fracture
l. fragment
l. intraarticular body
loosening
screw l.
Loosett maneuver
lop-ear
Lopez-Enriquez operation
Lord
L. dilation of hemorrhoid
L. hemorrhoidectomy
L. operation
lordosis
l. creation
l. preservation
lorentzian line
Lorenz procedure
Loreta operation
lorry-driver fracture
Lortat-Jacob approach
LOS
length of stay
Losee
L. modification
L. modification of MacIntosh technique
L. sling and reef technique
loss
anticipated blood l.
articular bone l.
blood l.
bone l.
cutaneous heat l.
dermal l.
discrimination l.
excessive blood l.
excessive weight l.
extreme hearing l.
insertion l.
intraoperative blood l.
memory l.
operative blood l.
percutaneous anesthetic l.
surgical weight l.
tissue l.
loss-of-resistance technique
loss-of-waist sign
lost wax pattern technique
Lotheissen
L. hernia repair
L. operation
Lothrop frontoethmoidectomy procedure
lotus position
Lougheed-White coccygectomy
Louis
L. angle
L. mastopexy
loupe magnification
Lovset maneuver
low
l. anterior resection (LAR)
l. central venous pressure anesthesia
l. cervical cesarean section
l. dose rate (LDR)
l. intermittent suction
l. lip line
l. lumbar spine fracture
l. rectal cancer
l. spinal anesthesia
l. thoracic level epidural anesthesia
l. transverse cesarean section
l. transverse incision
low-attenuation
l.-a. lesion
l.-a. mass
low-collar incision
low-current
l.-c. electrocautery
l.-c. monopolar coagulation
low-density mass
low-dose
l.-d. anesthetic
l.-d. irradiation
l.-d. radioiodine
LowDye taping technique
Lowell reduction
Löwenberg canal
low-energy fracture
Löwenstein operation
lower
l. body negative pressure
l. cervical spine fusion
l. cervical spine posterior stabilization
l. cervical spine procedure
l. esophageal sphincter (LES)
l. esophageal sphincter pressure
l. extremity
l. extremity edema
l. extremity nerve block

l. extremity noninvasive
l. extremity occlusive disease
l. extremity reconstruction
l. extremity revascularization
l. extremity surgery
l. gastrointestinal hemorrhage
l. genital tract infection
l. GI tract foreign body
l. incisor angulation
l. lateral quadrant
l. lid sling procedure
l. limb ischemia
l. medial quadrant
l. midclavicular line
l. motor neuron lesion
l. nephron syndrome
l. panendoscopy
l. plexus compression
l. pole laceration
l. quadrant abdominal incisional hernia
l. respiratory tract infection
l. thyroid artery
l. trapezius flap
l. uterine segment (LUS)
l. uterine segment incision
l. uterine segment transverse (LUST)
l. uterine segment transverse cesarean section
l. uterine segment transverse C-section

lower-extremity
l.-e. bypass
l.-e. fracture

Lowery method

lowest
l. lumbar artery
l. thyroid artery

low-flow
l.-f. anesthetic technique
l.-f. circuit

low-flux
l.-f. cellulose-based membrane
l.-f. cuprophane membrane
l.-f. dialysis membrane

low-frequency jet ventilation

low-grade
l.-g. dysplasia
l.-g. glioma
l.-g. MALT lymphoma
l.-g. squamous intraepithelial lesion
l.-g. suction unit

low-loop cutaneous ureterostomy

Lown
L. classification
L. technique
L. and Woolf method

low-pressure tamponade

low-resistance fundoplication

low-risk papillary cancer

Lowry method

low-segment transverse incision

Lowsley
L. lobar anatomy
L. ribbon gut method

low-speed rotational angioplasty

LPHR
laparoscopic paraesophageal hernia repair

LRD
living-related donor

LRLT
living-related liver transplantation

LRPH
laparoscopic repair of paraesophageal hernia

LRRFS
locoregional recurrence-free survival

LSG
lymphoscintigraphy
preoperative LSG

L-shaped capsular incision

LSV
left subclavian vein

LTCBDE
laparoscopic transcystic common bile duct exploration

LTCL
laparoscopic transcystic lithotripsy

LTO
laparoscopic total occlusion

LTP
laryngotracheoplasty

LTR
local twitch response

lubrication
skin l.

Lucas groove

lucent lung lesion

lückenschädel

Luc operation

Ludloff
L. bunionectomy

NOTES

Ludloff *(continued)*
L. incision
L. medial approach
L. osteotomy
L. technique
Ludwig
L. angle
L. ganglion
L. labyrinth
L. plane
Luke procedure
Lukes and Butler Hodgkin disease classification
Lukes-Collins classification
lumbale
lumbales
lumbalia
lumbalis
lumbalium
lumbar
l. accessory movement technique
l. anesthetic technique
l. approach
l. artery
l. branch
l. canal
l. cistern
l. diskectomy
l. disk herniation
l. epidural abscess
l. epidural anesthesia
l. epidural endoscopy
l. extension
l. extension test
l. facet injection
l. flexure
l. ganglion
l. gravitational line
l. hemilaminectomy
l. hernia
l. lordosis preservation
l. nephrectomy
l. nerve root injection
l. pedicle fixation
l. plexus
l. plexus block
l. port
l. puncture
l. region
l. rib
l. rotation
l. rotation test
l. segment
l. spinal cord lesion
l. spinal fusion
l. spine biopsy
l. spine burst fracture
l. spine fusion
l. spine kyphotic deformity
l. spine lesion
l. spine segmental fixation
l. spine stabilization
l. spine transpedicular fixation
l. spine vertebral osteosynthesis
l. spondylodiscitis
l. sympathectomy
l. sympathetic block
l. triangle
l. trunk
l. tumor
l. vein
l. vertebra
l. vertebral interbody fusion
l. vessel
lumbaria
lumbarization
lumbar-peritoneal shunting
lumbi (*pl. of* lumbus)
lumboabdominal
lumbocolostomy
lumbocolotomy
lumbocostale
lumbocostal ligament
lumbocostoabdominal triangle
lumbodorsal
l. fascia
lumboinguinal nerve
lumbo-ovarian
lumborum
lumbosacral
l. angle
l. canal
l. dislocation
l. fusion
l. joint
l. junction fracture
l. plexus
l. plexus lesion
l. root lesion
l. trunk
lumbosacralis
lumbrical muscle flap
lumbus, pl. **lumbi**
lumen, pl. **lumina**
bile duct l.
gut l.
irregularly widened l.
jejunal l.
luminal
l. content
l. factor
l. mass
l. side
lumpectomy
endoscopic aspiration l.
l. mastectomy

lunate
l. bone
l. dislocation
lunatum
lunatus
lung
l. biopsy
breathing l.
l. cancer
l. carcinoma
l. cavity
l. disease
essential brown induration of l.
fixed l.
human l.
inflated l.
Kolobow membrane l.
membrane artificial l.
nonventilated l.
oblique fissure of l.
pump l.
respirator l.
shock l.
l. transplant
l. transplantation
l. tumor
l. volume reduction (LVR)
l. volume reduction surgery
l. water
wet l.
lung-imaging fluorescent endoscopy
lunotriquetral
l. dissociation
l. fusion
lunula, pl. **lunulae**
azure l.
lupus
l. anticoagulant
l. erythematosus preparation
systemic l.
lupus-associated valve disease
Luque
L. instrumentation concave technique
L. instrumentation convex technique
L. loop fixation
L. rod fixation
L. sublaminar wiring technique
Luque-Galveston fixation
Luria-Delbruck fluctuation test
LUS
laparoscopic ultrasonography
lower uterine segment
LUS examination
LUS scanning technique
Luschka
L. cartilage
duct of L.
L. gland
L. joint
L. ligament
L. and Magendie foramen
L. sinus
lusitropism
LUST
lower uterine segment transverse
LUST C-section
luster
corneal l.
lustrous central yellow point
lutea
luteal
luteectomy
luteinization
luteinized thecoma
luteinoma
luteolysis
luteoma
pregnancy l.
luteus
luxatio erecta shoulder dislocation
luxation
habitual temporomandibular joint l.
rotatory l.
temporomandibular l.
luxurians
Luys
L. body
L. body syndrome
LVEDa
left ventricular end-diastolic area
LVESa
left ventricular end-systolic area
LVI
lymph vessel invasion
LVOT
left ventricular outflow tract
LVR
lung volume reduction
LVR procedure
Lyden-Lehman technique
Lyden technique
Lyme arthritis

L

NOTES

lymph
l. gland
l. nodal station
l. node basin
l. node biopsy
l. node dissection
l. node involvement
l. node metastasis
l. node sampling
l. node stage
l. node status
l. space
tissue l.
l. vessel
l. vessel invasion (LVI)
lymphadenectomy
axillary l.
bilateral l.
D2 l.
elective l.
endocavitary pelvic l. (ECPL)
extended pelvic l.
inguinal l.
Japanese-style l.
laparoscopic pelvic l.
mediastinal l.
Meigs pelvic l.
para-aortic l.
pelvic l.
prophylactic l.
regional l.
retroperitoneal l.
selective l.
sentinel l.
thoracoabdominal retroperitoneal l.
three-field l.
lymphadenocele
lymphadenoma
lymphadenopathy
axillary l.
en bloc l.
portal l.
lymphadenotomy
lymphangiectasis
lymphangiectomy
lymphangioendothelioma
lymphangiohemangioma
lymphangioleiomyomatosis
pulmonary l.
lymphangioma
lymphangiomyomatosis
end-stage l.
pulmonary l.
lymphangioplasty
Handley l.
lymphangiosarcoma
lymphangiotomy
Lymphapress compression therapy
lymphatic
l. canal
l. chain
l. dissection
l. drainage
l. drainage pattern
l. duct
l. edema
l. invasion
l. malformation
l. mapping
l. metastasis
parenchymal l.
l. pathway
l. permeation
l. plexus
l. spread
l. tissue
l. uptake
l. valvule
l. vessel
lymphatica
lymphatici
lymphaticostomy
lymphaticovenous
l. anastomosis
l. bypass
lymphatics
dermal l.
lymphaticum
lymphaticus
lymphatolysis
lymphedema
lymphoadenoma
lymphoblastoid cell line
lymphocelectomy
laparoscopic l.
pelvic l.
lymphocele drainage
lymphocyte
B phenotypic l.
l. cell
l. migration
phenotypic l.
T phenotypic l.
lymphocytic infiltration
lymphocytoma
lymphoepithelial lesion
lymphoepithelioma
lymphogenous metastasis
lymphogranuloma
lymphoid
l. infiltration
l. ring
l. tissue
lymphoidectomy

lymphoma
Ann Arbor Hodgkin l. stage I, IE, II, IIE, IIIE, IIIS, IIISE, IV
gastric MALT l.
gastric non-Hodgkin l.
high-grade MALT l.
low-grade MALT l.
MALT l.
mucosa-associated lymphoid tissue l.
node l.
primary gastric l. (PGL)
primary gastric non-Hodgkin l. (PGL)
l. relapse
small bowel l.
l. stage III
l. system
lymphomyeloma
lymphoplasty
lymphoproliferation
lymphoproliferative
l. disorder
l. lesion
lymphosarcoma
lymphoscintigraphy (LSG)
internal mammary l. (IML)
preoperative l.
lymphovascular invasion
Lynch
L. frontoethmoidectomy procedure
L. incision
L. operation
L. syndrome
Lynn technique
Lyon-Horgan procedure
lyophilization of bone
lyophilized
l. bone graft
l. dural patch
l. extract
lysate
melanoma cell l.
lyse
lysed
Lysholm
L. Knee Scale
L. score
lysing
lysis
l. of adhesion
adhesion l.
direct muscle l.
endothelial l.
muscle l.
lysogenic
l. induction
l. strain
lysosomal
l. enzyme disorder
l. membrane
l. storage disease
l. swelling
lyssa body
lytic
l. blockade
l. bone lesion
l. cocktail

NOTES

MAb
monoclonal antibody
MABP
mean arterial blood pressure
MAC
minimal anesthetic concentration
minimum alveolar anesthetic concentration
minimum alveolar concentration
monitored anesthesia care
MAC anesthesia
MAC ratio
1-MAC
1-minimum alveolar concentration
1-MAC halothane
MacAndrew Alcoholism Scale
MacAusland procedure
MAC-awake ratio
MacCallan classification
MacCarthy procedure
maceration
Macewen
M. classification
M. hernia operation
M. herniorrhaphy
M. triangle
Macewen-Shands osteotomy
MacFee incision
Machek-Blaskovics operation
Machek-Brunswick operation
Machek-Gifford operation
Machek ptosis operation
Mach line
MAC-hour
MacIntosh
M. extraarticular tenodesis
M. over-the-top ACL reconstruction
M. over-the-top repair
M. technique
MAC-intubation ratio
MACIS
metastasis, age, completeness of resection, local invasion, and tumor size
MACIS criteria
MACIS score
Mack-Brunswick operation
Mackenrodt
M. incision
M. ligament
Mackenzie point
MacNab
M. line
M. line for facet imbrication
M. operation
M. shoulder repair
MacNichol-Voutsinas classification
macroadenoma
macrocalcification
macrocirculation
macrocolon
macrocyst
multiple m.
macroelectrode
m. recording
m. recording technique
macrofollicular lesion
macroglossia
macro-Kjeldahl method
macronodular
macroorchidism
macropenis
macroperforation
macrophage
peritoneal m.
macrophagic migration
macrophallus
macroprolactinoma
macroprosopia
macroscopic
m. appearance
m. evidence
m. involvement
m. IPM
m. lesion
m. portal
m. sphincter
m. tumor removal
m. type
macrosigmoid
macrotraumatic insult
macrovascular coronary lesion
MAC-skin incision ratio
MAC-Surgical incision ratio
macula, pl. **maculae**
retinal m.
macular
m. ectopia
m. photocoagulation
macule
hypomelanotic m.
maculopapillary bundle
maculopapular bundle
maculopathy
Madden
M. incisional herniorrhaphy
M. repair
M. repair of incisional hernia
M. technique

M

Maddox
M. rod test
M. wing test
Madelung deformity
Madigan prostatectomy
Madlener operation
maduromycetoma
Maffucci syndrome
Magendie space
magenstrasse
Magerl
M. posterior cervical screw fixation
M. translaminar facet screw fixation technique
maggot
surgical m.
Magilligan measuring technique
Magitot keratoplasty operation
magna, pl. **magnae**
magnet
m. operation
m. therapy
magnetic
m. control suturing (MCS)
m. extraction
m. imaging guidance
m. induction
m. operation
m. radiation exposure
m. resonance (MR)
m. resonance angiography (MRA)
m. resonance cholangiopancreatography
m. resonance imaging (MRI)
m. resonance imaging cholangiography
m. resonance imaging scan
m. resonance spectroscopy
m. source imaging (MSI)
m. stimulation
magnetization
m. precession angle
magnetoelectric stimulation
magnification
electronic m.
loupe m.
relative spectacle m.
spot m.
magnitude preparation-rapid acquisition gradient echo (MP-RAGE)
magnum
foramen m.
magnus
M. operation
Magnuson-Stack
M.-S. operation
M.-S. procedure
M.-S. shoulder arthrotomy
Magnuson technique
MAGPI
MAGPI hypospadius repair
MAGPI operation
Ma-Griffith
M.-G. technique
M.-G. tendo calcaneus repair
Mahaim bundle
Mahan procedure
MAI
Mycobacterium avium-intracellulare
MAI infection
Maier sinus
maim
main
m. bundle
m. pancreatic duct (MPD)
mainstem intubation
maintainer cast space
maintenance
m. dialysis
m. fluid
insufficient airway m.
Mainz
M. pouch augmentation
M. pouch cutaneous urinary diversion
M. pouch operation
Maisonneuve fibular fracture
Maissiat band
Maitland technique
Majestro-Ruda-Frost tendon technique
Majewsky operation
major
m. abdominal surgery
m. amputation
m. artery
m. calix
m. duodenal papilla
m. fissure
m. histocompatibility complex (MHC)
m. liver resection (MLR)
m. manifestation
m. nonvascular abdominal surgery
m. operation
m. sinistral branch
trochanter m.
m. vascular injury
m. vascular structure
majores
majoris
majus
Maki pylorus-preserving gastrectomy
Makler insemination
mala
Malacarne space
malacotomy

Maladie de Graeffe operation
malar
m. fat pad
m. fold
m. foramen
m. fracture
m. node
malare
malaris
Malawer excision technique
Malbec operation
Malbran operation
maldistribution
male
m. breast
m. castration
m. gonad
m. urethra
malformation
angiographically occult intracranial vascular m. (AOIVM)
anorectal m.
Arnold-Chiari m.
arteriovenous m. (AVM)
atrioventricular m.
A-V m.
Bing-Siebenmann m.
bronchopulmonary foregut m.
capillary m.
cardiac valvular m.
cardiovascular m.
cavernous m.
central nervous system m.
cerebral arteriovenous m.
cerebral vascular m.
cerebrovascular m.
Chiari I–III m.
cloacal m.
clomiphene fetal m.
congenital brain m.
congenital cystic adenomatoid m.
congenital heart m.
congenital vascular m.
craniofacial m.
cutaneous m.
cystic adenomatoid m. (CAM)
Dandy-Walker m.
DeMyer system of cerebral m.
Dieulafoy vascular m.
dural arteriovenous m.
dysraphic m.
Ebstein m.
extremity m.
faciotelencephalic m.
fetal cystic adenomatoid m.
flocculonodular arteriovenous m.
foregut m.
frontal arteriovenous m.
frontoparietal arteriovenous m.
galenic venous m.
gastric arteriovenous m.
glomus arteriovenous m.
infratentorial arteriovenous m.
intracerebral arteriovenous m.
intracerebral vascular m.
intracranial arteriovenous m.
intracranial vascular m.
intramedullary arteriovenous m.
intramuscular venous m.
lymphatic m.
mermaid m.
Michel m.
mixed venous-lymphatic m.
Mondini-Alexander m.
Mondini pulmonary arteriovenous m.
neural axis vascular m.
neural crest m.
occipital m.
occult cerebrovascular m.
occult vascular m.
orbital arteriovenous m.
pulmonary arterial m.
pulmonary arteriovenous m.
radiculomeningeal spinal vascular m.
retinal arteriovenous m.
Scheibe m.
sink-trap m.
spinal vascular m.
split-cord m.
supratentorial arteriovenous m.
telencephalic m.
teratogen-induced m.
thalamocaudate arteriovenous m.
Uhl m.
vascular m.
vein of Galen m.
venous m.
malfunction
cuff m.
pacemaker m.
Malgaigne
M. fossa

NOTES

M

Malgaigne *(continued)*
M. hernia
M. pelvic fracture
M. triangle
malignancy
abdominal m.
digestive tract m.
gastric m.
gastrointestinal m.
gynecologic m.
hepatic m.
hereditary m.
metastatic m.
nonhereditary m.
pancreatic m.
primary m.
malignant
m. adenoma
m. angiomyolipoma
m. cell
m. degeneration
m. etiology
m. external otitis syndrome
m. fasciculation
m. glioma
m. hyperpyrexia
m. hypertension
m. hyperthermia (MH)
m. lesion
m. pancreatic disease
m. pituitary lesion
m. process
m. reading
m. renal mass
m. synovioma
m. transformation
m. tumor
malignant-appearing microcalcification
malingering questionnaire
malinterdigitation
Mallampati
M. oropharyngeal classification
M. pharyngeal visibility classification
Mallard incision
mallear
m. fold
m. ligament
m. process
m. prominence
mallei (*pl. of* malleus)
malleoincudal
malleolar
m. fracture
m. osteotomy
malleolus, pl. **malleoli**
medial m.
mallet
m. finger deformity
m. fracture
m. toe deformity
malleus, pl. **mallei**
Mallory technique
Mallory-Weiss
M.-W. lesion
M.-W. mucosal rupture
M.-W. procedure
M.-W. syndrome
M.-W. tear
malnutrition
malocclusion
Malone
M. ACE procedure
M. antegrade continence enema procedure
malpighian
m. body
m. pyramid
m. stigma
malposition
catheter m.
extension m.
strut m.
malpositioning
malpresentation
fetal m.
malrelation
malrotation
intestinal m.
renal m.
MALT
mucosa-associated lymphoid tissue
MALT lymphoma
malunion
humeral fracture m.
malunited
m. calcaneus fracture
m. forearm fracture
m. radial fracture
mamillaris
mamillary
m. body
m. duct
m. line
m. process
m. tubercle
mamillothalamic tract
mamma, pl. **mammae**
mammalian cell membrane
mammaplasty, mammoplasty
Aries-Pitanguy m.
augmentation m.
belly button augmentation m.
postreduction m.
reconstructive m.

reduction m.
Wise pattern m.
mammaria
mammariae
mammarii
mammarius
mammary
m. atrophy
m. branch
m. duct
m. duct ectasia
m. fistula
m. gland
m. line
m. node
m. node biopsy
m. plexus
m. region
m. tissue
mammectomy
mammilla, pl. **mammillae**
mammillaplasty
mammogram
abnormal m.
mammographer
mammographic
m. abnormality
m. appearance
m. evaluation
m. finding
m. lesion
m. malignant-appearing microcalcification
m. presentation
mammography
digital m.
screening m.
mammoplasty (*var. of* mammaplasty)
Mammotest Plus breast aspiration
mammotomy
management
airway m.
m. of anesthesia
anesthetic m.
anesthetic and fluid m.
aneurysm m.
emergency airway m.
endoscopic m.
expectant m.
fluid m.
foreign body m.
intraoperative fluid m.
laparoscopic m.
locoregional m.
mechanical endoscopic m.
medical m.
nonoperative m.
nonsurgical m.
obstetrical m.
operative m.
optimal intensive medical m.
pain m.
perioperative m.
postoperative m.
renal m.
selective nonoperative m.
m. strategy
surgical m.
ventilator m.
Manchester-Fothergill operation
Manchester operation
Mancini technique
mandatory
m. celiotomy
m. laparoscopy
Mandelbaum-Nartolozzi-Carney patellar tendon repair
mandible
mandibula, pl. **mandibulae**
mandibular
m. articulation
m. body fracture
m. canal
m. cartilage
m. centric relation
m. condyle
m. condylectomy
m. condyle fracture
m. disk
m. dislocation
m. equilibration
m. excess
m. fixation
m. foramen
m. fossa
m. head
m. hinge position
m. joint
m. nerve
m. nerve block
m. node
m. notch
m. osteotomy advancement
m. plane

NOTES

mandibular *(continued)*
m. ramus fracture
m. ramus osteotomy
m. reconstruction
m. rest position
m. space
m. surgery
m. swing operation
m. swing technique
m. symphysis
m. symphysis fracture
m. tongue
mandibularis
mandibulectomy
segmental m.
mandibulofacial dysotosis syndrome
mandibulomaxillary fixation
mandibulopharyngeal
mandibulotomy
mandibulum
mandrel graft
maneuver
Addison m.
Adson m.
Allen m.
Allis m.
alpha-loop m.
Apley m.
avoidance m.
Barlow m.
Bielschowsky m.
Bigelow m.
Bill m.
Bracht m.
Brandt-Andrews m.
bunching m.
Buzzard m.
Cairns m.
Carlo Traverso m.
circumduction m.
closed manipulative m.
Colanis m.
cold pressor testing m.
corkscrew m.
costoclavicular m.
Credé m.
Cushieri m.
Dandy m.
DeLee m.
Dix-Hallpike m.
doll's eye m.
doll's head m.
Duecollement m.
Ejrup m.
Epley m.
Finkelstein m.
flexion-extension m.
forceps m.
Fowler-Stephens m.
Frenzel m.
grunting m.
Hallpike m.
Halsted m.
Hampton m.
heel-to-ear m.
Heimlich m.
hemodynamic m.
Hillis-Müller m.
Hippocratic m.
Hodge m.
Hoguet m.
Hubscher m.
Hueter m.
hyperventilation m.
Jahss m.
jaw thrust m.
Jendrassik m.
Jonnson m.
J-type m.
jugular compression m.
key-in-lock m.
Ko-Airan m.
Kocher m.
Krackow m.
Kristeller m.
Lachman m.
Leadbetter m.
Lecompte m.
Levret m.
liver hanging m.
logrolling m.
Loosett m.
Lovset m.
Massini m.
Mattox m.
Mauriceau m.
Mauriceau-Levret m.
Mauriceau-Smellie-Veit m.
McDonald m.
McKenzie extension m.
McMurray circumduction m.
McRoberts m.
Mendelsohn m.
meticulous m.
midforceps m.
modified Ritgen m.
Mueller m.
Müller m.
Müller-Hillis m.
Munro-Kerr m.
notch-and-roll m.
Nylen-Barany m.
oculocephalic m.
Ortolani m.
osteoclasis m.
Pajot m.

peroral m.
Phalen m.
Pinard m.
postural fixation back m.
Prague m.
Prentiss m.
Pringle m.
Proetz m.
pull m.
push m.
recruitment m.
reexpansion m.
relative response attributable to the m.
reverse Bigelow m.
Ritgen m.
rotation-compression m.
Rubin m.
Saxtorph m.
scalene m.
Scanzoni m.
Scanzoni-Smellie m.
scarf m.
Schatz m.
Schreiber m.
Sellick m.
shoeshine m.
Slocum m.
Spurling m.
Steel m.
Stimson m.
straightening m.
surgical m.
Thorn m.
U-turn m.
Valsalva m.
Van Hoorn m.
wall push m.
Wigand m.
Woods screw m.
Wright m.
Zavanelli m.

mangled
m. extremity severity score
m. extremity syndrome

manifesta

manifestation
allergic m.
articular m.
cardiopulmonary m.
central nervous system m.
clinical m.
cutaneous m.
digestive m.
hepatobiliary m.
initial m.
major m.
minor m.
mucocutaneous m.
neurologic m.
neuroophthalmic m.
ocular m.
oral m.
otolaryngologic m.
presenting clinical m.
pulmonary m.
renal m.
vascular m.

manipulation
bile duct m.
catheter m.
cervical m.
contact m.
cranial nerve m.
digital m.
direct m.
fine m.
gamete m.
general thrust m.
gross m.
guidewire m.
Hippocrates m.
indirect m.
joint m.
laparoscopic dissection and m.
laser m.
Leadbetter hip m.
long- and short-lever rotational m.
myofascial m.
noncontact m.
opening wedge m.
pancreatic duct m.
passive joint m.
pharmacologic m.
physical m.
postureteroscopic m.
shunt m.
specific thrust m.
spinal m.
thrust m.

manipulative therapy

Mankin
M. resection
M. technique

NOTES

M

Manktelow transfer procedure
Mann-Bollman fistula
Mann-Coughlin-DuVries cheilectomy
Mann-Coughlin procedure
Mann-DuVries arthroplasty
Mann procedure
Mann-Whitney test
Mann-Williamson operation
manometer
saline m.
manometric
m. data
m. evaluation
m. finding
m. recording session
m. study
m. technique
manometry
anal m.
anorectal m.
esophageal m.
jejunal m.
laparoscopic transcystic sphincter of Oddi m.
small bowel m.
stationary m.
Mansfield Valvuloplasty Registry
Manske-McCarroll opponensplasty
Manske-McCarroll-Swanson centralization
Manske technique
mantle irradiation
Mantoux method
manual
m. extraction
m. method
m. pressure
m. push-pull technique
m. rotation
m. ventilation
manubriosternal
m. joint
m. junction
m. symphysis
manubriosternalis
manubrium, pl. **manubria**
manus
MAP
mean arterial pressure
maple leaf flap
maplike skull
mapping
activation-sequence m.
atrial activation m.
body surface Laplacian m.
breast lymphatic m.
catheter m.
dermatome m.
endocardial m.
intraoperative lymphatic m.
isosulfan blue-dye m.
lymphatic m.
retrograde atrial activation m.
SLN m.
Maquet
M. anteromedial osteoplasty
M. dome osteotomy
M. procedure
M. technique
Maragiliano body
marantic clot
Marbach-Weil technique
marbleization
Marcacci muscle
March
M. fracture
M. technique
Marchand adrenal
Marchi tract
Marcille triangle
Marckwald operation
Marcove-Lewis-Huvos shoulder girdle resection
Marcus-Balourdas-Heiple ankle fusion technique
Marcus Gunn phenomenon
Marcy
M. hernia repair
M. operation
mare's tail line
Marfan syndrome
margin
carious restoration m.
cavity m.
close m.
costal m.
dentate m.
dissection m.
falciform m.
free gastric m.
frontal m.
gastric m.
hepatic m.
interosseous m.
m. invasion
lacrimal m.
lambdoid m.
mastoid m.
mesovarian m.
negative m.
obtuse m.
occipital m.
parietal m.
positive resection m.
positive surgical m.

psoas m.
pupillary m.
m. resection
resection m.
m. resection involvement
squamous m.
superior m.
supraorbital m.
surgical m.
tumor-free m.

marginal
m. artery
m. excess
m. excision
m. incision
m. insertion
m. mandibular branch
m. myotomy
m. resection
m. ridge fracture
m. sinus rupture
m. sphincter
m. tentorial branch
m. tubercle
m. ulceration

margination
lesion m.
leukocytic m.

marginoplasty

margo, pl. **margines**

marian lithotomy

Marin Amat syndrome

Marion disease

Marion-Moschcowitz culdoplasty

mark
ecchymotic m.
port-wine m.
tape m.

marked
m. ascites
m. tenderness

marker
biologic m.
blood m.
genetic m.
histologic m.
immunohistochemical m.
prognostic m.
m. stitch
tumor m.
viral m.

Marks-Bayne technique for thumb duplication

Marlex
M. closure
M. hernial repair
M. plug technique

Marmo method

Marqez-Gomez conjunctival graft

Marquardt angulation osteotomy

Marquez-Gomez operation

Marriott method

marrow
m. ablation
allogenic bone m.
m. cavity
m. graft rejection
m. space
spinal m.

Marseille pancreatitis classification

Marshall
M. ligament repair technique
M. method
M. oblique vein
M. test

Marshall-Marchetti
M.-M. procedure
M.-M. test

Marshall-Marchetti-Krantz (MMK)
M.-M.-K. operation
M.-M.-K. procedure
M.-M.-K. urethropexy

Marshall-McIntosh technique

Marshall-Taylor vacuum extraction

marsupialization
renal cyst m.
Spence and Duckett m.
m. technique
transurethral m.

marsupium

MART
melanoma antigen reacting to T cell

Martin
M. anoplasty
M. incision
M. modification
M. osteotomy
M. patellar wiring technique
M. reduction technique

Martin-Gruber anastomosis

Martius
M. bulbocavernosus fat flap
M. procedure

masculina
vagina m.
masculinae
masculine
m. pelvis
m. uterus
masculinization
ovarian m.
masculinizing genitoplasty
masculinovoblastoma
mask
ecchymotic m.
m. leak
masking technique
Mason
M. abdominotranssphincteric resection
M. incision
M. operation
M. radial head fracture classification
M. vertical banded gastroplasty
Mason-Likar limb lead modification
masquerade technique
MASS
mitral valve prolapse, aortic anomalies, skeletal changes, and skin changes
MASS syndrome
mass
abdominal wall m.
abdominopelvic m.
adnexal m.
adrenal cystic m.
anterior mediastinal m.
appendiceal m.
apperceptive m.
asymptomatic m.
atomic m.
benign m.
body cell m.
bone m.
bony m.
brain m.
calcified renal m.
carbon gelatin m.
cardiac m.
cardiophrenic angle m.
cicatricial m.
circumscribed m.
colonic m.
complex chest m.
m. concentration
congenital nasal m.
congenital renal m.
conglomerate m.
cortical m.
critical m.
cul-de-sac m.
cystic m.
m. defect
dense brain m.
discrete m.
dominant m.
doughy m.
dumbbell m.
duodenal m.
dysplasia-associated m.
echodense m.
erythrocyte m.
esophageal m.
exchangeable m.
m. excision
exophytic gut m.
expansile abdominal m.
extracardiac m.
extramucosal m.
extrarenal m.
extrauterine pelvic m.
extravascular m.
extrinsic m.
fallopian tube m.
fat-free m.
filar m.
firm m.
flank m.
fluctuant m.
fungating m.
gastric m.
groin m.
hard m.
hilar m.
hyaline m.
ill-defined m.
m. infection
infraauricular m.
injection m.
inner cell m.
intraabdominal m.
intracardiac m.
intracranial m.
intradural extramedullary m.
intrasellar m.
intrathoracic m.
intravascular m.
intraventricular m.
intussuscepted m.
lacrimal m.
laminated acellular m.
lateral m.
lean body m.
m. lesion
limbus m.
liver m.
lobulated m.
low-attenuation m.
low-density m.

luminal m.
malignant renal m.
mediastinal high-attenuation m.
m. memory
mesenteric m.
mixed-density m.
molecular m.
mulberry-shaped m.
multiloculated renal m.
mushroom-shaped m.
mycelial m.
myocardial m.
neoplastic renal m.
noncalcified nodular m.
nonmobile m.
nonopaque intraluminal m.
ochre m.
ovarian m.
ovoid m.
oyster m.
palpable m.
parasellar m.
parovarian m.
pediatric m.
pelvic m.
periampullary m.
perirectal m.
perivascular m.
persistent ovarian m.
phlegmonous m.
plantar-hindfoot-midfoot bony m.
pleural m.
polypoid m.
posterior mediastinal m.
postmenopausal body m.
presacral m.
pulmonary m.
pulsatile m.
questionable m.
rectal m.
red blood cell m.
m. reflex
renal m.
retrobulbar m.
retrocardiac m.
retrosternal m.
rubbery m.
salivary m.
sclerotic cemental m.
scrotal m.
soft-tissue m.
solitary pulmonary m.
m. spectrometer
m. spectrometry
stellate m.
submucosal m.
suprasellar m.
testicular m.
thymic m.
tooth m.
transformary m.
traumatic renal m.
tubular excretory m.
tumor m.
umbilical m.
uncinate process m.
unit of m.
uterine m.
vaginal m.
vascular renal m.
vertebral bone m.
well-defined m.

massage
cardiac m.
connective tissue m.
external cardiac m.
hand m.
nerve-point m.
prostatic m.
soft-tissue m.

masse
reduction en m.

masseter
m. muscle
m. muscle flap
m. tendon

masseteri

masseteric
m. artery
m. fascia
m. nerve
m. space
m. tuberosity

masseterica

massetericus

masseter-mandibular-pterygoid space

Massie sliding graft

Massini maneuver

massive
m. ascites
m. autotransfusion
m. bowel resection
m. bowel resection syndrome
m. hemorrhage

NOTES

M

massive *(continued)*
m. incisional hernioplasty
m. lower GI bleeding
m. malignant infiltration
m. pulmonary hemorrhagic edema
Masson trichrome method
MAST
Michigan Abuse Screening Test
MAST technique
mastadenoma
mastectomy
Auchincloss modified radical m.
axillary node dissection m.
bilateral subcutaneous m.
breast-sparing m.
m. closure
complete skin-sparing m.
extended radical m.
m. for gynecomastia
Halsted radical m.
m. incision
lumpectomy m.
McKissock m.
McWhirter simple m.
modified radical m.
partial m.
Patey modified radical m.
preventive m.
prophylactic m.
quadrantectomy m.
radical m.
segmental m.
simple m.
skin-sparing m.
m. specimen
standard m.
subcutaneous m.
total m.
transverse m.
two-stage technique m.
master
m. gland
m. IG bundle
mastication
m. disorder
m. muscle
masticator
m. nerve
m. space
m. space infection
masticatorius
masticatory
m. fat pad
m. space
mastitis
granulomatous m.
periductal m.
mastoccipital
mastocytoma
mastoid
m. antrum
m. branch
m. canaliculus
m. cavity
m. cell
m. foramen
m. fossa
m. incision
m. margin
m. node
m. notch
m. obliteration operation
mastoidea
mastoidectomy
modified radical m.
radical m.
simple m.
tympanoplasty m.
mastoidei
mastoideum
mastoideus
mastopexy
anchor m.
areolar m.
Benelli lollipop m.
Biesenberger technique of m.
breast-lift m.
circumareolar m.
concentric m.
crescent m.
donut m.
double-skin m.
endoscopic m.
full m.
keyhole m.
Keystone m.
LeJour m.
lollipop m.
Louis m.
modified m.
periareolar m.
pursestring m.
reduction m.
Regnault type B m.
short-scar technique of m.
simple m.
vertical m.
Wise m.
mastoplasty
mastotomy
Mast-Spieghel-Pappas classification
Masuka modified thymic carcinoma classification
Matas
M. aneurysmectomy
M. operation

Matchett-Brown hip arthroplasty
matching
cross-modality m.
matchstick
m. graft
m. test
mater
arachnoid m.
pia m.
material
colloid m.
contrast m.
m. failure break point
hydatid m.
nonabsorbable m.
obstructive hydatid m.
osteosynthetic m.
maternal
m. abdominal pressure
m. anesthesia
m. birthing position
m. deprivation syndrome
m. fracture
m. hydration
m. infection
m. mercury exposure
m. rejection
m. tissue
m. venous (MV)
maternal-placental-fetal drug transfer
Mathews olecranon fracture classification
Mathieu
M. island onlay flap
M. procedure
M. technique
Mathieu-Horton-Devine flip-flap
matricectomy
matrilineal
matris
matrix, pl. **matrices**
bone m.
m. calculus
cartilage m.
distal nail m.
extracellular m.
germinal m.
glomerular extracellular m.
m. metalloproteinase (MMP)
nail m.
proximal nail m.
sterile m.
matrixectomy
chemical m.
partial m.
phenol m.
Steindler m.
Winograd partial m.
Zadik total m.
Matroc femoral head
Matsen procedure
Matsura preparation
Matta-Saucedo fixation
matted node
matter
white m.
Matti-Russe
M.-R. bone graft
M.-R. technique
Mattox maneuver
mattress
m. stitch
m. suture otoplasty
maturation
m. division
m. index
m. phase
mature teratoma
maturing the stoma
Mauchart ligament
Mauck procedure
Maudsley Mentation Test
Mauksch-Maumenee-Goldberg operation
Mauksch operation
Maumenee-Goldberg operation
Maunsell-Weir operation
Mau osteotomy
Mauriceau-Levret maneuver
Mauriceau maneuver
Mauriceau-Smellie-Veit maneuver
maxilla, pl. **maxillae**
maxillaris
maxillary
m. antrum
m. antrum closure
m. canal
m. excess
m. expansion
m. fracture
m. hiatus
m. nerve
m. nerve block

NOTES

maxillary *(continued)*
m. osteotomy
m. restoration
m. sinus carcinoma
m. sinus cavity
m. sinuscopy
m. sinus mucocele
m. surgery
m. tubercle
maxillectomy
Cocke m.
subtotal m.
maxillofacial
m. anomaly
m. fracture
m. surgery
maxillomandibular
m. fixation
m. relation
maxillotomy
extended m.
maximal
m. drug concentration
m. expiratory flow rate
m. expiratory flow volume
m. rectal diameter
m. ventilation rate
m. voluntary ventilation
Maximally Discriminative Facial Coding System
maximi
maximum
m. breathing capacity (MBC)
m. mouth opening
m. occipital point
m. permissible concentration
m. stimulation test
m. urethral closure pressure
m. voluntary ventilation (MVV)
maximum-intensity projection
Maxwell body
Maydl
M. hernia
M. procedure
M. ureterosigmoidostomy
Mayfield incision
May-Hegglin body
Maylard incision
Mayo
M. approach
M. carpal instability classification
M. hysterectomy
M. modified total elbow arthroplasty
M. operation
M. resection arthroplasty
M. rheumatoid elbow classification
Mayo-Fueth inversion procedure
Mayo-Heuter bunionectomy
Mayo-Robson
M.-R. incision
M.-R. position
Maze III procedure
Mazet
M. disarticulation
M. technique
mazolysis
mazopexy
MBC
maximum breathing capacity
MCA
middle cerebral artery
MCA occlusion
McAfee approach
McArthur incision
McBride
M. bunionectomy
M. procedure
McBurney
M. appendectomy
M. appendectomy incision
M. operation
M. point
McCall
M. culdoplasty
M. stitch
McCall-Schumann procedure
McCarroll-Baker procedure
McCauley technique
McConnell
M. extensile approach
M. median and ulnar nerve approach
M. technique
McCormick-Blount procedure
McCraw gracilis myocutaneous flap
McDonald
M. maneuver
M. procedure
McElfresh-Dobyns-O'Brien technique
McElvenny-Caldwell procedure
McElvenny technique
McFarland bone graft
McFarland-Osborne
M.-O. lateral approach
M.-O. technique
McFarlane
M. skin flap
M. technique
McGavic operation
McGill Pain Questionnaire (MPQ)
McGlamry-Downey procedure
McGoon technique
McGregor basal line
McGuire operation

mCi
millicurie
McIndoe
M. operation
M. procedure
M. vaginal creation
McIndoe-Hayes
M.-H. construction
M.-H. procedure
McKay-Simons clubfoot operation
McKee line
McKeever
M. and MacIntosh hemiarthroplasty
M. medullary clavicle fixation
M. open reduction
McKeever-Buck
M.-B. elbow technique
M.-B. fragment excision
McKenzie extension maneuver
McKissock mastectomy
McLaughlin
M. acromioplasty
M. approach
M. operation
M. procedure
McLaughlin-Hay technique
McLaughlin-Ryder incision
McLean
M. operation
M. technique
McMaster
M. bone graft
M. Quality of Life Scale
M. technique
McMurray circumduction maneuver
McNeer classification
McRae foramen magnum line
McReynolds
M. method
M. open reduction technique
M. operation
McRoberts maneuver
MCS
magnetic control suturing
McShane-Leinberry-Fenlin acromioplasty
McSpadden method
McVay
M. herniorrhaphy
M. incision
M. inguinal hernial repair
M. method
M. operation
M. procedure
M. technique
McVay-Cooper ligament repair
MCV Pain Questionnaire
McWhirter simple mastectomy
McWhorter posterior shoulder approach
M_0 disease
MDMQ
Menstrual Distress Management Questionnaire
mean
m. airway resistance
m. arterial blood pressure (MABP)
m. arterial pressure (MAP)
m. circulation time
m. diastolic left ventricular pressure
m. foundation plane
m. normalized systolic ejection rate
m. pulmonary artery wedge pressure
m. shunt index
m. systolic left ventricular pressure
m. UV/MV ratio
Meares-Stamey technique
Mears-Rubash approach
measure
nonpharmacologic m.
preventive m.
measurement
acoustic reflection m.
alveolar diffusion m.
ankle-brachial pressure m.
continuous intramucosal PCO_2 m.
diurnal intraocular pressure m.
endpoint m.
esophageal m.
facial excursion m.
Fick cardiac output m.
four-cuff technique segmental pressure m.
hematocrit m.
intrauterine pressure m.
invasive pressure m.
muscle m.
near-infrared m.
negative inspiratory pressure m.
oxygen saturation m.
pH m.
pressure m.
pulse-echo distance m.
serial hematocrit m.

NOTES

measurement *(continued)*
skin m.
skin-temperature gradient m.
tissue pressure m.
total exchangeable potassium m.
transcutaneous oxygen pressure m.
transstenotic pressure gradient m.
tympanic membrane m.
urethral pressure m.
vasodilator-stimulated rCBF single photon emission computed tomographic m.
voiding urethral pressure m.
meatal
m. advancement and glansplasty
m. cartilage
meatoplasty
V-flap m.
meatorrhaphy
meatoscopy
meatotomy
ureteral m.
meatus, pl. **meatus**
anterior nasal m.
external auditory m.
inferior m.
middle m.
superior m.
ureteral m.
meaty appearance
MEC
minimum effective concentration
mechanical
m. anastomosis
m. endoscopic management
m. esophagojejunostomy
m. extrahepatic obstruction
m. leech
m. lithotripsy
m. occlusion
m. perforation
m. pulp exposure
m. stimulation
m. thrombectomy
m. ureteral dilation
m. variceal compression
m. ventilation
m. ventilation anesthetic technique
m. ventilatory support
mechanism
antireflux flap-valve m.
association m.
central extensor m.
cholinergic m.
clotting m.
countercurrent m.
digital extensor m.
extensor hood m.
extrinsic m.
fascial shutter m.
flap-valve m.
hematogenous m.
hemolytic m.
immune m.
inhibitory-excitatory m.
noradrenergic m.
obstructive m.
renal m.
screw-home m.
surveillance m.
urethral closure m.
mechanoactivation
mechanogram
mechanomyography
mechanoreflex
mèche
Meckel
M. band
M. cartilage
M. cave
M. cavity
M. diverticulectomy
M. diverticulum
M. ganglion
M. ligament
M. scan
M. space
M. sphenopalatine ganglionectomy
meconium
m. aspiration
m. aspiration syndrome
m. plug syndrome
media (*pl. of* medium)
mediae
medial
m. aspect
m. aspiration
m. basal segment
m. canthus
m. capsular imbrication
m. capsulorrhaphy
m. clear space
m. condyle
m. crus
m. cutaneous branch
m. displacement osteotomy
m. dissection
m. extradural approach
m. flap
m. malleolar network
m. malleolar subcutaneous bursa
m. malleolus
m. malleolus fixation
m. malleolus resection
m. mammary branch
m. parapatellar capsular approach

m. parapatellar incision
m. process
m. repair
m. rotation
m. rotation procedure
m. rotator
m. sector
mediale
mediales
medialis
medialization
silicone elastomer m.
medial-sector pedicle
median
m. biopsy volume
m. corpectomy
m. detection threshold
m. episiotomy
m. glossoepiglottic fold
m. groove
m. jaw relation
m. labiomandibular glossotomy
m. line
m. lithotomy
m. longitudinal raphe
m. mandibular point
m. nerve
m. nerve compression
m. section
m. sternotomy
m. sternotomy incision
m. strumectomy
m. thoracotomy
mediana
mediani
medianum
medianus
mediastinal
m. artery
m. branch
m. CTD
m. enlargement
m. esophagojejunostomy
m. hemorrhage
m. high-attenuation mass
m. irradiation
m. lymphadenectomy
m. lymph node biopsy
m. lymph node dissection
m. pleura
m. shed blood (MSB)
m. space
m. tumor
m. vein
m. wedge
mediastinale
mediastinales
mediastinalis
mediastinitis
mediastinoscopic examination
mediastinoscopy
Chamberlain m.
video m.
mediastinoscopy-assisted transhiatal esophagectomy
mediastinotomy
mediastinum
anterior m.
inferior m.
middle m.
posterior m.
superior m.
upper m.
mediate transfusion
mediator
proinflammatory m.
medical
m. care
m. care evaluation
m. chemoprevention
m. diathermy
m. dilation
m. illness
m. intervention
m. management
m. oncologist
m. ophthalmoscopy
m. problem
m. record
m. systemic condition
m. therapy
m. treatment
m. treatment option
m. vagotomy
medication
aerosolized m.
antalgic m.
anticholinergic m.
antiepileptic m.
antiinflammatory m.
base m.
beta-blocker m.
m. bezoar
concomitant m.

NOTES

medication *(continued)*
dopaminergic m.
intravenous m.
iodide-containing m.
levodopa dopaminergic m.
nonsteroidal antiinflammatory m.
oral antibiotic m.
over-the-counter m.
parenteral m.
preanesthetic m.
pressor m.
prophylactic m.
psychopharmacologic m.
psychotropic m.
M. Quantification Scale
teratogenic m.
vasoactive m.
medication-induced injury
medicinal preparation
medicine
alternative m.
anesthesiology critical care m.
complementary and alternative m.
critical care m. (CCM)
emergency m.
evidence-based m. (EBM)
fetal m.
herbal m.
nuclear m.
vascular m.
medicochirurgical
medicolegal aspect
medii
Medina infection
mediocarpea
medioccipital
medioclavicularis
mediocolic sphincter
mediolateral episiotomy
medisect
Mediterranean exanthematous fever
medium, pl. **media**
adhesive otitis media
contrast m.
culture m.
m. lesion
medium-scale integration
medium-sized artery
medius
medulla, pl. **medullae**
renal m.
rostral ventrolateral m.
suprarenal m.
medullar
medullare
medullaris
medullary
m. adenocarcinoma
m. bone graft
m. canal
m. carcinoma
m. cavity
m. nail fixation
m. oxygenation
m. pyramid
m. pyramidotomy
m. ray
m. space
m. spinal artery
m. spinothalamic tractotomy
m. sponge kidney
m. substance
m. tube
medullated
medullation
medullectomy
medullization
medulloblastoma
desmoplastic m.
melanotic m.
m. metastasis
medulloepithelioma
medullomyoblastoma
medullostomy
tarsal m.
medullovasculosa
meduloblastoma
medusae
Medusa head
Meek operation
Mees line
mefenamic acid
megacalycosis
megacolon
megacystic syndrome
megacystis
megacystis-megaureter
m.-m. association
m.-m. syndrome
megacystis-microcolon-intestinal hypoperistalsis syndrome
megadolichovertebrobasilar anomaly
megaloureter
megalourethra
megarectum
megasigmoid
megaureter
Mehn-Quigley technique
Meibom gland
meibomian
m. gland
m. gland carcinoma
Meigs
M. pelvic lymphadenectomy
M. suture technique
Meigs-Okabayashi procedure

Meigs-Werthein hysterectomy
Meissner plexus
melanization
melanoacanthoma
melanoameloblastoma
melanoblastoma
melanocarcinoma
melanocytic conjunctival lesion
melanocytoma
melanoma
acral lentiginous m. (ALM)
anorectal m.
m. antigen reacting to T cell (MART)
axial m.
m. cell lysate
CTL immunity against m.
cutaneous m.
extremity m.
familial atypical mole and m. (FAM-M)
lentigo m.
node-negative m.
node-positive m.
thick cutaneous m. (TCM)
m. transferrin
truncal m.
melanoma-associated
m.-a. antigen GD2
m.-a. antigen GD3
m.-a. antigen GM2
melanosarcoma
melanotic
m. carcinoma
m. lesion
m. medulloblastoma
m. whitlow
MELAS
mitochondrial myopathy, encephalopathy, lactic acidosis, and stroke-like syndrome
Meleney
M. gangrene
M. infection
Meller operation
mellitus
diabetes m.
melocervicoplasty
melolabial flap
Melone distal radius fracture classification
melonoplasty
melon seed body
meloplasty
meloschisis
melting point
Meltzer method
membrana, pl. **membranae**
membranaceae
membrane
acute inflammatory m.
acute pyogenic m.
adamantine m.
alveolar-capillary m.
alveolocapillary m.
alveolodental m.
amniotic m.
antibasement m.
antiglomerular basement m.
antitubular basement m.
antral m.
arachnoid m.
m. artificial lung
asymmetric unit m.
atlantooccipital m.
Barkan m.
basal cell m.
basement m.
basilar m.
basolateral m.
Bichat m.
bilaminar m.
Bowman m.
m. bridge
Bruch m.
brush-border m.
m. catheter technique
cell m.
cellulose-based m.
chorioallantoic m.
choroidal neovascular m.
cloacal m.
collodion m.
congenital pyloric m.
conjunctival m.
connective tissue m.
cricothyroid m.
cricotracheal m.
cricovocal m.
croupous m.
cuprophane m.
m. current
cuticular m.
cyclitic m.

NOTES

membrane *(continued)*
cytoplasmic m.
Debove m.
decidual m.
Demours m.
dentinoenamel m.
Descemet m.
dialyzer m.
diphtheritic m.
drum m.
dry mucous m.
Duddell m.
dysmenorrheal m.
egg m.
enamel m.
endothelial cell basement m.
epipapillary m.
epiretinal m.
epithelial basement m.
erythrocyte m.
exocelomic m.
m. expansion theory
false m.
fenestrated m.
fetal m.
fibroproliferative m.
Fielding m.
m. filtration method
filtration-slit m.
Fresnel m.
germinal m.
glassy m.
gliotic m.
Golgi m.
Haller m.
Hemophan m.
Henle elastic m.
Henle fenestrated m.
Heuser m.
high-flux dialysis m.
hourglass m.
Hovius m.
hyaline basement m.
hyalitis anterior m.
hyaloid posterior m.
hymenal m.
hyoglossal m.
idiopathic preretinal m.
inflammatory m.
inner limiting m.
m. instability
intact m.
intercostal m.
intermuscular m.
interposition m.
intraosseous m.
invaginated m.
ivory m.
Jackson m.
Jacob m.
m. of Liliequist
limiting m.
low-flux cellulose-based m.
low-flux cuprophane m.
low-flux dialysis m.
lysosomal m.
mammalian cell m.
microvillous m.
moist mucous m.
mucous m.
NaK-ATPase m.
Nasmyth m.
neovascular m.
neuronal m.
nictitating m.
onion skin-like m.
otolithic m.
outer limiting m.
Payr m.
m. peeling
peridental m.
perineal m.
periodontal m.
periorbital m.
m. permeability
phrenoesophageal m.
pial-glial m.
placental m.
plasma m.
polyacrylonitrile m.
porous filter m.
postsynaptic m.
m. potential
preretinal m.
presynaptic m.
prophylactic m.
pseudoserous m.
pulpodentinal m.
pupillary m.
purpurogenous m.
pyogenic m.
quadrangular m.
Reichert m.
Reissner m.
reticular m.
retrocorneal m.
rolling m.
m. rupture
Ruysch m.
ruyschian m.
salpingopalatine m.
salpingopharyngeal m.
sarcolemmal m.
schneiderian respiratory m.
secondary m.
semiimpermeable m.

semipermeable m.
serous m.
Shrapnell m.
Slavianski m.
small intestinal m.
spiral m.
statoconic m.
stripping m.
stylomandibular m.
subepithelial m.
subimplant m.
submucous m.
subretinal neovascular m.
suprapleural m.
surface m.
synovial m.
tarsal m.
tectorial m.
Tenon m.
thickened synovial m.
thin basement m.
thyrohyoid m.
Toldt m.
Tourtual m.
trabecular m.
m. trafficking
tubular basement m.
tympanic m.
undulating m.
unit m.
urea-impermeable m.
urogenital m.
urorectal m.
urothelial basement m.
vernix m.
vestibular m.
virginal m.
vitelline m.
vitreal m.
vitreous m.
Wachendorf m.
wrinkling m.
yolk m.
Zinn m.

membrane-coating granule
membranectomy
membranocartilaginous
membranoproliferative glomerulonephritis
membranotomy
transcardiac m.
membranous
m. acute inflammation
m. adhesion
m. obstruction
m. septum
m. urethra
Memford-Gurd arthroplasty
Memorial Pain Assessment Card (MPAC)
memory
explicit m.
m. guidance saccade test
implicit m.
indirect m.
m. loss
mass m.
m. recall
scratch-pad m.
MEN
multiple endocrine neoplasia
MEN syndrome
MEN-2a
multiple endocrine neoplasia type 2a
MEN-2a, -2b syndrome
MEN-2b
multiple endocrine neoplasia type 2b
Mendelsohn maneuver
Mendelson syndrome
Menghini
M. biopsy technique
M. technique for percutaneous liver biopsy
Ménière
M. disease
M. syndrome
meningeae
meningeal
m. branch
m. carcinoma
m. groove
m. hernia
m. layer
m. plexus
m. vein
meningei
meningeorrhaphy
meninges
meningeus
meningioma
meningioma-en-plaque
meningiomatosis
meningitic respiration
meningitis
meningocele

NOTES

meningoencephalitis
meningoencephalocele
meningomyelocele
meningoosteophlebitis
meningorrhagia
meningosis
meninguria
meniscal
m. excision
m. repair
meniscectomy
arthroscopic m.
lateral m.
partial m.
Patel medial m.
subtotal lateral m.
total m.
meniscofemorale
meniscoplasty
meniscus, pl. **menisci**
Dickhaut-DeLee classification of discoid m.
Watanabe classification of discoid m.
Mensor-Scheck
M.-S. hanging hip operation
M.-S. technique
menstrual
m. aspiration
m. cycle induction
M. Distress Management Questionnaire (MDMQ)
m. extraction
m. extraction abortion
menstruation
reflux m.
mental
m. artery
m. block injection
m. branch
m. canal
m. foramen
m. nerve
m. nerve block
m. point
m. process
m. projection
m. region
m. spine
m. status evaluation
m. status examination
m. symphysis
m. tubercle
mentale
mentalis
m. muscle
menti (*pl. of* mentum)
mentoanterior position
mentolabial
m. furrow
m. sulcus
mentolabialis
mentoplasty
mentoposterior position
mentotransverse position
mentum, pl. **menti**
m. anterior position
m. posterior position
m. transverse position
Menzies method
MEP
motor-evoked potential
myogenic motor-evoked potential
MER
motor-evoked response
meralgia paresthetica
Mercator projection
Mercier
M. bar
mercurial line
Mercurio position
mercuroscopic expansion
mercury pressure
Merendino technique
meridian
corneal m.
meridional aberration
Merindino operation
Merkel
M. cell cancer
M. cell carcinoma
M. fossa
M. muscle
mermaid malformation
Méry gland
mesangial matrix expansion
mesangiolysis
mesangium
extraglomerular m.
mesareic
mesatipellic pelvis
mesencephalic
m. cistern
m. hemorrhage
m. low-density lesion
m. reticular formation
m. tractotomy
mesencephalotomy
mesenchymal
m. lesion
m. tissue
mesenchymoma
mesenteriale
mesenteric
m. angiogram

m. angiography
m. arterial system
m. arteriovenous fistula
m. artery
m. border
m. bypass graft
m. circulation
m. cyst
m. gland
m. hematoma
m. hernia
m. insufficiency
m. ischemia (MI)
m. lymph node (MLN)
m. mass
m. nodal disease
m. node
m. portion
m. rupture
m. tear
m. vascular lesion
m. vasodilator
m. vasodilator infusion
m. vein
m. venoconstriction

mesenterici
mesentericoparietal
m. fossa
m. recess
mesentericoportal axis
mesenterii
mesenteriolum processus vermiformis
mesenteriopexy
mesenteriorrhaphy
mesenteriplication
mesenteritis
mesenterium
mesentery
m. abscess
edematous m.
mesethmoid bone
mesh
m. herniorrhaphy
m. implantation
m. inguinodynia
m. plug hernioplasty
m. removal
m. repair
mesial
mesioangular position
mesiobuccal
m. canal
m. line angle
mesiobuccoocclusal point angle
mesiodistal
m. fracture
m. plane
mesiolabial
m. bilobed transposition flap
m. line angle
mesiolabioincisal point angle
mesiolingual line angle
mesiolinguoincisal point angle
mesiolinguo-occlusal point line angle
mesioocclusal line angle
mesioocclusodistal (MOD)
mesoappendix
mesoatrial shunt
mesocaval
m. anastomosis
m. H-graft
mesocecal
mesocecum
mesocolic
m. hernia
m. involvement
m. tenia
mesocolica
mesocolici
mesocolon
ascending m.
descending m.
sigmoid m.
transverse m.
mesocolopexy
mesocoloplication
mesoderm
extraembryonic m.
intermediate m.
mesoduodenal
mesoduodenum
mesoenteriolum
mesoepididymis
mesoesophageal dissection
mesohepatectomy
mesoileum
mesojejunum
mesolepidoma
mesolimbic-mesocortical tract
mesonephric
m. adenocarcinoma
m. duct

NOTES

M

mesonephric *(continued)*
m. ridge
m. tubule
mesonephricus
mesonephroma
mesonephros
mesoneuritis
mesopexy
mesophryon
mesorchium
mesorectal
m. excision
mesorectum
residual m.
mesorrhaphy
mesosigmoid
mesosigmoidopexy
mesostenium
mesosternum
mesostructure
implant m.
mesotendineum
mesotendon
mesothelial
m. cell
m. cell layer
m. tissue
mesothelioma
benign m.
mesothelium
mesovarian
m. margin
mesovarium
Messerklinger technique
metabolic
m. acidosis
m. change
m. coma
m. complication
m. disorder
m. evaluation
m. heat production
m. rate
m. response
metabolism
pyruvate m.
metabolite
metacarpal
m. bone
m. neck fracture
m. osteotomy
metacarpi (*pl. of* metacarpus)
metacarpophalangeae
metacarpophalangeal
m. articulation
m. joint arthroplasty
metacarpus, pl. **metacarpi**
metachronous emergence
metadiaphysis
metafacial angle
metal-ceramic restoration
metallic
m. cranioplasty
m. foreign body
m. fragment
m. restoration
m. rod fixation
metalloproteinase
matrix m. (MMP)
metalloscopy
metamorphosing respiration
metanephric
m. cap
m. duct
metaphysial
m. abscess
m. osteotomy
m. tibial fracture
metaphysis, pl. **metaphyses**
distal m.
femoral m.
fibular m.
funnelization of m.
rachitic m.
tibial m.
metaplasia
apocrine m.
Barrett m.
columnar m.
squamous m.
metaplastic epithelium
metastasectomy
pulmonary m.
metastasis, pl. **metastases**
adnexal m.
adrenal m.
m., age, completeness of resection, local invasion, and tumor size (MACIS)
aortic node m.
axillary node m.
bilobar liver m.
biochemical m.
biopsy-proven m.
blastic m.
bone m.
bony m.
brain m.
breast m.
calcareous m.
calcified liver m.
calcifying m.
cardiac m.
cavitating m.
celiac lymph node m.
cerebral m.

cervical m.
chiasmal m.
choroidal m.
clivus m.
colonic m.
colorectal m.
contact m.
contralateral axillary m.
cutaneous m.
cystic m.
diffuse m.
distal m.
distant m.
drop m.
duodenal m.
echopenic liver m.
extracapsular m.
extrahepatic m.
extralymphatic m.
extrathoracic m.
fallopian tube m.
floxuridine in hepatic m.
gastric bed m.
gastrointestinal m.
hematogenic m.
hematogenous m.
hematopoietic m.
hemorrhagic m.
hepatic colorectal m.
hernia m.
implantation m.
incisional m.
inguinal lymph node m.
intracapsular m.
intrahepatic m.
intramucosal m.
in-transit m.
intrapulmonary m. (IPM)
laparoscopic port site m.
lateroaortic m.
leptomeningeal m.
liver m.
lymphatic m.
lymph node m.
lymphogenous m.
medulloblastoma m.
necrotic m.
neoplasm m.
nodal m.
noncolorectal liver m. (NCRLM)
nonneuroendocrine m.
occult m.
ocular m.
omental m.
orbital m.
osseous m.
osteoblastic m.
ovarian cancer m.
paracardiac m.
parasellar m.
parenchymal brain m.
periesophagogastric lymph node m.
peritoneal m.
placental m.
port site m.
pulmonary m.
regional m.
resectable liver m.
retrobulbar orbital m.
satellite m.
serosal m.
serosal-peritoneal m.
skeletal m.
skip m.
soft-tissue m.
sphenoid sinus m.
spinal m.
stomach cancer m.
synchronous hepatic m.
testicular m.
tumor, node, m. (TNM)
unique noncolorectal liver m.
unresectable m.
uterine sarcoma m.
uveal m.
vascular m.
Virchow m.

metastatic
m. abscess
m. adenocarcinoma
m. adenopathy
m. colorectal cancer
m. colorectal carcinoma
m. contamination
m. disease
m. implantation
m. involvement
m. lesion
m. malignancy
m. nodule
m. prostatic carcinoma
m. renal cell carcinoma
m. spread

NOTES

metastatic *(continued)*
m. tumor
m. tumor removal
metasternum
metasynchronous bacterial urinary tract infection
metatarsal
m. artery
m. bone
m. fracture
m. head
m. head resection
m. pad
m. Reverdin osteotomy
m. V-shaped osteotomy
metatarsi (*pl. of* metatarsus)
metatarsocuneiform articulation
metatarsophalangeae
metatarsophalangeal
m. articulation
m. joint disarticulation
m. joint dislocation
metatarsus, pl. **metatarsi**
metathesis
meter-kilogram-second (mks)
methacholine bronchoprovocation challenge
methamphetamine exposure
methanol freezing method
methemoglobin
methemoglobinemia
method
Abbott m.
Abell m.
Abell-Kendall m.
acid anhydride m.
acid guanidine thiocyanate-phenol-chloroform m.
acoupedic m.
acoustic m.
acridine orange m.
agar diffusion m.
Allain m.
analytic m.
Anderson-Keys m.
Anel m.
antegrade m.
anthrone m.
antibody linkage m.
Antyllus m.
area-length m.
aristotelian m.
artificial m.
Arvidsson dimension-length m.
Ashby differential agglutination m.
Astrand 30-beat stopwatch m.
atrial extrastimulus m.
Attwood staining m.
auditory m.
Autenrieth and Funk m.
avidin-biotin-peroxidase complex m.
Ayoub-Shklar m.
bacterial agar m.
Baker Sudan black m.
bandage m.
Barnett-Bourne acetic alcohol-silver nitrate m.
barostat m.
Barraquer m.
barrier m.
Barrnett-Seligman dihydroxydinaphthyl disulfide m.
Barrnett-Seligman indoxyl esterase m.
Barroso-Moguel and Costero silver m.
Bass m.
Bassini m.
Batch least-squares m.
Baumgartner m.
Beaver direct smear m.
Beck m.
Belsey fundoplication m.
Benedict-Talbot body surface area m.
Bengston m.
Bennett sulfhydryl m.
Bennhold Congo red m.
Bensley aniline-acid fuchsin-methyl green m.
benzo sky blue m.
Berg chelate removal m.
Bielschowsky m.
Bier m.
bilateral inguinal hernia repair m.
Billings m.
Billroth I m.
bimodal m.
bisensory m.
black periodic acid m.
Bland-Altman m.
Bleck m.
Bobath m.
Bodian m.
Bohr isopleth m.
Bonnaire m.
Borchgrevink m.
Borggreve m.
Brasdor m.
breast-conserving m.
breathing m.
Brecher-Cronkite m.
brine flotation m.
Brisbane m.
Brown-Dodge m.

Brown and Wickham pressure profile m.
Bruhn m.
Buck m.
Budin-Chandler m.
Buist m.
bulkhead m.
Burch bladder suspension m.
Burgess m.
Burkhalter-Reyes m. of phalangeal fracture
Burow quantitative m.
bypass m.
Byrd-Drew m.
Cajal gold-sublimate m.
Cajal uranium silver m.
Caldwell-Moloy m.
Callahan root canal filling m.
Camp-Gianturco m.
Carpue m.
catheter introduction m.
Celermajer m.
cellophane tape m.
Chang aniline-acid fuchsin m.
Charters m.
Chayes m.
chewing m.
Chiffelle and Putt m.
chloranilate m.
chromate m.
chrome alum hematoxylin-phloxine m.
chromogenic m.
chromolytic m.
Ciaccio m.
cinefluoroscopic m.
Clark-Collip m.
Clausen m.
clean-catch collection m.
closed circuit m.
cobaltinitrite m.
Cockroft m.
Colcher-Sussman m.
cold knife m.
collagen staining m.
Collis-Nissen fundoplication m.
combined m.
composite pelvic resection m.
computer-assisted design-controlled alignment m.
confrontation m.
Con-Lish polishing m.
consonant-injection m.
constitutive heterochromatin m.
contact m.
contoured adduction trochanteric-controlled alignment m.
contraceptive m.
conventional m.
cooled-knife m.
Cope m.
copper sulfate m.
Corning m.
correlational m.
Craigie tube m.
Crawford m.
Credé m.
Cribier m.
Crippa lead tetraacetate m.
cross-consonant injection m.
cross-sectional m.
crown-contouring m.
Cryolife Single Step dilution m.
Cuignet m.
cup-and-cone m.
Cutler-Ederer m.
cyanogen bromide m.
cysteic acid m.
Dale-Laidlaw clotting time m.
Dane m.
Danielson m.
Defares rebreathing m.
definitive m.
depth caliper-meter stick m.
Devereux-Reichek m.
diazo staining m.
Dick m.
Dieffenbach m.
Dieterle m.
diffusion root canal filling m.
digitonin m.
direct m.
disk diffusion m.
disk sensitivity m.
Distress Risk Assessment M. (DRAM)
Dixon fat suppression m.
Döderlein m.
Dodge area-length m.
Doppler m.
Dor fundoplication m.
double antibody m.
double-stapled ileoanal reservoir m.
Douglas bag collection m.

NOTES

method *(continued)*
Dow m.
downstream sampling m.
dye-dilution m.
dyed starch m.
dye scattering m.
dynamic traction m.
edge-detection m.
Eggleston m.
Eicken m.
ellipsoid m.
Elmslie-Trillat patellar realignment m.
encu m.
endorectal ileoanal pull-through m.
endoscopic mucosal resection m.
end-to-end reconstruction m.
ensu m.
enucleation m.
Epstein m.
estimated Fick m.
Eve m.
excisional biopsy m.
experimental m.
extension block splinting m.
extraanatomic bypass m.
extracorporeal m.
Fahraeus m.
Fallat-Buckholz m.
Ferguson scoliosis measuring m.
fiberoptic intubation m.
fibrinogen m.
fibrin plate m.
Fick oxygen extraction m.
field m.
filtration m.
Fite m.
fixed sediment m.
flat substrate m.
floppy Nissen fundoplication m.
flow convergence m.
fluorescence polarization m.
fluoroscopic m.
flush m.
Folin and Wu m.
Fones m.
Fontana-Masson staining m.
Foot reticulin m.
formal m.
formaldehyde-induced fluorescence m.
formalin-ether sedimentation m.
forward triangle m.
four-port m.
freehand m.
freeze-cleave m.
freeze-etch m.
freeze-fracture-etch m.
French m.
frozen section m.
Gabastou hydraulic m.
Galanti-Giusti colorimetric m.
Gärtner m.
gas clearance m.
gaseous laparoscopy m.
gasless laparoscopy m.
gastric valve tightening m.
Gerbert-Mellilo m.
German m.
glass-bead retention m.
glucose oxidase m.
glycerin m.
Gohil-Cavolo m.
gradient m.
gradient-echo m.
gradient-reversal fat suppression m.
grammatic m.
Granger m.
Gräupner m.
Greenwald and Lewman m.
Grimelius argyrophil m.
Grocott-Gomori methenamine-silver m.
guidance m.
Hagedorn and Jansen m.
half-time m.
Hall m.
Hamilton m.
Hammerschlag m.
hanging chain m.
Hanley-McNeil m.
Harrison m.
Hatle m.
Hawkins m.
head-tilt m.
Heinecke m.
helium dilution m.
hemidouble stapling m.
Hetzel forward triangle m.
heuristic m.
hexokinase m.
Hilton m.
Hirschberg m.
Hirschfeld m.
histochemical m.
Hoechst dye m.
hold-relax m.
hole preparation m.
Holmes m.
Holmgren m.
Holzer m.
Howard m.
Howe silver precipitation m.
H.P. Wright m.
Hugenholtz m.
hydrogen washout m.

Ilizarov m.
imaging m.
Imanaga m.
immersion m.
immobilization m.
immunodiagnostic m.
immunofluorescence m.
immunohistochemical m.
immunometric sandwich m.
immunoperoxidase m.
impedance m.
Indian m.
indirect restorative m.
indocyanine green m.
indophenol m.
informal m.
inhalation m.
injection m.
injection-molded m.
Insall patella alta m.
install m.
intraoperative imaging m.
intraperitoneal m.
introspective m.
Israel m.
Italian m.
Ito m.
Jahss ninety-ninety m.
jejunoileal bypass reversal m.
Jena m.
Jenckel m.
Jendrassik-Grof m.
Johnson root canal filling m.
Johnston m.
Kaplan-Meier m.
Karr m.
Kasser-Kennedy m.
Keating-Hart m.
Kendrick m.
Kennedy area-length m.
Kety-Schmidt m.
keyhole m.
kinesthetic m.
King biopsy m.
Kinzie m.
Kirby-Bauer disk diffusion m.
Kirstein m.
Kjeldahl m.
Kluge m.
Kocher m.
Konno biopsy m.
Krause m.
Krimsky m.
Kristeller m.
LaBorde m.
Lamaze m.
Langendorff m.
laparoscopic lymph node dissection m.
laparoscopic Nissen fundoplication m.
laparoscopic paraaortic lymph node sampling m.
laser m.
Laurell m.
Leboyer m.
Lee-White clotting time m.
Levaditi m.
Levy, Rowntree, and Marriott m.
Lewis and Benedict m.
Lewissohn m.
Liang and Pardee m.
life table m.
Lillie allochrome m.
limb-saving m.
Lindsjö m.
Lison-Dunn m.
Lister m.
logical m.
longitudinal m.
loop gastric bypass m.
Lowery m.
Lown and Woolf m.
Lowry m.
Lowsley ribbon gut m.
macro-Kjeldahl m.
Mantoux m.
manual m.
Marmo m.
Marriott m.
Marshall m.
Masson trichrome m.
McReynolds m.
McSpadden m.
McVay m.
Meltzer m.
membrane filtration m.
Menzies m.
methanol freezing m.
Metzer-Boyce m.
Meyerding m.
microinjection m.
micro-Kjeldahl m.
microsurgery m.

NOTES

method *(continued)*
microwave-assisted streptavidin-biotin peroxidase m.
minimal-access m.
modified band lid m.
Monte Carlo multiway sensitivity analysis m.
Moore m.
Morison m.
mother m.
Movat pentachrome m.
Mueller m.
Mueller-Walle m.
multiple cone root canal filling m.
multiple-port incision m.
Murphy m.
nail length gauge m.
Narula m.
natural m.
Needles split cast m.
needle thoracentesis m.
Neufeld dynamic m.
Nichols m.
Nikiforoff m.
ninety-ninety m.
Nissen fundoplication m.
Nissen-Rosseti fundoplication m.
Nitchie m.
noninvasive m.
nonresectional m.
non-rib-spreading thoracotomy incision m.
nonsurgical m.
numerical cipher m.
odd-even m.
Ogata m.
O'Hara two-clamp m.
Okamoto m.
Oliver-Rosalki m.
Ollier m.
one-inclinometer m.
open circuit m.
optical density m.
oral-aural m.
Orsi-Grocco m.
Ouchterlony m.
oxygen step-up m.
Pachon m.
Palmer m.
Papanicolaou m.
Paris m.
Parker-Kerr closed m.
pause-squeeze m.
Pavlov m.
Payr clamp m.
pedicle m.
Penaz volume-clamp m.
Penfield m.
Penn m.
percutaneous sampling m.
Pfeiffer-Comberg m.
Pfiffner and Myers m.
pharmacologic m.
phosphotungstic acid-magnesium chloride precipitation m.
Pichlmayer m.
pin-and-plaster m.
pinprick m.
Pizzolato peroxide-silver m.
plasma thrombin clot m.
plateau m.
plosive-injection m.
polarographic m.
Politzer m.
Pólya m.
prick-test m.
Pringle vascular control m.
prism m.
Prochownik m.
Puchtler alkaline Congo red m.
Puchtler Sirius red m.
Purmann m.
Puzo m.
pyramid m.
Quick m.
m. of Quinones
Rackley m.
Raff-Glantz derivative m.
rag-wheel m.
Ranawat-Dorr-Inglis m.
Ranawat triangle m.
Read rebreathing m.
reconstruction m.
Reddick-Saye m.
reduction m.
Rees-Ecker m.
reference m.
Rehfuss m.
Reichel-Pólya m.
relaxation m.
retrofilling m.
retrograde root canal filling m.
Reverdin m.
rhythm m.
Rideal-Walker m.
Risser m.
Riva-Rocci m.
Rochester m.
Rodeck m.
Russe-Gerhardt m.
Sahli m.
Salzman m.
Sandler-Dodge area-length m.
Sargenti m.
Satterthwaite m.
Scarpa m.

Schäfer m.
Schede m.
Schick m.
Schiller m.
Schober m.
Schüller m.
Schwartz m.
scientific m.
Scudder m.
sectional root canal filling m.
segmentation root canal filling m.
Seldinger m.
Sengstaken-Blakemore m.
shadowing m.
Shaffer-Hartmann m.
Shimazaki area-length m.
sigma m.
silver cone m.
silver point root canal filling m.
Silvester m.
simultaneous m.
single cone root canal filling m.
single-stick m.
sliding scale m.
Smellie m.
Smellie-Veit m.
sniff m.
Somogyi m.
special reference m.
sperm washing insemination m.
sphincter-saving m.
sphincter-sparing m.
split-cast m.
Stammer m.
standard radioenzymatic m.
Stanford biopsy m.
stapled reconstruction m.
static m.
Stegemann-Stalder m.
stereotactic core biopsy m.
Stillman m.
Stimson gravity m.
Stovall-Black m.
Strauss m.
Stroganoff m.
suction m.
surgical enucleation m.
swallow m.
Sweet m.
symptothermal m.
synthetic m.
systematic m.
Tajima m.
Tarkowski m.
tetanic stimulation m.
Thal fundoplication m.
Thane m.
Theden m.
thermally active m.
thermodilution m.
Thiersch m.
Thom flap laryngeal
  reconstruction m.
Thompson-Hatina m.
three-dimensional FATS m.
threshold shift m.
Thrombo-Wellcotest m.
Tilden m.
total fundoplication m.
Toupe m.
Towako m.
traditional m.
trapezoid m.
triangulation stapling m.
triphenyltetrazolium staining m.
trocar drainage m.
Tweed m.
twin m.
twirling m.
two-dye m.
two-inclinometer m.
two-microphone acoustic
  reflection m.
ultropaque m.
uncut Collis-Nissen
  fundoplication m.
unilateral inguinal hernia repair m.
Vecchietti m.
verbotonal m.
vertical condensation root canal
  filling m.
vertical-cut m.
Victor Gomel m.
visual m.
Vogel m.
volumetric m.
von Claus chronometric m.
von Kossa m.
V-slope m.
Wardill four-flap m.
Wardill-Kilner advancement flap m.
Wardrop m.
Warthin-Starry staining m.
Waterston m.

NOTES

method *(continued)*
- Watson m.
- Watson-Crick m.
- Weiss logarithmic m.
- Welcker m.
- Westergren sedimentation rate m.
- Wheeler m.
- Willett-Stampfer m.
- Wilson-White m.
- Winston-Lutz m.
- Wintrobe and Landsberg m.
- Wintrobe sedimentation rate m.
- Wolfe m.
- Woolf m.
- Wroblewski m.
- xenon m.
- x-line m.
- zeta sedimentation ratio m.
- zinc-sulfate flotation m.
- Z-track intramuscular injection m.

methylation
methylene blue dye localization
methyl-*tert*-butyl ether (MTBE)
meticulous
- m. hemostasis
- m. maneuver

metopic
- m. point

metopica
metopion
metopoplasty
metoposcopy
metrectomy
metric ophthalmoscopy
metrofibroma
metromalacoma
metroperitoneal fistula
metroplasty
- Strassman m.

metrotomy
Metzer-Boyce method
Meuli arthroplasty
Meyer
- M. cartilage
- M. incision
- M. line
- M. operation

Meyerding
- M. method
- M. spondylolisthesis classification line

Meyerding-Van Demark technique
Meyer-Overton
- M.-O. rule
- M.-O. theory of narcosis

Meyer-Schwickerath
- M.-S. light coagulation
- M.-S. operation

Meyers-McKeever tibial fracture classification
Meyers quadratus muscle-pedicle bone graft
Meynert
- M. decussation
- M. retroflex bundle

Meyn reduction
mg
- milligram

MH
- malignant hyperthermia

MHA-TP
- microhemagglutination *Treponema pallidum*
  - MHA-TP test

MHC
- major histocompatibility complex

MI
- mesenteric ischemia
- myocardial infarction
  - occlusive MI

Miami pouch
micelle formation
Michaelson
- M. counter pressure
- M. operation

Michal
- M. I, II procedure
- M. II technique

Michel
- M. anomaly
- M. deformity
- M. malformation

Michele vertebral aspiration
Michigan Abuse Screening Test (MAST)
microadenoma
- pituitary m.

microadenomectomy
- selective m.

microaerosol
microamperage
- m. electrical nerve stimulation
- m. neural stimulation

microanastomosis
- laser-assisted m. (LAMA)

microaneurysm
microaspiration
microatheroma
microbic dissociation
microbiliary inflammation
microbubble
microcalcification
- diffuse m.
- malignant-appearing m.

mammographic malignant-appearing m.
suspicious m.
microcavitation
microchromoendoscopy
microcirculation
native myocardial m.
pulp m.
microcirculatory
m. disturbance
m. failure
microcolon
microcolpohysteroscopy
microcorneal
microcurrent therapy
microcystic disease
microdialysis
microdiffusion
microdiskectomy, microdiscectomy
arthroscopic m.
uniportal arthroscopic m.
microdissection
microelectrode
m. recording
m. recording technique
microembolization
microfilament bundle
microfistulous communication
microfollicle
microfollicular
microgastria
microgenia
microgenitalism
microglioma
micrograms per kilogram per minute
micrograph
microhamartoma
microhemagglutination *Treponema pallidum* (MHA-TP)
microincineration
microincision
microinjection method
microinvasion
microinvasive
m. carcinoma
m. carcinoma classification
m. technique
micro-Kjeldahl method
microlaparoscopic
m. cholecystectomy
m. Nissen fundoplication
microlaparoscopy
microlaryngoscopy
Thornell m.
micro liquid extraction
microlith
microlithiasis
microlumbar
m. diskectomy
m. disk excision
micromanipulation
gamete m.
oocyte m.
m. technique
micrometastasis, pl. **micrometastases**
hematogenous m.
micrometastatic peritoneal disease
micromyelia
micron
microneurography
sympathetic m.
microneurolysis
microneurorrhaphy
microneurovascular anastomosis
microoperative procedure
microorganism
gram-negative m.
gram-positive m.
micropapillary
m. carcinoma
m. subtype
micropenis
microperforation
microprolactinoma
microproliferation
micropuncture
microscopic
m. absence
m. diagnosis
m. disease
m. epididymal sperm aspiration
m. invasion
m. IPM
m. multifocal medullary carcinoma
m. resection
m. sphincter
microscopically controlled surgery
microscopy
binocular m.
cryoelectron m.
dark-field m.
electron m.
epifluorescent m.
fluorescence m.

NOTES

M

microscopy *(continued)*
fundus m.
immersion m.
immune electron m.
immunofluorescence m.
intravital m.
light m.
paraffin-section light m.
polarization m.
rotary shadowing electron m.
scanning electron m.
scanning force m.
specular m.
television m.
transmission electron m.
microspectrofluorometry
microspectroscopy
microsphere
radioactive m.
microstomia
microsurgery
m. method
m. procedure
m. technique
transanal endoscopic m. (TEM)
videoendoscopic-assisted m.
microsurgical
m. diskectomy
m. epididymal sperm aspiration
m. epididymal sperm aspiration procedure
m. free flap
m. inguinal varicocelectomy
m. technique
m. tubocornual anastomosis
microtia
microtrabecular hepatocellular carcinoma
microtransducer technique
microtraumatic insult
micro-tubulotomy technique
microvascular
m. decompression (MVD)
m. free flap
m. free flap transfer
m. surgical anastomosis
m. technique
microvessel
microvillous membrane
microwave
m. coagulation
m. fixation
m. radiation injury
m. therapy
m. thermotherapy
microwave-assisted streptavidin-biotin peroxidase method
microwelding
micrurgical
micturition pain
midabdominal transverse incision
midaxillary
m. line
m. line incision
midazolam-induced excitatory reaction
midbody tumor
midbrain reticular formation
MIDCAB
minimally invasive direct coronary artery bypass
midcarpal
m. arthroscopy
m. dislocation
midclavicular
m. line
m. port
midcoronal plane
middle
m. cerebral artery (MCA)
m. cerebral artery occlusion
m. ear infection
m. meatus
m. mediastinum
m. phalanx
midesophageal traction diverticulum
midexpiratory/midinspiratory flow ratio
midface
m. degloving technique
m. fracture
midfoot fracture
midforceps maneuver
midfrontal
m. plane
m. plane coronal section
midgastric transverse sphincter
midgut volvulus
midheel line
midhumeral line
midlateral approach
midline
m. abdominal crease
m. aponeurotic closure
m. disk herniation
m. exposure
m. forehead flap
m. incisional hernia
m. incisional hernioplasty
m. lower abdominal incision
m. medial approach
m. myelotomy
m. oblique incision
m. position
m. spinal approach
m. upper abdominal incision
midmalleolar line
midoccipital
midpalatal suture opening

midpalmar
m. abscess
m. space
midpapillary
anterior m. (AM)
m. longitudinal (MP-L)
m. transverse (MP-T)
midpelvis
midpoint to meatal line
midriff
midsagittal
m. plane
m. section
midscapular line
midsection
midshaft fracture
midsigmoid sphincter
midsternal line
midsternum
midthalamic plane
Mielke bleeding time
MIGET
multiple inert gas elimination technique
migraine
abdominal m.
m. abortive therapy
basilar artery m.
familial hemiplegic m.
retinal m.
vertiginous m.
migrating abscess
migration
m. abnormality
calculus m.
cell m.
cellular m.
electrode m.
embolus m.
epithelial m.
fibroblast m.
gallstone m.
graft m.
implant m.
instrument m.
intragastric prosthesis m.
intravesical m.
lymphocyte m.
macrophagic m.
neural crest m.
neuronal m.
neutrophil m.
phagocyte m.
physiologic mesial m.
pigmentary m.
placental m.
rod m.
stage m.
tooth m.
trochanteric m.
tube m.
m. velocity
mika operation
Mikulicz
M. colostomy
M. incision
M. operation
M. pyloroplasty
M. sac
Milch
M. condylar fracture classification
M. cuff resection of ulna technique
M. elbow fracture classification
M. elbow technique
M. humeral fracture classification
mild traumatic brain injury (mTBI)
Miles
M. abdominoperineal resection
M. operation
Milford mallet finger technique
miliary
m. abscess
m. aneurysm
m. granulomatous inflammation
military
m. brace position
m. tuck position
milk
m. duct
m. gland
m. spot
milk-ejection reflex
milk-filled cyst
milkmaid elbow dislocation
milkman fracture
milky ascites
Millard
M. advancement rotation flap reconstruction
M. rotation-advancement lip repair
Millender arthroplasty
Millen-Read modification
Millen technique
mille pattes technique

NOTES

Miller
M. flatfoot operation
M. procedure
Miller-Galante knee arthroplasty
Millesi
M. interfascicular graft
M. modified technique
M. nerve graft
millibar
millicurie (mCi)
Milligan-Morgan hemorrhoidectomy
milligram (mg)
milligram-hour
millimeters partial pressure
millimicrogram
milliosmole/kilogram
Miltner-Wan calcaneus resection
mimetic muscle
MIN
multiple intestinal neoplasia
mineral
m. oil aspiration
m. oil foreign body
mineralized tissue
Ming gastric carcinoma classification
miniature
m. end-plate potential
m. uterine cavity
minicholecystostomy
surgical-radiologic m.
minification
minikeratoplasty
Castroviejo m.
minilaparoscopic cholecystectomy
minilaparotomy
m. incision
m. technique
minimae
minimal
m. access general surgery
m. air
m. alveolar concentration
m. anesthetic concentration (MAC)
m. bactericidal concentration
m. leak technique
m. transurethral resection
minimal-access
m.-a. method
m.-a. procedure
m.-a. technique
minimal-change
m.-c. disease
m.-c. nephrotic syndrome
minimal-incision pubovaginal suspension
minimal-lesion nephrotic syndrome
minimally
m. displaced fracture
m. invasive approach
m. invasive biopsy
m. invasive direct coronary artery bypass (MIDCAB)
m. invasive esophagectomy
m. invasive mitral valve repair
m. invasive nature
m. invasive parathyroidectomy
m. invasive procedure
m. invasive robotic heart valve surgery
m. invasive surgical access
m. invasive surgical technique
m. invasive video-assisted parathyroidectomy (MIVAP)
minimi
minimum
m. alveolar anesthetic concentration (MAC)
m. alveolar concentration (MAC)
m. audible pressure
m. bactericidal concentration
m. detectable concentration
m. effective analgesic concentration
m. effective concentration (MEC)
m. lethal concentration
m. local analgesic concentration (MLAC)
minimus
Minkoff-Jaffe-Menendez posterior approach
Minkoff-Nicholas procedure
Minnesota EKG classification
minor
m. amputation
m. calix
m. duodenal papilla
m. fissure
m. injury
m. manifestation
m. operation
m. splenic injury
m. sublingual duct
m. surgery
trochanter m.
minorem
minores
minoris
Minsky operation
minus
minute
alveolar ventilation per m. (V_A)
micrograms per kilogram per m.
physiological dead space ventilation per m.
m. polypoid lesion
m. ventilation (V_E)
m. volume
mirabile

Mirizzi syndrome
mirror-image
m.-i. breast biopsy
m.-i. interpretation
m.-i. laryngoscopy
m.-i. reflection
misarticulation
misdirection phenomenon
mismatch
ventilation/perfusion m.
misregistration
chemical shift m.
flow m.
oblique flow m.
missed fracture
missile
m. injury
m. track abscess
m. trajectory
missionary position
mistranslation
Mital elbow release technique
Mitchell osteotomy
miter technique
mitochondrial myopathy, encephalopathy, lactic acidosis, and stroke-like syndrome (MELAS)
mitomycin transarterial embolization treatment
mitosis
mitotic activity
mitral
m. balloon commissurotomy
m. balloon valvotomy
m. regurgitation murmur
m. valve
m. valve aneurysm
m. valve anulus
m. valve area
m. valve closure index
m. valve disorder
m. valve gradient
m. valve homograft graft
m. valve insufficiency
m. valve leaflet
m. valve prolapse, aortic anomalies, skeletal changes, and skin changes (MASS)
m. valve prolapse syndrome
m. valve repair
m. valve replacement
m. valve-transverse (MV-T)
m. valve valvotomy
m. valvuloplasty
mitralis
mitralization
Mitrofanoff
M. appendicovesicostomy
M. conduit
M. continent urinary diversion technique
M. principle
M. procedure
M. stoma
mittelschmerz
MIVAP
minimally invasive video-assisted parathyroidectomy
mixed
m. acid fermentation
m. chancre
m. connective-tissue disease
m. connective tissue disorder
m. fat-water density lesion
m. fungal/bacterial infection
m. fungal organism
m. hemorrhoid
m. malignant glioma
m. nail infection
m. nerve
m. nodule
m. sclerotic and lytic bone lesion
m. tumor
m. venous-lymphatic malformation
m. venous oxygen content
m. venous oxygen saturation
mixed-density mass
mixture
anesthetic gas m.
epinephrine-anesthetic m.
racemic m.
Mize-Bucholz-Grogen approach
Mizuno-Hirohata-Kashiwagi technique
Mizuno technique
mks
meter-kilogram-second
MLAC
minimum local analgesic concentration
M line
MLN
mesenteric lymph node
MLR
major liver resection

NOTES

M

MMK
Marshall-Marchetti-Krantz
MMK procedure
MMP
matrix metalloproteinase
Moberg
M. advancement flap
M. key-pinch procedure
Moberg-Gedda
M.-G. fracture
M.-G. open reduction
mobile
m. arc
m. sternum
mobilis
mobility
abdominal wall m.
impaired m.
muscle tissue m.
rotation m.
translation m.
mobilization
circumferential m.
colonic m.
dorsal thyroid m.
esophageal m.
grade 1–5 m.
intraperitoneal m.
joint m.
lateral band m.
localized leukocyte m.
nonthrust m.
rectal m.
soft-tissue m.
spinal joint m.
stapes m.
stem cell m.
m. test
thoracoscopic esophageal m.
m. with impulse
MOD
mesioocclusodistal
multiple organ dysfunction
modality
adjuvant diagnostic m.
diagnostic m.
imaging m.
implantable pain m.
nonexcisional m.
therapeutic m.
treatment m.
mode
Bernse Coping M.'s (BeCoMo)
tumor dormancy m.
model
corpectomy m.
Emory Pain Estimate M. (EPEM)
Gail m.
guidance-cooperation m.
implant m.
mutual participation m.
tumor kinetic m.
Zimmerman-Brittin exchange m.
modeling-derivation
moderate
m. hyperplasia
m. pain
m. resuscitative hypothermia
moderator band
modification
activator m.
Al-Ghorab m.
appliance m.
A-V nodal m.
Bloom-Raney m.
Bonfiglio m.
bracket m.
Burch m.
Burwell-Scott m. of Watson-Jones incision
C-D screw m.
Clark-Southwick-Odgen m.
Deller m.
Duncan-Lovell m.
environment m.
fiber tip m.
Gesell test with Knobloch m.
glutathione m.
Gunderson-Sosin m.
Harriluque sublaminar wiring m.
interference m.
Kelly-Kennedy m.
Kleinert m.
Losee m.
Martin m.
Mason-Likar limb lead m.
Millen-Read m.
Mullins m.
Muzsnai m.
Neer m.
Pereyra-Lebhertz m.
posttranslation m.
racemic m.
Raz m.
Rosch m.
Schoemaker m.
Seddon m.
Sequeira-Khanuja m.
Smith m.
Soper m.
Stauffer m.
Strickland m.
thiol m.
Van Herick m.
Youngwhich m.

modified
m. band lid method
m. Bassini herniorrhaphy
m. Belsey fundoplication
m. Belsey fundoplication procedure
m. Belsey fundoplication technique
m. brachial technique
m. Cantwell technique
m. Child technique
m. dorsalis pedis myofascial flap
m. Essed-Schroeder corporoplasty
m. flap operation
m. Gibson incision
m. Hassan open technique
m. Heller esophagomyotomy
m. Hoke-Miller flatfoot procedure
m. Irving-type tubal ligation
m. Konno procedure
m. lithotomy position
m. mastopexy
m. McVay herniorrhaphy
m. method of Pugh
m. mold and surface replacement arthroplasty
m. Norfolk procedure
m. piggyback (MPB)
m. piggyback technique
m. Pomeroy technique
m. radical hysterectomy
m. radical mastectomy
m. radical mastoidectomy
m. radical neck dissection
m. Raynaud phenomenon
m. Ritgen maneuver
m. Sacks-Vine push-pull technique
m. Seldinger procedure
m. Seldinger technique
m. Shouldice hernioplasty
m. Sugiura procedure
m. TAPP hernioplasty
The M. Somatic Pain Questionnaire
m. Toupe procedure
m. Toupe technique
m. two-portal endoscopic carpal tunnel release
m. ultrafiltration
m. Van Lint anesthesia
m. V-Y advancement technique
m. Weber-Fergusson procedure
m. Whitehead hemorrhoidectomy
m. Wies procedure
m. Young urethroplasty
M. Zung Depression Scale

modiolus, pl. **modioli**

MODS
multiple organ dysfunction syndrome

modulation
amplitude m.
antigenic m.
autonomic m.
biochemical m.
brightness m.
frequency m.
immune m.
obstruction-induced m.
pain m.
m. potential
pressure amplitude m.
sex steroid m.
specific m.

module
dialysate preparation m.

Moebius anomaly

Moe scoliosis technique

MOF
multiorgan failure
multiple organ failure

Mogensen procedure

Mohrenheim
M. fossa
M. space

Mohr syndrome

Mohs
M. fresh tissue chemosurgery technique
M. micrographic surgery
M. microsurgery technique
M. microsurgical resection

moist
m. gangrene
m. mucous membrane

moisture exchanger

molar
anchor m.
m. teeth
m. tooth fracture
m. tube

mold acetabular arthroplasty

molding
compression m.
injection m.
tissue m.

NOTES

molecular
m. biology
m. external layer
m. genetics
m. lesion
m. mass
m. sieve
m. technique
Molesworth-Campbell elbow approach
Molesworth osteotomy
Moll gland
molluscíformis
Moloney
M. hernia repair
M. line
Molteno
M. drainage
M. episcleral explant
moment
activation m.
three-point bending m.
Monakow
M. bundle
M. tract
Moncrieff operation
Mondini
M. anomaly
M. deformity
M. pulmonary arteriovenous malformation
Mondini-Alexander malformation
Mondor disease
Monfort operation
monilial infection
monitor
intraoperative m.
monitored
m. anesthesia care (MAC)
m. anesthesia care anesthesia
m. anesthesia care anesthetic technique
m. anesthesia control
monitoring
airway gas m.
anesthetic m.
anticoagulant m.
anticoagulation m.
blood pressure m.
central venous pressure m.
close m.
depth of anesthesia m.
ECoG m.
electrophysiologic m.
epicardial m.
esophageal pH m.
evoked external urethral sphincter potential m.
external fetal m.
fetal heart rate m.
hemodynamic m.
hospital m.
intracranial pressure m.
intraoperative neurophysiologic m. (IOM)
intraoperative parathyroid hormone m.
intraoperative transcranial Doppler m.
invasive hemodynamic m.
laboratory m.
neuromuscular blockade m.
outcome m.
posttetanic count m.
radiation m.
screw position perioperative m.
standard patient m.
m. technique
tissue pH m.
transcutaneous oxygen m.
two-dimensional m.
vigilance m.
water vapor m.
monoamine reuptake-inhibitor
monochromatic aberration
monoclonal
m. adenoma
m. antibody (MAb)
m. component
m. expansion
m. growth
monoclonality
monocular fixation
monodermoma
monodisperse
monofixation syndrome
monoinfection
monomalleolar ankle fracture
mononuclear cell infiltration
monopolar
m. coagulation
m. electrocautery
m. electrocoagulation
monorchidic
monorchidism
monorecidive chancre
monospherical total shoulder arthroplasty
monotherapy
oral m.
monotypic lesion
monoxide
carbon m. (CO)
dinitrogen m.
nitrogen m.
Monro
bursa of M.

M. foramen
M. line
Monro-Richter line
mons, pl. **montes**
m. plasty
m. pubis
Monte Carlo multiway sensitivity analysis method
Monteggia
M. dislocation
M. equivalent lesion
M. forearm fracture
Montercaux fracture
montes (*pl. of* mons)
Montgomery
M. gland
M. tracheostomy
Monticelli-Spinelli distraction technique
mood state
Moore
M. fracture
M. method
M. osteotomy-osteoclasis
M. posterior approach
M. technique
M. tibial plateau fracture classification
Moran operation
Morax
M. keratoplasty
M. operation
morbidity
cumulative operative m.
m. excess
febrile m.
intraoperative m.
long-term m.
m. and mortality
perioperative m.
postoperative m.
morbidly obese patient
morcel
morcellation
m. operation
Robinson m.
Robinson-Chung-Farahvar clavicular m.
m. technique
morcellement
morcellized
m. bone graft
Moreland-Marder-Anspach femoral stem removal
Morel-Fatio-Lalardie operation
Morel-Lavele lesion
Morgagni
M. cartilage
M. caruncle
M. crypt
M. foramen
M. fossa
M. fovea
M. frenum
M. hernia
M. lacuna
M. retinaculum
M. sinus
M. tubercle
M. ventricle
Morgagni-Larrey type hernia
Morgan-Casscells meniscus suturing technique
Morganella morganii
morganii
Morganella m.
Morgan line
moribund
Morinaga hemorrhoidectomy
Morison
M. incision
M. method
M. pouch
morning glory optic disk anomaly
morphallactic regeneration
morpheaform basal cell carcinoma
morphea-like lesion
morphine narcotic analgesic therapy
morphogenesis
branching m.
morphological difference
morphologic classification
morphology
endometrial m.
gram-stain m.
lesion m.
Morquio syndrome
Morrey-Bryan total elbow arthroplasty
Morris hepatoma cell line
Morrison
M. neurovascular free flap
M. technique
Morse head

NOTES

mortality
cause-specific m.
cumulative operative m.
disease-associated m.
hospital m.
morbidity and m.
operative m.
perioperative m.
postoperative m.
m. rate
mortar kidney
mortification
Morton plane
Moschcowitz procedure
Mose technique
Mosher operation
Mosher-Toti operation
Moss
M. classification
M. operation
Motais operation
moth-eaten
m.-e. appearance
m.-e. bone destruction
mother
m. cyst
m. method
moth patch
motilin
m. effect
m. level
motility
contractile m.
cyclic · fasting m.
m. disturbance
jejunal m.
postoperative m.
upper jejunal m.
motion
abdominal respiratory m.
angulation m.
m. barrier
osteokinematic m.
pattern of m.
range of m. (ROM)
m. segment
translation m.
motion-preserving procedure
motivating operation
motor
m. activity
m. change
m. decussation
m. disturbance
m. examination
m. fusion
m. nerve
m. oil peritoneal fluid
m. paraplegia
m. pattern
m. perseveration
m. point
m. point block
m. point block anesthetic technique
m. recording
m. response
motor-evoked
m.-e. potential (MEP)
m.-e. response (MER)
m.-e. response to transcranial stimulation (tc-MER)
Mott body
mottled appearance
Mouchet fracture
Mould arthroplasty
mounted point stone
mouse
joint m.
peritoneal m.
mouth preparation
mouth-to-mouth
m.-t.-m. respiration
m.-t.-m. resuscitation
m.-t.-m. ventilation
movable
m. joint
m. kidney
m. spleen
m. testis
Movat pentachrome method
movement
anterosuperior external ilium m.
border tissue m.
bowel m.
m. disorder
dissociation m.
external ilium m.
extraneous m.
extraocular m.
fetal body m.
head m.
posteroinferior external m.
primary rotation m.
saccadic eye m.
segmentation m.
sound-stimulated fetal m.
vocal cord m.
movement-related pain
Moynihan
M. operation
M. position
MPAC
Memorial Pain Assessment Card
MPB
modified piggyback
MPB technique

MPD
main pancreatic duct
MPGR
multiple planar gradient-recalled
MPGR technique
MPI
Multidimensional Pain Inventory
MP-L
midpapillary longitudinal
MP-L image
MPQ
McGill Pain Questionnaire
MP-RAGE
magnitude preparation-rapid acquisition gradient echo
MP-RAGE technique
MP-T
midpapillary transverse
MP-T image
MPT
multidisciplinary pain treatment
MR
magnetic resonance
MR spectroscopy
MRA
magnetic resonance angiography
MRI
magnetic resonance imaging
MRI cholangiography
intraoperative MRI
MSB
mediastinal shed blood
MSI
magnetic source imaging
MSOF
multisystem organ failure
MTBE
methyl-*tert*-butyl ether
MTBE therapy
mTBI
mild traumatic brain injury
Mubarak-Hargens decompression technique
mucilaginous gland
mucinous
m. adenocarcinoma
m. ascites
m. cystadenocarcinoma
muciparous gland
mucobuccal
m. fold
m. reflection
mucocele
appendix m.
breast m.
frontal sinus m.
frontoethmoidal m.
maxillary sinus m.
orbital m.
paranasal m.
retention m.
sinus m.
sphenoid m.
mucociliary function
mucocutaneous
m. hemorrhoid
m. junction
m. lesion
m. lymph node syndrome
m. manifestation
m. muscle
m. pigmentation of Peutz-Jeghers syndrome
mucoepidermal carcinoma
mucoepidermoid carcinoma
mucogingival
m. line
m. surgery
mucoid ascites
mucoperichondrial flap
mucoperiosteal
m. periodontal flap
m. periodontal graft
m. sliding flap
mucopolysaccharidosis
mucopurulent exudate
mucopyocele
mucor infection
mucormycosis
mucosa
bursa m.
colorectal m.
ectopic gastric m.
endocervical m.
gastric m.
gastroduodenal m.
inlet patch m.
lingual m.
multifocal ectopic gastric m.
oral m.
pharyngeal m.
ulcerated m.
upper respiratory tract m.

NOTES

mucosa-associated
m.-a. lymphoid tissue (MALT)
m.-a. lymphoid tissue lymphoma
mucosae
mucosal
m. ablation
m. abnormality
m. advancement
m. atrophy
m. barrier
m. biopsy
m. bridge
m. destruction
m. esophageal ring
m. hernia
m. homeostasis
m. inflammation
m. invasion
m. lesion
m. line
m. needle aspiration
m. neuroma syndrome
m. patch replacement
m. periodontal flap
m. periodontal graft
m. proctectomy
m. reconditioning
m. relaxing incision technique
m. remnant
m. tunic
m. ulceration
m. vascular dilation
m. web
m. weight
mucosa-to-mucosa
m.-t.-m. anastomosis
m.-t.-m. Roux-en-Y hepaticojejunostomy
mucosectomy
endoanal m.
rectal m.
transabdominal m.
transanal m.
mucositis
radiation m.
mucous
m. colic
m. desiccation
m. fistula
m. gland
m. membrane
m. membrane graft
m. membrane lesion
m. membrane ulceration
m. patch
m. plug syndrome
m. sheath
mucronate
mucus
excess m.
mud bed
Muehrcke line
Mueller
M. femoral supracondylar fracture classification
M. hip arthroplasty
M. intertochanteric varus osteotomy
M. maneuver
M. method
M. operation
M. patellar tendon graft
M. technique
M. tibial fracture classification
M. transposition osteotomy
Mueller-type femoral head replacement
Mueller-Walle method
MUGA
multiple gated acquisition
MUGA exercise stress test
mulberry
m. calculus
m. lesion
mulberry-shaped mass
Mules
M. graft
M. operation
Mulholland sphincterotomy
muliebre
muliebris
Müller
M. capsule
M. duct
M. duct body
M. maneuver
Müller-Hillis maneuver
müllerian
m. duct anomaly
m. duct derivation syndrome
m. duct fusion
m. inhibiting substance
Mullins
M. blade technique
M. modification
multangular
m. bone
m. ridge fracture
multiaxial
m. classification
m. joint
multicentricity
multicentric study
Multidimensional Pain Inventory (MPI)
multidisciplinary
m. approach
m. pain treatment (MPT)
multidose vial

multifactorial
multifetal pregnancy reduction
multifetation
multifidus
m. muscle
multifocal
m. change
m. ectopic gastric mucosa
m. enhancing lesion
m. inflammation
m. tumor
m. variety
multifocal-extensive
m.-e. DCIS
m.-e. disease
multiforme
multigated angiogram
multigland
m. disease
m. hyperplasia
multiglandular
m. disease
m. parathyroid hyperplasia
multi-infection
multilamellar body
multilevel
m. atherosclerotic arterial occlusive disease
m. fracture
m. laminectomy
multilocular
m. cyst
m. cystic lesion
multiloculated renal mass
multimerization
multimodal
m. adjuvant therapy
m. analgesia
multimodality therapy
multinodular goiter
multiorgan
m. failure (MOF)
m. hernia
m. system dysfunction
m. system failure
multiparameter sensor
multiplanar image
multiple
m. calcification
m. cone root canal filling method
m. core biopsy
m. endocrine neoplasia (MEN)
m. endocrine neoplasia syndrome
m. endocrine neoplasia type 2a (MEN-2a)
m. endocrine neoplasia type 2a, 2b syndrome
m. endocrine neoplasia type 2b (MEN-2b)
m. endocrinopathy
m. exostoses
m. fracture
m. gated acquisition (MUGA)
m. gland hyperplasia
m. hamartoma syndrome
m. hepatitis virus infection
m. hydatid disease
m. inert gas elimination technique (MIGET)
m. inert gas exchange
m. intestinal neoplasia (MIN)
m. line scan imaging
m. macrocyst
m. mechanism inhaled anesthetic
m. mucosal neuroma syndrome
m. myeloma staging
m. organ dysfunction (MOD)
m. organ dysfunction syndrome (MODS)
m. organ failure (MOF)
m. organ failure syndrome
m. organ system failure
m. planar gradient-recalled (MPGR)
m. pterygium syndrome
m. ray amputation
m. sensitive point
m. shunt levels
m. site
m. site inhaled anesthetic
m. spin-echo imaging
m. system atrophy
m. system organ failure
m. therapy
multiple-balloon valvuloplasty
multiple-echo imaging
multiple-plane imaging
multiple-point sacral fixation
multiple-port
m.-p. incision
m.-p. incision method
m.-p. incision procedure
m.-p. incision technique
multiple-punch resection
multiple-stage approach

M

NOTES

multipolar
m. coagulation
m. electrocautery
m. electrocoagulation
multipotential stem cell
multiray fracture
multisegmental resection
multistaged carrier flap
Multistage Maximal Effort exercise stress test
multisystem
m. disorder
m. failure
m. organ failure (MSOF)
multivessel PTCA
multiviscera
multivisceral graft
Muma Assessment Program
Mumford
M. procedure
M. resection
Mumford-Gurd arthroplasty
mummification
m. necrosis
pulp m.
Munro
M. and Parker laparoscopic hysterectomy classification
M. point
Munro-Kerr maneuver
mu receptor
murine
m. graft
m. mesangial cell line
murmur
aortic regurgitation m.
Austin Flint m.
diamond ejection m.
ejection m.
endocardial m.
exit block m.
exocardial m.
expiratory m.
extracardiac m.
mitral regurgitation m.
reduplication m.
systolic ejection m.
Murphy method
muscarinic
m. agonist
m. receptor
muscle
abdominal external oblique m.
abdominal internal oblique m.
abductor digiti minimi m.
abductor hallucis m.
abductor longus m.
abductor magnus m.
abductor pollicis brevis m.
abductor pollicis longus m.
accessory flexor m.
Aeby m.
airway smooth m. (ASM)
Albinus m.
anconeus m.
antagonistic m.
anterior auricular m.
anterior cervical intertransverse m.
anterior rectus m.
anterior scalene m.
anterior serratus m.
anterior tibial m.
antigravity m.
antitragicus m.
appendicular m.
aryepiglottic m.
arytenoid m.
auricular m.
axial m.
Bell m.
belt m.
m. biopsy
bipennate m.
Bovero m.
brachial m.
brachioradial m.
branchiomeric m.
Braune m.
m. breakdown
broadest m.
bronchoesophageal m.
buccinator m.
bulbocavernosus m.
m. cachexia
Casser perforated m.
ceratocricoid m.
cervical rotator m.
cheek m.
chin m.
chondroglossus m.
circular pharyngeal m.
coccygeal m.
coccygeus m.
Coiter m.
compressor naris m.
coracobrachial m.
coracobrachialis m.
corrugator cutis m.
corrugator supercilii m.
cowl m.
cremaster m.
cremasteric m.
cricoarytenoid m.
cricopharyngeus m.
cricothyroid m.
cruciate m.

crus m.
cutaneomucous m.
cutaneous m.
dartos m.
de-epithelialized rectus abdominis m. (DRAM)
deltoid m.
detrusor m.
digastric m.
dilator m.
m. dissection
m. distraction
dorsal sacrococcygeal m.
Duverney m.
m. dystonia
elevator m.
m. energy technique
epicranial m.
epicranius m.
erector spinae m.
extensor carpi radialis brevis m.
extensor carpi radialis longus m.
extensor carpi ulnaris m.
extensor digiti minimi m.
extensor digiti quinti m.
extensor digitorum brevis m.
extensor digitorum communis m.
extensor digitorum longus m.
extensor hallucis brevis m.
extensor hallucis longus m.
extensor indicis proprius m.
extensor pollicis brevis m.
extensor pollicis longus m.
extraocular m.
extrinsic m.
facial m.
femoral m.
fibularis brevis m.
fibularis longus m.
fibularis tertius m.
fixator m.
m. flap
flexor hallucis brevis m.
frontalis m.
Gavard m.
genioglossal m.
geniohyoid m.
glossopalatine m.
gluteus maximus m.
greater rhomboid m.
Guthrie m.
hamstring m.
m. hernia
Horner m.
Houston m.
hyoglossal m.
hyoid m.
hypothenar m.
iliac m.
iliococcygeal m.
iliocostal m.
iliohypogastric m.
iliopsoas m.
infrahyoid m.
interosseous m.
interspinal m.
intertransverse m.
intrinsic m.
ischiocavernous m.
Jung m.
Klein m.
Kohlrausch m.
Krause m.
laryngeal m.
lateral m.
longus capitis m.
longus colli m.
m. lysis
Marcacci m.
masseter m.
mastication m.
m. measurement
mentalis m.
Merkel m.
mimetic m.
mucocutaneous m.
multifidus m.
muscular fascia
mylohyoid m.
nasal m.
oblique abdominal m.
oblique arytenoid m.
oblique auricular m.
occipitofrontal m.
occipitofrontalis m.
ocular m.
omohyoid m.
orbicular m.
orbital m.
orbitalis m.
palatoglossus m.
palatopharyngeal sphincter m.
palatopharyngeus m.
palpebral m.

NOTES

M

muscle *(continued)*

pectoralis m.
pectorodorsal m.
pennate m.
perineal m.
peroneal m.
peroneus brevis m.
peroneus longus m.
peroneus tertius m.
piriform m.
plantar interosseous m.
plantar quadrate m.
platysma m.
pleuroesophageal m.
popliteal m.
posterior cricoarytenoid m.
procerus m.
pronator quadratus m.
pronator teres m.
m. proteolysis
psoas major m.
psoas minor m.
pubococcygeal m.
puboprostatic m.
puborectal m.
pubovaginal m.
pubovesical m.
pupillae sphincter m.
pupillary m.
pyramidal auricular m.
quadrate m.
radial dilator m.
rectococcygeal m.
rectourethral m.
rectouterine m.
rectovesical m.
rectus abdominis m.
red m.
Reisseisen m.
m. relaxant
m. repositioning
m. resection
rhomboid major m.
rhomboid minor m.
ribbon m.
Riolan m.
risorius m.
rotator cuff m.
salpingopharyngeal m.
scalenus anterior m.
scalenus medius m.
scalenus minimus m.
scalenus posterior m.
scalp m.
scapular m.
Sebileau m.
second tibial m.
semimembranosus m.
semispinal m.
semispinalis capitis m.
semispinalis cervicis m.
semitendinosus m.
serratus anterior m.
serratus posterior inferior m.
serratus posterior superior m.
shunt m.
Sibson m.
skeletal m.
m. sliding operation
smooth m.
Soemmerring m.
sphincter m.
spinal m.
stapedius m.
sternal m.
sternochondroscapular m.
sternoclavicular m.
sternocleidomastoid m.
sternohyoid m.
sternomastoid m.
sternothyroid m.
strap m.
striated m.
styloauricular m.
styloglossus m.
stylohyoid m.
stylopharyngeal m.
subclavian m.
subcostal m.
suboccipital m.
subscapular m.
subscapularis m.
supinator m.
supraclavicular m.
suprahyoid m.
supraspinalis m.
supraspinatus m.
supraspinous m.
suspensory m.
synergistic m.
temporal m.
temporoparietal m.
tensor fascia lata m.
teres major m.
Theile m.
thenar m.
thoracic interspinal m.
thoracic intertransverse m.
thoracic longissimus m.
thoracic rotator m.
thyroarytenoid m.
thyroepiglottic m.
thyrohyoid m.
thyroid m.
m. tissue mobility
Tod m.

toe extensor m.
Toynbee m.
trachealis m.
tracheloclavicular m.
tragicus m.
transverse abdominal m.
transverse arytenoid m.
transverse rectus abdominis m. (TRAM)
transversospinal m.
transversus abdominis m.
Treitz m.
triangular m.
true m.
two-bellied m.
unipennate m.
unstriated m.
uvular m.
Valsalva m.
ventral sacrococcygeus m.
vestigial m.
visceral m.
vocal m.
vocalis m.
m. wasting
m. weakness
white m.
Wilson m.
wrinkler m.
zygomaticus major m.
zygomaticus minor m.

muscle-balancing procedure
muscle-periosteal flap
muscle-plasty
Speed V-Y m.-p.
muscle-sparing thoracotomy
muscle-splitting
m.-s. incision
m.-s. technique
muscle-tendon transplantation
muscular
m. anesthesia
m. artery
m. atrophy
m. change
m. coat
m. contraction
m. esophageal ring
m. fascia
m. pulley
m. substance
m. tissue
m. triangle
m. tunic
musculare
muscularis
m. tunnel closure
musculature
musculi (*pl. of* musculus)
musculoaponeurotic
musculocutaneous
m. free flap
m. nerve
musculocutaneus
musculomembranous
musculophrenic
m. artery
m. vein
musculophrenica
musculophrenicae
musculoplasty
Rambo m.
musculoskeletal
m. disorder
m. infection
m. system
m. tissue
m. tumor
musculospiral
m. groove
m. nerve
musculotendinous
m. cuff
m. flap
musculotubal canal
musculotubarius
musculus, pl. **musculi**
mushroom
corneal m.
m. corneal graft
mushroom-shaped mass
mussitation
Mustard
M. intraatrial procedure
M. operation
Mustardé
M. graft
M. operation
M. otoplasty procedure
M. rotational cheek flap
mutation
m. analysis
breast cancer-related m.
m. carrier

NOTES

mutation *(continued)*
m. carrier status
factor V Leiden m.
somatic m.
true m.
mutator gene
mutilation
mutual participation model
Muzsnai modification
MV
maternal venous
MV blood
MVD
microvascular decompression
MV-T
mitral valve-transverse
MV-T image
MVV
maximum voluntary ventilation
mycelial mass
mycobacterial infection
Mycobacterium
M. avium complex infection
M. avium-intracellulare (MAI)
M. avium-intracellulare infection
***Mycoplasma* infection**
mycotic
m. aneurysm
m. club nail
m. infection
m. pseudoaneurysm
myectomy
anorectal m.
m. operation
rectal m.
septal m.
myectopy
myelination
nerve fiber m.
optic pathway m.
myelinization
myelinolysis
central pontine m.
pontine m.
myelitis
myeloablation
myeloblastoma
myelocele
myelocystocele
myelocystomeningocele
myelocytoma
myelodiastasis
myelodysplasia
myeloid tissue
myelolipoma
myelolysis
myeloma
myelomalacia
myelomeningocele
m. operation
m. repair
myelomonocytic cell line
myelonic
myelopathic symptom
myelopathy
cervical spondylitic m.
radiation m.
spondylitic m.
myelophthisic
myelophthisis
myelopoiesis
extramedullary m.
myelorrhagia
myelorrhaphy
commissural m.
myelosarcoma
myeloschisis
myeloscopy
flexible fiberoptic m.
myelotomy
Bischof m.
commissural m.
midline m.
T m.
myenteric
m. plexus
m. reflex
myentericus
myenteron
mylohyoid
m. artery
m. bridge
m. fossa
m. groove
m. line
m. muscle
m. nerve
m. ridge
mylohyoidea
mylohyoideus
mylopharyngeus
myoablative therapy
myoarchitectonic
myoblastoma
myocardial
m. contusion
m. cytochrome
m. hibernation
m. infarction (MI)
m. inflammation
m. ischemia
m. mass
m. perforation
m. protection
m. revascularization

m. rupture
m. tissue
myocardiorrhaphy
myocarditis
myocardium
postischemic stunned m.
m. retrograde
stunned m.
myocele
myocutaneous
m. flap
m. graft
myocytolysis
coagulative m.
myocytoma
myodegeneration
myodermal flap
myodesis
myodiastasis
myoelastic-aerodynamic theory of phonation
myoepithelioma
myofascial
m. flap
m. manipulation
m. pain
m. pain syndrome
m. trigger point
myofibroblastoma
myofibroma
myofunctional therapy
myogenic motor-evoked potential (MEP)
myoglobin tubular obstruction
myoid cyst
myoides
myolipoma
myolysis
cardiotoxic m.
myoma
myomatectomy
myomectomy
abdominal m.
laparoscopic esophageal m.
vaginal m.
myomedulloblastoma
myometrial
myometrium
myomotomy
myonecrosis
clostridial m.
myoneural blockade
myoneurectomy
myoneuroma
myoneurotization
myopathy
myopectineal orifice
myopia
space m.
myoplastic muscle stabilization
myoplasty
myorrhaphy
myorrhexis
myosalpinx
myosarcoma
myositis
myosteoma
myotenontoplasty
myotenotomy
myotomy
circular m.
cricoid m.
cricopharyngeal m.
diverticulectomy with m.
esophageal m.
Heller m.
laparoscopic Heller m.
Livadatis circular m.
longitudinal m.
marginal m.
m. operation
septal m.
Z m.
myotomy-myectomy-septal resection
myotonia fluctuans
myotonic dystrophy
myotoxicity
myovascular sphincter
myovenous sphincter
myringoplasty
myringostapediopexy
myringotomy
m. with aspiration
myrtiformis
myxadenoma
myxedema
m. ascites
m. coma
myxochondrofibrosarcoma
myxochondroma
myxofibroma
myxofibrosarcoma
myxolipoma
myxoliposarcoma
myxoma sarcomatosum

M

NOTES

myxomatosis
myxoneuroma
myxopapilloma
myxosarcoma

N
newton
nabothian cyst
Naclerio
V-sign of N.
NACS
Neurologic and Adaptive Capacity Score
nadir pressure
Naffziger operation
Nagamatsu incision
nail
anteroposterior n.
beak n.
n. bed
boat n.
brittle n.
cannulated n.
n. change
closed n.
clubbed n.
n. clubbing
condylocephalic n.
convex n.
digital n.
n. disorder
Dooley n.
dystrophic n.
egg shell n.
n. fold
n. groove
half-and-half n.
hooked intramedullary n.
n. horn
ingrown n.
left-sided n.
n. length gauge method
n. matrix
mycotic club n.
nested n.
onychocryptosis n.
open-section n.
parrot-beak n.
pincer n.
n. pit
pitted n.
n. pitting
racket n.
ram horn n.
reamed n.
reedy n.
n. root
shell n.
sliding n.
telescoping n.
thickened n.
n. wall
yellow n.
nail-fold
n.-f. capillaroscopy
n.-f. removal
nailing
antegrade n.
femoral n.
intramedullary n.
reamed femoral n.
retrograde n.
tibiocalcaneal medullary n.
unreamed n.
nail-patella-elbow syndrome
nail-patella syndrome
nail-plate
n.-p. fixation
n.-p. removal
nail-to-nail bed angle
naive recipient
NaK-ATPase membrane
Nakayama anastomosis
Nalebuff classification
Nalebuff-Millender lateral band mobilization technique
nana
Nance leeway space
nanogram (ng)
napkin-ring
n.-r. annular lesion
n.-r. carcinoma
n.-r. compression
n.-r. defect
narcosis
adsorption theory of n.
colloid theory of n.
lipoid theory of n.
Meyer-Overton theory of n.
nitrogen n.
oxygen deprivation theory of n.
permeability theory of n.
surface tension theory of n.
thermodynamic theory of n.
narcotic
n. analgesic
n. reversal
narcotism
naris, pl. **nares**
narrowed pulse pressure
narrow-field laryngectomy
narrowing
disk space n.
eccentric n.
joint space n.
narrow internal ring

narrow-slit illumination
Narula method
nasal
- n. airway
- n. antrostomy
- n. border
- n. canal
- n. cavity
- n. cavity cancer
- n. concha
- n. crest
- n. deformity
- n. dissection
- n. endoscopic surgery
- n. endoscopy
- n. foramen
- n. fracture
- n. height
- n. hemorrhage
- n. index
- n. intubation
- n. mucosal identification
- n. mucosal ulceration
- n. muscle
- n. oxygen (NO)
- n. pharynx
- n. placode
- n. port
- n. provocation test
- n. pyramid
- n. reconstruction
- n. respiration
- n. septal perforation
- n. septum
- n. tip
- n. tract
- n. trumpet
- n. vestibule
- n. wall

nasale
nasalis
NASCET
North American Symptomatic Carotid Endarterectomy Trial
nasi
nasioiniac
nasion-alveolar point line
nasion soft tissue
Nasmyth membrane
nasobasilar line
nasobregmatic arc
nasociliary
- n. ganglion
- n. nerve

nasoendoscopy
nasofrontal
- n. duct
- n. vein

nasofrontalis
nasogastric (NG)
- n. intubation
- n. suction
- n. tonometry

nasoileal
nasojejunal
nasojugal fold
nasolabial
- n. groove
- n. line
- n. rotation flap

nasolacrimal
- n. canal
- n. sac

nasomandibular fixation
nasomaxillaris
nasomaxillary suture
nasooccipital arc
nasooral
nasoorbital fracture
nasopalatine injection
nasopharyngeal
- n. airway
- n. biopsy
- n. carcinoma
- n. groove
- n. hematoma
- n. hemorrhage
- n. passage
- n. suction

nasopharyngoscopy
nasopharynx
nasorostral
nasotracheal
- n. intubation (NTI)
- n. intubation anesthetic technique
- n. suction

nasovesicular catheter technique
natal cleft
natatorium
nates (*pl. of* natis)
Nathan-Trung modification of Krukenberg hand reconstruction
National
- N. Cancer Data Base (NCDB)
- N. Cancer Institute (NCI)
- N. Football Head and Neck Injury Registry
- N. Marrow Donor Program
- N. Pediatric Trauma Registry (NPTR)
- N. Surgical Adjuvant Breast and Bowel Project (NSABP)

natis, pl. **nates**
native
- n. caudate lobe
- n. coronary anatomy

n. liver
n. myocardial microcirculation
n. portal vein
n. renal biopsy

natriuresis
pressure n.

naturales

natural method

nature
benign n.
dense n.
minimally invasive n.
n. root canal filling

navel

navicular
n. abdomen
n. bone
n. fracture

naviculare

navicularis

naviculocapitate
n. fracture
n. fracture syndrome

naviculocuneiform fusion

navigated
n. brain tumor surgery
n. neurosurgery

navigation
surgical microscope n. (SMN)

navigational surgery

NCDB
National Cancer Data Base

NCI
National Cancer Institute

NCJ
needle catheter jejunostomy

NCPB
neurolytic celiac plexus block

NCRLM
noncolorectal liver metastasis
isolated NCRLM
unique NCRLM

NDSA
nondermatomal sensory abnormality

Nd:YAG
neodymium:yttrium-aluminum-garnet
Nd:YAG cyclophotocoagulation
Nd:YAG laser ablation
Nd:YAG laser irradiation
Nd:YAG laser therapy

Nealon technique

near
n. fixation
n. visual point

near-anatomic position

near-and-far suture technique

near-infrared (NIR)
n.-i. measurement
n.-i. spectrophotometry
n.-i. spectroscopy

near-point relative

near-total
n.-t. esophagectomy
n.-t. gastrectomy
n.-t. laryngectomy
n.-t. pancreatectomy
n.-t. thyroidectomy

NEB
New England Baptist
NEB hip arthroplasty

nebula, pl. **nebulae**
corneal n.

nebulization

nebulizer
spinning disk n.
ultrasonic n.

NEC
necrotizing enterocolitis

neck
anterolateral n.
aortic n.
deep anterior n.
N. Disability Index
n. dissection
n. exploration
n. extension position
n. flap
n. fracture
gallbladder n.
implant n.
implant superstructure n.
innervation of head and n.
pancreatic n.
residual n.
superficial n.
surgical n.
virgin n.

necrectomy

necrolysis
epidermal n.
toxic epidermal n.

necropsy

necroscopy

NOTES

necrosectomy
initial n.
operative n.
reoperative n.
necrosis
acute tubular n. (ATN)
aminoglycoside tubular n.
avascular n.
bloodless zone of n.
caseation n.
centrilobular n.
cerebral radiation n. (CRN)
cheesy n.
coagulation n.
cumarin n.
cystic medial n.
diffuse n.
electrocoagulation n.
Erdheim cystic medial n.
ethanol-induced tumor n.
fat n.
flap n.
frank n.
hepatic n.
infected n.
liquefaction n.
mummification n.
pancreatic n.
periodontal membrane n.
peripancreatic n.
pressure n.
radiation n.
skin flap n.
soft-tissue n.
splenic n.
strangulation n.
subcutaneous n.
thermal n.
tissue n.
tumor n.
necrotic
n. abscess
n. flap
n. focus
n. hemorrhoid
n. hyalinized tissue
n. inflammation
n. metastasis
n. remain
n. ulceration
necrotic/fibrotic tissue
necrotizing
n. angiitis
n. enterocolitis (NEC)
n. granulomatous inflammation
n. infection
n. pancreatitis (NP)
necrotomy
osteoplastic n.
needle
n. ablation
n. arthroscopy
n. aspiration
n. aspiration cytology
n. catheter jejunostomy (NCJ)
n. core biopsy
n. laparoscopy
n. localization
n. prick
n. reaction
n. suspension procedure
n. thoracentesis
n. thoracentesis method
n. thoracentesis procedure
n. thoracentesis technique
n. tracheoesophageal puncture
n. tract
n. tract implantation
n. tract tumor seeding
needle-free system
needleholder
needle-knife
n.-k. papillotomy
n.-k. sphincterotomy
n.-k. technique
needleless
n. intravenous administration system
n. suturing
needle-localized open biopsy (NLOB)
needlepoint electrocautery
needlescopic laparoscopic cholecystectomy
needlescopy
Needles split cast method
needlestick injury
needle-through-needle single interspace technique
Neer
N. acromioplasty
N. capsular shift procedure
N. hemiarthroplasty
N. modification
N. open reduction
N. posterior shoulder reconstruction
N. shoulder fracture classification
N. unconstrained shoulder arthroplasty
Neer femur fracture classification
Neer-Horowitz humeral fracture classification
negative
n. abdominal pressure
n. appendectomy
n. aspiration
axillary node n.

n. breast biopsy
n. celiotomy
n. control enzyme induction
n. correlation
n. cytology
n. effect
n. end-expiratory pressure
false n.
n. inotropy
n. inspiratory breathing
n. inspiratory pressure measurement
n. laparotomy
n. margin
n. peritoneal cytology (NPC)
n. predictive value (NPV)
n. pressure therapy
true n.
tumor receptor protein n.

negative-pressure
neglected rupture
neglect-like phenomena
Neher operation
Nehra-Mack operation
Neill-Mooser body
neisserial infection
Nélaton
N. ankle dislocation
N. fiber
N. fold
N. line
N. sphincter

nematode infection
neoadjuvant
n. therapy
n. total androgen ablation

neobladder
neocartilage formation
neocystostomy
neodymium:YAG laser therapy
neodymium:yttrium-aluminum-garnet (Nd:YAG)
neoesophagus
neoformation
neoglottic reconstruction
neointima formation
neonatal
n. anesthesia
N. Facial Pain Inventory (NFCS)
N. Infant Pain Scale (NIPS)
n. infection
n. intracranial hemorrhage
n. intraventricular hemorrhage
n. line
n. pulmonary transplantation
n. resuscitation
n. ring
n. severe hyperparathyroidism
n. thymectomy

neonate
n. examination
surgical n.
n. ventilation

neoplasia
multiple endocrine n. (MEN)
multiple endocrine n. type 2a (MEN-2a)
multiple endocrine n. type 2b (MEN-2b)
multiple intestinal n. (MIN)
thyroid n.

neoplasm
asymptomatic n.
brain n.
colonic n.
follicular n.
hepatic n.
intraaxial parenchymal brain n.
n. metastasis
parenchymal brain n.
pediatric n.
vascular n.

neoplastic
n. dissemination
n. fracture
n. lesion
n. pathology
n. port site implant
n. renal mass
n. tissue
n. transformation

neorectal function
neosalpingostomy
terminal n.

neostigmine toxicity
neostomy
neovagina
skin graft n.

neovascular
n. bundle
n. membrane
n. network

neovascularization
choroidal n.
corneal n.

NOTES

neovascularization *(continued)*
disk n.
disseminated asymptomatic unilateral n.
interstitial n.
iris n.
pathologic n.
preretinal n.
retinal quadrant n.
stromal n.
subretinal n.
vitreous n.
neovasculature
tumor n.
nephradenoma
nephralgia
nephralgic
nephratonia
nephrectomy
abdominal n.
adjuvant n.
anterior n.
apical polar n.
Balkan n.
extracorporeal partial n.
extraperitoneal laparoscopic n.
hand-assisted laparoscopic live-donor n.
laparoscopic n.
laparoscopic-assisted living donor n.
laparoscopic donor n. (LDN)
laser partial n.
live donor n.
living donor n.
lumbar n.
paraperitoneal n.
partial n.
perifascial n.
posterior n.
radical n.
retroperitoneoscopic n.
transperitoneal laparoscopic n.
transplant n.
unilateral n.
nephredema
nephrelcosis
nephric
nephritic
n. calculus
n. colic
n. syndrome
nephritis
interstitial n.
nephritogenic
nephroblastoma
nephrocalcinosis
nephrocapsectomy
nephrocardiac
nephrocele
nephrogenetic
nephrogenic
n. cord
n. tissue
nephrogenous
nephrohydrosis
nephroid
nephrolith
nephrolithiasis
nephrolithotomy
anatrophic n.
percutaneous n.
simultaneous bilateral percutaneous n.
nephrolithotripsy
percutaneous n. (PCNL)
nephrology
nephrolysis
nephrolytic
nephroma
nephron
nephronia
lobar n.
nephronic loop
nephron-sparing surgery
nephropathic
nephropathy
nephropexy
nephrophthisis
nephroptosis
nephropyeloplasty
nephropyosis
nephrorrhaphy
nephros
nephrosclerosis
nephroscopic fulguration
nephroscopy
anatrophic n.
flexible n.
percutaneous n.
nephrosis
nephrospasia
nephrostolithotomy
caliceal n.
percutaneous n. (PCNL)
nephrostomy
circle wire n.
n. drainage
percutaneous n.
n. puncture
nephrotic edema
nephrotomic cavity
nephrotomy
anatrophic n.
nephrotoxic
nephrotoxicity
nephrotoxin

nephrotrophic
nephrotropic
nephrotuberculosis
nephroureterectomy
bilateral n.
radical n.
transperitoneal laparoscopic n.
nephroureterocystectomy
nephroureteroscopy
nerve
abdominopelvic splanchnic n.
abducens n.
accelerator n.
accessory n.
acoustic n.
n. allografting
n. anastomosis
Andersch n.
ansa cervicalis n.
anterior auricular n.
anterior cutaneous n.
anterior ethmoidal n.
anterior labial n.
anterior scrotal n.
anterior supraclavicular n.
Arnold n.
articular recurrent n.
auditory tube n.
augmentor n.
auriculotemporal n.
autonomic n.
axillary n.
baroreceptor n.
Bell respiratory n.
n. biopsy
n. block
n. block anesthesia
n. block infusion
Bock n.
brachial plexus n.
buccal n.
buccinator n.
caroticotympanic n.
cavernous n.
centrifugal n.
centripetal n.
cervical splanchnic n.
chorda tympani n.
ciliary n.
circumflex n.
n. coaptation
coccygeal n.
cochlear n.
common peroneal n.
n. compression anesthesia
n. compression-degeneration syndrome
corneal n.
cranial n.
cranial n. (I–XII)
n. cross section
cutaneous cervical n.
n. decompression
deep peroneal n.
deep petrosal n.
deep temporal n.
dental n.
descending n.
dorsal interosseous n.
dorsal rami n.
dorsal scapular n.
eighth cranial n.
eleventh cranial n.
entrapped n.
esodic n.
ethmoidal n.
n. excitability test
excitor n.
excitoreflex n.
exodic n.
external nasal n.
external saphenous n.
external spermatic n.
extrinsic n.
facial n.
femoral n.
n. fiber bundle
n. fiber bundle layer
n. fiber myelination
fifth cranial n.
first cranial n.
fold of laryngeal n.
fourth cranial n.
fourth lumbar n.
furcal n.
Galen n.
gangliated n.
genitocrural n.
genitofemoral n.
glossopharyngeal n.
great auricular n.
n. growth factor receptor
hemorrhoidal n.
Hering n.

NOTES

N

nerve *(continued)*
hypogastric n.
iliohypogastric n.
ilioinguinal n.
n. implantation
inferior alveolar n.
inferior hemorrhoidal n.
inferior palpebral n.
inferior rectal n.
inferior vesical n.
infraorbital n.
infratrochlear n.
inhibitory n.
n. injury
intercarotid n.
intercostal n.
intercostohumeral n.
intermediary n.
internal rectal n.
Jacobson n.
jugular n.
lacrimal n.
Latarget n.
lingual n.
lumboinguinal n.
mandibular n.
masseteric n.
masticator n.
maxillary n.
median n.
mental n.
mixed n.
motor n.
musculocutaneous n.
musculospiral n.
mylohyoid n.
nasociliary n.
ninth cranial n.
obturator n.
occipital n.
oculomotor n.
olfactory n.
olivocochlear n.
Oort n.
ophthalmic n.
optic n.
palatine n.
n. paralysis
parasympathetic n.
pericardiophrenic n.
perineal n.
peripheral n.
peritonsillar n.
peroneal communicating n.
petrosal n.
phrenic n.
plantar digital n.
pneumogastric n.
popliteal communicating n.
presacral n.
pterygoid n.
pterygopalatine n.
pudendal n.
pudic n.
recurrent meningeal n.
n. regeneration
right common iliac n.
n. root
n. root compression
n. root injection
n. rootlet ablation
n. root sleeve injection
sacral splanchnic n.
second cranial n.
secretory n.
sensory n.
seventh cranial n.
sinocarotid n.
sinuvertebral n.
sixth cranial n.
somatic n.
sphenopalatine n.
spinal accessory n.
splanchnic n.
statoacoustic n.
n. stimulator anesthetic technique
subclavian n.
subcostal n.
suboccipital n.
subscapular n.
supraclavicular n.
supraorbital n.
suprascapular n.
supratrochlear n.
n. suture technique
sympathetic n.
temporomandibular n.
tenth cranial n.
tentorial n.
third cranial n.
third occipital n.
thoracic cardiac n.
thoracic spinal n.
thoracoabdominal n.
thoracodorsal n.
Tiedemann n.
n. tract
trifacial n.
trigeminal n.
trochlear n.
n. trunk
twelfth cranial n.
upper subscapular n.
vaginal n.
vagus n.
vascular n.

vasomotor n.
vestibular n.
vestibulocochlear n.
vidian n.
visceral n.
vomeronasal n.
Wrisberg n.
zygomatic n.
nerve-containing plate
nerve-point massage
nerve-sparing
n.-s. dissection
n.-s. radical retropubic prostatectomy
nervi (*pl. of* nervus)
nervorum
nervosa
foramina n.
nervosum
nervosus
nervous
n. damage
n. exhaustion
n. respiration
n. system
n. system involvement
nervus, pl. **nervi**
Nesbit
N. operation
N. plication
N. tuck procedure
nesidiectomy
nesidioblastoma
nest
Brunn n.
choristoma n.
nested nail
net
vascular n.
network
acromial arterial n.
articular vascular n.
calcaneal arterial n.
Cancer Genetics N.
cytokine n.
medial malleolar n.
neovascular n.
neural n.
patellar n.
peritarsal n.
plantar venous n.
Purkinje n.
trabecular n.
Neubauer artery
Neufeld dynamic method
Neugebauer-LeFort procedure
neural
n. arch
n. arch resection technique
n. axis vascular malformation
n. canal
n. crest malformation
n. crest migration
n. lesion
n. network
n. plasticity
n. spine
n. tissue
n. tube
n. tube defect
neuralgia
geniculate n.
inguinal n.
intercostal n.
laparoscopic-induced n.
petrosal n.
postherpetic n.
posttraumatic gustatory n.
secondary n.
Sluder n.
trigeminal n.
vidian n.
neurapophysis
neurasthenia
experimental n.
neuraxial
n. medication trial
n. neurolytic block
neurectasis
neurectomy
cochleovestibular n.
Cotte presacral n.
Eggers n.
genitofemoral n.
iliohypogastric n.
ilioinguinal n.
obturator n.
occipital n.
opticociliary n.
peripheral n.
pharyngeal plexus n.
Phelps n.
presacral n.

N

NOTES

neurectomy *(continued)*
retrogasserian n.
retrolabyrinthine-retrosigmoid vestibular n.
retrolabyrinthine vestibular n.
Sonnenberg n.
transcochlear cochleovestibular n.
transcochlear vestibular n.
transtympanic n.
tympanic n.
ulnar motor n.
vestibular n.
neurenteric canal
neurilemmosarcoma
neurilemoma, neurilemmoma
neurilemosarcoma
neurinoma
neuritic plaque
neuritis
vibration n.
neuroablation
neuroablative technique
neuroadenolysis
pituitary n.
neuroanastomosis
neuroanatomy
neuroanesthesia
neuroastrocytoma
neuroaugmentation
neuroaxial opioid
neuroblastoma
neurocele
neurocentral
n. joint
n. suture
neurochronaxic theory of phonation
neurocirculation
neurocladism
neurocognitive change
neurocranium
neurocutaneous island flap
neurocytolysis
neurocytoma
neurodiagnostic evaluation
neuroectomy
neuroeffector junction
neuroelectric event
neuroendocrine
n. cancer
n. skin carcinoma
n. tumor
neuroepithelioma
neuroepithelium
neurofibroma
neurofibromatosis
neurofibrosarcoma
neuroganglion
neurogastric
neurogenic
n. bladder
n. fracture
n. hypertension
n. incontinence
n. pulmonary edema (NPE)
neurogliomatosis
neurohypophysial
neurohypophysis
neuroimaging
neuroleptanalgesia
n. anesthesia
n. anesthetic technique
neuroleptanesthesia
neuroleptic
n. agent
n. malignant syndrome (NMS)
neurologic
N. and Adaptive Capacity Score (NACS)
n. complication
n. deficit
n. disease
n. disorder
n. evaluation
n. examination
n. function
n. injury
n. manifestation
n. recovery
n. surgery
n. symptom
neurological
n. nerve conduction velocity examination
n. surgery
neurology
surgical n.
neurolysis
distal n.
internal n.
intrathecal n.
neurolytic celiac plexus block (NCPB)
neuroma
acoustic n.
n. relocation surgery
neuroma-in-continuity
neuromatosis
neuromodulation
neuromotor dysfunction
neuromuscular
n. block
n. blockade (NMB)
n. blockade monitoring
n. blocking agent
n. electrical stimulation
n. facilitation
n. pedicle graft

n. relaxant
n. system electric induction
n. transmission
neuron
inspiratory bulbospinal n.
nondopaminergic n.
neuronal
n. cell line
n. membrane
n. migration
n. regeneration
neuronavigational system
neuronephric
neuronoma
neuroophthalmic manifestation
neuroophthalmologic examination
neuropathic
n. bladder
n. fracture
n. pain
n. ulcer
neuropathicum
papilloma n.
neuropathologist
neuropathology
neuropathophysiology
normalization of n.
neuropathy
optic n.
neurophysiologic examination
neuroplasticity
neuroplasty
epidural n.
neuropsychological deficit
neuroradiologic evaluation
neurorrhaphy
epineurial n.
perineurial n.
neurosarcocleisis
neurosarcoma
neuroschwannoma
neurostimulating procedure
neurostimulation trial
neurosurgeon
pediatric n.
neurosurgery
functional stereotactic n.
image-guided interactive n.
navigated neurosurgery
stereotactic n.
neurosurgical
n. anesthesia
n. approach
n. intensive care unit (NICU)
n. intervention
n. procedure
neurosuture
neurotendinous
neurothekeoma
neurotic excoriation
neurotization
neurotize
neurotologic examination
neurotomy
opticociliary n.
retrogasserian n.
neurotoxicology
neurotransmitter system
neurotrauma
neurotripsy
neurotrosis
neuroureterectomy
neurourology
neurovaricosis
neurovascular
n. anatomy
n. bundle
n. complication
n. compression syndrome
n. cross compression
n. free flap
n. island graft
n. island pedicle flap
n. lesion
n. sheath
neuroxanthoendothelioma
neutral
n. hip position
n. point
n. rotation
n. spine position
neutralization
n. plate fixation
serum n.
n. test
neutron
n. activation analysis
n. beam therapy
n. capture therapy
neutropenia-related bacterial infection
neutrophil
n. migration
polymorphonuclear n. (PMN)

NOTES

N

neutrophilic
n. infiltration
n. inflammation
nevi (*pl. of* nevus)
Neviaser
N. acromioclavicular technique
N. operation
Neviaser-Wilson-Gardner technique
nevocarcinoma
nevoid
n. anomaly
n. basal cell carcinoma syndrome
nevolipoma
nevoxanthoendothelioma
juvenile n.
nevus, pl. **nevi**
bathing trunk n.
new
N. England Baptist (NEB)
N. York Heart Association heart disease classification
newborn
n. anesthesia
n. examination
n. resuscitation
Newman
N. procedure
N. radial neck and head fracture classification
newton (N)
newtonian
n. aberration
n. body
NFCS
Neonatal Facial Pain Inventory
NG
nasogastric
NG suction
ng
nanogram
NHBD
non-heart-beating donor
NIBP
noninvasive blood pressure
Nicholas
N. five-in-one reconstruction technique
N. ligament technique
Nichols
N. method
N. procedure
N. sacrospinous fixation
nick
skin n.
nickel-and-dime lesion
Nicks procedure
Nicola
N. incision
N. shoulder procedure
Nicoll
N. cancellous bone graft
N. cancellous insert graft
N. classification
N. fracture operation
N. fracture repair procedure
nicotinic receptor
nictation, nictitation
nictitating membrane
NICU
neurosurgical intensive care unit
Nida nicking operation
nidus, pl. **nidi**
cellular n.
Niebauer-King technique
Niebauer trapeziometacarpal arthroplasty
Niemeier
N. classification
N. gallbladder perforation
nightstick fracture
nigroid body
nigrostriatal tract
Nikaidoh-Bex technique
Nikiforoff method
nil disease
ninety-ninety method
ninth cranial nerve
nipple
accessory n.
aortic n.
n. aspiration cytology
n. line
n. reconstruction
n. retraction
n. stimulation test
nipple-areolar reconstruction
nippled stoma
nipple-flat duct resection
NIPS
Neonatal Infant Pain Scale
NIR
near-infrared
Nirschl
N. operation
N. technique
Nissen
N. antireflux operation
N. 360-degree wrap fundoplication
N. fundoplasty
N. fundoplication method
N. fundoplication operation
N. fundoplication procedure
N. fundoplication technique
N. fundoplication wrap
N. repair

Nissen-Rosseti
N.-R. fundoplication method
N.-R. fundoplication procedure
N.-R. fundoplication technique
Nissen-Rossetti fundoplication
Nitchie method
nitrate-induced venodilation
nitric
n. oxide bioavailability
n. oxide blocked sphincter relaxation
n. oxide signaling
nitrogen
expiratory n.
n. monoxide
n. narcosis
n. partial pressure
nitrous
n. oxide (NO)
n. oxide-opioid-barbiturate anesthetic technique
n. oxide-oxygen-opioid anesthetic technique (N_2O-O_2-opioid anesthetic technique)
nitrovasodilator
Nizetic operation
NLOB
needle-localized open biopsy
NMB
neuromuscular blockade
NMR
nuclear magnetic resonance
NMR spectroscopy
NMS
neuroleptic malignant syndrome
NO
nasal oxygen
nitrous oxide
no
no infection-no rejection
no rejection
no signs of life
Noble
N. bowel plication
N. position
N. surgical plication of bowel
Noble-Mengert perineal repair
nocebo
nociception
nociceptive stimulation
nociceptor afferent peripheral terminal
nocturia
nocturnal
n. enuresis
n. painful tonic spasm (NPTS)
nodal
n. disease
n. extirpation
n. involvement
n. metastasis
n. plane
n. point
n. recurrence
n. tissue
n. yield
node
n. of Aschoff and Tawara
atrioventricular n.
n. biopsy
buccinator n.
Cloquet n.
companion lymph n.
coronary n.
cystic n.
diaphragmatic n.
n. dissection
foraminal n.
free n.
gastroomental n.
hot sentinel n.
internal mammary n.
intramammary sentinel n.
n. involvement
juguloomohyoid n.
n. lymphoma
n. lymphoma system
malar n.
mammary n.
mandibular n.
mastoid n.
matted n.
mesenteric n.
mesenteric lymph n. (MLN)
nonsentinel n.
occipital n.
paratracheal n.
parietal n.
parotid n.
perigastric n.
prelaryngeal n.
pretracheal n.
radiolabeled sentinel n.
Ranvier n.
regional n.

NOTES

N

node *(continued)*
retroauricular n.
retroperitoneal n.
retropharyngeal n.
retropyloric n.
Rosenmüller n.
n. of Rouviere
sentinel n.
sentinel lymph n. (SLN)
sinoatrial n.
n. station
subdigastric n.
submandibular n.
submental n.
subpyloric n.
suprapyloric n.
Tawara n.
tracheal n.
tracheobronchial n.
visceral n.
node-negative
n.-n. disease
n.-n. melanoma
node-positive
n.-p. breast cancer
n.-p. disease
n.-p. melanoma
nodi (*pl. of* nodus)
nodo-hisian bypass tract
nodose ganglion
nodoventricular tract
nodular
n. chondrodermatitis
n. hidradenoma
n. lesion
nodulation
nodule
cold n.
hot n.
hyperfunctioning n.
metastatic n.
mixed n.
posterior n.
subependymal brain n.
thyroid n.
nodulectomy
nodule-in-nodule lesion
nodulus, pl. **noduli**
nodus, pl. **nodi**
noise
n. detection threshold
n. exposure
no-leak technique
nomenclature
Anglo-Saxon n.
Couinaud n.
linnaean system of n.
NOMI
nonocclusive mesenteric ischemia
nomogram
Radford n.
nonabsorbable material
nonadherent
nonanatomic
n. renal bypass
n. wedge resection
nonanesthetic gas
nonaneurysmal perimesencephalic subarachnoid hemorrhage
nonappendiceal carcinoid
nonarticular distal radial fracture
nonaxillary location
nonbacterial thrombotic endocardial lesion
nonbench surgery
nonblanchable, abnormally colored lesion
nonbullous emphysema
noncalcified nodular mass
noncancer death
noncardiac surgery
noncausal association
noncemented total hip arthroplasty
noncircumferential antireflux procedure
noncirrhotic metabolic liver disease
nonclassic nodal basin
noncolorectal
n. liver metastasis (NCRLM)
n. primary
noncontact manipulation
noncontiguous fracture
nondepolarizer
nondepolarizing
n. block
n. blockade
n. muscle relaxant
n. relaxant
nondermatomal sensory abnormality (NDSA)
nondermatophyte fungal infection
nondiabetic
nondiagnostic FNA
nondismembered anastomosis
nondisplaced fracture
nondistended abdomen
nondominant gland
nondopaminergic neuron
nondysgerminoma
nonencapsulated
nonerosive gastric mucosal lesion
nonexcisional modality
nonfamilial
n. malignant endocrine tumor
n. multiglandular disease
n. untreated HPT

nonfatal
n. complication
n. stroke
nonfenestrated Fontan procedure
nonfunction
primary graft n.
nonfunctional
n. malignant tumor
non-heart-beating donor (NHBD)
nonhereditary malignancy
nonideal solution
nonimmunologic complication
noninfective extraabdominal complication
noninhalation
noninvasive
n. assessment
n. blood pressure (NIBP)
n. diagnosis
n. evaluation
n. infestation
n. localization study
lower extremity n.
n. method
n. positive-pressure ventilation (NPPV)
n. procedure
n. programmed stimulation
n. recurrence
n. technique
n. venous study
nonisometric graft
nonkeratinization
nonlaparoscopic
n. series
n. technique
nonmalignant
chronic n.
n. disease
nonmeningiomatous malignant lesion
nonmobile mass
nonmucosal hemorrhoidectomy
nonmutagenic
nonnecrotizing granulomatous inflammation
nonneoplastic tumor-like lesion
nonneuroendocrine metastasis
nonocclusive
n. mesenteric ischemia (NOMI)
n. mesenteric ischemia syndrome
nonopaque intraluminal mass
nonoperative
n. approach
n. closure
n. diagnosis
n. management
n. reduction
n. staging
nonoperatively
nonophthalmologic surgical specialty
nonopportunistic infection
nonoptimal technique
nonorganic stridor
nonpalpable
n. invasive breast cancer
n. mammographic abnormality
nonparametric test
nonpathologic scar
nonpenetrating
n. keratoplasty
n. rupture
n. wound
nonperforative lesion
nonpharmacologic measure
nonphysial fracture
nonphysiologic position
nonplicated appendicocystostomy
nonprosthetic closure
nonpulmonary route of elimination (NPE)
nonrebreathing anesthesia
nonresectional method
non-rib-spreading
n.-r.-s. thoracotomy incision
n.-r.-s. thoracotomy incision method
n.-r.-s. thoracotomy incision procedure
n.-r.-s. thoracotomy incision technique
nonrotation
nonrotational burst fracture
nonsecretory sigmoid cystoplasty
nonseminomatous testicular tumor
nonsentinel node
nonseptate cavity
nonsevered injury
nonshivering thermogenesis
nonspecific
n. symptom
n. therapy
nonstereospecific action
nonsteroidal
n. antiinflammatory drug (NSAID)
n. antiinflammatory medication

NOTES

nonsurgical
n. clinician
n. management
n. method
n. therapy
n. treatment
nonsurvivor
nonsympathetically mediated pain
nontherapeutic
nonthoracotomy
nonthrust mobilization
nontraumatic hernia
nontuberculous mycobacterial infection
nontumoral gastric wall
nonunion
n. fracture
nonunited fracture
nonvascular
n. abdominal surgery
nonventilated lung
nonviable tissue
nonvisualization
nonvital tissue
N_2O-O_2-opioid anesthetic technique
noose
Dormia n.
n. suture technique
noradrenergic mechanism
Norfolk technique
norma, pl. **normae**
normal
n. anatomic alignment
n. anatomic position
n. base deficit
n. body temperature
n. CI
n. colon
n. intravascular pressure
n. ovariotomy
n. planar MR anatomy
n. saline
n. saline solution
n. serum lactate
n. tissue
n. transformation zone
normalization
assay n.
n. of neuropathophysiology
normalizing lactate
normal-pressure hydrocephalus
Norman Miller vaginopexy
normocalcemia
normocalcemic
normocapnia
normocephalic
normotensive
normothermia
intraoperative n.
normothermic
n. ischemia
n. temperature
normoventilation
normovolemic
North American Symptomatic Carotid Endarterectomy Trial (NASCET)
Northern blot technique
Norton operation
Norwood
N. operation
N. univentricular heart procedure
no-scalpel vasectomy
nose
n. anesthesia
artificial n.
cleft n.
external n.
nosocomial
n. fire
n. fungal infection
n. gangrene
n. pneumonia
nostril
notal
notancephalia
notch
acetabular n.
n. of acetabulum
anacrotic n.
angular n.
auricular n.
costal n.
craniofacial n.
ethmoidal n.
frontal n.
greater sciatic n.
inferior thyroid n.
inferior vertebral n.
infraorbital n.
interarytenoid n.
interclavicular n.
intercondyloid n.
intervertebral n.
Kernohan n.
lacrimal n.
lesser sciatic n.
mandibular n.
mastoid n.
pancreatic n.
parietal n.
parotid n.
preoccipital n.
presternal n.
pterygoid n.
scapular n.
sternal n.
superior thyroid n.

superior vertebral n.
supraorbital n.
suprascapular n.
suprasternal n.
tentorial n.
tympanic n.
umbilical n.
vertebral n.
notch-and-roll maneuver
notching
rib n.
notchplasty procedure
notencephalocele
notha
notochord
no-touch technique
noxious stimulus
Noyes flexion rotation drawer test
NP
necrotizing pancreatitis
NPC
negative peritoneal cytology
NPE
neurogenic pulmonary edema
nonpulmonary route of elimination
NPPV
noninvasive positive-pressure ventilation
NPTR
National Pediatric Trauma Registry
NPTS
nocturnal painful tonic spasm
NPV
negative predictive value
NSABP
National Surgical Adjuvant Breast and Bowel Project
NSAID
nonsteroidal antiinflammatory drug
NSAID analgesic
N2-Sargenti technique
N-shaped sigmoid loop
NTI
nasotracheal intubation
nub
fibrotic n.
nucha
nuchae
nuchal
n. fascia
n. ligament
n. line
n. plane
n. region
nuchalis
Nuck canal
nuclear
n. atypia
n. external layer
n. grade
n. magnetic resonance (NMR)
n. medicine
n. tissue
nucleation time
nucleolysis
percutaneous laser n.
nucleus, pl. **nuclei**
n. ambiguus lesion
Edinger-Westphal n.
external cuneate n.
extrapyramidal n.
ossifying n.
n. pulposus herniation
n. rotator
Nuhn gland
nulliparity
null point
numbness
numerary renal anomaly
numerical cipher method
nummular lesion
nummulation
nurse
n. anesthetist
visiting n.
nutcracker fracture
nutmeg
n. appearance
n. liver
nutricium
nutricius
nutrient
n. absorption
n. artery
n. canal
n. flap
n. foramen
hepatotrophic n.
n. vessel
nutrition
enteral n.
parenteral n.
tissue n.
total parenteral n. (TPN)

NOTES

nutritional
 n. assessment
 n. status
Nuttall operation
nycturia
Nyhus classification
Nylen-Barany maneuver
nympha
nymphal
nymphectomy
nymphocaruncularis
nymphocaruncular sulcus
nymphohymenal sulcus
nymphotomy
nystagmogram
nystagmoid-like oscillation
nystagmus
nyxis

O_2
oxygen
OA
open appendectomy
Oakley-Fulthorpe technique
oat cell carcinoma
OAV
oculoauriculovertebral
OAV syndrome
obcecation
O'Beirne sphincter
Ober
O. incision
O. tendon technique
Ober-Barr
O.-B. procedure for brachioradialis transfer
O.-B. transfer technique
Obersteiner-Redlich line
obese
o. patient
obesity-hypoventilation syndrome
obex
object
O. Classification Test
fixation o.
o. program
o. space
objective
O. Pain Scale
surgical treatment o.
object-space focus
obliqua
oblique
o. abdominal muscle
o. aberration
o. arytenoid muscle
o. auricular muscle
o. base-wedge osteotomy
o. cord
o. coronal plane
o. displacement osteotomy
external o.
o. facial cleft
o. fissure of lung
o. flap
o. flow misregistration
o. fracture
o. head
o. hernia
o. illumination
left anterior o. (LAO)
o. pericardial sinus
o. projection
right anterior o. (RAO)
o. sagittal gradient-echo MR imaging
o. section
obliquum
obliquus
obliterans
arteriosclerosis o. (ASO)
thromboangiitis o.
obliteration
balloon-occluded retrograde transvenous o. (B-RTO)
endoscopic extirpation cicatricial o.
fibrous o.
percutaneous transhepatic o.
radiographic o.
subdeltoid fat plane o.
total ear o.
obliterative
o. bronchiolitis
o. inflammation
o. scarring
oblongata
rostral ventrolateral medulla o.
O'Brien
O. akinesia technique
O. anesthesia
O. capsular shift procedure
O. pelvic halo operation
obscuration
transient visual o.
observation
o. period
o. ward
observer-dependent criteria
obstetric
o. anesthesia
o. pain
o. position
obstetrical
o. complication
o. hysterectomy
o. management
o. operation
o. traction injury
obstetrics
International Federation of Gynecology and O. (FIGO)
obstipation
obstipum
obstructed
o. bowel
o. liver
obstructing
o. colorectal cancer
o. pathology

obstruction
acute intestinal o.
adherence o.
airway o.
anorectal outlet o.
ball-valve o.
biliary tract o.
bowel o.
catheter o.
closed-loop intestinal o.
clot-induced urinary tract o.
colon o.
colonic o.
common duct o.
complete o.
complex left ventricular outflow tract o.
ductal o.
esophageal o.
extrahepatic bile duct o.
extrahepatic biliary o.
extrahepatic binary o.
extrahepatic portal vein o. (EHPO)
extramural upper airway o.
hepatic venous outflow o.
intermittent subclavian vein o.
intestinal o.
ipsilateral portal vein o.
left-sided colorectal o.
longer-segment o.
mechanical extrahepatic o.
membranous o.
myoglobin tubular o.
outflow tract o.
partial mechanical o.
portal vein o.
postoperative airway o.
shunt o.
site of o.
stop-valve airway o.
upper airway o.
ureteropelvic o.
ureterovesical o.
urinary tract o.
vein o.
ventricular inflow tract o.
ventricular outflow tract o.

obstruction-induced modulation

obstructive
o. apnea
o. esophagogastric cancer
o. hydatid material
o. hydrocephalus
o. jaundice
o. mechanism
o. pulmonary dysfunction
o. uropathy

obstruent

obtainer space

obtundation

Obtura injectable technique

obturation
canal o.
intermittent self-o.
retrograde o.
root canal filling technique o.

obturator
o. artery
o. avulsion fracture
o. bypass
o. canal
o. crest
o. fascia
o. foramen
o. groove
o. hernia
o. line
o. lymphatic chain
o. nerve
o. nerve block
o. nerve damage
o. nerve injury
o. neurectomy
o. shelf cystourethropexy
o. test
o. tubercle

obturatoria

obturatoriae

obturatorii

obturatorium

obturatorius

obtuse margin

obviate

OC
operative cholangiography

occipital
o. angle
o. artery
o. belly
o. bone
o. border
o. branch
o. cephalocele
o. cerebral vein
o. condyle
o. condyle fracture
o. condyle syndrome
o. emissary vein
o. fontanelle
o. groove
left anterior o. (LAO)
o. malformation
o. margin
o. nerve
o. neurectomy
o. node

o. plane
o. plexus
o. point
right anterior o.
o. sinus
o. suture
o. triangle

occipitale
occipitales
occipitalis
occipitalization
occipitis
occipitoanterior position
occipitoatlantal dislocation
occipitoatlantoaxial anomaly
occipitoatloid
occipitoaxial
occipitobregmatic
occipitocervical

o. fixation
o. fusion
o. stabilization

occipitocollicular tract
occipitofacial
occipitofrontalis muscle
occipitofrontal muscle
occipitomastoidea
occipitomastoid suture
occipitomental projection
occipitoparietal suture
occipitopontine tract
occipitoposterior position
occipitosphenoid suture
occipitotectal tract
occipitotemporal
occipitothalamic radiation
occipitotransverse position
occiput
occluded segment
occluding

o. centric relation record
o. relation

occlusal

o. cavity
o. correction
o. equilibration
o. plane
o. plane angle
o. position
o. pressure
o. projection
o. relation
o. therapy

occlusion

angioplasty-related vessel o.
aortic o.
arterial o.
artery o.
carotid artery o.
centric relation o.
clip o.
contralateral carotid artery o.
eccentric o.
endovascular balloon o.
graft o.
hemihepatic vascular o.
inflow o.
intermittent inflow o.
IVC o.
laparoscopic total o. (LTO)
MCA o.
mechanical o.
middle cerebral artery o.
plastic stent o.
o. pressure
rapid o.
subclavian artery o.
o. therapy
tourniquet o.
two-plane o.
vascular o.
vein o.
venous o.

occlusive

o. carotid artery disease
o. coronary artery disease
o. ileus
o. MI
o. patch test
o. therapy

occult

o. bleeding
o. blood
o. cerebrovascular malformation
o. diaphragmatic injury
o. enterotomy
o. extrahepatic disease
o. fracture
o. hepatic disease
o. irresectable disease
o. metastasis
o. systemic disease

NOTES

occult *(continued)*
o. talar lesion
o. vascular malformation
occulta
occupational
o. therapy
o. toxin exposure
ochre
o. hemorrhage
o. mass
Ochsenbein gingivectomy
Ockerblad-Boari flap
O'Connor operation
O'Connor-Peter operation
OCR
oculocardiac reflex
ocryptosis
octanol/water coefficient
octogenarian
octreotide
ocular
o. adnexa
o. adnexal lesion
o. barrier
o. cul-de-sac
o. inflammation
o. manifestation
o. metastasis
o. motility disorder
o. muscle
o. oscillation
o. radiation therapy
o. tumor
ocular-mucous membrane syndrome
oculi (*pl. of* oculus)
oculoauriculovertebral (OAV)
o. dysplasia
oculobuccogenital syndrome
oculocardiac reflex (OCR)
oculocephalic
o. maneuver
o. vascular anomaly
oculofacial
oculogyration
oculomandibulofacial syndrome
oculomotor
o. decussation
o. foramen
o. ganglion
o. nerve
oculomotorii
oculopharyngeal muscular dystrophy
oculoplastic
o. surgeon
o. surgery
oculovertebral syndrome
oculozygomatic
oculus, pl. **oculi**
odansetron
odd-even method
Oddi sphincter
O'Donnell operation
O'Donoghue
O. ACL reconstruction
O. facetectomy
O. procedure
odontectomy
odontoameloblastoma
odontoblastoma
odontocele
odontoclastoma
odontogenic infection
odontoid
o. condyle fracture
o. fracture internal fixation
o. fracture stabilization
o. neck fracture
o. perpendicular line
o. process osteosynthesis
o. screw fixation
o. screw placement
odontoidectomy
odontoideum
odontolysis
odontoplasty
odontoscopy
odontosteophyte
odontotomy
prophylactic o.
odoriferous gland
ODQ
Owestry Disability Questionnaire
O'Dwyer intubation
OFD
orofaciodigital
OFD syndrome
off-center isoperistaltic technique
off-label use
off-pump coronary artery bypass (OPCAB)
off-set V-osteotomy
Ogata
O. method
O. technique
Ogden
O. epiphysial fracture classification
O. knee dislocation classification
Ogilvie
O. operation
O. syndrome
Ogston-Luc operation
Ogura operation
O'Hara two-clamp method
Ohngren line
OHS
open heart surgery

OI
oxygenation index
oil
o. drop lesion
o. gland
iodized o.
joint o.
oil-aspiration pneumonia
Okamoto method
Okamura technique
Okuda transhepatic obliteration of varix
old posterior cyst
O'Leary lesser curvature gastroplasty
olecrani
olecranization
olecranon
o. fracture
o. process
oleogranuloma
oleoma
olfactoria
olfactory
o. anesthesia
o. bulb
o. bundle
o. nerve
o. tract
oligoanalgesia
oligoastrocytoma
recurrent vermian o.
oligoclonal growth
oligodendroblastoma
oligodendroglioma
oligomerization
oligosegmental correction
oligospermia
oligozoospermatism
oliguresia
oliguria
olisthesis
olivae
olivary body
Oliver-Rosalki method
olivocerebellar tract
olivocochlear
o. bundle
o. nerve
olivospinal tract
Ollier
O. arthrodesis approach
O. incision
O. lateral approach
O. method
O. technique
O. thick split free graft
Ollier-Thiersch graft
Olshausen
O. procedure
O. suspension
OLT
orthotopic liver transplant
orthotopic liver transplantation
OLT recipient
OLV
one-lung ventilation
Olympus gastrostomy
Ombrédanne operation
omega-shaped incision
omenta (*pl. of* omentum)
omental
o. appendage
o. branch
o. bursa
o. cyst
o. enterocleisis
o. flap
o. hernia
o. J-pexy
o. metastasis
o. nodal disease
o. patch
o. pedicle
o. pedicle wrapping
o. pouch
o. reinforcement
o. sac
o. spread
o. tenia
o. tuber
omentale
omentales
omentalis
omentectomy
greater o.
lesser o.
omentitis
omentofixation
omentopexy
omentoplasty
pedicled o.
omentorrhaphy
omentosplenopexy
omentotomy

NOTES

omentovolvulus
omentulum
omentum, pl. **omenta**
colic o.
gastrocolic o.
gastrohepatic o.
gastrosplenic o.
greater o.
lesser o.
o. majus flap procedure
pancreaticosplenic o.
permanent mesh o.
splenogastric o.
omentumectomy
Omer-Capen
O.-C. carpectomy
O.-C. technique
omniplane scan
omocervical flap
omoclavicular
o. fossa
o. triangle
omoclaviculare
omohyoidei
omohyoideus
omohyoid muscle
omothyroid
omotracheale
omotracheal triangle
omphalectomy
omphalic
omphalocele
infraumbilical o.
omphalomesenteric
omphalos
omphalospinous
omphalotomy
omphalotripsy
omphalovesical
omphalus
oncho-osteodysplasia
oncocytoma
oncogene
tumor suppressor o.
oncologic
o. clearance
o. consideration
oncologist
medical o.
radiation o.
surgical o.
oncology
GI o.
surgical o.
urologic o.
oncolysate
polyvalent melanoma o.
vaccinia melanoma o. (VMO)
oncoma
oncometric
oncoplastic surgery
oncotic pressure
oncotomy
Ondine curse
one-flight exertional dyspnea
one-handed knot
one-hour office pad test
one-inclinometer method
oneirogmus
oneiroscopy
one-lung
o.-l. anesthesia
o.-l. ventilation (OLV)
o.-l. ventilation anesthetic technique
one-minute endoscopy room test
one-part fracture
one-phase subperiosteal implant technique
one-piece ostomy pouch
one-plane
o.-p. deformity
o.-p. instability
o.-p. view
one-pour technique
one-session removal
one-sitting endodontics
one-snip punctum operation
one-stage
o.-s. amputation
o.-s. hypospadias repair
o.-s. left colectomy
o.-s. operation
o.-s. posterior mediastinal esophagoplasty
o.-s. procedure
oneuropathy
ONF
open Nissen fundoplication
onion
o. peel appearance
o. scale lesion
o. skin-like membrane
onion-bulb changes on biopsy
onlay
o. island flap
o. island-flap urethroplasty
o. patch anastomosis
o. technique
onlay-tube-onlay urethroplasty technique
on-line data
onset of blockade
on-table irrigation
onychectomy
onychocryptosis nail
onychogryposis
onycholysis

onychoma
onychomycosis
onycho-osteodysplasia
onychoplasty
onychotomy
oocyte
o. extrusion
o. micromanipulation
oophorectomy
prophylactic o.
oophorocystectomy
oophorohysterectomy
oophoroma
oophoropeliopexy
oophoropexy
oophoroplasty
oophororrhaphy
oophorosalpingectomy
oophorostomy
oophorotomy
Oort nerve
opacification
opacity
OPCAB
off-pump coronary artery bypass
open
o. adjustable silicone gastric banding
o. adrenalectomy
o. amputation
o. anesthesia system
o. anti-reflux surgery
o. appendectomy (OA)
o. application test
o. bone graft epiphysiodesis
o. brain biopsy
o. cavity
o. cholecystectomy
o. circuit method
o. colectomy
o. common bile duct exploration
o. disk surgery
o. diverticulectomy
o. drainage
o. drop anesthesia
o. drop technique
o. endarterectomy
o. esophagectomy
o. esophagomyotomy
o. flap
o. flap technique
o. fundoplication
o. Hasson technique
o. head injury
o. heart surgery (OHS)
o. hemorrhoidectomy
o. hernia operation
o. herniorrhaphy
o. intraoperative ultrasonography
o. laparoscopic approach
o. laparoscopic technique
o. laparoscopy
o. laparotomy
o. liver biopsy
o. loop
o. lung biopsy
o. Nissen fundoplication (ONF)
o. Nissen operation
o. osteotomy
o. palm technique
o. patch test
o. pinning
o. pneumothorax
o. pyelolithotomy
o. pyelotomy
o. reconstruction
o. reconstructive procedure
o. reduction
o. reduction and internal fixation
o. repair
o. retroperitoneal high ligation
o. skull fracture
o. splenectomy
o. stereotactic craniotomy
o. surgical biopsy
o. surgical cordotomy
o. surgical therapy
o. surgical treatment
o. thoracotomy
o. venous channel
o. vertical banded gastroplasty
o. wedge
o. wound
open-book fracture
open-break fracture
open-end ostomy pouch
open-gloving technique
opening
appendiceal o.
o. flap
ileocecal o.
maximum mouth o.
midpalatal suture o.
o. pressure

O

NOTES

opening *(continued)*
saphenous o.
tendinous o.
urethral o.
vaginal o.
o. wedge manipulation
open-section nail
open-sky
o.-s. cryoextraction operation
o.-s. technique
o.-s. trephination
o.-s. vitrectomy
operable
opera-glass deformity
operant
o. conditioning
o. procedure
operating
o. room (OR)
o. theater
o. time
operation
Abbe o.
Abbe-Estlander o.
Abbott-Lucas shoulder o.
Abernethy o.
ab externo filtering o.
Adams hip o.
Adler o.
Agnew o.
Agrikola o.
Alexander o.
Allen o.
Allport o.
Alsus-Knapp o.
Alvis o.
Ammon o.
Amsler o.
Amussat o.
Anagnostakis o.
anastomotic o.
Anel o.
Angelucci o.
annular corneal graft o.
Anson-McVay o.
antiperistaltic o.
antireflux o.
Appolito o.
Argyll-Robertson o.
Aries-Pitanguy o.
Arion o.
Arlt o.
Arlt-Jaesche o.
Armistead ulnar lengthening o.
Arrowhead o.
Arroyo o.
Arruga o.
Arruga-Berens o.
arterial switch o.
Ashford retracted nipple o.
atrial baffle o.
Auchincloss o.
Aylett o.
Babcock o.
Bacon-Babcock o.
Badal o.
Baker patellar advancement o.
Baker translocation o.
Baldy o.
Baldy-Webster o.
Ball o.
Ball-Hoffman o.
Band-Aid o.
Bangerter pterygium o.
Bankart o.
Bankart-Putti-Platt o.
bariatric o.
Barkan-Cordes linear cataract o.
Barkan double cyclodialysis o.
Barkan goniotomy o.
Barnard o.
Barraquer enzymatic zonulolysis o.
Barraquer keratomileusis o.
Barrie-Jones canaliculodacryorhinostomy o.
Barrio o.
Barr tendon transfer o.
Bassini o.
Bateman modification of Mayer transfer o.
Battle o.
Baudelocque o.
Bauer-Tondra-Trusler o.
Baynton o.
Beard o.
Beard-Cutler o.
Beck I, II o.
Beer o.
Belsey Mark IV antireflux o.
Benedict orbit o.
Berens pterygium transplant o.
Berens sclerectomy o.
Berens-Smith o.
Berger o.
Berke o.
Berke-Motais o.
Bernard o.
Bethke o.
Bielschowsky o.
biliary-enteric anastomosis o.
Billroth I, II o.
Bircher o.
Birch-Hirschfeld entropion o.
Blair o.
Blalock-Hanlon o.
Blalock-Taussig o.

Blasius lid flap o.
Blaskovics canthoplasty o.
Blaskovics dacryostomy o.
Blaskovics lid o.
Blatt o.
Bloch-Paul-Mikulicz o.
bloodless o.
Böhm o.
Bonaccolto-Flieringa vitreous o.
Bonnet enucleation o.
Bonzel o.
Bora o.
Bose o.
Bossalino blepharoplasty o.
Bowman o.
Boyd o.
Bozeman o.
Brailey o.
Brenner o.
Bricker o.
Bridge o.
bridge pedicle flap o.
Briggs strabismus o.
Bristow o.
Brock o.
Bromley foreign body o.
Bronson foreign body removal o.
Brophy o.
Brunschwig o.
Bryant o.
Budinger blepharoplasty o.
Burch eye evisceration o.
Burow flap o.
Butler fifth toe o.
buttonhole o.
Buzzi o.
bypass o.
Byron Smith ectropion o.
Cairns o.
Caldwell-Luc o.
Calhoun-Hagler lens extraction o.
Callahan o.
Camey I, II o.
Campodonico o.
capital o.
Carmody-Batson o.
Carrel o.
Carter o.
Casanellas lacrimal o.
Casey o.
Castroviejo o.
Castroviejo-Scheie cyclodiathermy o.
cataract extraction o.
Cattell o.
cautery o.
Cawthorne o.
Celsus-Hotz o.
Celsus spasmodic entropion o.
cerclage o.
cesarean o.
Chandler-Verhoeff o.
Chandler vitreous o.
Chaput o.
Chaput anal o.
Charles o.
Cheyne o.
Child o.
Cibis o.
cinching o.
Clagett o.
clean o.
clean-contaminated o.
Cleasby iridectomy o.
Cloward o.
cluster o.
Collin-Beard o.
Collis antireflux o.
colorectal o.
Comberg foreign body o.
commando o.
comparison o.
complete wrap Nissen o.
Conn o.
Conrad orbital blowout fracture o.
conventional o.
Cooper o.
corneal graft o.
Cotte o.
Cotting toenail o.
Counsellor-Davis artificial vagina o.
Crawford sling o.
crescent o.
Crespo o.
Crile-Matas o.
Critchett o.
Crock encircling o.
cryoextraction o.
cryotherapy o.
Csapody orbital repair o.
Cupper-Faden o.
curative-intent o.
curative sphincter-saving o.
Cushing o.
Cusick o.

NOTES

operation *(continued)*
Cusick-Sarrail ptosis o.
Cutler o.
Cutler-Beard o.
cyclodiathermy o.
Czermak pterygium o.
Czerny o.
dacryoadenectomy o.
dacryocystectomy o.
dacryocystorhinotomy o.
dacryocystostomy o.
Dailey o.
Dalgleish o.
Dallas o.
Damus-Kaye-Stansel o.
Dana o.
Dandy o.
Danforth fetal o.
Daviel o.
day-case o.
debulking o.
de Grandmont o.
Deiter o.
DeKlair o.
de Lapersonne o.
Delorme rectal prolapse o.
Del Toro o.
Denker sinus o.
Derby o.
Desmarres o.
de Vincentiis o.
DeWecker o.
Diamond-Gould syndactyly o.
Dianoux o.
diathermy o.
Dickey o.
Dickey-Fox o.
Dickson-Wright o.
Dieffenbach o.
DKS o.
Döderlein roll-flap o.
Dohlman o.
D'ombrain o.
Donald-Fothergill o.
Doyle o.
Drummond-Morison o.
Duhamel colon o.
Duke-Elder o.
Dunnington o.
Dupuy-Dutemps o.
Durham flatfoot o.
Durr o.
Duverger-Velter o.
Dwyer clawfoot o.
Eagleton o.
Eaton-Malerich fracture-dislocation o.
Edlan-Mejchar o.
effector o.
Ekehorn o.
Elliot o.
Elschnig canthorrhaphy o.
Ely o.
emergency o.
emergent o.
Emmet o.
equilibrating o.
Erbakan inferior fornix o.
Escapini cataract o.
Esser inlay o.
Estes o.
Estlander o.
Eversbusch o.
eversion o.
evisceration o.
Ewing o.
exploratory o.
extraabdominal o.
extracapsular cataract extraction o.
Faden o.
Falk-Shukuris o.
Fanta cataract o.
Farmer o.
Fasanella o.
Fasanella-Servat ptosis o.
fenestrated Fontan o.
fenestration o.
Fergus o.
Filatov o.
Filatov-Marzinkowsky o.
filtering o.
Fink o.
Finney o.
Flajani o.
flap o.
floating forehead o.
Föerster o.
Foley o.
Fontan o.
Fothergill o.
Fothergill-Donald o.
Fothergill-Hunter o.
Fould entropion o.
Fox o.
Franceschetti coreoplasty o.
Franceschetti corepraxy o.
Franceschetti deviation o.
Franceschetti keratoplasty o.
Franceschetti pupil deviation o.
Franke tabes o.
Frazier-Spiller o.
Fredet-Ramstedt o.
French supracondylar fracture o.
Freund o.
Fricke o.
Friede o.

Friedenwald o.
Friedenwald-Guyton o.
Frost-Lang o.
Fuchs canthorrhaphy o.
Fuchs iris bombe transfixation o.
Fukala o.
Furlow-Fisher modification of Virag 1 o.
Galeazzi patellar o.
Gallie o.
Gardner o.
Gauderer-Ponsky PEG o.
Gayet o.
Gifford delimiting keratotomy o.
Gigli o.
Gilles o.
Gilliam o.
Gilliam-Doleris o.
Gillies scar correction o.
Gil-Vernet o.
Giordano o.
Girard keratoprosthesis o.
Gittes o.
Glenn o.
Goldmann-Larson foreign body o.
Goldsmith o.
gold weight and wire spring o.
Gomez-Marquez lacrimal o.
Gonin cautery o.
goniotomy o.
Goodall-Power o.
Gradle keratoplasty o.
Graefe o.
Grant-Ward o.
Greaves o.
Grimsdale o.
Grondahl-Finney o.
Gross o.
Grossmann o.
Gussenbauer o.
Gutzeit dacryostomy o.
Guyton ptosis o.
Halpin o.
Halsted o.
Hampton o.
Handley o.
hanging hip o.
hanging toe o.
Harmon o.
Harms-Dannheim trabeculotomy o.
Hartmann o.
Hasner o.
Hassab o.
Haultain o.
Heaney o.
Heaton o.
Heine o.
Heineke o.
Heisrath o.
Heller o.
Heller-Belsey o.
Heller-Dor o.
Heller-Nissen o.
hemi-Fontan o.
Henry o.
Herbert o.
Hess eyelid o.
Hess ptosis o.
Hiff o.
Hill antireflux o.
Hinsberg o.
Hippel o.
Hirst o.
Hochenegg o.
Hofmeister o.
Hogan o.
Hoguet o.
Holth o.
Hopkins o.
Horay o.
Horvath o.
Hotz-Anagnostakis o.
Hotz entropion o.
Huggins o.
Hughes o.
Hummelsheim o.
Hunt o.
Hunter o.
Hunt-Transley o.
Hutch ureteral reflux o.
I-beam hip o.
Iliff o.
Imre lateral canthoplasty o.
indentation o.
Indian o.
initial o.
interval o.
intracapsular cataract extraction o.
iridectomy o.
iridencleisis o.
iridodialysis o.
iridotasis o.
iridotomy o.
Irvine o.

NOTES

operation *(continued)*
Italian o.
Ivalon sponge-wrap o.
Jaboulay-Doyen-Winkleman o.
Jackson-Babcock o.
Jaesche o.
Jaesche-Arlt o.
Jaime lacrimal o.
Jameson o.
Japanese standard o.
Japanese-style o.
Jensen o.
Johnson o.
Kader-Senn o.
Kasai o.
Katzin o.
Kazanjian o.
Keen o.
Keller-Madlener o.
Kelman o.
Kennedy-Pacey o.
keratectomy o.
keratocentesis o.
keratomileusis o.
keratoplasty o.
keratotomy o.
Key o.
kidney-sparing o.
King o.
Kirby o.
Knapp o.
Knapp-Wheeler-Reese o.
Kochs o.
Koffler o.
Kondoleon o.
Konno o.
Kraske o.
Kraupa o.
Kreiker o.
Krempen-Silver-Sotelo nonunion o.
Krönlein o.
Krönlein-Berke o.
Kropp o.
Kuhnt eyelid o.
Kuhnt-Helmbold o.
Kuhnt-Thorpe o.
Kwitko o.
Ladd o.
Lagleyze-Trantas o.
Lagrange o.
Lahey o.
laissez-faire lid o.
Lancaster o.
Lanchner o.
Landolt o.
Lane o.
Langenbeck o.
laparoscopic Hassab o.
Laroyenne o.
laryngeal keel o.
Lash o.
Lawson o.
Leahey o.
Le Fort o.
Le Fort-Neugebauer o.
Leriche o.
Lester-Jones o.
Lester Martin modification of Duhamel o.
Levine dislocation o.
Lewis o.
Lexer o.
Lichtenstein o.
limb-sparing o.
Lincoff o.
Lindesmith o.
Lindner o.
Lindsay o.
Linton o.
lip adhesion o.
liver o.
logical o.
Löhlein o.
Londermann o.
Longmire o.
Lopez-Enriquez o.
Lord o.
Loreta o.
Lotheissen o.
Löwenstein o.
Luc o.
Lynch o.
Macewen hernia o.
Machek-Blaskovics o.
Machek-Brunswick o.
Machek-Gifford o.
Machek ptosis o.
Mack-Brunswick o.
MacNab o.
Madlener o.
Magitot keratoplasty o.
magnet o.
magnetic o.
Magnus o.
Magnuson-Stack o.
MAGPI o.
Mainz pouch o.
Majewsky o.
major o.
Maladie de Graeffe o.
Malbec o.
Malbran o.
Manchester o.
Manchester-Fothergill o.
mandibular swing o.
Mann-Williamson o.

Marckwald o.
Marcy o.
Marquez-Gomez o.
Marshall-Marchetti-Krantz o.
Mason o.
mastoid obliteration o.
Matas o.
Mauksch o.
Mauksch-Maumenee-Goldberg o.
Maumenee-Goldberg o.
Maunsell-Weir o.
Mayo o.
McBurney o.
McGavic o.
McGuire o.
McIndoe o.
McKay-Simons clubfoot o.
McLaughlin o.
McLean o.
McReynolds o.
McVay o.
Meek o.
Meller o.
Mensor-Scheck hanging hip o.
Merindino o.
Meyer o.
Meyer-Schwickerath o.
Michaelson o.
mika o.
Mikulicz o.
Miles o.
Miller flatfoot o.
minor o.
Minsky o.
modified flap o.
Moncrieff o.
Monfort o.
Moran o.
Morax o.
morcellation o.
Morel-Fatio-Lalardie o.
Mosher o.
Mosher-Toti o.
Moss o.
Motais o.
motivating o.
Moynihan o.
Mueller o.
Mules o.
muscle sliding o.
Mustard o.
Mustardé o.
myectomy o.
myelomeningocele o.
myotomy o.
Naffziger o.
Neher o.
Nehra-Mack o.
Nesbit o.
Neviaser o.
Nicoll fracture o.
Nida nicking o.
Nirschl o.
Nissen antireflux o.
Nissen fundoplication o.
Nizetic o.
Norton o.
Norwood o.
Nuttall o.
O'Brien pelvic halo o.
obstetrical o.
O'Connor o.
O'Connor-Peter o.
O'Donnell o.
Ogilvie o.
Ogston-Luc o.
Ogura o.
Ombrédanne o.
one-snip punctum o.
one-stage o.
open hernia o.
open Nissen o.
open-sky cryoextraction o.
optical iridectomy o.
orbital implant o.
orthotopic hemi-Koch o.
outpatient thyroid o.
Owen o.
Pagenstecher o.
palliative o.
Palma o.
Palomo o.
Panas o.
pancreatic o.
parallel o.
parathyroid o.
Partsch o.
Patey o.
pattern cut corneal graft o.
Payne o.
pedicle flap o.
Peet o.
Pemberton o.
peripheral iridectomy o.

NOTES

operation *(continued)*
Peter o.
Physick o.
Pico o.
Pirogoff o.
plastic o.
plombage o.
pocket o.
Pollock o.
Pólya o.
Polyak o.
Pomeroy o.
Porro o.
portacaval shunt o.
Portmann interposition o.
Potts o.
Poulard o.
Power o.
Preziosi o.
probing lacrimonasal duct o.
protective antireflux o.
pubovaginal o.
Puestow-Gillesby o.
pull-through o.
pulsed-mode o.
Putenney o.
Quaglino o.
Ramstedt o.
Ransohoff o.
Rashkind o.
Rastan o.
Rastelli o.
Raverdino o.
Ray-Brunswick-Mack o.
Ray-McLean o.
Récamier o.
reconstructive o.
Redmond-Smith o.
Reese-Cleasby o.
Reese-Jones-Cooper o.
Reese ptosis o.
repeat o.
resectional phase of o.
resurfacing o.
Richet o.
Ripstein rectal prolapse o.
Rizzoli o.
Rosenburg o.
Rosengren o.
Roux-en-Y o.
Roux-Goldthwait dislocation o.
Roveda o.
Rovsing o.
Rowbotham o.
Rowinski o.
Rubbrecht o.
Ruedemann o.
Rycroft o.
sacrofixation o.
Saemisch o.
Saenger o.
Safar o.
Sanders o.
Sato o.
Savin o.
Sawyer o.
Sayoc o.
Scarpa o.
Schauta vaginal o.
Scheie o.
Schepens o.
Schimek o.
Schirmer o.
Schlatter o.
Schmalz o.
Schönbein o.
Schroeder o.
Schuchardt o.
scleral buckling o.
scleral fistulectomy o.
scleral shortening o.
scleroplasty o.
sclerotomy o.
Scott o.
scrotal pouch o.
Scudder o.
second-look o.
sector iridectomy o.
Selinger o.
semielective o.
Senn o.
Senning o.
sensor o.
serial o.
seton o.
sex change o.
Shaffer o.
Shirodkar o.
Shugrue o.
Sichi o.
Silva-Costa o.
Silver-Hildreth o.
single-stage o.
slant muscle o.
Smith-Boyce o.
Smith eyelid o.
Smith-Gibson o.
Smith-Indian o.
Smith-Kuhnt-Szymanowski o.
Smith-Robinson o.
Snellen ptosis o.
Soave o.
Soria o.
Soriano o.
Sorrin o.
Sourdille keratoplasty o.

Sourdille ptosis o.
Spaeth cystic bleb o.
Spaeth ptosis o.
Speas o.
Spencer-Watson Z-plasty o.
sphincter-saving o.
Spinelli o.
splitting lacrimal papilla o.
staging o.
Stallard eyelid o.
Stallard flap o.
Stallard-Liegard o.
Stamey o.
State o.
step graft o.
stereotactic o.
Stetta o.
Stock o.
Stocker o.
Stoffel o.
Stookey-Scarff o.
Straith eyelid o.
Strampelli-Valvo o.
Streatfield o.
Streatfield-Fox o.
Streatfield-Snellen o.
Sturmdorf o.
Suarez-Villafranca o.
subcutaneous o.
Sugarbaker o.
Summerskill o.
suprapubic urethrovesical suspension o.
suspensory sling o.
switch o.
symmetry o.
synchrocyclotron o.
Szymanowski o.
Szymanowski-Kuhnt o.
tagliacotian o.
talc o.
Tanner o.
Tansini o.
Tansley o.
Tasia o.
Taussig o.
Taussig-Morton o.
Teale-Knapp o.
TeLinde o.
tenotomy o.
Terson o.
Tessier craniofacial o.
Thal fundic patch o.
Thiersch anal incontinence o.
Thiersch graft o.
Thomas o.
Thomson o.
three-snip punctum o.
thyroid o.
Tillett o.
tongue-in-groove o.
Torek o.
total excisional o.
Toti o.
Toti-Mosher o.
Townley-Paton o.
trabeculectomy o.
Trainor o.
Trainor-Nida o.
transsphenoidal o.
Trantas o.
Trendelenburg o.
Treves o.
Tripier o.
Troutman o.
Truc o.
Tudor-Thomas o.
tumbling technique o.
Turnbull multiple ostomy o.
Turner o.
Ulloa o.
unattended laboratory o.
Urban o.
urologic o.
Uyemura o.
van Buren o.
Van Milligen o.
Vecchietti o.
Verhoeff o.
Verhoeff-Chandler o.
Vermale o.
Verneuil o.
Verwey eyelid o.
Viers o.
Virag o.
Vogt o.
Von Ammon o.
von Blaskovics-Doyen o.
von Graefe o.
von Hippel o.
Waldhauer o.
Walter Reed o.
Waters o.
Waterston o.

O

NOTES

operation *(continued)*
Watson o.
Watzke o.
Waugh o.
Way o.
Webster o.
Weeker o.
Weeks o.
Weir o.
Weisinger o.
Wendell Hughes o.
Werb o.
Wertheim o.
Wertheim-Schauta o.
West o.
Weve o.
Wharton-Jones o.
Wheeler o.
Wheeler-Reese o.
Wheelhouse o.
Whipple o.
Whitehead o.
Whitnall sling o.
Wicherkiewicz eyelid o.
Wiener o.
Wies o.
Williams copulating pouch o.
Wilmer o.
Winiwarter o.
Wise o.
Witzel o.
Wolfe ptosis o.
Worst o.
Worth ptosis o.
Wright o.
Young o.
Young-Dees o.
Young-Dees-Leadbetter o.
Zickel subtrochanteric fracture o.
Ziegler o.
Zimmerman o.
Zylik o.
operational homeostasis
operative
o. approach
o. arthroscopy
o. arthrotomy
o. biliary bypass
o. blood loss
o. cholangiography (OC)
o. choledochoscopy
o. correction
o. débridement
o. diagnosis
o. drainage
o. excision
o. exposure
o. field
o. finding
o. intervention
o. management
o. mortality
o. mortality rate
o. necrosectomy
o. perforation
o. procedure
o. reconstruction
o. reexploration
o. result
o. site complication
o. specimen
o. stress
o. technique
o. therapy
o. time
o. treatment
operatively stabilized
operator exposure
operculectomy
operculum, pl. **opercula**
O'Phelan technique
ophryon
ophryospinal angle
ophthalmectomy
ophthalmic
o. anesthesia
o. artery
o. ctivating solution
o. cul-de-sac
o. examination
o. nerve
o. vein
ophthalmocarcinoma
ophthalmocele
ophthalmologic anesthesia
ophthalmomyotomy
ophthalmopathy
ophthalmophlebotomy
ophthalmoplasty
ophthalmoplegia
ophthalmoscopy
binocular indirect o.
direct o.
indirect o.
medical o.
metric o.
slit-lamp o.
ophthalmospectroscopy
ophthalmostasis
ophthalmotomy
opiate
opioid
o. agonist
o. analgesia
o. analgesic
o. anesthesia

o. anesthetic
endogenous o.
epidural o.
esterase-metabolized o.
lipophilic o.
neuroaxial o.
o. prescreening
o. receptor
o. rotation
o. system

opioid-insensitive pain
opisthion
opisthionasial
opisthotonos
o. position
opisthotonus
OPO
organ procurement organization
opponensplasty
abductor digiti minimi o.
abductor digiti quinti o.
Bunnell o.
Huber adductor digiti quinti o.
Manske-McCarroll o.
opportunistic
o. complication
o. organism
o. systemic fungal infection
opposition respiration
opposure
opsonization
optic
o. canal
o. chiasm compression
o. cul-de-sac
o. cup
o. cup-to-disc ratio
o. decussation
o. disk
o. evagination
o. foramen
o. ganglion
o. iridectomy
o. keratoplasty
o. nerve
o. nerve atrophy
o. nerve head
o. nerve tumor
o. neuropathy
o. papilla
o. papilla cavity
o. pathway myelination
o. radiation
o. sheath
o. tract
o. tract compression
o. tract syndrome
o. vesicle
optical
o. aberration
o. biopsy
o. correction
o. density method
o. iridectomy
o. iridectomy operation
o. keratoplasty
o. nodal point
o. rotation
o. system
o. tracking
optici
opticociliary
o. neurectomy
o. neurotomy
opticum
optimal
o. intensive medical management
O. Observation Score
o. technique
o. therapy
opting
o. in
o. out
option
interventional o.
medical treatment o.
surgical treatment o.
therapeutic o.
treatment o.
optode
optometrist
OR
operating room
OR technician
ora, pl. **orae**
orad
O'Rahilly limb deficiency classification
oral
o. administration
o. analgesic
o. anesthetic
o. anesthetic technique
o. anomaly
o. antibiotic medication

O

NOTES

oral *(continued)*
- o. anticoagulant
- o. anticoagulation
- o. antimotility agent
- o. aphthous ulcer
- o. cavity
- o. cavity abnormality
- o. cavity cytology
- o. cavity tumor
- o. cephalocele
- o. complication
- o. condyloma planus
- o. endotracheal intubation
- o. feeding
- o. fissure
- o. infection
- o. irrigation
- o. lighted-stylet intubation
- o. manifestation
- o. and maxillofacial surgery
- o. monotherapy
- o. mucosa
- o. peripheral examination
- o. pharyngeal airway
- o. pharynx
- o. reconstruction
- o. region
- o. respiration
- o. tissue
- o. ulceration

oral-aural method
oral-facial-digital
oralis
Orandi technique
orbicular
- o. muscle
- o. zone

orbiculare
orbicularis
orbit
- deep o.
- lateral o.
- superficial o.
- superior o.

orbita, pl. **orbitae**
orbital
- o. adipose tissue
- o. anesthesia
- o. angioma
- o. apex syndrome
- o. arteriovenous malformation
- o. blow-out fracture
- o. branch
- o. canal
- o. cavity
- o. decompression
- o. eminence
- o. exenteration
- o. exenteration gastroscopic access technique
- o. extension
- o. fascia
- o. fat pad
- o. floor fracture
- o. height
- o. hematoma
- o. hernia
- o. implant operation
- o. index
- o. layer
- o. lesion
- o. line
- o. metastasis
- o. mucocele
- o. muscle
- o. phlebogram
- o. plane
- o. pyramid
- o. region
- o. rim fracture
- o. rim reconstruction
- o. section
- o. septum
- o. surface
- o. surgery
- o. tumor
- o. vein
- o. wall
- o. wall fracture

orbitale
orbitales
orbitalis muscle
orbitofrontal artery
orbitomaxillectomy
orbitomeatal line
orbitonasal
- o. index
- o. tissue

orbitopalpebralis
orbitosphenoid
orbitotomy
- Berke-Krönlein o.
- Krönlein o.

orbitozygomatic
- o. mandibular osteotomy
- o. temporopolar approach

orchalgia
orchectomy
orchialgia
orchichorea
orchidectomy
- partial o.
- radical o.

orchidic
orchiditis
orchidoblastoma

orchidoptosis
orchidorraphy
orchiectomy
prophylactic o.
radical inguinal o.
orchiepididymitis
orchioblastoma
orchiocele
orchiodynia
orchioneuralgia
orchiopathy
orchiopexy
Bevan o.
Cabot-Nesbit o.
eversion o.
Fowler-Stephens o.
laparoscopic o.
Prentiss o.
scrotal pouch o.
staged o.
Torek o.
transseptal o.
two-step o.
orchioplasty
orchiorrhaphy
orchiotherapy
orchiotomy
orchis, pl. **orchises**
orchitic
orchitis
orchotomy
ordinal classification
organ
o. ablation
o. allograft
o. compromise
Corti o.
o. donation
o. donor
o. dysfunction
effector o.
external female genital o.
external male genital o.
o. failure criteria
floating o.
genital o.
o. harvest
internal female genital o.
internal male genital o.
intraabdominal o.
intromittent o.
o. perfusion
o. procurement organization (OPO)
O. Procurement Program
ptotic o.
o. of Rosenmüller
secondary retroperitoneal o.
solid o.
supernumerary o.
o. system
o. transplantation
urinary o.
wandering o.
Weber o.
organa (*pl. of* organum)
organic
o. articulation disorder
o. lesion
o. short bowel syndrome
organism
aerobic gram-negative o.
colonizing o.
commensal o.
enteric o.
fungal o.
gram-negative aerobic o.
gut-derived gram-negative aerobic o.
mixed fungal o.
opportunistic o.
pure fungal o.
organization
organ procurement o. (OPO)
World Health O. (WHO)
organized
o. clot
o. hematoma
organizing inflammation
organoaxial rotation
organology
organopexy
organoscopy
organ-specific
o.-s. pattern
o.-s. pattern of injury
organum, pl. **organa**
Oriental
O. cholangiohepatitis
O. V-Y flap
orientation
angle of o.
limbal parallel o.
phalangeal articular o.

NOTES

O

orientation *(continued)*
temporal o.
visual o.
orifice
anal o.
appendiceal o.
esophagogastric o.
eustachian tube o.
exocranial o.
external urethral o.
gastroduodenal o.
golf-hole ureteral o.
ileocecal o.
internal urethral o.
myopectineal o.
pharyngeal o.
pulmonary o.
pyloric o.
renal artery o.
root canal o.
vaginal o.
vein o.
orificium, pl. **orificia**
origin
aberrant bronchial o.
biliodigestive o.
ectal o.
flexor-pronator o.
pancreatic head o.
pectoralis major muscle o.
primary o.
sternocleidomastoid muscle o.
tumor o.
oris
Ormond disease
oroantral fistula
orocutaneous fistula
oroendotracheal
orofacial
o. carcinoma
o. fistula
orofaciodigital (OFD)
o. syndrome
orogastric
o. pathway
o. suction
oromandibular
o. defect
o. reconstruction
oronasal fistula
oropharyngeal
o. airway
o. anesthesia
o. approach
o. carcinoma
o. hemorrhage
o. passage
o. reconstruction
oropharynx
ororespiratory tract
orostoma
orotracheal intubation
Orr
O. incision
O. rectal prolapse repair
Orr-Loygue transabdominal proctopexy
Orsi-Grocco method
orthodontia
surgical o.
orthodontic
o. procedure
o. therapy
orthodontics
surgical o.
orthodox procedure
orthognathic surgery
orthogonal
o. plane
o. projection
orthokeratinization
Orthopaedic Trauma Association classification
orthopedic, orthopaedic
o. anesthesia
o. anomaly
o. problem
o. surgical procedure
o. traumatologist
orthoptic transplantation
orthoradioscopy
orthoscopy
orthosis drop-lock ring
orthotopic
o. appendicocystostomy
o. bladder
o. graft
o. heart transplantation
o. hemi-Koch operation
o. liver transplant (OLT)
o. liver transplantation (OLT)
o. liver transplant recipient
o. ureterocele
o. urinary diversion
Orticochea
O. procedure
O. scalping technique
Ortolani maneuver
os, pl. **ossa**
o. calcis osteotomy
external o.
Osborne-Cotterill
O.-C. elbow technique
O.-C. procedure
Osborne posterior approach
oscheal
oscheitis

oschelephantiasis
oscheohydrocele
oscheoplasty
oscillation
grade I, II o.
high-frequency o.
laryngeal o.
nystagmoid-like o.
ocular o.
oscillatory ventilation
oscillometric calibration
oscillometry
Osgood
O. modified technique
O. rotational osteotomy
Osgood-Schlatter lesion
osmication
osmification
Osmond-Clarke technique
osmotic pressure
ossa (*pl. of* os)
osseointegration
osseoligamentous ring
osseous
o. anomaly
o. fixation
o. labyrinth
o. lesion
o. metastasis
o. ring of Lacroix
o. surgery
o. tissue
osseus
ossicle
ossicular chain reconstruction
ossiculectomy
ossiculoplasty
tympanoplasty o.
ossiculum, pl. **ossicula**
ossification
ossificationis
ossifying
o. epiphysis
o. inflammation
o. nucleus
ossium
ostectomy
buccal o.
fibular o.
partial o.
periodontal o.
osteitis
bone flap o.
osteoaneurysm
osteoarthritis disease
osteoarthropathy
osteoarticular
o. allograft
o. allograft transplantation
o. defect
o. graft
osteoblast
osteoblastic
o. bone regeneration
o. lesion
o. metastasis
osteoblastoma
osteobunionectomy
osteocachexia
osteocarcinoma
osteocartilaginous
o. graft
o. loose body
osteocementum
osteochondral
o. allograft
o. defect
o. fragment
o. graft
o. injury
o. lesion
o. loose body
o. prominence
o. ridge
osteochondritis
osteochondrodesmodysplasia
osteochondrodysplasia
osteochondrodystrophy
familial o.
osteochondrofibroma
osteochondrolysis
osteochondroma
osteochondromatosis
osteochondropathy
osteochondrophyte
osteochondrosarcoma
osteochondrosis
osteochrondral slice fracture
osteoclasia
osteoclasis
Blount technique for o.
o. maneuver
osteoclastic

NOTES

O

osteoclastoma
osteoconduction
osteocranium
osteocutaneous flap
osteocystoma
osteocyte
osteocytic lacuna
osteocytoma
osteodentin
osteodentinoma
osteodermatopoikilosis
osteodermatous
osteodermia
osteodiastasis
osteodysplasty
osteodystrophia
osteodystrophy
osteoectasia
osteoectomy
osteoenchondroma
osteoepiphysis
osteofibrochondrosarcoma
osteofibroma
osteofibromatosis
osteofibrosis
osteogenesis
- distraction o.
- o. imperfecta
- o. imperfecta congenita syndrome

osteogenetic fiber
osteogenic
osteohalisteresis
osteohypertrophy
osteoid osteoma
osteoinduction
osteointegration phenomenon
osteokinematic motion
osteokinematics
osteolathyrism
osteolipochondroma
osteolipoma
osteologia
osteologist
osteology
osteolysis
osteolytic bone lesion
osteoma
- extraspinal osteoid o.
- osteoid o.

osteomalacia
osteomalacic pelvis
osteomatoid
osteomatosis
osteomeatal
osteomere
osteomesopyknosis
osteometry
osteomized
osteomusculocutaneous flap
osteomyelitic sinus
osteomyelitis
osteomyelodysplasia
osteomyelofibrosis
osteomyelofibrotic syndrome
osteomyelosclerosis
osteomyocutaneous flap
osteon
osteonal
- o. bone union
- o. lamellar bone

osteoncus
osteonecrosis
osteonectin
osteoneogenesis
osteoneuralgia
osteopathia striata syndrome
osteopathic lesion
osteopathy
osteopedion
osteopenia
osteoperiosteal
- o. bone graft
- o. flap

osteoperiostitis
osteopetrosis
- cranial o.

osteopetrotic scar
osteophlebitis
osteophyma
osteophyte formation
osteophytosis
osteoplastic
- o. bone flap
- o. craniotomy
- o. frontal sinus procedure
- o. necrotomy
- o. reconstruction

osteoplasty
- Maquet anteromedial o.

osteopoikilosis
osteopontin
osteoporosis pseudoglioma syndrome
osteoporotic
- o. bone
- o. fracture
- o. spine

osteopsathyrosis
osteopulmonary arthropathy
osteoradionecrosis
osteosarcoma
osteosarcomatosis
osteosclerotic lesion
osteosis
osteospongioma
osteosteatoma
osteosynovitis

osteosynthesis
anterior column o.
cranial o.
facial o.
lumbar spine vertebral o.
odontoid process o.
plate-screw o.
posterior column o.
thoracic spine vertebral o.
thoracolumbar spine vertebral o.
vertebral o.
wire o.
osteosynthetic material
osteotabes
osteotelangiectasia
osteothrombophlebitis
osteothrombosis
osteotomize
osteotomy
Abbott-Gill o.
abduction o.
abductor o.
abductory wedge o.
adduction o.
Agliette supracondylar o.
Akin proximal phalangeal o.
Amspacher-Messenbaugh closing wedge o.
Amstutz-Wilson o.
Anderson-Fowler calcaneal displacement o.
angular o.
angulation o.
anterior calcaneal o.
anterior innominate o.
Austin o.
Axer lateral opening wedge o.
Axer varus derotational o.
Bailey-Dubow o.
Baker-Hill o.
Balacescu closing wedge o.
ball-and-socket trochanteric o.
base-of-the-neck o.
base wedge o.
basilar o.
Bellemore-Barrett closing wedge o.
Berman-Gartland metatarsal o.
bifurcation o.
biplane trochanteric o.
blind o.
block o.
Blount displacement o.
Brackett o.
Brett-Campbell tibial o.
calcaneal L o.
Campbell o.
Canale o.
canal innominate o.
Carstan reverse wedge o.
Cartam-Treander reverse wedge o.
cervical o.
C-form o.
Chambers o.
chevron o.
Chiari innominate o.
Chiari-Salter-Steel pelvic o.
closed intramedullary o.
closed wedge o.
closing abductory wedge o.
closing base wedge o.
Cole o.
compensatory basilar o.
controlled rotational o.
countersinking o.
Coventry distal femoral o.
Coventry vagal o.
craniofacial o.
Crego femoral o.
crescentic calcaneal o.
C sliding o.
cuneiform o.
cup-and-ball o.
cylindrical o.
Dega pelvic o.
delayed femoral o.
derotational o.
dial pelvic o.
dial periacetabular o.
diaphysial o.
Dickinson-Coutts-Woodward-Handler o.
Dickson geometric o.
Diebold-Bejjani o.
Dillwyn-Evans o.
Dimon-Hughston intertrochanteric o.
displacement o.
dome o.
dome-shaped o.
dorsal closing wedge o.
dorsal proximal metatarsal o.
dorsal-V o.
dorsiflexory wedge o.
double o.
Dunn o.

O

NOTES

osteotomy *(continued)*
Dunn-Hess trochanteric o.
Dwyer o.
Elizabethtown o.
Emmon o.
epiphysial-metaphysial o.
Eppright dial o.
Estersohn o.
ethmoidal o.
Evans anterior calcaneal o.
eversion o.
extension o.
failed femoral o.
femoral o.
Fernandez o.
flexion o.
French lateral closing wedge o.
frontonasomaxillary o.
frontoorbital o.
geometric supracondylar extension o.
Gerbert o.
Giannestras oblique metatarsal o.
Gibson-Piggott o.
glabellar exposure o.
Gleich o.
glenoid o.
Golden closing wedge o.
Grant-Small-Lehman supracondylar extension o.
Greenfield o.
Green-Reverdin o.
greenstick dorsal proximal metatarsal o.
Green-Watermann o.
Gudas scarf Z-plasty o.
Haber-Kraft o.
Haddad metatarsal o.
Herman-Gartland o.
high tibial o.
hinge o.
Hirayma o.
horizontal o.
iliac o.
Ingram-Canle-Beaty epiphysial-metaphysial o.
innominate o.
intertrochanteric varus o.
intraarticular o.
intracapsular o.
intraepiphysial o.
inverted L-form o.
Irwin o.
Japas o.
Johnson chevron o.
Kalish o.
Kaplan o.
Kawamura dome o.
Kawamura pelvic o.
Kelly-Keck o.
Kempf-Grosse-Abalo Z-step o.
Kessel-Bonney extension o.
Kitaoka-Leventen medial displacement metatarsal o.
Koutsogiannis calcaneal displacement o.
Koutsogiannis-Fowler-Anderson o.
Kramer-Craig-Noel basilar femoral neck o.
Lambrinudi o.
lateral closing wedge o.
Leach-Igou step-cut medial o.
Le Fort o.
Lelièvre o.
Lichtblau o.
Lindseth o.
linear o.
Ludloff o.
Macewen-Shands o.
malleolar o.
mandibular ramus o.
Maquet dome o.
Marquardt angulation o.
Martin o.
Mau o.
maxillary o.
medial displacement o.
metacarpal o.
metaphysial o.
metatarsal Reverdin o.
metatarsal V-shaped o.
Mitchell o.
Molesworth o.
Mueller intertochanteric varus o.
Mueller transposition o.
oblique base-wedge o.
oblique displacement o.
open o.
orbitozygomatic mandibular o.
os calcis o.
Osgood rotational o.
Pauwels proximal o.
Pauwels valgus o.
peg-in-hole o.
Peimer reduction o.
pelvic o.
Pemberton pericapsular o.
perforation o.
pericapsular o.
phalangeal o.
Platou o.
posterior iliac o.
posterior spinal wedge o.
Pott eversion o.
radial wedge o.
Ranawat-DeFiore-Straub o.

Rappaport o.
reduction o.
Reverdin o.
Reverdin-Laird o.
reverse Dillwyn-Evans calcaneal o.
reverse wedge o.
Root-Siegal varus derotational o.
rotational o.
sagittal-split mandibular o.
Sakoff o.
Salter innominate o.
Salter pelvic o.
Samilson crescentic calcaneal o.
Sarmiento intertrochanteric o.
scarf o.
Schanz angulation o.
Schanz femoral o.
Schwartz dorsiflexory o.
segmental alveolar o.
Siffert intraepiphysial o.
Siffert-Storen intraepiphysial o.
Simmonds-Menelaus metatarsal o.
Simmonds-Menelaus proximal phalangeal o.
Simmons o.
o. site
sliding oblique o.
Smith-Petersen o.
Sofield o.
Southwick biplane trochanteric o.
spinal o.
Sponsel oblique o.
Stamm metatarsal o.
Steel triple innominate o.
step o.
step-cut o.
stepdown o.
Stren intraepiphysial o.
subcapital o.
subcondylar oblique o.
subtrochanteric o.
Sugioka transtrochanteric rotational o.
supracondylar varus o.
supramalleolar varus derotation o.
Sutherland-Greenfield o.
tarsal wedge o.
Tessier o.
Thompson telescoping V o.
through-and-through V-shaped horizontal o.
tibial tuberosity o.
transtrochanteric rotational o.
trapezoidal o.
Trethowan metatarsal o.
triplane o.
triple innominate o.
trochanteric o.
tubercle o.
unplanned valgus o.
valgus wedge-prop o.
valgus Y-shaped prop o.
varus rotation shortening o.
vertical o.
V-shaped o.
Waterman o.
Weber humeral o.
Weber subcapital o.
wedge o.
wedge-shaped o.
Whitman o.
Wilson oblique displacement o.
Wiltse ankle o.
Wiltse varus supramalleolar o.
Yancey o.
Yu o.

osteotomy-bunionectomy
scarf o.-b.

osteotomy-osteoclasis
Moore o.-o.

osteotripsy

osteotrite

osteotympanic bone conduction

ostial
o. lesion
o. sphincter

ostium, pl. **ostia**
abdominal o.
celiac o.

ostomate

ostomy
o. loop
o. skin

Ostrum-Furst syndrome

Ostrup
O. harvesting technique
O. vascularized rib graft

Osypka rotational angioplasty

otic
o. ganglion
o. periotic shunt procedure
o. vesicle

oticum

otitis

NOTES

otoconia
degenerating o.
otolaryngologic manifestation
otolaryngologist
otolaryngology
pediatric o.
otolith
otolithic membrane
otomandibular syndrome
otomicrosurgical transtemporal approach
otoplasty
mattress suture o.
otorhinolaryngology
otorrhea
clear o.
otosclerosis
otoscopy
pneumatic o.
Otto pelvis dislocation
ouabain
Ouchterlony
O. gel diffusion technique
O. method
O. technique
Oudard procedure
out
opting o.
outcome
clinical o.
cosmetic o.
final o.
long-term o.
o. monitoring
perioperative o.
short-term o.
surgical o.
outer
o. limiting membrane
Outerbridge classification
outermost
outflow
cerebrospinal fluid o.
o. control
craniosacral o.
thoracolumbar o.
o. tract
o. tract obstruction
venous o.
outlet
o. strut fracture
out-of-phase endometrial biopsy
outpatient
o. anesthesia
o. biopsy
o. dialysis
o. dialysis clinic
o. endoscopy
o. physical therapy
o. setting
o. surgical setting
o. thyroidectomy
o. thyroid operation
output
cardiac o. (CO)
chest tube o. (CTO)
intraoperative urine o.
o. layer
pacemaker o.
radiation o.
saturation o.
thermodilution cardiac o. (TDCO)
outside-to-outside arthroscopy technique
outward rotation
ova (*pl. of* ovum)
oval
o. cup erysiphake
o. window
ovale
foramen o.
patent foramen o. (PFO)
ovalis
oval-shaped crushing
ovarian
o. ablation
o. artery
o. branch
o. bursa
o. cancer
o. cancer metastasis
o. carcinoma
o. carcinoma debulking
o. clear cell adenocarcinoma
o. cortex
o. cystectomy
o. dermoid cyst
o. fimbria
o. follicle exhaustion
o. hernia
o. hyperstimulation syndrome
o. incision
o. masculinization
o. mass
o. overstimulation syndrome
o. plexus
o. stimulation
o. surface
o. thecoma
o. tumor
O. Tumor Registry
o. vein
o. vein syndrome
o. wedge resection
ovarica
ovaricae
ovaricus
ovariectomy

ovarii
ovariocele
ovariohysterectomy
ovariosalpingectomy
ovariostomy
ovariotomy
  Beatson o.
  normal o.
ovary
  premenopausal o.
  right o.
overall sound level
over-and-over suture technique
overangulation
overbite
overcirculation
  pulmonary o.
overcompensation
overcorrected position
overcorrection
overdetermination
overdilation
overfilled canal
overflow incontinence
overgrafting
overgrowth
  bacterial o.
  cartilage o.
  fungal o.
overhang
overhanging restoration
Overhauser technique
Overholt procedure
overinflation
overinstrumentation
overlap
  o. midline incisional hernioplasty
  suture o.
overlapping
  o. incision
  o. suture technique
overlay restoration
overload
  circulatory o.
  compression o.
  pressure o.
overprojecting nasal tip
overrotation
oversedation
oversewing
  early o.
oversewn
overshoot
  calibration o.
overstimulation
over-the-counter medication
over-the-top position
over-the-wire technique
Overton dowel graft
overventilation
overwhelming postsplenectomy infection
oviduct
oviductal
ovoidalis
ovoid mass
ovotestis
ovular transmigration
ovulation
  estimated time of o. (ETO)
  o. induction
  o. rate
  o. stimulation
ovum, pl. **ova**
Owen
  interglobular space of O.
  O. line
  O. operation
Owestry Disability Questionnaire (ODQ)
owl eye inclusion body
oxalate calculus
Oxford technique
oxidation
  o. of solution
  o. state
oxidation-reducing potential
oxide
  ethylene o. (ETO)
  nitrous o. (NO)
oximetry
  oxygen saturation as measured using pulse o.
  pulse o.
oxycarbonate
oxycardiorespirogram
oxycephalia
oxycephalic
oxycephaly
oxygen (O_2)
  o. administration
  o. in air
  o. concentration in pulmonary capillary blood
  o. consumption
  o. debt

O

NOTES

oxygen *(continued)*
- o. deprivation theory of narcosis
- o. desaturation
- o. dissociation curve
- o. effect
- o. extraction rate
- flow-dependent o.
- hyperbaric o.
- nasal o. (NO)
- partial pressure of o. (PO_2)
- partial pressure of alveolar o.
- partial pressure of arterial o.
- o. poisoning
- rapid recompression-high pressure o.
- o. reduction product
- o. saturation
- o. saturation as measured using pulse oximetry
- o. saturation of the hemoglobin of arterial blood
- o. saturation index
- o. saturation measurement
- o. step-up method
- supplementary o.
- o. supply line
- o. tension
- o. therapy
- o. toxicity
- transcutaneous partial pressure of o.
- o. under high pressure
- o. utilization

oxygenation
- apneic o.
- bubble o.
- cell o.
- disk o.
- extracorporeal membrane o. (ECMO)
- fetal scalp o.
- film o.
- hyperbaric o.
- o. index (OI)
- medullary o.
- pump o.
- rotating disk o.
- screen o.
- splanchnic o.
- tissue o.
- tumor o.

oxygen-carrying resuscitative fluid
oxygen-enriched atmosphere
oxygen-hemoglobin dissociation curve
oxyhemoglobin dissociation curve
oxyhemogram
oyster mass
ozonization
ozonolysis

P2 prolongation
p53 tumor suppressor gene analysis
PA
prophylactic antibiotic
pulmonary artery
pulmonary autograft
PA filling pressure
PA projection
PA therapy
pacchionian granulation
pacemaker
p. adaptive rate
p. artifact
p. burst pacing
p. capture
p. escape interval
p. failure
p. impedance
p. lead fracture
p. malfunction
p. output
p. pocket
p. potential
p. syndrome
p. threshold
p. undersensing
pacemaker-mediated tachycardia
Pacey technique
Pachon
P. method
P. test
pachydermatocele
pachymeningitis
pachyperitonitis
pachyvaginalitis
pacing
implantable cardioverter-defibrillator/atrial tachycardia p.
pacemaker burst p.
transesophageal atrial p. (TEAP)
transesophageal echocardiography with p.
transesophageal ventricular p. (TEVP)
packed red blood cells (PRBC)
Pack-Ehrlich deep iliac dissection
Pack technique
$PaCO_2$
partial pressure of arterial carbon dioxide
Pacquin ureterolysis
PACU
postanesthesia care unit
PAD
percutaneous abscess drainage
pad
abdominal fat p.
adenoid p.
adenoidal p.
antimesenteric fat p.
artificial fat p.
axillary fat p.
Bichat fat p.
branch p.
buccal fat p.
bulbocavernosus fat p.
buttocks p.
digital p.
epicardial fat p.
esophagogastric fat p.
fat p.
heel fat p.
herniated presacral fat p.
Hoffa fat p.
ileocecal fat p.
infrapatellar fat p.
ischiorectal fat p.
labial p.
malar fat p.
masticatory fat p.
metatarsal p.
orbital fat p.
patellar fat p.
pericardial fat p.
pubic p.
retrodiskal p.
retromolar p.
retropatellar fat p.
PAF
paroxysmal atrial fibrillation
pulmonary arteriovenous fistula
Pagenstecher
P. circle
P. operation
P. suture technique
Paget
P. carcinoma
P. extramammary disease
Paget-Eccleston stain
Paget-von Schrötter syndrome
PAG/PVG
periaqueductal-periventricular
PAG/PVG region
PAH
pulmonary artery hypertension
PAI
Pain Appraisal Inventory
pain
p. anxiety symptoms scale
P. Appraisal Inventory (PAI)

pain *(continued)*
back p.
p. behavior
bone p.
burning p.
cancer p.
p. catastrophizing scale
cementum p.
central p.
central poststroke p. (CPSP)
chronic p.
colicky p.
colorectal distention p.
P. Coping Questionnaire (PCQ)
cyclic p.
deafferentation p.
dentin p.
diffuse abdominal p.
dysesthetic p.
dystonic p.
Edmonton Staging System for Cancer P.
epigastric p.
exacerbation of p.
existential p.
experimental p.
expulsive p.
exquisite p.
herpes zoster p.
IASP Classification of Chronic P.
incisional p.
p. induction
inflammatory p.
International Association for the Study of P. (IASP)
intractable p.
joint line p.
labor p.
limb ischemia p.
p. management
micturition p.
moderate p.
p. modulation
movement-related p.
myofascial p.
neuropathic p.
nonsympathetically mediated p.
obstetric p.
opioid-insensitive p.
palliation of p.
pancreatic cancer p.
pediatric p.
p. perception profile
phantom foot p.
phantom limb p.
postherniorrhaphy p.
postoperative cesarean section p.
poststroke p.
postsurgical truncal p.
postthoracotomy p.
referred trigger-point p.
P. Relief Scoring System
p. sensitivity range
shortcut sciatic p.
somatic p.
spinal cord injury p.
stump p.
sympathetically maintained p. (SMP)
sympathetically mediated p.
p. syndrome
temporomandibular p.
thalamic p.
p. threshold reduction
p. tolerance level
tourniquet-induced p.
tourniquet ischemic p.
visceral p.

painful
p. anesthesia
p. point

painless rectal bleeding

Painter colic

paired
p. electrical stimulation
p. vasomotor response

Pais fracture

PAJB
primary antecubital jump bypass

Pajot maneuver

palatal
p. expansion
p. flap
p. index
p. lengthening procedure
p. vein

palate
Byzantine arch p.
cleft p.
hard p.
itchy soft p.
p. reconstruction
soft p.

palati

palatina

palatine
p. bone
p. canal
p. foramen
p. gland
p. nerve
p. suture

palatini

palatinum

• **palatoethmoidalis**

palatoethmoidal suture

palatoglossal fold
palatoglossus muscle
palatomaxillaris
palatomaxillary
p. canal
p. index
p. suture
palatooccipital line
palatopharyngeal
p. closure
p. fold
p. ring
p. sphincter
p. sphincter muscle
palatopharyngeus muscle
palatopharyngoplasty
palatopharyngorrhaphy
palatoplasty
palatorrhaphy
palatosalpingeus
palatostaphylinus
palatovaginal
p. canal
p. groove
Paley classification
Palfyn
P. sinus
P. suture technique
palliation of pain
palliative
p. bypass
p. cerebrospinal shunt procedure
p. esophagostomy
p. exeresis
p. gastrostomy
p. hepatojejunostomy
p. intent
p. operation
p. resection
p. surgery
p. surgical procedure
p. technique
p. therapy
p. total gastrectomy
pallidectomy
pallidoamygdalotomy
pallidoansotomy
pallidotomy
posteroventral p.
stereotactic p.
unilateral p.
VPL p.
pallor
Palma operation
palmar
p. advancement flap
p. angulation
p. approach
p. branch
p. crease
p. cross-finger flap
p. incision
p. interosseous artery
p. synovectomy
palmaria
palmaris
palmate fold
palmatus
Palmer
P. method
P. technique
P. transscaphoid perilunar dislocation
Palmer-Dobyns-Linscheid ligament repair
Palmer-Widen shoulder technique
palmoscopy
palm space
Palomo
P. operation
P. procedure
P. technique
palpable
p. mass
p. rib diastasis
palpation
bimanual p.
p. testing
palpatory examination
palpebra, pl. **palpebrae**
levator palpebrae
palpebral
p. artery
p. branch
p. fascia
p. fissure
p. ligament
p. muscle
p. rim
palpebrales
palpebralis
palpebrarum
palpebration
palpebronasal fold
palpebronasalis

NOTES

palpitation
paroxysmal p.
premonitory p.
palsy
Bell p.
temporary p.
vocal cord p.
pampiniform
p. body
p. plexus
pampiniforme
pampiniformis
pampinocele
Panas operation
panclavicular dislocation
Pancoast
P. suture technique
P. tumor
pancolectomy
pancolonoscopy
pancreas
aberrant p.
accessory p.
annular p.
artificial endocrine p.
Aselli p.
p. cancer
distal p.
ectopic p.
endocrine p.
exocrine p.
lesser p.
retroperitoneal p.
small p.
p. transplant (PTX)
p. transplantation
uncinate p.
Willis p.
Winslow p.
pancrease-specific amylase isoenzyme
pancreas-kidney transplantation
pancreatectomy
Child radical p.
complete laparoscopic distal p. (C-LDP)
conventional distal p.
distal p. (DP)
distal laparoscopic p.
donor p.
en bloc distal p.
laparoscopic distal p.
left-to-right subtotal p.
limited p.
near-total p.
partial p.
proximal subtotal p.
spleen-preserving distal p.
subtotal distal p.
total p.
transduodenal p.
Whipple p.
pancreatemphraxis
pancreatic
p. abscess
p. adenocarcinoma
p. anastomosis
p. artery
p. autotransplantation
p. bacterial infection
p. biopsy
p. body
p. branch
p. bypass
p. calculus
p. cancer pain
p. capsule
p. carcinoma
p. colic
p. complication
p. cutaneous fistula
p. cyst
p. cystoduodenostomy
p. disease
p. duct
p. duct dilatation
p. duct manipulation
p. duct pressure
p. duct sphincterotomy
p. endocrine tumor
p. endoscopy
p. enzyme
p. enzyme secretion
p. extract
p. fascia
p. fluid
p. fluid collection
p. fungal detection
p. fungus
p. head
p. head cancer
p. head origin
p. imaging
p. intraluminal radiation therapy
p. islet
p. lithiasis
p. malignancy
p. neck
p. necrosis
p. necrosis prognostic score
p. notch
p. operation
p. parenchyma
p. plexus
p. pseudocyst
p. pseudocystogastrostomy
p. sphincter

p. sphincteroplasty
p. stump
p. stump closure
p. stump leak
p. surgeon
p. surgery
p. tail
p. tail resection
p. tissue
p. transplantation
p. transplantation alone (PTA)
p. trauma
p. tumor localization
p. vein

pancreatica

pancreaticae

pancreatici

pancreaticobiliary

p. endoscopy
p. tract

pancreaticoblastoma

pancreaticocystostomy

pancreaticoduodenal

p. allograft
p. arcade vessel
p. arterial arcade
p. artery
p. transplantation
p. vein

pancreaticoduodenales

pancreaticoduodenectomy

pylorus-preserving p.
pylorus-sparing p.
Whipple p.

pancreaticoduodenostomy

Child p.
Dennis-Varco p.
Waugh-Clagett p.
Whipple p.

pancreaticoenterostomy

pancreaticogastric anastomosis

pancreaticogastrointestinal anastomosis

pancreaticogastrostomy

p. anastomosis (PGA)
p. reconstruction

pancreaticojejunal anastomosis

pancreaticojejunostomy

p. anastomosis (PJA)
Cattell-Warren p.
caudal p.
distal p.
duct-to-mucosa p.
Duval p.
end-to-end intussuscepted p.
end-to-end inverting p.
Frey p.
longitudinal p.
Puestow p.
Roux-en-Y p.

pancreaticopleural fistula

pancreaticosplenectomy

pancreaticosplenic

p. ligament
p. omentum

pancreatic-preserving total gastrectomy

pancreatic-renal

simultaneous p.-r. (SPR)

pancreaticus

pancreatis

pancreatitis

acute p. (AP)
biliary p.
centrilobular p.
chronic p.
clinical acute p.
diffuse hemorrhagic p.
p. dysfunction
gallstone p.
necrotizing p. (NP)

pancreatitis-related hemorrhage

pancreatobiliary canal

pancreatoblastoma

pancreatocholecystostomy

pancreatoduodenectomy

Billroth II p.
conventional p.
extended p.
Kausch-Whipple p.
partial p.
pylorus-preserving p. (PPPD)
radical p.
subtotal p.
two-step p.
Whipple p.

pancreatoduodenostomy

pancreatoenterostomy

pancreatogastrostomy

pancreatography

pancreatojejunostomy

cystolateral p.
retrocolic end-to-end p.

pancreatolith

pancreatolithectomy

pancreatolithiasis

NOTES

pancreatolithotomy
pancreatologist
pancreatolysis
pancreatolytic
pancreatomy
pancreatoscopy
peroral p.
pancreatotomy
pancreectomy
pancreolith
pancreolithotomy
pancreoprivic
pancreoscopy
infragastric p.
pancreticolienales
pandiculation
panel
bleeding time coagulation p.
clot retraction coagulation p.
clotting time coagulation p.
partial thromboplastin time coagulation p.
plasma assay coagulation p.
prediluted antibody p.
prothrombin time coagulation p.
panendoscopy
fiberoptic p.
lower p.
primary p.
upper gastrointestinal p.
panhysterectomy
panmetatarsal head resection
panmucosal inflammatory cell infiltration
panni (*pl. of* pannus)
pannicular hernia
panniculectomy
panniculus, pl. **panniculi**
abdominal p.
p. retraction
pannus, pl. **panni**
p. formation
panoramic surface projection
PANP
pelvic autonomic nerve preservation
panphotocoagulation
panproctocolectomy
panretinal
p. ablation
p. argon laser photocoagulation
pantalar fusion
pantaloon
p. hernia
p. patch
pants-over-vest
p.-o.-v. capsulorrhaphy
p.-o.-v. hernial repair
p.-o.-v. herniorrhaphy
p.-o.-v. technique
Panum fusion area
PAO_2
alveolar oxygen partial pressure
PaO_2
arterial oxygen partial pressure
PAOD
popliteal artery occlusive disease
PAOP
pulmonary artery occlusion pressure
PAP
positive airway pressure
pulmonary artery pressure
Papanicolaou method
Papavasiliou olecranon fracture classification
paper point
papilla, pl. **papillae**
bile p.
circumvallate p.
foliate p.
inferior lacrimal p.
interdental p.
lacrimal p.
lenticular p.
major duodenal p.
minor duodenal p.
optic p.
renal p.
retrocuspid p.
retromolar p.
sublingual p.
superior lacrimal p.
urethral p.
vallate p.
Vater p.
papillaris
papillary
p. adenoma
p. cancer
p. cystadenocarcinoma
p. duct
p. ectasia
p. foramen
p. gastric carcinoma
p. hidradenoma
p. hyperplasia
p. lesion
p. muscle rupture
p. muscle tip
p. pedicle graft
p. process
p. projection
p. reconstruction
p. subtype
papillectomy
papillitis

papilloadenocystoma
papillocarcinoma
papillogram
papilloma
choroid plexus p.
p. neuropathicum
papillomacular nerve fiber bundle
papillomatosis
diffuse p.
papillomavirus infection
Papillon-Léage and Psaume syndrome
papillotomy
accessory p.
endoscopic p.
laparoscopic transcystic p.
needle-knife p.
precut p.
Papineau
P. bone graft
P. technique
papulation
papulopustular lesion
papulosis
papulosquamous lesion
papulovesicular lesion
papyracea
Paquin technique
para-aortic
p.-a. hematoma
p.-a. lymphadenectomy
p.-a. lymph node dissection
p.-a. node irradiation
para-aortica
paraaortic region
para-appendicitis
parabiosis
parabiotic flap
paracancerous tissue
paracanthoma
paracardiac metastasis
paracentesis
abdominal p.
paracentetic
paracentral
p. lobe
p. nerve fiber bundle
paracentralis
paracervical
p. block
p. block anesthesia
p. injection
paracervix
parachroma
parachute
p. deformity
p. jumper dislocation
paraclavicular thoracic outlet decompression
paracoagulation
paracolic
p. gutter
p. recess
paracolici
paracollicular biopsy
paracolpium
paracystic pouch
paracystitis
paracystium
paradidymal
paradidymis
paradoxical
p. embolism
p. extensor reflex
p. incontinence
p. reaction
p. respiration
p. technique
paraduodenal
p. fossa
p. hernia
p. recess
paraduodenalis
paraesophageal
p. diaphragmatic hernia
p. hiatal hernia
paraesophagogastric devascularization
paraexstrophy skin flap
paraffin graft
paraffinoma
paraffin-section light microscopy
paraganglioma
paragenital tubule
paraglenoid groove
paraglottic
p. area
p. space
paragranuloma
parahepatic
parahiatal hernia
parahypophysis
paraileostomal hernia
parainfluenza virus infection
parainguinal incision
parajejunal fossa

NOTES

P

parajejunalis
parakeratinization
parakeratosis
paralaryngeal space
parallel
p. operation
p. technique
paralleling
p. cone position
p. technique
parallelism
paralysis
compression p.
cord p.
hernia p.
laryngeal nerve p.
long-term p.
nerve p.
permanent p.
pharmacologic p.
pharmacologically induced p.
pressure p.
recurrent nerve p.
soft-palate p.
tourniquet p.
unilateral laryngeal p.
vocal cord p. (VCP)
paralytic
p. ileus
p. strabismus
paralyzant
paramagnetic
p. contrast injection
p. enhancement accentuation by chemical shift imaging
p. shift relaxation
paramammarii
paramedial incision
paramedian
p. approach
p. incision
p. pontine reticular formation
p. sagittal plane
p. sheath
paramedical personnel
paramesonephric duct
paramesonephricus
parameter
canonical univariate p.
clinical p.
clotting p.
conventional p.
effect p.
laboratory p.
postprandial motor p.
parametrectomy
radical p.
parametrial
parametric test
parametritis
posterior p.
parametrium
paramuscular incision
paranalgesia
paranasal
p. cell
p. mucocele
p. sinus
paranasales
paraneoplastic ectopic ACTH production
paranephric
p. abscess
p. body
paranephros, pl. **paranephroi**
paranesthesia
paraneural infiltration
paraomphalic
paraoperative
paraoral tissue
paraorbital lesion
paraovarian
parapancreatic
paraparesis
parapatellar
p. arthrotomy
p. incision
paraperitoneal
p. hernia
p. nephrectomy
parapharyngeal
p. space
p. space abscess
paraphasia
extended jargon p.
paraphimosis
paraphysis
parapineal
paraplegia
complete motor p.
p. in extension
motor p.
postoperative p.
paraproctium
paraprostatitis
parapubic hernia
pararectal
p. fistula
p. fossa
p. line
p. pouch
pararectales
pararectus
p. approach
p. incision
pararenal space
parasaccular hernia

parasacral
parasagittal
p. incision
p. lesion
p. plane
p. section
parascapular
p. flap
p. incision
parasellar
p. mass
p. metastasis
p. syndrome
parasinoidal
parasitic
p. castration
p. cyst
p. flap
p. infection
paraspinal
p. approach
p. line
p. rod application
paraspinous aspect
parasternal
p. examination
p. line
parasternales
parasternalis
parastomal
p. hernia
p. infection
p. irritation
parasympathectomy
sinoatrial nodal p.
parasympathetic
p. ganglion
p. nerve
p. projection
paraterminal body
parathyroid
p. adenoma
p. artery
p. autograft
p. biopsy
p. carcinoma
p. extract
p. gland
p. hormone (PTH)
p. hormone chemiluminescent assay
p. hormone level
p. hyperplasia
p. operation
p. remnant
superior p.
p. surgeon
p. surgery
p. tissue
p. tumor
p. tumor ablation
parathyroidea
parathyroidectomy
endoscopic p.
2-1/2 gland p.
incidental p.
minimally invasive p.
minimally invasive video-assisted p. (MIVAP)
radioguided p.
reoperative p.
subtotal p.
total p.
unilateral p.
paratonsillar vein
paratracheal
p. node
p. tissue stripe
paratracheales
paratrachoma
paratrigeminal syndrome
paratrooper fracture
paraumbilical
p. hernia
p. incision
p. vein
paraumbilicales
paraurethral
p. duct
p. gland
paraurethrales
parauterini
paravaccinia virus infection
paravaginal
p. defect repair
p. hysterectomy
p. incision
p. soft tissue
paravaginales
paravariceal
p. injection
p. sclerotherapy
paravertebral
p. anesthesia
p. ganglion

NOTES

P

paravertebral *(continued)*
p. gutter
p. line
p. lumbar sympathetic block
paravertebralis
paravesical
p. fossa
p. pouch
paravesicalis
paravesiculares
parectasis
parencephalia
parencephalocele
parencephalous
parenchyma
breast p.
cirrhotic liver p.
damaged p.
functional p.
hepatic p.
liver p.
pancreatic p.
parenchymal
p. brain metastasis
p. brain neoplasm
p. cell
p. change
p. dissection
p. hematoma
p. laceration
p. lymphatic
p. route of injection
p. sparing surgery
p. tissue
p. transection
parenchymatous intracerebral hemorrhage
parenteral
p. administration
p. analgesia
p. analgesic
p. anesthesia
p. hyperalimentation
p. medication
p. nutrition
p. nutritional support
p. therapy
parent vessel
parepicele
parepididymis
Pare reduction
paresis
elevation p.
paresthesia anesthetic technique
paresthetica
meralgia p.
postlaparoscopy meralgia p.
Paré suture technique
paries, pl. **parietes**
parietal
p. angle
p. artery
p. bone
p. border
p. branch
p. cell vagotomy
p. defect
p. eminence
p. emissary vein
p. fistula
p. foramen
p. hernia
p. layer
p. margin
p. node
p. notch
p. pelvic fascia
p. pericardiectomy
p. pericardium
p. peritoneum
p. pleura
p. region
p. suture
p. tuber
p. wall
parietale
parietales
parietalis
parietes (*pl. of* paries)
parietofrontal
parietography
parietomastoidea
parietomastoid suture
parietooccipital
p. approach
p. artery
parieto-occipitalis
parietopontine tract
parietosphenoid
parietosplanchnic
parietosquamosal
parietotemporal
parietovisceral
Paris
P. classification
P. method
park-bench position
Parker incision
Parker-Kerr
P.-K. closed method
P.-K. suture technique
Parkinson disease
parkinsonian tremor
Parks
P. hemorrhoidectomy

P. ileoanal anastomosis
P. method of anal fistulotomy
P. partial sphincterotomy
P. staged fistulotomy

Parks-Bielschowsky three-step, head-tilt test
paroccipital process
parolivary
paromphalocele
Parona space
paronychial infection
parorchidium
parorchis
parosteal
parotic
parotid

p. bed
p. branch
p. carcinoma
p. dissection
p. duct
p. duct ligation
p. fascia
p. gland
p. node
p. notch
p. papilla
p. plexus
p. recess
p. resection
p. sheath
p. space
p. vein

parotidea
parotidectomy

facial nerve-preserving p.
superficial p.

parotidei
parotideomasseterica
parotideomasseteric fascia
parotideus
parotidoauricularis
parotis
parovarian mass
parovariotomy
parovarium
paroxysmal

p. atrial fibrillation (PAF)
p. nocturnal hemoglobinuria
p. palpitation

Parrish-Mann hammertoe technique
Parrish procedure
parrot-beak nail
Parry-Jones vulvectomy
pars, pl. **partes**
Parsonnet score
partial

p. alveolectomy
p. atrioventricular canal
p. breech extraction
p. central hypophysectomy
p. colectomy
p. cricotracheal resection
p. cystectomy
p. diskectomy
p. dislocation
p. duplication
p. encircling endocardial ventriculotomy
p. ethmoidectomy
p. facetectomy
p. fasciectomy
p. fibulectomy
p. gastrectomy (PG)
p. gastric resection
p. glossectomy
p. hemilaminectomy
p. hepatectomy
p. hepatic vascular exclusion (PHVE)
p. ileal bypass
p. inferior retrocolic end-to-side gastrojejunostomy
p. internal hemipelvectomy
p. keratoplasty
p. laryngectomy
p. laryngopharyngectomy
p. lateral internal sphincterotomy
p. left ventriculectomy
p. liquid ventilation
p. mastectomy
p. matrixectomy
p. mechanical obstruction
p. meniscectomy
p. mesh excision
p. nephrectomy
p. orchidectomy
p. ostectomy
p. pancreatectomy
p. pancreatoduodenectomy
p. patellectomy
p. pericystectomy
p. pressure
p. pressure of alveolar oxygen

NOTES

partial *(continued)*
p. pressure of arterial carbon dioxide ($PaCO_2$)
p. pressure of arterial oxygen
p. pressure of carbon dioxide (PCO_2)
p. pressure of CO_2 gas
p. pressure of intramuscular carbon dioxide ($PiCO_2$)
p. pressure of mesenteric venous carbon dioxide ($PmvCO_2$)
p. pressure of oxygen (PO_2)
p. pressure of water vapor
p. proctectomy
p. pulpectomy
p. pulpotomy
p. saturation
p. saturation spin-echo
p. superior retrocolic end-to-side gastrojejunostomy
p. thromboplastin time coagulation panel
p. zonal dissection
partial-breast irradiation
partial-thickness
p.-t. burn
p.-t. craniectomy
p.-t. flap
partial-throw surgeon knot
particle
p. beam radiation therapy
free-floating p.
p. reposit
particulate cancellous bone graft
Partipilo gastrostomy
partition
Partsch operation
parturient canal
parumbilical
paruresis
parva
Parvin
P. gravity technique
P. reduction
PAS
peripheral access system
PAS port
PAS technique
passage
nasopharyngeal p.
oropharyngeal p.
p. pressure
transforaminal p.
transperineurial p.
wire p.
Passavant
P. bar
P. fold
P. ridge
passé
coma dé p.
passive
p. clot
p. gliding technique
p. incontinence
p. joint manipulation
p. reciprocation
p. tissue cooling
Pastia line
patch
achromic p.
p. amnesia
aortic p.
p. aortoplasty
ash-leaf p.
autologous pericardial p.
blood p.
butterfly p.
cardiac p.
p. clamp electrophysiology
colic p.
colonic p.
cotton-wool p.
eczematous p.
electrodispersive skin p.
epidural blood p.
p. esophagoplasty
glue p.
gray p.
herald p.
Hutchinson p.
p. lesion
lyophilized dural p.
moth p.
mucous p.
omental p.
pantaloon p.
pericardial p.
peritoneal p.
Peyer p.
pigskin p.
prosthetic p.
pruritic erythematous p.
salmon p.
sandwich p.
sclerotic calvarial p.
shagreen p.
soldier p.
p. stage
p. technique
p. testing
p. test scarring
vein p.
venous sheath p.
white p.

patch-graft angioplasty
patchplasty
patchy
p. colonic ulceration
p. infiltration
patefaction
patella, pl. **patellae**
p. turndown approach
patellapexy
patellar
p. fat pad
p. intraarticular dislocation
p. network
p. retinaculum
p. sleeve fracture
p. tendon graft donor site (PTGDS)
p. tendon repair
patellectomy
partial p.
total p.
West-Soto-Hall p.
patelliform
patellofemoral articulation
Patel medial meniscectomy
patency
biliary stent p.
catheter p.
graft p.
shunt p.
stent p.
valve p.
patent
p. ductus arteriosus (PDA)
p. foramen ovale (PFO)
p. iridectomy
p. portal vein
Paterson
P. procedure
P. technique
Patey
P. modified radical mastectomy
P. operation
path
p. of insertion
p. of removal
pathogen
fungal p.
initial primary p.
primary p.
pathogenesis
pathologic
p. amputation
p. barrier
p. breast discharge
p. cause
p. characteristic
p. diagnosis
p. dislocation
p. entity
p. examination
p. fracture
p. lesion
p. neovascularization
p. perforation
p. retraction ring
p. specimen
p. sphincter
pathological anatomy
pathology
adrenal p.
anatomic p.
clinical p.
colorectal p.
p. examination
experimental p.
inciting p.
intracranial p.
intrahepatic p.
intrathyroidal p.
neoplastic p.
obstructing p.
p. scarring
surgical p.
synchronous p.
thyroid p.
venous p.
pathomechanics
kyphotic deformity p.
spinal fusion p.
pathophysiologic factor
pathophysiology
pathostimulation
pathway
beta-oxidation p.
coagulation p.
effector p.
extrapyramidal p.
extrinsic p.
lymphatic p.
orogastric p.
proteolytic p.
receptor-mediated endocytosis p.

NOTES

P

pathway *(continued)*
shunt p.
somatosensory p.
spinothalamic p.
taste p.
visual p.
PATI
penetrating abdominal trauma index
patient
adult p.
asymptomatic p.
brain-dead p.
diabetic p.
dialysis-dependent p.
disease-free p.
endoscopically normal p.
head-injured p.
hemodialysis-dependent p.
high-risk p.
inoperable p.
morbidly obese p.
obese p.
pediatric p.
poor-risk p.
p. population
surgically treated p.
symptomatic p.
trauma p.
tube-fed p.
vascular access p.
patient-controlled
p.-c. analgesia (PCA)
p.-c. analgesia anesthetic technique
p.-c. epidural analgesia (PCEA, PEA)
p.-c. epidural anesthesia
p.-c. intranasal analgesia (PCINA)
p.-c. intravenous anesthesia
patient-dependent factor
patocyte growth factor
patrilineal
pattern
abdominal wall venous p.
airway p.
p. arborization
architectural p.
p. of breathing
butterfly p.
chromatin p.
p. cut corneal graft operation
distribution p.
p. of distribution
p. of drainage
drainage p.
flow p.
histologic p.
lymphatic drainage p.
p. of motion
motor p.
organ-specific p.
p. recognition
spider-web p.
p. of staining
upper jejunal motor p.
pattern-cut corneal graft
patulous
Pauchet procedure
paucity
Paufique
P. keratoplasty
P. synechiotomy
Pauli exclusion principle
Pauling
P. theory
Paul-Mikulicz resection
Paulos ligament technique
Pauly point
pause-squeeze method
Pauwels
P. femoral neck fracture classification
P. fracture
P. proximal osteotomy
P. technique
P. valgus osteotomy
P. Y-osteotomy
PAV
proportional assist ventilator
Pavlov method
Payne-DeWind jejunoileal bypass
Payne operation
Payr
P. clamp method
P. membrane
PBS
phosphate buffered saline
PCA
patient-controlled analgesia
PCC
propagating clustered contraction
PCEA
patient-controlled epidural analgesia
PCINA
patient-controlled intranasal analgesia
PCIRV
pressure control inverse ratio ventilation
PCNA
proliferating cell nuclear antigen
PCNL
percutaneous nephrolithotripsy
percutaneous nephrostolithotomy
PCO_2
partial pressure of carbon dioxide
PCQ
Pain Coping Questionnaire

PCV
pressure control ventilation
PDA
patent ductus arteriosus
PDPH
postdural puncture headache
PDT
photodynamic therapy
PE
pulmonary embolism
submassive PE
PEA
patient-controlled epidural analgesia
Peabody-Mitchell bunionectomy
Peacock transposing technique
peak
p. exercise oxygen consumption
p. expiratory flow
p. expiratory flow rate
p. inspiratory ventilator pressure
p. pressure analysis
p. systolic aortic pressure
p. systolic gradient
p. systolic gradient pressure
p. transaortic valve gradient
Péan incision
pearl
cholesteatoma p.
perineal p.
PEBB
percutaneous excisional breast biopsy
Pecquet
P. cistern
P. duct
pecqueti
pecten
anal p.
p. band
pectinata
pectinate
p. body
p. line
p. zone
pectinatum
pectinea
pectineal
p. fascia
p. hernia
p. ligament
pectineale
pectineus
pectiniform septum
pectoral
p. branch
p. fascia
p. groove
pectoralis
p. fascia
p. major muscle origin
p. major myocutaneous flap
p. muscle
p. myocutaneous esophagoplasty
p. myofascial flap
pectus
p. carinatum deformity
p. excavatum deformity
p. index
PED
percutaneous external drainage
pedes (*pl. of* pes)
pediatric
p. airway
p. analgesic
p. anesthesia system
p. anesthetic
p. cardiovascular surgery
p. circle
p. colonoscopy
p. endoscopy
p. esophagogastroduodenoscopy
p. esophagoplasty
p. hepatojejunostomy
p. hernia
p. hypothermia
p. injury
p. intussusception
p. laparoscopic surgical procedure
p. mass
p. neoplasm
p. neurosurgeon
P. Oncology Group (POG)
p. ophthalmic surgery
p. otolaryngology
p. pain
p. patient
p. population
p. portal hypertension
p. radiotherapy anesthesia
p. surgeon
p. trauma scale (PTS)
p. urologist
p. urology
p. vaginoscopy
pedicellation

NOTES

pedicle
p. anatomy
p. entrance point
p. evaluation
p. fat graft
Filatov-Gillies tubed p.
p. flap operation
p. flap urethroplasty
p. fracture
glissonian p.
p. groin flap
hepatic p.
p. landmark
lateral-sector p.
p. ligation
p. localization
medial-sector p.
p. method
omental p.
portal p.
posterior p.
p. screw hardware prominence
p. screw path length
p. screw plating
p. screw-rod fixation
sectoral p.
vascular p.
vasculobiliary p.
p. wrapping
pedicled
p. jejunal reconstruction
p. myocutaneous flap
p. omentoplasty
pedicolaminar fracture-dislocation
pedicular fixation
pediculation
pediculus, pl. **pediculi**
pediphalanx
pedis
pedodontic endodontics
peduncle
peduncular loop
pedunculated loose body
pedunculation
pedunculotomy
peeling
membrane p.
PEEP
positive end-expiratory pressure
PEEP/CPAP
positive end-expiratory pressure/continuous positive airway pressure
PEEPi
intrinsic positive end-expiratory pressure
Peet
P. operation
P. splanchnic resection
P. Z-plasty
PEG
percutaneous endoscopic gastrostomy
PEG insertion
peg
p. bone graft
p. flap
peg-and-socket
p.-a.-s. articulation
p.-a.-s. joint
p.-a.-s. technique
peg-in-hole osteotomy
Peimer reduction osteotomy
PEJ
percutaneous endoscopic jejunostomy
pelidnoma
pelioma
peliosis hepatitis
Pell and Gregory classification
pellucidum
pelma
pelmatic
peltation
pelves (*pl. of* pelvis)
pelvic
p. abscess
p. adhesive disease
p. appendix
p. aspiration biopsy
p. autonomic nerve preservation (PANP)
p. autonomic plexus
p. avulsion fracture
p. axis
p. brim
p. canal
p. cavity
p. colonic surgery
p. diaphragm
p. direction
p. examination
p. exenteration
p. fascia
p. fixation
p. floor dysfunction
p. ganglion
p. girdle
p. hematocele
p. ileal reservoir construction
p. inclination
p. infection
p. inflammation
p. irradiation
p. kidney
p. laparoscopy
p. limb
p. lymphadenectomy

p. lymph node dissection (PLND)
p. lymphocelectomy
p. mass
p. node dissection
p. osteotomy
p. peritonectomy
p. plane
p. pouch
p. pouchoscopy
p. pouch procedure
p. promontory
p. relaxation
p. ring
p. ring fracture
p. rotation
p. sidewall
p. skeleton
p. stimulation
p. straddle fracture

pelvica
pelvicaliceal
pelvifixation
pelvilithotomy
pelvinus
pelviolithotomy
pelvioplasty
pelvioscopy
pelviotomy
pelvirectal sphincter
pelvis, pl. **pelves**

android p.
anthropoid p.
assimilation p.
axis p.
brachypellic p.
contracted p.
cordate p.
Deventer p.
dolichopellic p.
dwarf p.
extrarenal renal p.
false p.
flat p.
funnel-shaped p.
greater p.
gynecoid p.
heart-shaped p.
inclinatio p.
inverted p.
juvenile p.
large p.
lesser p.
longitudinal oval p.
masculine p.
mesatipellic p.
osteomalacic p.
platypellic p.
platypelloid p.
pseudoosteomalacic p.
renal p.
reniform p.
Robert p.
round p.
small p.
spider p.
transverse oval p.
true p.
ureteric p.

pelvisacral
pelviscopic

p. clip ligation technique
p. intrafascial hysterectomy

pelviscopy
pelvitomy
pelvivertebral angle
pelvoscopy
Pemberton

P. acetabuloplasty
P. operation
P. pericapsular osteotomy

PEMF

pulsed electromagnetic field
PEMF therapy

pemphigoid
pemphigus
penalization
Penaz volume-clamp method
pencil-in-cup deformity
Penduloff incision
pendulous abdomen
pendulum
penectomy
penes (*pl. of* penis)
penetrance
penetrating

p. abdominal trauma index (PATI)
p. corneal transplant
p. fracture
p. keratoplasty
p. liver injury
p. rupture
p. thoracoabdominal injury
p. trauma

NOTES

P

penetrating *(continued)*
- p. ulcer
- p. wound

penetration
- peritoneal p.
- serosal p.
- p. test

Penfield method
penial
penicillary
penicillate
penicillus
penile
- p. amputation
- p. block
- p. cancer
- p. carcinoma
- p. deformity
- p. erection
- p. extensibility
- p. incarceration
- p. injection testing
- p. injection therapy
- p. island flap
- p. raphe
- p. revascularization
- p. rupture
- p. urethra
- p. vein occlusion therapy
- p. venous ligation surgery

penile-brachial pressure index
penis, pl. **penes**
- bifid p.
- buried p.
- clubbed p.
- concealed p.
- deep p.
- dorsal p.
- glans p.
- webbed p.

penischisis
peniscopy
penitis
Pennal classification
pennate muscle
Penn method
penoid tissue
penoplasty
penoscrotal transposition
penotomy
pentadactyl
pentagonal block excision
pentane excretion level
penumbral region
Peptavlon stimulation test
peptic
- p. aspiration pneumonitis
- p. gland
- p. stricture
- p. ulcer
- p. ulcer disease

peptide
- atrial natriuretic p.
- brain natriuretic p. (BNP)
- connective tissue activating p.
- endogenous opioid p.
- fusion p.

per
- p. anum
- p. contiguum
- p. continuum

peraxillary
perceived
- p. exertion
- p. quality of life (PQOL)

perceptual expansion
percolation
Percoll technique
percussion
- hard p.
- p. therapy

percutaneous
- p. abscess drainage (PAD)
- p. access
- p. alcohol injection
- p. anesthetic loss
- p. anterior gastropexy
- p. appendectomy
- p. arterial cannulation
- p. aspirate
- p. aspiration thromboembolectomy
- p. balloon angioplasty
- p. balloon aortic valvuloplasty
- p. balloon aspiration
- p. balloon dilation
- p. balloon mitral valvuloplasty
- p. balloon pericardiotomy
- p. balloon pulmonic valvuloplasty
- p. bone marrow infection
- p. catheter cecostomy
- p. catheter drainage
- p. catheter insertion
- p. cholangioscopic lithotomy
- p. cholecystectomy
- p. cholecystolithotomy
- p. cholecystostomy
- p. cordotomy
- p. coronary rotational atherectomy
- p. corticotomy
- p. CT-guided aspiration
- p. dilational tracheostomy
- p. embolization therapy
- p. endofluoroscopy
- p. endopyeloureterotomy
- p. endoscopic gastrojejunostomy
- p. endoscopic gastrostomy (PEG)

p. endoscopic gastrostomy insertion
p. endoscopic jejunostomy (PEJ)
p. endoscopic removal
p. endoscopy
p. endovascular treatment
p. enterostomy
p. epididymal sperm aspiration
p. ethanol ablation
p. ethanol injection
p. ethanol injection therapy
p. excisional breast biopsy (PEBB)
p. external drainage (PED)
p. fetal cystoscopy
p. fetal tissue sampling
p. fine-needle aspiration
p. fine-needle aspiration biopsy
p. fine-needle pancreatic biopsy
p. fixation
p. FNA
p. gastroenterostomy
p. glycerol rhizolysis
p. injury (PI)
p. insertion technique
p. interventional technique
p. intraaortic balloon counterpulsation
p. laser nucleolysis
p. line
p. liver biopsy
p. localization
p. low-stress angioplasty
p. lumbar diskectomy
p. microwave coagulation therapy
p. mitral balloon commissurotomy
p. mitral balloon valvotomy
p. native renal biopsy
p. needle liver biopsy
p. needle puncture
p. nephrolithotomy
p. nephrolithotripsy (PCNL)
p. nephroscopy
p. nephrostolithotomy (PCNL)
p. nephrostomy
p. nephrostomy tube placement
p. pancreas biopsy
p. patent ductus arteriosus closure
p. pin insertion
p. pinning
p. plantar fasciotomy
p. portocaval anastomosis
p. pressure ureteral perfusion test
p. radical cryosurgical ablation
p. radiofrequency catheter ablation
p. radiofrequency dorsal rhizotomy
p. radiofrequency gangliolysis
p. radiofrequency rhizolysis
p. radiofrequency rhizotomy
p. reduction
p. renal puncture
p. retrogasserian glycerol chemoneurolysis
p. retrogasserian glycerol rhizolysis
p. rotational thrombectomy
p. sampling method
p. stimulation
p. stone removal
p. stricture dilatation (PSD)
p. tenotomy
p. transatrial mitral commissurotomy
p. transcatheter therapy
p. transhepatic approach
p. transhepatic biliary drainage (PTBD)
p. transhepatic biliary procedure
p. transhepatic cardiac catheterization
p. transhepatic cholangiography (PTC)
p. transhepatic cholangioscopic lithotomy (PTCSL)
p. transhepatic cholangioscopy
p. transhepatic cholecystoscopy
p. transhepatic obliteration
p. transhepatic obliteration of esophageal varix
p. transluminal angioscopy
p. transluminal balloon valvuloplasty
p. transluminal coronary angioplasty (PTCA)
p. transluminal coronary revascularization
p. transluminal renal angioplasty
p. transtracheal jet ventilation (PTV)
p. transvenous mitral commissurotomy
p. tumor ablation
p. venoablation

Pereyra
P. bladder neck suspension
P. needle suspension
P. procedure

NOTES

P

Pereyra-Lebhertz
P.-L. modification
P.-L. modification of Frangenheim-Stoeckel procedure
Pereyra-Raz cystourethropexy
perflation
perforans
perforantes
perforata
perforated
p. cancer
p. cholecystitis
p. peptic ulcer
p. space
perforating
p. abscess
p. branch
p. keratoplasty
p. wound
perforation
advanced tumor p.
amebic p.
appendiceal p.
bladder p.
bowel p.
cardiac p.
colon p.
colonic p.
corneal p.
cortical p.
diaphragm p.
ductal system p.
duodenal p.
esophageal p.
frank p.
gallbladder p.
gastric p.
guidewire p.
ileal p.
inflammatory p.
instrumental p.
intestinal p.
intraperitoneal p.
lateral p.
mechanical p.
myocardial p.
nasal septal p.
Niemeier gallbladder p.
operative p.
p. osteotomy
pathologic p.
peritoneal p.
p. peritonitis
prepyloric p.
retroduodenal p.
retroperitoneal p.
p. risk
root p.
sealing p.
septal p.
strip p.
sublabial p.
tooth p.
ureteral p.
uterine p.
vascular p.
ventricular p.
perforative lesion
performance status
perfrigeration
perfusion
aortic p.
blood p.
cerebral p.
continuous hyperthermic peritoneal p.
continuous sanguineous p.
distal aortic p.
distal visceral p.
extracorporeal liver p.
ex vivo p.
p. flow rate
hepatic p.
hyperthermic isolated limb p. (HILP)
p. hypothermia technique
hypothermic hepatic p.
in-line p.
intramural blood p.
intraperitoneal hyperthermic p.
isolated hepatic p.
isolated limb p. (ILP)
Langendorff p.
p. measurement technique
organ p.
p. pressure
sanguineous p.
in situ hypothermic p.
splanchnic p.
superficial renal cortical p. (SRCP)
p. system
systemic p.
p. therapy
tissue p.
visceral p.
perfusion/ventilation
periadventitial tissue
periampullary
p. cancer
p. carcinoma
p. mass
perianal
p. anorectal space
p. condyloma
p. fistula
p. fistula abscess

p. hematoma
p. incision
p. infection
perianesthetic thermoregulation
perianeurysmal hemorrhage
periangiocholitis
periaortic mediastinal hematoma
periaortitis
periapical
p. curettage
p. infection
p. pressure
p. surgery
p. tissue
p. tooth repair
periappendiceal abscess
periappendicitis
periappendicular
periaqueductal gray matter stimulation
periaqueductal-periventricular (PAG/PVG)
p.-p. region
p.-p. stimulation
periareolar
p. incision
p. mastopexy
periarterial
p. plexus
p. sympathectomy
periarterialis
periarticular
p. fluid collection
p. fracture
p. tissue
periauricular
periaxial
periaxillary
peribronchial
peribronchiolar lymphocyte infiltration
peribuccal
peribulbar
p. anesthesia
p. anesthetic technique
p. injection
peribursal
pericallosa
pericallosal artery
pericanalicular connective tissue
pericapsular
p. fat infiltration
p. osteotomy
pericardectomy
pericardiaca
pericardiacae
pericardiacophrenic
p. artery
p. vein
pericardiacophrenica, pl. **pericardiacophrenicae**
pericardial
p. biopsy
p. branch
p. decompression
p. fat pad
p. flap
p. fluid examination
p. hematoma
p. patch
p. pressure
p. puncture
p. reflection
p. reflex
p. reinforcement
p. sac
p. vein
p. window
pericardiectomy
parietal p.
thoracoscopic p.
visceral p.
pericardii
pericardiocentesis
pericardiophrenic nerve
pericardioplasty in pectus excavatum repair
pericardiorrhaphy
pericardioscopy
pericardiostomy
pericardiotomy, pericardotomy
percutaneous balloon p.
subxiphoid limited p.
p. syndrome
pericarditis
constrictive p.
pericardium
parietal p.
visceral p.
pericardotomy (*var. of* pericardiotomy)
pericecal
pericholecystic
p. edema
p. fluid collection
pericholecystitis

NOTES

P

perichondral, perichondrial
p. circulation
p. ring
p. sheath
perichondrium
perichoroidal space
pericolic membrane syndrome
pericolonitis
pericolostomy
p. area
p. hernia
pericorneal plexus
pericoronal flap
pericostal suture technique
pericranial temporalis flap
pericranium
pericystectomy
partial p.
total p.
pericystic
pericystitis
pericystium
peridectomy
peridental
p. ligament
p. membrane
p. space
peridentinoblastic space
peridesmic
peridesmium
peridiaphragmatic hematoma
perididymis
perididymitis
periductal
p. fibrosis
p. mastitis
peridural anesthesia
perienteric
periependymal
periesophageal
p. abscess
p. blood vessel
p. fat
p. lymph node dissection
p. structure
p. tissue
periesophagogastric lymph node metastasis
perifascial nephrectomy
periganglionic
perigastric
p. node
p. node station
perigenicular vascular injury
perigraft hematoma
perihepatic
p. abscess
p. lymph nodal station
p. space
perihepatitis
gonococcal p.
perihernial
periimplant
p. space
p. tissue
periimplantation
perikaryon
perilaryngeal
perilenticular space
periligamentous
perilimbal
p. incision
p. suction
perilobular connective tissue
perilunar transscaphoid dislocation
perilunate
p. carpal dislocation
p. fracture-dislocation
perilymphatic
p. cavity
p. duct
p. fistula
p. fluid
p. space
perilymphatica
perilymphaticum
perilymphaticus
perilymph fistula
perimesencephalic cistern
perimeter
p. corneal reflex test
p. projection
perimetric
perimetrium
perimyelis
perimylolysis
perimysium
perinatal
p. infection
p. torsion
perinea (*pl. of* perineum)
perineal
p. abscess
p. analgesia
p. anesthesia
p. artery
p. body
p. defect
p. flap
p. flexure
p. hernia
p. impact trauma
p. incision
p. infection
p. laceration

p. lithotomy
p. membrane
p. muscle
p. nerve
p. nerve terminal motor latency test
p. pearl
p. polyp
p. proctectomy
p. prostatectomy
p. raphe
p. region
p. repair
p. scar
p. section
p. sinus
p. sinus tract
p. space
p. urethrostomy
p. urethrotomy
p. urinary fistula

perineales

perinealis

perinei

perineocele

perineoplasty

perineorrhaphy
vaginal p.

perineoscrotal

perineostomy

perineosynthesis

perineotomy

perineovaginal fistula

perinephrial

perinephric
p. abscess
p. fluid collection
p. hematoma
p. space hemorrhage
p. tissue

perinephritis

perinephrium

perineum, pl. **perinea**

perineural
p. anesthesia
p. infiltration
p. invasion
p. tissue

perineurial neurorrhaphy

perineurium

perinodal tissue

perinuclear
p. cisterna
p. space

periocular injection

period
early postoperative p.
immediate postoperative p.
interdigestive p.
later postoperative p.
observation p.
postoperative p.
postprandial p.
postresuscitation p.
preoperative p.
resuscitation p.

periodic respiration

periodontal
p. disease
p. flap
p. inflammation
p. lesion
p. ligament
p. ligament anesthesia
p. membrane
p. membrane necrosis
p. ostectomy
p. therapy

periodontium

periodontolysis

periomphalic

perioperative
p. analgesia
p. antibiotic
p. antibiotic prophylaxis
p. antibiotic therapy
p. bacteremia
p. complication
p. corneal abrasion
p. death
p. management
p. morbidity
p. mortality
p. outcome
p. reduction
p. risk factor
p. shock
p. standardized protocol
p. stroke
p. transfusion

perioptic subarachnoid space

NOTES

periorbital
p. infection
p. membrane
periostea (*pl. of* periosteum)
periosteal
p. elevation
p. flap
p. implantation
p. new bone formation
p. tissue
periosteoma
periosteophyte
periosteotomy
periosteous
periosteum, pl. **periostea**
posterior p.
periostoma
periotic
p. bone
p. duct
p. space
peripancreatic
p. abdominal drainage
p. fat plane
p. infection
p. necrosis
p. tissue
peripartum endoscopy
peripenial
peripharyngeal space
peripharyngeum
peripheral
p. access system (PAS)
p. aneurysm
p. arterial aneurysmal disease
p. arterial line
p. balloon angioplasty
p. bruit
p. capillary filtration slit length
p. cavity wall
p. chemoreflex loop
p. circulation
p. extremity edema
p. fusion
p. hepatojejunostomy
p. hyperalimentation
p. hyperinsulinemia
p. insulin resistance
p. intravenous alimentation
p. iridectomy
p. iridectomy operation
p. laceration
p. laser angioplasty
p. lymphoid tissue
p. nerve
p. nerve allografting
p. nerve block
p. nerve block anesthesia
p. nerve block anesthetic technique
p. nerve injury
p. nerve lesion
p. nerve regeneration
p. neurectomy
p. panretinal ablation
p. pressure
p. pulse
p. thrombus
p. vascular disease
p. vascular surgery
p. vein
p. venous cannulation
peripherally inserted central catheter
peripherica
periporoma
periportal
p. sinusoidal dilatation
p. sinusoidal dilation
periproctic
periprostatic tissue
periprostatitis
periprosthetic
p. fracture
p. leak
peripylephlebitis
peripylic
peripyloric
perirectal
p. abscess
p. inflammation
p. mass
p. pelvic dissection
perirenal
p. fascia
p. hematoma
p. insufflation
p. space
perisalpinx
periscapular incision
periscleral space
perisellar vascular lesion
perisinusoidal space
perisplanchnic
perisplenic
perispondylic
peristalsis
absent p.
peristaltic
peristasis
peristomal
p. infection
p. varix
peritarsal network
peritectomy
peritendineum
perithelioma
perithoracic

peritomist
peritomy
peritonea (*pl. of* peritoneum)
peritoneal
p. access
p. adenocarcinoma
p. adhesion
p. anatomy
p. aspiration
p. band
p. biopsy
p. cancer
p. carcinomatosis
p. cavity
p. cavity abscess
p. cavity fluid
p. cytological assessment
p. cytology
p. cytology sample
p. defect
p. dialysis
p. disease
p. dissemination
p. drainage
p. encapsulation
p. envelope
p. equilibration test
p. fluid examination
p. friction rub
p. fungal infection
p. hernia
p. incision
p. insufflation
p. irritation
p. lavage
p. macrophage
p. membrane permeability
p. metastasis
p. mouse
p. patch
p. penetration
p. perforation
p. pocket
p. reconstruction
p. recurrence
p. reflection
p. reinforcement
p. sac
p. seeding
p. sepsis
p. soilage
p. space
p. spill
p. spread
p. studding
p. surface
p. tap
p. toilet
p. transfusion
p. tuberculosis
p. vein
ventricular p. (VP)
p. villus
p. violation
p. washing
p. washout
p. window
peritoneales
peritonealis
peritonectomy
left upper quadrant p.
pelvic p.
right upper quadrant p.
peritonei
peritoneocentesis
peritoneoclysis
peritoneopericardial diaphragmatic hernia
peritoneopexy
peritoneoplasty
peritoneoscopy
peritoneotomy
inverted-V p.
peritoneovenous shunt patency scan
peritoneum, pl. **peritonea**
abdominal p.
parietal p.
visceral p.
peritonitis
adhesive p.
amebic p.
aseptic p.
barium p.
chemical p.
diffuse p.
focal p.
gastric perforation p.
generalized p.
perforation p.
purulent p.
P. Severity Score (PSS)
talc p.
peritonization
peritonize

NOTES

P

peritonsillar
p. nerve
p. space
peritracheal
peritrochanteric fracture
peritubal syndrome
peritumoral site
perityphlic
periumbilical
p. abscess
p. hernia
p. incision
p. port
periureteral abscess
periureteric venous ring
periurethral abscess
periurethritis
periuterine
perivascular
p. canal
p. mass
peri-vaterian therapeutic endoscopic procedure
periventricular
p. hyperintense lesion
p. white matter lesion
periventricular-intraventricular hemorrhage
perivertebral
perivesical
perivisceral
perivitelline space
Perkins vertical line
permanent
p. anticoagulant therapy
p. bipolar magnet placement
p. end colostomy
p. hypoparathyroidism
p. loop ileostomy
p. mesh omentum
p. pacemaker placement
p. paralysis
p. pedicle flap
p. proctectomy
p. restoration
p. section
p. stoma
permanganate
permeability
membrane p.
peritoneal membrane p.
p. theory of narcosis
permeation
analgesia p.
lymphatic p.
permissive hypercapnia (PHC)
permutation
perone
peroneal
p. artery
p. brevis tendon
p. communicating nerve
p. compartment syndrome
p. dislocation
p. groove
p. longus tendon
p. muscle
p. muscle atrophy
p. nerve entrapment
p. nerve injury
p. phenomenon
p. pulley
p. retinaculum
p. somatosensory evoked potential
p. spastic flatfoot
p. tendon sheath injection
p. vein
peronealis
peroneus
p. brevis muscle
p. longus muscle
p. tertius muscle
peroral
p. approach
p. cholangiopancreatoscopy
p. cholangioscopy
p. endoscopy
p. esophageal dilation
p. intestinal biopsy
p. maneuver
p. pancreatoscopy
peroxidation
lipid p.
perpendicular
p. of ethmoid plate
p. fashion
p. plane
perpendicularis
Perry
P. extensile anterior approach
P. technique
Perry-Nickel technique
Perry-O'Brien-Hodgson technique
Perry-Robinson cervical technique
perseveration
infantile p.
motor p.
persistent
p. anovulation
p. breast abnormality
p. common atrioventricular canal
p. fetal circulation
p. hypercalcemia
p. müllerian duct syndrome
p. occiput posterior position

p. ovarian mass
p. tolerant infection
personnel
paramedical p.
perspective
surgical p.
p. volume rendering (pVR)
perspiratory gland
Perthes
P. incision
P. lesion
P. procedure
P. test
pertubation
hemodynamic p.
perversus
pes, pl. **pedes**
p. planus deformity
PET
positron emission tomography
$PETCO_2$
extrapolated end-tidal carbon dioxide tension
petechia, pl. **petechiae**
petechial hemorrhage
Peter operation
Peters anomaly
PET-guided biopsy
petiolus
Petit
P. aponeurosis
P. canal
P. hernia
P. herniotomy
P. ligament
P. lumbar triangle
P. suture technique
petrobasilar suture
petroccipital
petroclinoid ligament
petromastoid
petrooccipital
p. fissure
p. joint
petropharyngeus
petrosa, pl. **petrosae**
petrosal
p. approach
p. artery
p. bone
p. branch
p. foramen
p. fossa
p. fossula
p. ganglion
p. nerve
p. neuralgia
p. vein
p. venous sinus
petrosalpingostaphylinus
petrosectomy
total p.
petrosi
petrositis
petrosomastoid
petrosphenoid ligament
petrospheno-occipital suture
petrosquamosa
petrosquamosal
petrosquamous
p. fissure
p. suture
p. venous sinus
petrostaphylinus
petrosum
petrotympanic
p. fissure
p. suture
p. tissue
petrotympanica
petrous
p. apex cell
p. pyramid
p. pyramid air cell exploration
p. pyramid exenteration
p. pyramid fracture
p. ridge
petrousitis
petrous-to-supraclinoid bypass
Peutz-Jeghers syndrome
Peyer
P. gland
P. patch
Peyman
P. full-thickness eyewall resection
P. iridocyclochoroidectomy
Peyronie disease
Peyrot thorax
Pfannenstiel
P. incision
P. transverse approach
Pfeiffer-Comberg method
Pfiffner and Myers method

NOTES

P

PFO
patent foramen ovale
PG
partial gastrectomy
PGA
pancreaticogastrostomy anastomosis
PGA afferent
PGA efferent
PGL
primary gastric lymphoma
primary gastric non-Hodgkin lymphoma
pH
pH electrode placement
esophageal pH
gastric mucosal pH
intramural pH
pH measurement
phaco-anaphylactic-endophthalmitis
phacocele
phacocystectomy
phacoemulsification
phacoexcavation
phacofragmentation
phacoglaucoma
phacolysis
phacoma, phakoma
retinal p.
phacomatosis
phacoscopy
phagocyte migration
phagolysis
phakomatosis
phalangeal
p. articular orientation
p. diaphysial fracture
p. dislocation
p. fracture fixation
p. malunion correction
p. osteotomy
phalangealization
phalangectomy
intermediate p.
phalangis
phalangization
phalanx, pl. **phalanges**
distal p.
middle p.
proximal p.
Phalen
P. maneuver
P. position
phallalgia
phallectomy
phallic
phallica
phalliform
phallitis
phallocampsis
phallocrypsis
phallodynia
phalloid
phalloncus
phalloplasty
phallotomy
Phaneuf-Graves repair
phantasmoscopia
phantasmoscopy
phantom
p. aneurysm
p. foot pain
p. limb
p. limb pain
pharmacodynamics
pharmacologic
p. immunosuppression
p. manipulation
p. method
p. paralysis
pharmacologically
p. induced erection
p. induced paralysis
pharyngeal
p. airway
p. anesthesia
p. branch
p. bursa
p. canal
p. cell
p. exudate
p. flap
p. fornix
p. gland
p. gonococcal infection
p. hypophysis
p. mucosa
p. orifice
p. plexus
p. plexus neurectomy
p. pouch
p. pouch syndrome
p. raphe
p. recess
p. region
p. residue
p. ridge
p. space
p. tissue
p. tubercle
p. vein
p. wall carcinoma
pharyngealis
pharyngectomy
pharyngei
pharynges (*pl. of* pharynx)

pharyngeum
pharyngeus
pharyngis
pharyngobasilar fascia
pharyngobasilaris
pharyngocutaneous fistula
pharyngoepiglottic fold
pharyngoesophageal
p. diverticulectomy
p. reconstruction
pharyngoesophagogastroduodenoscopy
pharyngoesophagoplasty
pharyngoglossal
pharyngoglossus
pharyngolaryngeal
pharyngolaryngectomy
pharyngomaxillary space
pharyngonasal cavity
pharyngooral
pharyngopalatine
pharyngopalatinus
pharyngoplasty
Hynes p.
Wardill p.
pharyngoscleroma
pharyngoscopy
pharyngostaphylinus
pharyngostoma
pharyngotomy
transhyoid p.
pharyngotympanic
p. groove
pharynx, pl. **pharynges**
laryngeal p.
nasal p.
oral p.
posterior p.
phase
eclipse p.
ejection p.
end-expiratory p.
excitement p.
exponential p.
extradural p.
granulation p.
p. I, II block
implantation p.
maturation p.
posthepatic resection p.
prehepatic resection p.
preinduction p.
presensitization p.
prolonged expiratory p.
resectional p.
reservoir p.
transverse magnetization p.
vector p.
phase-encoding direction
phase-sensitive gradient-echo MR imaging
phasic pressure wave
PHC
permissive hypercapnia
PHCA
profoundly hypothermic circulatory arrest
Pheasant elbow technique
Phelps
P. neurectomy
P. partial resection
P. scapulectomy
Phemister
P. acromioclavicular pin fixation
P. incision
P. medial approach
P. onlay bone graft
P. onlay bone graft technique
Phemister-Bonfiglio technique
phenol
p. cauterization
p. matrixectomy
phenolization
angular p.
phenol-preserved extract
phenomenon, pl. **phenomena**
all-or-nothing p.
Ascher glass-rod p.
common cavity p.
declamping p.
doll's head p.
entry p.
extinction p.
extravasation p.
glass-rod negative p.
glass-rod positive p.
Goldblatt p.
hesitation p.
identification p.
Marcus Gunn p.
misdirection p.
modified Raynaud p.
neglect-like phenomena
osteointegration p.
peroneal p.
referred trigger-point p.

NOTES

P

phenomenon *(continued)*
relaxation p.
staircase p.
steal p.
temporary cavity p.
tip-of-the-tongue p.
truncation p.
yo-yo weight fluctuation p.
phenotypic lymphocyte
phenozygous
phenylethylbarbituric acid
pheochromoblastoma
pheochromocytoma
adrenal p.
philtrum, pl. **philtra**
phimosis, pl. **phimoses**
phimotic
phincterotomy
phlebectomy
greater saphenous p.
phlebitis
phlebogram
orbital p.
phlebolite
phlebolith
phlebophlebostomy
phlebophthalmotomy
phleboplasty
phleborrhagia
phleborrhaphy
phleborrhexis
phlebostasis
phlebostrepsis
phlebotomy
bloodless p.
therapeutic p.
phlegmon
phlegmonous
p. abscess
p. gastritis
p. mass
Phocas syndrome
phonation
hypervalvular p.
myoelastic-aerodynamic theory of p.
neurochronaxic theory of p.
reverse p.
ventricular p.
voice disorder of p.
phonophoresis
phonoscopy
phosphatase
serum alkaline p.
phosphatase-antiphosphatase
alkaline p.-a.
phosphate
p. buffered saline (PBS)
p. excretion index
primary sodium p.
phosphotungstic acid-magnesium chloride precipitation method
photic stimulation
photoablation
laser p.
photoactivation
photocoagulation
argon laser p.
infrared p.
laser p.
macular p.
panretinal argon laser p.
retinal scatter p.
scatter p.
in situ p.
transendoscopic laser p.
p. treatment
xenon arc p.
photodisintegration
photodissociation
photodocumentation
photodynamic therapy (PDT)
photoexcitation
photography
cross-polarization p.
endoscopic p.
laparoscopic p.
photoinactivation
photoirradiation
photolysis
flash p.
photomicrograph
photomicroscopy
photon-deficient bone lesion
photoonycholysis
photopatch
photophore
photoplethysmography
photoradiation therapy
photorefractive
p. keratectomy (PRK)
p. keratoplasty
photoresection
photoscopy
photosensitive cell
phototherapeutic keratectomy
photothermal laser ablation
photothermolysis
selective p.
photovaporization
laser p.
phrenectomy
phrenemphraxis
phrenic
p. ganglion
p. nerve

p. nerve block
p. nerve block anesthetic technique
p. pleura
p. plexus
p. vein
phrenica
phrenicectomy
phrenici
phreniclasia
phrenicoabdominal branch
phrenicocolic ligament
phrenicocolicum
phrenicocostal sinus
phrenicoexeresis
phrenicogastric
phrenicoglottic
phrenicohepatic
phrenicolienale
phrenicolienal ligament
phrenicomediastinalis
phrenicomediastinal recess
phreniconeurectomy
phrenicopleural fascia
phrenicopleuralis
phrenicosplenic ligament
phrenicosplenicum
phrenicotomy
phrenicotripsy
phrenicus
phrenocolic
phrenocolopexy
phrenoesophageal
p. ligament
p. membrane
phrenogastric ligament
phrenohepatic
phrenosplenic ligament
phrictopathic
phrygian
p. cap
p. cap deformity
PHVE
partial hepatic vascular exclusion
phyllode
cystosarcoma p.
phyllodes tumor
physial
p. fracture
p. line
physical
p. barrier
p. capacity evaluation
p. examination
p. finding
p. manipulation
p. problem
p. restoration
p. therapy
p. therapy index
Physick operation
physicochemical basis of gallstone formation
physiologic
p. aspect
p. barrier
p. breast discharge
p. change
p. dose
p. excavation
p. mesial migration
p. pattern release
p. rest position
p. retraction ring
p. saline solution
p. salt solution
physiological
p. dead space
p. dead space ventilation per minute
p. sphincter
physiology
colorectal p.
exercise p.
flap p.
physiolysis
central p.
physis
physocele
phytobezoar
PI
percutaneous injury
pial-glial membrane
pia mater
piano-wire adhesion
PIC
plasmin-inhibitor complex
Pichlmayer
P. method
P. procedure
P. technique
Pick bundle
Pickerill
imbrication line of P.
P. imbrication line

NOTES

pickling solution
$PiCO_2$
partial pressure of intramuscular carbon dioxide
Pico operation
Picot incision
picrotoxin
picture
clinical p.
p. frame vertebra
pie-crusting skin graft
Piedmont fracture
Pierre Robin anomalad
Pierrot-Murphy
P.-M. advancement insertion
P.-M. tendon technique
Piersol point
piezoelectric lithotripsy
pigeon-breast deformity
piggyback
p. liver transplantation
modified p. (MPB)
pigment
p. cell transplantation
p. epithelial lesion
pigmentary
p. demarcation line
p. migration
pigmented lesion
pigskin
p. graft
p. patch
pigtail
pileus
pili (*pl. of* pilus)
pilimiction
pillar rib
pill-induced esophagitis
pillion fracture
pillow fracture
piloerection
pilojection
piloleiomyoma
pilomatricoma
pilomatrixoma
pilon ankle fracture
pilonidal
p. abscess
p. cyst
p. cystectomy
p. fistula
pilorum
arrectores p.
pilot application
pilus, pl. **pili**
arrector p.
pimobendan
pin
cranial p.
p. retention
p. site
p. suture technique
p. track
p. tract infection
pin-and-plaster
p.-a.-p. fixation
p.-a.-p. method
Pinard maneuver
pin-bone interface
pincer nail
pinch
p. biopsy
p. restoration
p. skin graft
pinch-grasp injection technique
pin-cushion distortion
pineal
p. body
p. eye
p. gland
p. recess
p. region
p. teratocarcinoma
pinealcytoma
pinealectomy
pinealoblastoma
pinealocytoma
pinealoma
pineoblastoma
pineocytoma
ping-pong
p.-p. ball deformity
p.-p. fracture
piniform
pin-index safety system
pink frothy sputum
pinning
closed p.
hip p.
Knowles p.
open p.
percutaneous p.
Sherk-Probst percutaneous p.
Sofield p.
Wagner closed p.
pinpoint
p. electrocoagulation
p. gastric mucosal defect
p. gastric mucosal defect bleeding
pinprick method
pin-supported restoration
pinworm preparation
PIP
prolactin inducible protein
pipe bone

Pipelle biopsy
Pipkin
P. femoral fracture classification
P. posterior hip dislocation classification
P. subclassification of Epstein-Thomas classification
PIPP
Premature Infant Pain Profile
Pirie bone
piriform
p. fossa
p. muscle
p. recess
p. sinus
piriformis
p. syndrome
Pirogoff
P. amputation
P. angle
P. operation
P. triangle
pisiform
p. bone
p. fracture
pisiforme
pisiformis
pisohamatum
pisometacarpeum
pisotriquetral arthritis
pit
p. of atlas for dens
commissural lip p.
costal p.
p. and fissure cavity
gastric p.
granular p.
herniation p.
inferior articular p.
inferior costal p.
nail p.
pterygoid p.
sublingual p.
superior costal p.
suprameatal p.
pitted
p. keratolysis
p. nail
pitting
nail p.
pituicytoma
pituitaria
pituitary
p. ablation
p. adenoma
p. body
p. endocrine disorder
p. fossa
p. gland
p. gland transplantation
p. microadenoma
p. neuroadenolysis
p. stalk section
p. tumor
p. tumor cell
pituitectomy
pituitous
pivot
p. joint
p. point
Pizzolato peroxide-silver method
PJA
pancreaticojejunostomy anastomosis
PJA afferent
PJA efferent
PKD
polycystic kidney disease
place of articulation
placebo therapy
placement
aortic graft p.
band p.
biliary sphincterotomy and stent p.
bone graft p.
bur-hole p.
catheter tip p.
clip p.
dilator p.
electrode p.
endoscopic biliary stent p.
endotracheal tube p.
feeding tube p.
filter p.
five-port fan p.
fluoroscopic p.
four-port diamond p.
graft p.
implant p.
infrarenal endograft p.
intrapleural catheter p.
Kirschner wire p.
K-wire p.
long-term central venous access catheter p.

NOTES

P

placement *(continued)*
- odontoid screw p.
- percutaneous nephrostomy tube p.
- permanent bipolar magnet p.
- permanent pacemaker p.
- pH electrode p.
- plate p.
- posterolateral bone graft p.
- radiologic biliary stent p.
- rod p.
- sacral screw p.
- screw p.
- shunt p.
- stent p.
- suprarenal filter p.
- surgical p.
- temporary pacemaker p.
- T-tube p.
- tube p.
- ureteral stent p.
- variable screw p.
- ventriculoperitoneal shunt p.
- wire-guided p.

placenta, pl. **placentae**
- endotheliochorial p.
- endothelio-endothelial p.
- extrachorial p.
- premature separation of p.

placental
- p. barrier
- p. circulation
- p. extrusion
- p. fragment
- p. hemangioma syndrome
- p. hemorrhage
- p. implantation
- p. localization
- p. membrane
- p. metastasis
- p. migration
- p. respiration
- p. tissue
- p. tissue transplant
- p. transfer
- p. uptake

placentation bleeding

placentoma

Placido ring

placode
- nasal p.

pladaroma

plafond fracture

plagiocephaly

plain
- p. abdominal film
- p. abdominal radiography

plana (*pl. of* planum)

plane
- Aeby p.
- alveolar point-meatus p.
- anatomic p.
- auriculoinfraorbital p.
- axial p.
- axiobuccolingual p.
- axiolabiolingual p.
- axiomesiodistal p.
- base p.
- bite p.
- Broca visual p.
- buccolingual p.
- Camper p.
- cleavage p.
- coronal p.
- cove p.
- cusp p.
- datum p.
- Daubenton p.
- diffuse p.
- p. of dissection
- equatorial p.
- equivalent refracting p.
- eye-ear p.
- facet p.
- facial p.
- fascial p.
- fat p.
- first parallel pelvic p.
- flexion-extension p.
- focal p.
- fourth parallel pelvic p.
- Frankfort horizontal p.
- French p.
- frontal p.
- guide p.
- guiding p.
- Hensen p.
- His p.
- Hodge p.
- horizontal p.
- internervous p.
- interspinal p.
- intertubercular p.
- ischiorectal fossa p.
- p. joint
- labiolingual p.
- lens p.
- Listing p.
- Ludwig p.
- mandibular p.
- mean foundation p.
- mesiodistal p.
- midcoronal p.
- midfrontal p.
- midsagittal p.
- midthalamic p.

Morton p.
nodal p.
nuchal p.
oblique coronal p.
occipital p.
occlusal p.
orbital p.
orthogonal p.
paramedian sagittal p.
parasagittal p.
pelvic p.
peripancreatic fat p.
perpendicular p.
preglenoid p.
primary movement p.
principal p.
sagittal p.
scan p.
second parallel pelvic p.
sensitive p.
short-axis p.
slant of occlusal p.
spectacle p.
spinous p.
sternal p.
sternoxiphoid p.
subcostal p.
subcutaneous p.
subpectoral p.
supracrestal p.
supracristal p.
suprasternal p.
symmetry p.
temporal p.
terminal p.
thalamic p.
third parallel pelvic p.
thoracic p.
tooth p.
transaxial scan p.
transection p.
transpyloric p.
transtubercular p.
transverse p.
umbilical p.
varus-valgus p.
vertical p.
visual p.
wide p.

planimetry

planithorax

planned
p. awakening
p. extracapsular cataract extraction
p. reoperation

planning
image-integrated surgery treatment p.

planta, pl. **plantae**

plantar
p. angulation
p. approach
p. aspect
p. compartmental anatomy
p. condylectomy
p. digital nerve
p. fasciotomy
p. flexion-inversion deformity
p. interosseous muscle
p. longitudinal incision
p. plate release
p. pressure
p. quadrate muscle
p. space
p. tendon sheath
p. venous network

plantare

plantar-hindfoot-midfoot bony mass

plantaria

plantaris
p. tendon

planum, pl. **plana**

planuria

planus
condyloma p.
oral condyloma p.

plaque
atheromatous p.
atherosclerotic p.
augmentation p.
carotid p.
echogenic p.
echolucent p.
eczematoid pruritic p.
p. fracture
p. incision
neuritic p.
Randall p.
p. rupture
senile p.
p. technique

NOTES

P

plaque-like
p.-l. hamartoma
p.-l. lesion
plaquing
plasma
p. assay coagulation panel
p. atrial natriuretic protein
p. cell portal infiltration
p. clotting time
p. colloid osmotic pressure
p. concentration
p. endotoxin concentration
p. exchange
p. exchange therapy
expanded p.
extracellular p.
fresh frozen p.
p. gastrin concentration
p. half-life
p. iron concentration
p. level
p. membrane
p. norepinephrine concentration
p. oncotic pressure
p. renin concentration
p. separation rate
target p.
p. thrombin clot method
p. urea concentration
p. volume expansion
plasmacytoma
plasmapheresis
plasmin coagulation
plasmin-inhibitor complex (PIC)
plasminogen plasma level
plasmocytoma
plasmolysis
plaster
p. cast application burn
plastic
p. bowing fracture
p. clot
p. induration
p. matrix technique
p. operation
p. reconstruction
p. and reconstructive surgery
p. repair
p. section
p. stent occlusion
p. surgeon
p. suture technique
plastica
plasticity
connective tissue p.
neural p.
plastron
plasty
Coleman p.
Durham p.
endoventricular circular patch p.
Foley Y-V p.
mons p.
posterior bladder flap p.
rotation p.
skin p.
sliding p.
V-Y p.
Y-V p.
plate
p. of Arantius
cribriform p.
p. fixation
gallbladder p.
hilar p.
nerve-containing p.
perpendicular of ethmoid p.
p. placement
pterygoid p.
tarsal p.
umbilical p.
vessel-containing p.
plateau
alveolar p.
p. method
platelet
p. aggregation
p. concentrate
p. nucleotide content
plateletpheresis
intraoperative p.
plate-screw
p.-s. fixation
p.-s. osteosynthesis
plating
compression p.
pedicle screw p.
Platou osteotomy
platybasia
platycephaly
platycrania
platyhieric
platymeric
platyopia
platyopic
platypellic pelvis
platypelloid pelvis
platyrrhine
platyrrhiny
platysma, pl. **platysmas, platysmata**
p. muscle
p. myocutaneous flap
platyspondylia
platystencephaly
Pleatman sac

pledgeted
pleoptics
Bangerter method of p.
Cüppers method of p.
plethysmography
forearm p.
impedance p.
venous-occlusion volume p.
volume p.
pleura, pl. **pleurae**
cervical p.
costal p.
diaphragmatic p.
mediastinal p.
parietal p.
phrenic p.
pulmonary p.
visceral p.
pleuracentesis
pleuracotomy
pleural
p. biopsy
p. calculus
p. cavity
p. cupula
p. effusion
p. fluid
p. fluid aspiration
p. fluid collection
p. fluid examination
p. line
p. mass
p. patch reinforcement
p. recess
p. reflection
p. sac
p. sinus
p. space
p. symphysis
p. villus
p. violation
pleurales
pleuralis
pleurapophysis
pleurectomy
thorascopic apical p.
pleurisy
pleurobiliary fistula
pleurocele
pleurocentesis
pleurocentrum
pleuroclysis
pleurodesis
talc p.
pleuroesophageal
p. fistula
p. line
p. muscle
pleuroesophageus
pleurolith
pleuroparietopexy
pleuropericardial
pleuropericarditis
pleuroperitoneal
p. canal
p. fold
p. foramen
p. hernia
p. hiatus
p. shunting
p. space
pleuropneumonectomy
pleuropulmonary
pleuroscopy
pleurotomy
pleurovisceral
plexectomy
plexiform
p. external layer
p. lesion
plexopathy
idiopathic brachial p.
postradiation p.
plexus, pl. **plexuses, plexus**
abdominal aortic p.
ascending pharyngeal p.
Auerbach p.
autonomic p.
axillary p.
basilar venous p.
Batson p.
brachial p.
cardiac p.
carotid venous p.
cavernous p.
celiac nervous p.
cervical p.
choroid p.
coccygeal p.
colic p.
colonic mesenteric p.
common carotid p.
coronary p.

NOTES

P

plexus *(continued)*
- Cruveilhier p.
- deep cardiac p.
- deferential p.
- enteric p.
- esophageal p.
- Exner p.
- external carotid p.
- external iliac p.
- external maxillary p.
- extrapancreatic nerve p.
- facial p.
- femoral p.
- gastroesophageal variceal p.
- Haller p.
- Heller p.
- hemorrhoidal p.
- hepatic p.
- hypoglossal canal venous p.
- iliac p.
- inferior hemorrhoidal p.
- inferior hypogastric p.
- inferior mesenteric p.
- inferior rectal p.
- inferior thyroid p.
- inferior vesical p.
- infraclavicular part of brachial p.
- inguinal p.
- intermesenteric p.
- internal carotid venous p.
- internal mammary p.
- internal maxillary p.
- internal thoracic lymphatic p.
- intracavernous p.
- intraparotid p.
- ischiadic p.
- Jacques p.
- jugular p.
- lingual p.
- lumbar p.
- lumbosacral p.
- lymphatic p.
- mammary p.
- Meissner p.
- meningeal p.
- myenteric p.
- occipital p.
- ovarian p.
- pampiniform p.
- pancreatic p.
- parotid p.
- pelvic autonomic p.
- periarterial p.
- pericorneal p.
- pharyngeal p.
- phrenic p.
- popliteal p.
- posterior auricular p.
- posterior coronary p.
- prostaticovesical p.
- prostatic venous p.
- pterygoid p.
- pulmonary p.
- Quénu hemorrhoidal p.
- rectal venous p.
- Remak p.
- renal p.
- sacral venous p.
- Santorini p.
- Sappey p.
- sciatic p.
- solar p.
- spermatic p.
- splenic p.
- subclavian periarterial p.
- submucosal p.
- suboccipital venous p.
- superficial cardiac p.
- superficial temporal p.
- superior hemorrhoidal p.
- superior hypogastric p.
- superior mesenteric p.
- superior rectal p.
- superior thyroid p.
- suprarenal p.
- testicular p.
- thoracic aortic p.
- tympanic p.
- ureteric p.
- uterine venous p.
- uterovaginal p.
- vaginal venous p.
- vascular p.
- venous p.
- vertebral venous p.
- vesical p.
- vesicular venous p.
- Walther p.

plica, pl. **plicae**

plicated appendicocystostomy

plicating suture technique

plication
- buccinator p.
- Child-Phillips bowel p.
- disk p.
- fundal p.
- Graham p.
- Kelly p.
- Nesbit p.
- Noble bowel p.
- Rehne-Delorme p.
- retractor p.
- soft-tissue p.
- suture p.
- tongue p.

transgastric p.
transmesenteric p.
plicectomy
plicotomy
PLIF
posterior lumbar interbody fusion
PLIF procedure
PLND
pelvic lymph node dissection
ploidy
tumor p.
plombage operation
plop
cardiac tumor p.
tumor p.
plosive-injection method
plot
load-displacement p.
pressure-flow p.
plug
p. flow
p. prosthetic mesh repair
plumb line
plume
laser p.
plyometric exercise
PMN
polymorphonuclear neutrophil
$PmvCO_2$
partial pressure of mesenteric venous carbon dioxide
pneumatic
p. bag esophageal dilation
p. balloon catheter dilation
p. bone
p. compression
p. dilatation
p. otoscopy
p. reduction
p. retinopexy
p. space
pneumaticum
pneumatinuria
pneumatization
pneumatocele
pneumatorrhachis
pneumaturia
pneumectomy
pneumobulbar
pneumocardial
pneumocele
pneumocentesis
pneumocephalus
pneumococcal infection
pneumococcolysis
pneumoconiosis, pl. **pneumoconioses**
pneumocystography
pneumocystosis
pneumodissection
laparoscopic p.
pneumoencephalos
pneumogastric nerve
pneumography
impedance p.
retroperitoneal p.
pneumohydroperitoneum
pneumolysis
pneumonectomy chest
pneumonia
aspiration p.
congenital aspiration p.
endogenous lipid p.
extensive bilateral p.
gram-negative p.
inhalation p.
nosocomial p.
oil-aspiration p.
postoperative p.
ventilator-associated p.
pneumonic
pneumonitis
acute radiation p.
aspiration p.
peptic aspiration p.
radiation p.
pneumonocele
pneumonocentesis
pneumonopexy
pneumonoresection
pneumonorrhaphy
pneumonotomy
pneumoorbitography
pneumopericardium
tension p.
ventilator-induced p.
pneumoperitoneum
ambulatory p.
CO_2 p.
hospital p.
positive-pressure p.
preoperative p.
stent-induced p.
pneumopexy
pneumopleuroparietopexy

NOTES

pneumopyelography
pneumoresection
pneumoretroperitoneum
unilateral p.
pneumostatic dilation
pneumotachogram
pneumotachograph
pneumothorax, pl. **pneumothoraces**
delayed p.
extrapleural p.
iatrogenic tension p.
induced tension p.
open p.
posttraumatic persistent p. (PPP)
pressure p.
spontaneous p.
tension p.
ventilator-induced p.
pneumotomy
PNPB
positive-negative pressure breathing
PO_2
partial pressure of oxygen
pocket
circulating air p.
elimination p.
ionization chamber p.
p. operation
pacemaker p.
peritoneal p.
subpectoral p.
pocketed calculus
POD
postoperative day
podalic extraction
PODVT
postoperative deep venous thrombosis
POG
Pediatric Oncology Group
Pog
point P.
pogonion
Pogrund lateral approach
point
p. A
abrasive p.
p. of abscess
absorbent p.
Addison p.
alveolar p.
anchoring p.
p. angle
anterior focal p.
APACHE-II p.
apophysary p.
apophysial p.
p. of Arrhigi
associated myofascial trigger p.
auricular p.
axial p.
p. B
B p.
bleeding p.
blur p.
Boas p.
Bolton p.
bounce p.
Boyd p.
break p.
Brinell hardness indenter p.
Broadbent registration p.
p. B, supramentale
Cannon p.
Capuron p.
cardinal p.
Castellani p.
central-bearing p.
central yellow p.
p. centric
change p.
Chauffard p.
choroid p.
Clado p.
condenser p.
conjugate p.
contact area p.
convenience p.
convergence p.
copular p.
corresponding p.
craniometric p.
Crowe pilot p.
cut p.
D p.
de Mussy p.
Desjardins p.
disparate p.
dorsal p.
E p.
electrodesiccated bleeding p.
end p.
entry p.
equivalence p.
Erb p.
ethmoid registration p.
exit p.
eye p.
far p.
faulty contact p.
F2 focal p.
fibromyalgia trigger p.
fixation p.
fixed p.
focal bleeding p.
focal image p.
freezing p.

fusing p.
gingival p.
glenoid p.
growing p.
Guéneau de Mussy p.
gutta-percha p.
Halle p.
Hartmann p.
hinge-axis p.
ice p.
identical p.
ignition p.
image p.
p. imaging
impaction p.
incident p.
incisal p.
incisor p.
p. of inflection
insertion p.
isoelectric p.
isometric p.
isosbestic p.
J p.
jugal p.
jugomaxillary p.
Keen p.
Knoop hardness indenter p.
Kocher p.
Krackow p.
lacrimal p.
Lanz p.
Legat p.
lustrous central yellow p.
Mackenzie p.
material failure break p.
p. of maximum impulse
maximum occipital p.
McBurney p.
median mandibular p.
melting p.
mental p.
metopic p.
motor p.
multiple sensitive p.
Munro p.
myofascial trigger p.
near visual p.
neutral p.
nodal p.
null p.
occipital p.
optical nodal p.
painful p.
paper p.
Pauly p.
pedicle entrance p.
Piersol p.
pivot p.
p. Pog
posterior focal p.
power p.
preauricular p.
pressure inversion p.
primary myofascial trigger p.
principal p.
purchase p.
radix p.
Ramond p.
referred p.
respiratory inversion p.
restoration p.
retention p.
retrograde insertion p.
retromandibular p.
Robson p.
root canal p.
rotary mounted p.
sacral brim target p.
satellite myofascial trigger p.
p. scanning
secondary focal p.
secondary myofascial trigger p.
sensitive p.
separation p.
set p.
p. source
spinal p.
Starlite p.
stereo-identical p.
Sudeck critical p.
sulfur and silver p.
supraauricular p.
supraorbital p.
sylvian p.
tender p.
thermal death p.
trial p.
trigger p.
triple p.
Trousseau p.
Valleix p.
virtual p.
visual p.

NOTES

point *(continued)*
- Weber p.
- white p.
- William Dixon Cratex p.
- wood p.
- yellow p.
- Z p.
- zygomaxillary p.

point-counting image
pointed condyloma
point-in-space stereotactic biopsy
Poirier
- P. gland
- P. line
- space of P.

Poiseuille space
poisoning
- oxygen p.
- radiation p.

Poland
- P. anomaly
- P. epiphysial fracture classification
- P. physical injury classification

polariscopy
polarization microscopy
polarographic method
pole
- inferior p.
- lateral p.
- p. ligation
- superior p.

poli (*pl. of* polus)
poliomyelitis
Politano-Leadbetter
- P.-L. anastomosis
- P.-L. reimplantation
- P.-L. tunnel creation
- P.-L. ureterolysis
- P.-L. ureteroneocystostomy

Politzer method
pollakiuria
pollex, pl. **pollices**
pollicis
pollicization
- Buck-Gramcko p.
- index p.
- Riordan p.

pollination
Pollock operation
polus, pl. **poli**
poly
Pólya
- P. anastomosis
- P. gastrectomy
- P. gastroenterostomy
- P. method
- P. operation
- P. procedure
- P. technique

polyacrylonitrile membrane
polyadenous
polyadenylation
polyagglutination
Polyak operation
polyaxial joint
polycentric rotation
polychondritis
- relapsing p.

polyclonal
- p. growth
- p. hyperplasia

polycystic
- p. kidney disease (PKD)
- p. liver

polydactylous
polydactyly
polydysplasia
polyembryoma
polyganglionic
polyglandular
polymer anesthetic
polymicrobial infection
polymorphism
polymorphonuclear neutrophil (PMN)
polymyalgia rheumatica
polyorchism
polyp
- adenomatous p.
- cellular p.
- colon p.
- colorectal p.
- cystic p.
- dental p.
- diffuse GI hamartoma p.
- endocervical p.
- endometrial p.
- hyperplastic p.
- juvenile p.
- perineal p.

polypapilloma
polypectomy
- colonoscopic p.
- duodenal endoscopic p.
- electrosurgical snare p.
- endoscopic sessile p.
- gastric p.
- incomplete p.
- intranasal p.

polypeptide growth factor
polypoid
- p. lesion
- p. mass
- p. superficial gastric carcinoma
- p. tissue

polypoidal lesion

polyposis
carpet-like p.
diffuse mucosal p.
familial adenomatous p. (FAP)
polyradiculoneuropathy
chronic inflammatory demyelinating p. (CIDP)
polyradiculopathy
polysinusectomy
polyspermia
polysyndactyly
polythelia
polyuria
polyvalent
p. melanoma oncolysate
p. VMO
Pomeroy
P. operation
P. tubal ligation
Poncet perineal urethrostomy
pond fracture
Ponka
P. herniorrhaphy
P. technique for local anesthesia
pons, pl. **pontes**
p. hepatis
Ponsky pull or guidewire insertion technique
Pontén fasciocutaneous flap
ponticulus hepatis
pontile
pontine
p. artery
p. cistern
p. hemorrhage
p. myelinolysis
p. paramedian reticular formation
p. spinothalamic tractotomy
pontis
PONV
postoperative nausea and vomiting
pool
abdominal p.
p. therapy
poorly compliant bladder
poor-risk patient
poplitea
popliteal
p. artery
p. artery occlusive disease (PAOD)
p. artery trifurcation
p. communicating nerve
p. fascia
p. fossa
p. groove
p. incision
p. muscle
p. plexus
p. region
p. space
p. vein
p. web syndrome
popliteales
popliteus
p. tendon
population
adult p.
patient p.
pediatric p.
p. sample
population-based registry
porcelain
p. cervical ditching technique
p. condensation
p. fracture
p. gallbladder
p. jacket restoration
porcelain-bonded restoration
porcelain-fused-to-metal restoration
porcine
pori (*pl. of* porus)
porocarcinoma
porocele
poroid hidradenoma
poroma
porotomy
porous
p. filter membrane
p. ingrowth fixation
porphyria
acute intermittent p.
intermittent acute p.
Porro
P. cesarean section
P. operation
Porstmann technique
port
chest p.
p. displacement
implantable infusion p.
p. incision
infusion p.
inlet p.

NOTES

P

port *(continued)*
lumbar p.
midclavicular p.
nasal p.
PAS p.
periumbilical p.
side p.
p. site
p. site hernia
p. site metastasis
subcostal p.
subcutaneous implanted injection p.
subxiphoid p.
suprapubic p.
umbilical p.
velopharyngeal p.
p. vitrectomy
porta, pl. **portae**
portable C-arm image intensifier fluoroscopy
portacaval
p. anastomosis
p. H graft
p. shunt
p. shunt operation
port-access
p.-a. coronary artery bypass grafting
p.-a. technique for coronary bypass surgery
portae (*pl. of* porta)
portal
arthroscopic entry p.
aspiration p.
p. bifurcation
p. collateral
p. decompression
p. decompression surgery
p. delta
p. drainage
p. eosinophilic inflammation
p. fissure
p. hypertension
p. hypertensive bleeding
p. inflow
p. infusion
p. lymphadenopathy
p. lymph node basin
macroscopic p.
p. mesenteric shunting
p. nodal involvement
p. pedicle
p. shunt index
p. space
p. steal
p. thrombosis
p. tract
p. tract inflammation
p. triad
p. triad clamping
p. tumor thrombus
p. vein
p. vein catheterization
p. vein obstruction
p. vein reconstruction
p. vein resection
p. vein tumor thrombus (PVTT)
p. venous pressure
p. vessel
portal-collateral circulation
portal-hypophysial circulation
portalis
portal-systemic
p.-s. anastomosis
p.-s. collateral
p.-s. collateral vein
p.-s. encephalopathy (PSE)
p.-s. shunt
p.-s. shunt surgery
Porter fascia
Porter-Richardson-Vainio
P.-R.-V. synovectomy
P.-R.-V. technique
portio, pl. **portiones**
portion
distal p.
intrapancreatic p.
lateral p.
mesenteric p.
proximal p.
subcutaneous p.
portiplexus
Portmann interposition operation
portmanteau procedure
portobilioarterial
portoenterostomy
Kasai p.
portography
computed tomography arterial p. (CTAP)
CT p.
indirect p.
portoportal anastomosis
portopulmonary venous anastomosis
portosystemic
p. anastomosis
p. collateral circulation
p. shunt
p. shunting
port-site wound recurrence
port-wine
p.-w. hemangioma
p.-w. mark
p.-w. stain
porus, pl. **pori**
Posada fracture

position

abdominal brace p.
Adams p.
airplane p.
p. ametropia
anatomic p.
anatomical p.
angular p.
anomalous p.
antecolic p.
anterior oblique p.
antiembolic p.
arch-and-slouch p.
arm p.
arm-extension p.
asynclitic p.
back-up p.
backward p.
barber chair p.
batrachian p.
bayonet fracture p.
beach chair p.
Bertel p.
birthing p.
bisecting angle cone p.
body p.
Bonner p.
Boyce p.
Bozeman p.
Brickner p.
brow p.
brow-anterior p.
brow-down p.
brow-posterior p.
brow-up p.
Buie p.
calcaneal stance p.
cardiac p.
cardinal p.
Casselberry p.
catheter p.
centric p.
cervical p.
chin p.
condylar hinge p.
consonant p.
convergence p.
corrected sternal p.
cottonloader p.
curved flank p.
cuspid-molar p.
decubitus p.
dissociated p.
distoangular p.
dorsal elevated p.
dorsal inertia p.
dorsal lithotomy p.
dorsal recumbent p.
dorsal rigid p.
dorsal supine p.
dorsosacral p.
Duncan p.
eccentric jaw p.
Edebohls p.
electrical heart p.
Elliot p.
emprosthotonos p.
en face p.
English p.
equinus p.
exaggerated sniffing p.
extraabdominal p.
extrathoracic p.
face-down p.
face-to-pubes p.
Feist-Mankin p.
fetal head p.
Fick p.
figure-four p.
final cone p.
final consonant p.
first cone p.
flank p.
flexed p.
forehead-nose p.
French p.
frogleg p.
frontoanterior p.
frontoposterior p.
frontotransverse p.
Fuchs p.
fusion-free p.
Gaynor-Hart p.
genucubital p.
genufacial p.
genupectoral p.
gingival p.
greater curve p.
head dependent p.
head-up tilt p.
heart p.
heterophoric p.
hinge p.
hook-lying p.

NOTES

P

position *(continued)*
horizontal p.
hornpipe p.
infraumbilical p.
initial consonant p.
intercuspal p.
intraperitoneal p.
intrathoracic p.
intrinsic minus p.
jackknife p.
James p.
jaw-to-jaw p.
jet pilot p.
Jones p.
jumper-knee p.
kidney p.
knee-chest p.
knee-elbow p.
kneeling p.
kneeling-squatting p.
Kraske p.
LAO p.
lateral decubitus p.
lateral prone p.
lateral recumbent p.
leapfrog p.
left anterior oblique p.
left decubitus p.
left lateral decubitus p.
left-side-down p.
levo-transposed p.
lithotomy p.
Lloyd Davis modified lithotomy p.
lotus p.
mandibular hinge p.
mandibular rest p.
maternal birthing p.
Mayo-Robson p.
mentoanterior p.
mentoposterior p.
mentotransverse p.
mentum anterior p.
mentum posterior p.
mentum transverse p.
Mercurio p.
mesioangular p.
midline p.
military brace p.
military tuck p.
missionary p.
modified lithotomy p.
Moynihan p.
near-anatomic p.
neck extension p.
neutral hip p.
neutral spine p.
Noble p.
nonphysiologic p.
normal anatomic p.
obstetric p.
occipitoanterior p.
occipitoposterior p.
occipitotransverse p.
occlusal p.
opisthotonos p.
overcorrected p.
over-the-top p.
paralleling cone p.
park-bench p.
persistent occiput posterior p.
Phalen p.
physiologic rest p.
posterior border p.
postural resting p.
prayer p.
premuscular p.
primary p.
Proetz p.
prone split-leg p.
protrusive occlusal p.
proximal bow p.
pterygoid p.
pulmonary p.
quasistatic stressed p.
RAO p.
reclining p.
rectus p.
recumbent p.
rest p.
retrocolic p.
retromuscular p.
retruded p.
reverse Trendelenburg p.
Rhese p.
right acromiodorsoposterior p.
right anterior oblique p.
right-side-down p.
Robson p.
Rose p.
sacroanterior p.
sacroposterior p.
sacrotransverse p.
Samuel p.
scapuloanterior p.
scapuloposterior p.
Schuller p.
scissor-leg p.
Scultetus p.
semi-Fowler p.
semilateral p.
semioblique p.
semiprone p.
semireclining p.
semirecumbent p.
semiupright p.
shock p.

shoe-and-stocking p.
Simon p.
Sims p.
sitting p.
ski p.
sniffing p.
p. in space
spinal fusion p.
static p.
steep Trendelenburg p.
sternal p.
subcostal p.
sulcus fixated p.
supine p.
terminal hinge p.
tooth p.
tooth-to-tooth p.
translational p.
Trendelenburg p.
tricuspid p.
tuck p.
upright p.
Valentine p.
vertex p.
vertical divergence p.
Walcher p.
Waters-Waldron p.
W-sitting p.
Zanelli p.

positional
p. release therapy
p. vertigo

positioning
surgical p.

positive
p. airway pressure (PAP)
p. control enzyme induction
p. correlation
p. cytology
p. end-airway pressure
p. end-expiratory pressure (PEEP)
p. end-expiratory pressure/continuous positive airway pressure (PEEP/CPAP)
p. expiratory pressure
extradomain A p.
false p.
p. inspiratory pressure
p. peritoneal cytology (PPC)
p. predictive value (PPV)
p. resection margin
p. surgical margin
true p.

positive-negative pressure breathing (PNPB)

positive-pressure
p.-p. pneumoperitoneum
p.-p. ventilation (PPV)

positron
p. emission tomography (PET)
p. emission tomography-guided biopsy
p. emission tomography scanning

post
p. herniorrhaphy inguinodynia
P. total shoulder arthroplasty

postactivation
p. exhaustion
p. facilitation

postadrenalectomy syndrome

postage stamp skin graft

postanal repair

postanesthesia care unit (PACU)

postanesthetic central nervous system dysfunction

postangioplasty
p. intimal flap
p. restenosis

postaugmentation

postauricular incision

postautoclave contamination

postaxial

postaxillaris

postaxillary line

postballoon angioplasty restenosis

postbiopsy
p. renal A-V fistula
p. vascular complication

postbrachial

postbulbar ulceration

postburn
p. bone marrow failure
p. hypermetabolic response

postcardiotomy
p. shock (PS)
p. syndrome

postcatheterization

postcavales

postcaval ureter

postcementation

postcentral
p. gyrectomy
p. sulcal artery

NOTES

P

postcentralis
postcesarean anesthesia
postcholecystectomy
p. flatulent dyspepsia
p. syndrome
postclavicular
post-coiling
postcoital
p. bleeding
p. test
postcolonoscopy distention syndrome
postcommissurotomy syndrome
postcondensation
postcordial
postcore restoration
postcoronary angioplasty
postcostal
postcricoid web
postdiagnosis
postdischarge
postdrug latency
postductal coarctation
postdural puncture headache (PDPH)
postembolization syndrome
postendoscopy
posterior
p. alveolar artery
p. antebrachial region
anterior and p. (A&P)
p. anterior jugular vein
p. arch
p. arch fracture
p. arm
p. articular aorta
p. aspect
p. auricular artery
p. auricular groove
p. auricular plexus
p. auricular vein
p. basal branch
p. basal segment
p. belly
p. bladder flap plasty
p. border jaw relation
p. border position
p. brachial region
p. capsular zonular barrier
p. capsulorrhaphy
p. capsulotomy
p. cecal artery
p. cerebral artery
p. cervical fixation
p. cervical fusion
p. cervical space
p. choroidal artery
p. circulation aneurysm
p. circumflex humeral artery
p. clinoid process
p. colporrhaphy
p. column
p. column cordotomy
p. column fracture
p. column osteosynthesis
p. communicating artery
p. condyloid foramen
p. coronary plexus
p. costotransversectomy approach
p. cranial fossa
p. cricoarytenoid muscle
p. crus
p. cyst
p. diaphragmatic gastropexy
p. element fracture
p. explant
p. facial vein
p. flap
p. flap technique
p. flap vaginoplasty
p. focal point
p. fontanelle
p. fornix of vagina
p. fossa circulation
p. fossa decompression
p. fracture-dislocation
p. fundoplasty
p. glenoplasty
p. great vessel
p. hemicircular incision
p. hip dislocation
p. humeral circumflex artery
p. iliac osteotomy
p. inferior cerebellar artery
p. inferior iliac spine
p. innominate rotation
p. intercostal artery 1–11
p. intercostal vein
p. intermuscular septum
p. interosseous artery
p. interosseous nerve compression syndrome
p. interosseous vein
p. intraoccipital joint
p. inverted-U approach
p. knee
p. knee region
p. labial artery
p. labial commissure
p. labial vein
p. laparoscopic approach
p. larynx
p. layer
p. leg
p. limiting ring
p. lobule
p. longitudinal bundle
p. lower cervical spine surgery

p. lumbar approach
p. lumbar interbody fusion (PLIF)
p. lumbar interbody fusion procedure
p. lumbar interbody fusion surgery
p. lumbar spine and sacrum surgery
p. mediastinal artery
p. mediastinal mass
p. mediastinum
p. meningeal artery
p. midline approach
p. mitral valve leaflet
p. neck region
p. nephrectomy
p. nodule
p. occipitocervical approach
p. oropharyngeal wall
p. pancreaticoduodenal artery
p. parametritis
p. parietal artery
p. parotid vein
p. pedicle
p. pelvic exenteration
p. periosteum
p. pharynx
p. Pólya procedure
p. primary division
p. proctotomy
p. radicular artery
p. rectopexy
p. rectus sheath
p. rectus sheath wall
p. repair
p. rhizotomy
p. ring fracture
p. root
p. sclerotomy
p. screw fixation
p. scrotal vein
p. segmental fixation
p. shoulder dislocation
p. side
p. spinal artery
p. spinal fusion
p. spinal wedge osteotomy
p. spinocerebellar tract
p. stomach
p. superior alveolar artery
p. superior iliac spine
superior labrum anterior and p. (SLAP)
p. surface
p. synechia formation
p. temporal artery
p. thermal sclerostomy
p. thigh
p. tibialis tendon
p. tibial recurrent artery
p. tibiotalar
p. translation
p. transolecranon approach
p. transthoracic incision
p. truncal vagotomy
p. ulnar recurrent artery
p. upper cervical spine surgery
p. urethra
p. uveitis
p. vaginal fornix
p. vaginal hernia
p. vaginal trunk
p. vertical canal
p. vitrectomy
p. wall fracture

posteriora
posterior-anterior pressure
posteriores
posterior-interbody lumbar spinal fusion
posterioris
posterior-lateral
p.-l. lobule
p.-l. lumbar spinal fusion
posterior-superior oblique projection
posterius
posteroanterior projection
posteroinferior
p. external
p. external movement
posterolateral
p. approach
p. aspect
p. bone graft placement
p. bundle
p. central artery
p. costotransversectomy incision
p. costotransversectomy technique
p. herniation
p. interbody fusion
p. lumbosacral fusion
posterolateralis
posteromedial
p. approach
p. central artery
p. dislocation

NOTES

P

posterosuperior segment
posteroventral pallidotomy
postesophageal
postevacuation
postexcision cavity
postextraction hemorrhage
postextubation
p. croup
p. laryngospasm
p. stridor
postfixation radiography
postfracture lesion
postfundoplication syndrome
postganglionic
p. parasympathetic fiber
p. sympathetic fiber
postgastrectomy
p. bleed
p. cancer
p. dysfunction
p. hemorrhage
p. syndrome
posthemorrhagic
posthepatic resection phase
postherniorrhaphy pain
postherpetic neuralgia
posthetomy
posthioplasty
posthitis
postholith
posthyoid
posthyperventilation apnea
posticus
postinfection lipoatrophy
postinflammatory hypopigmentation
postinjury immunologic defect
post-injury level
postinsufflation
postintervention
postirradiation
p. fracture
p. study
p. syndrome
postischemic
p. administration
p. stunned myocardium
postischial
postkeratoplasty
postlaminectomy
p. kyphosis
p. syndrome
postlaparoscopy meralgia paresthetica
postlumpectomy skin thickening
postlymphangiography abdomen
postmastectomy
postmastoid
postmedian
postmediastinal
postmediastinum
postmembrane
p. pressure
p. rupture
postmenopausal
p. bleeding
p. body mass
postmortem
p. clot
p. examination
p. hypostasis
p. suggillation
postnatal therapy
postocular
postoperative
p. abscess
p. airway obstruction
p. analgesia
p. analgesic
p. anastomotic leak
p. anesthesia
p. anisocoria
p. antibiotic
p. anticoagulation therapy
p. apnea
p. bleeding
p. cesarean section pain
p. chemotherapy
p. choledochoscopy
p. course
p. CT scan
p. day (POD)
p. death
p. deep venous thrombosis (PODVT)
p. diagnosis
p. dialysis
p. ductal dilation
p. dysphagia
p. ERCP
p. extubation
p. fatigue
p. followup evaluation
p. fracture
p. hemorrhage
p. hepatic failure
p. hernia
p. hour
p. hydrocele
p. hypocalcemia
p. ileus
p. immobilization
p. infection
p. irradiation
p. irrigation-suction
p. irrigation-suction drainage
p. liver failure
p. management

p. morbidity
p. mortality
p. motility
p. nausea and vomiting (PONV)
p. paraplegia
p. pelvic radiation
p. period
p. pleurobiliary fistula
p. pneumonia
p. recovery
p. regimen for oral early feeding (PROEF)
p. renal dysfunction
p. repair
p. respiratory complication
p. result
p. supplementation
p. survival
p. survival probability (PSP)
p. symptom
p. systemic chemotherapy
p. tetany
p. ventilation

postpartum
p. hemorrhage
p. infection

postpericardiotomy syndrome
postpharyngeal space
postphlebitic syndrome
postpneumonectomy tuberculous empyema
postpolypectomy
p. bleed
p. coagulation syndrome
p. hemorrhage

postprandial
p. AUC
p. distention
p. hour
p. motor activity
p. motor parameter
p. motor result
p. period
p. value

postprostatectomy incontinence
postpyloric sphincter
postradiation
p. change
p. fistula
p. kyphosis
p. plexopathy
p. therapy

postradical neck dissection
postreduction mammaplasty
postrema
postresection
p. defect
p. filling
p. filling technique

postresuscitation period
postreversal
postsacral
postscapular
postsclerotherapy ulcer
postsensation
postshunt
postsphenoid bone
postsphincterotomy ERCP cannulation
postsplenectomy
p. complication
p. infection
p. sepsis

postsplenic
poststenotic
p. dilatation
p. dilation

poststroke pain
post-subarachnoid hemorrhage hydrocephalus
postsulcal
postsurgical
p. abdomen
p. disturbance
p. endoscopy
p. motor anomaly
p. motor change
p. nervous damage
p. truncal pain

postsynaptic membrane
posttecta
posttetanic
p. count
p. count monitoring
p. facilitation

postthoracotomy
p. change
p. pain

posttranslation modification
posttransplant
p. day
p. immunosuppression therapy
p. lymphoproliferative disease (PTLD)

NOTES

P

posttransplant *(continued)*
p. lymphoproliferative disorder (PTLD)
posttransverse
posttraumatic
p. autotransplantation
p. cervical dystonia
p. chondrolysis
p. gustatory neuralgia
p. hemorrhage
p. intradiploic pseudomeningocele
p. pancreatic-cutaneous fistula
p. persistent pneumothorax (PPP)
p. renal failure
p. seizure
p. spinal deformity
p. stress disorder
p. subcapsular hepatic fluid collection
posttreatment hemorrhage
posttubal ligation syndrome
postural
p. deformity
p. drainage
p. fixation back maneuver
p. reduction
p. resting position
p. therapy
posture
compensatory head p.
forward head p.
head p.
postureteral ligation
postureteroscopic manipulation
postuterine
postvagotomy
p. dysphagia
p. gastroparesis
p. syndrome
postvalvar
postvasectomy
postvesiculares
postvitrectomy fibrin
postzygomatic space
potassium space
potato tumor
potency
anesthetic p.
sphincteric p.
potential
compound muscle action p. (CMAP)
curative p.
demarcation p.
denervation p.
electrode p.
endogenous event-related p.
excitatory junction p.
excitatory postsynaptic p.
extreme somatosensory evoked p.
fasciculation p.
fibrillation p.
laser-evoked p.
membrane p.
miniature end-plate p.
modulation p.
motor-evoked p. (MEP)
myogenic motor-evoked p. (MEP)
oxidation-reducing p.
pacemaker p.
peroneal somatosensory evoked p.
reduction p.
regeneration motor unit p.
resting membrane p.
somatosensory evoked p. (SEP, SSEP)
standard electrode p.
standard reduction p.
potentially
p. curative procedure
p. lethal x-ray damage repair
p. resectable lesion
potentiation
potentiometric titration
Pott
P. aneurysm
P. ankle fracture
P. eversion osteotomy
P. gangrene
Potter
P. classification
P. facies
Potts
P. anastomosis
P. operation
P. procedure
Potts-Smith anastomosis
pouch
anal p.
antibiotic bead p.
arachnoid retrocerebellar p.
bead p.
p. biopsy
bladder replacement urinary p.
blind rectal p.
blind upper esophageal p.
Broca p.
colonic p.
coloplasty p.
continent ileal p.
continent urinary p.
copulating p.
deep perineal p.
dermal p.
p. development
p. dilatation

double-loop p.
Douglas p.
drainable ostomy p.
endorectal ileal p.
p. failure
gastric p.
Hartmann p.
haustral p.
heat-seal p.
hepatorenal p.
hernia p.
ileal neobladder urinary p.
p. ileitis
ileoanal p.
ileocecal p.
ileocolonic p.
inflamed synovial p.
intraluminal p.
intravaginal p.
inverted-U p.
jejunal p.
J-shaped ileal p.
J versus S versus W pelvic ileal p.
kangaroo p.
Koch p.
labioperineal p.
laryngeal p.
lateral-lateral p.
Miami p.
Morison p.
omental p.
one-piece ostomy p.
open-end ostomy p.
paracystic p.
pararectal p.
paravesical p.
pelvic p.
pharyngeal p.
Prussak p.
p. reconstruction
rectal blind p.
rectouterine p.
rectovaginal p.
rectovaginouterine p.
rectovesical p.
renal p.
self-seal p.
sigma rectum p.
sigmoid rectum p.
superficial perineal p.
suprapatellar p.
terminal ileal p.
three-loop ileal p.
triple loop p.
two-loop J-shaped ileal p.
two-piece ostomy p.
U p.
U-shaped jejunal p.
uterovesical p.
VBG p.
vertical banded gastroplasty p.
vesicouterine p.
visceral p.
wallaby p.
Willis p.
Zenker p.

pouched ileostomy

pouchitis

pouchoscopy
pelvic p.

Poulard operation

Poupart line

powdered bone graft

power
p. Doppler imaging
P. operation
p. point
p. spectral analysis

Pozzi procedure

PPC
positive peritoneal cytology

PPG
pylorus-preserving gastrectomy

PPH
primary pulmonary hypertension

PPI
proton pump inhibitor

PPP
posttraumatic persistent pneumothorax

PPPD
pylorus-preserving pancreatoduodenectomy

PPS
presurgical psychological screening

PPT
pressure pain threshold

PPV
positive predictive value
positive-pressure ventilation

PQOL
perceived quality of life

practitioner
alternative p.

NOTES

Prague maneuver
Pratt
P. open reduction
P. technique
prayer position
PRBC
packed red blood cells
preadaptation
preadventitial dissection
preanal
preanesthetic
p. medication
p. skin-surface warming
preantiseptic
preaortic
preaseptic
preauricular
p. cyst
p. fistula
p. fossa
p. groove
p. incision
p. point
p. sulcus
preauriculares
preauricularis
preaxial
preaxillaris
preaxillary line
precancerous lesion
precapillary anastomosis
precatheterization
precaution
radiation p.
prececales
precentral
p. cortical stimulation
p. gyrectomy
p. gyrus
p. sulcal artery
precentralis
prechiasmal
p. compression
p. optic nerve lesion
precipitate in solution
precipitating
p. lesion
p. noxious event
precise dissection
preclotted graft
precommissural bundle
preconditioning
ischemic p. (IPC)
precordial wound
precordium, pl. **precordia**
precorneal
precostal
precuneal artery
precunealis
precursor lesion
precut
p. incision
p. papillotomy
p. sphincterotomy
predental space
predialysis plasma phosphate concentration
prediction
breast cancer risk p.
Gail model of breast cancer risk p.
predictive value
prediluted antibody panel
predisposing
p. condition
p. factor
predisposition
hereditary p.
predorsal bundle
preeclamptic liver disease
preemergence
preemptive
p. analgesia
p. anesthesia
preendoscopy
preepiglottic
p. soft tissue
p. space
preexcitation
p. syndrome
ventricular p.
preexisting lesion
prefabrication
prefrontal
p. leukotomy
p. lobotomy
preganglionic
p. cardiac sympathetic blockade
p. parasympathetic fiber
p. sympathectomy
p. sympathetic block
p. sympathetic denervation
p. sympathetic fiber
preglenoid plane
pregnancy
abdominal p.
p. complication
ectopic p.
p. luteoma
pregnancy-induced anesthesia
prehepatic resection phase
prehospital resuscitation
prehyoid gland
preincision
preincubation
preinduction phase

preinsufflation
preinterparietal bone
preintervention
preischemic administration
Preiser disease
prelabor membrane rupture
prelaryngeal
p. node
prelaryngeales
prelimbic
preliminary iridectomy
preload
decreased p.
p. reduction
premalignant lesion
premasseteric
p. space
p. space abscess
premature
p. airway closure
p. amnion rupture
p. ductus arteriosis closure
P. Infant Pain Profile (PIPP)
p. membrane rupture
p. separation of placenta
premaxilla
premedicate
premedication
premembrane
p. pressure
p. rupture
premenopausal ovary
premicturition pressure
premolar teeth
premonitory palpitation
premorbid performance status
premuscular
p. mesh technique
p. position
p. prosthetic repair
prenatal
p. diethylstilbestrol exposure
p. dislocation
p. therapy
Prentiss
P. maneuver
P. orchiopexy
preoccipital notch
preoperative
p. analgesia
p. anesthetic
p. biopsy
p. chemoradiotherapy
p. diagnosis
p. dose
p. ERCP
p. evolution time
p. factor
p. fasting
p. feature
p. FNA specimen
p. imaging
p. induction chemotherapy
p. investigation
p. jaundice
p. lesion
p. liver function
p. localization
p. localization signal
p. LSG
p. lymphoscintigraphy
p. percutaneous aspiration
p. period
p. pneumoperitoneum
p. preparation
p. retrograde cholangiogram
p. scoring
p. scoring system
p. skin-surface warming
p. staging
p. staging evaluation
p. study
p. systemic chemotherapy
p. therapy
p. ultrasound
preoperatively donated autologous blood
preoxygenation
prepancreatic arch
prepapillary sphincter
preparation
access p.
biomechanical p.
bone-patellar tendon-bone p.
bowel p.
Brown dietary method for colon p.
cavity p.
chamfer p.
corrosion p.
crush p.
p. and draping
facet joint p.
facial butt joint p.
figure-eight p.
fortified topical p.

NOTES

P

preparation *(continued)*
full shoulder p.
galenic p.
graft p.
heart-lung p.
impression p.
incisal p.
initial p.
insulin p.
intraoperative bowel p.
Langendorff heart p.
lavage bowel p.
liposomal p.
lupus erythematosus p.
Matsura p.
medicinal p.
mouth p.
pinworm p.
preoperative p.
renal proximal tubule p.
rod contour p.
shoulder with bevel p.
skin p.
slice p.
slot p.
slot-type p.
Spälteholz p.
step p.
surgical p.
unfiltered p.
vertical versus horizontal p.
wire contour p.
preparatory iridectomy
prepared
p. cavity
p. cavity impression
p. large bowel
prepatellar
p. bursa
p. bursa inflammation
prepatellaris
prepericardiales
preperitoneal
p. anesthesia
p. approach
p. fat
p. space
preplacental hemorrhage
prepontine
p. cistern
p. white epidermoidoma
prepped and draped
preprostate urethral sphincter
preprosthetic surgery
prepubic fascia
prepuce
preputial
p. calculus
p. continent vesicostomy
p. gland
p. sac
preputiales
preputii
preputiotomy
prepyloric
p. perforation
p. sphincter
p. vein
prepylorica
prepyramidal tract
prerecruitment
prerectal lithotomy
prerenal
prerepair
preretinal
p. hemorrhage
p. membrane
p. neovascularization
pre-rolandic artery
presacral
p. anesthesia
p. anomaly
p. cystic lesion
p. fascia
p. insufflation
p. mass
p. nerve
p. neurectomy
p. rectopexy
p. resection
p. space
p. sympathectomy
presacralis
presaturation technique
presbyopia
presbyopic vision
prescreening
opioid p.
presence
arteriographic p.
presensitization phase
presentation
acute p.
chronic p.
clinical p.
p. of cord
mammographic p.
presenting
p. clinical manifestation
p. symptom
preseptal space
preservation
autonomic nerve p. (ANP)
breast p.
cadaver renal p.
carotid p.

extracorporeal renal p.
extremity p.
lordosis p.
lumbar lordosis p.
pelvic autonomic nerve p. (PANP)
renal p.
simple cold storage p.
sphincter p.
spleen p.
p. technique
p. time
tissue p.
visual p.

preservative solution
presigmoid-transtransversarium intradural approach
presphenoid bone
prespinal
presplenic fold
pressoreceptor
pressor medication
pressure

abdominal p.
acoustic p.
airway p.
p. alopecia
alveolar carbon dioxide p.
alveolar oxygen partial p. (PAO_2)
alveolar partial p.
p. amaurosis
p. amplitude modulation
anal resting p.
anal sphincter squeeze p.
p. anesthesia
aortic blood p.
aortic dicrotic notch p.
aortic pullback p.
applanation p.
p. area
arterial blood p.
arterial carbon dioxide p.
arterial dicrotic notch p.
arterial oxygen partial p. (PaO_2)
arterial partial p.
ascending aortic p.
atmospheres of p.
atrial filling p.
p. atrophy
average mean p.
barometric p.
basal anal canal p.
basal anal sphincter p.
bile duct p.
bilevel positive airway p.
biliary tract p.
BiPAP nasal continuous positive airway p.
biting p.
bladder p.
bleeding controlled with direct p.
p. blister
blood p.
bone marrow p.
capillary wedge p.
carbon dioxide p.
cardiovascular p.
carotid artery stump p.
central posterior-anterior p.
central venous p. (CVP)
cerebral perfusion p.
cerebrospinal fluid p. (CSFP)
choledochal basal p.
closing p.
closure p.
coaxial p.
colloidal osmotic p.
colloid osmotic p. (COP)
compartmental p.
compliance, rate, oxygenation, and p. (CROP)
p. condensation
continuous distending airway p.
continuous negative airway p.
continuous positive airway p. (CPAP)
p. control inverse ratio ventilation (PCIRV)
p. control ventilation (PCV)
p. conversion
coronary perfusion p.
coronary venous p.
cricoid p.
critical closing p.
CSF p.
detrusor p.
diastolic blood p. (DBP)
diastolic filling p.
differential blood p.
digital p.
direct p.
disk p.
Donders p.
downstream venous p.
dynamic closure p.

NOTES

pressure *(continued)*
elastic recoil p.
end-diastolic left ventricular p.
end-expiratory intragastric p.
end-systolic left ventricular p.
p. epiphysis
esophageal peristaltic p.
esophageal sphincter p.
expiratory positive airway p.
external direct p.
free hepatic venous p.
p. gangrene
gastric p.
glomerular capillary p.
p. gradient
p. half-time technique
high blood p.
high-frequency positive p.
high intraluminal p.
hydrostatic p.
hyperbaric p.
increased p.
p. increment rate
inferior vena cava p. (IVCP)
inspiratory occlusion p.
inspiratory positive airway p.
insufflation p.
intermittent positive p. (IPP)
interstitial p.
intraabdominal p. (IAP)
intraanal p.
intracardiac p.
intracholedochal p.
intracranial p. (ICP)
intradiscal p.
intraductal p.
intraesophageal peristaltic p.
intraesophageal variceal p.
intragastric p.
intraglomerular p.
intraluminal esophageal p.
intraluminal urethral p.
intramyocardial p.
intraneural p.
intraocular p.
intraoral p.
intrapericardial p.
intraperitoneal p.
intrapleural p.
intrapulpal p.
intrathoracic p.
intraurethral p.
intravariceal p.
intravascular p.
intravesical p.
intrinsic end-expiratory p.
intrinsic positive end-expiratory p. (PEEPi)
p. inversion point
IVC p.
jugular venous p.
juxtacardiac pleural p.
labile blood p.
leak point p.
left atrial p. (LAP)
left ventricular end-diastolic p.
left ventricular systolic p.
LES p.
lower body negative p.
lower esophageal sphincter p.
manual p.
maternal abdominal p.
maximum urethral closure p.
mean arterial p. (MAP)
mean arterial blood p. (MABP)
mean diastolic left ventricular p.
mean pulmonary artery wedge p.
mean systolic left ventricular p.
p. measurement
mercury p.
Michaelson counter p.
millimeters partial p.
minimum audible p.
nadir p.
narrowed pulse p.
p. natriuresis
p. necrosis
negative abdominal p.
negative end-expiratory p.
nitrogen partial p.
noninvasive blood p. (NIBP)
normal intravascular p.
occlusal p.
occlusion p.
oncotic p.
opening p.
osmotic p.
p. overload
oxygen under high p.
PA filling p.
p. pain threshold (PPT)
pancreatic duct p.
p. paralysis
partial p.
passage p.
peak inspiratory ventilator p.
peak systolic aortic p.
peak systolic gradient p.
perfusion p.
periapical p.
pericardial p.
peripheral p.
plantar p.
plasma colloid osmotic p.
plasma oncotic p.
p. pneumothorax

portal venous p.
positive airway p. (PAP)
positive end-airway p.
positive end-expiratory p. (PEEP)
positive end-expiratory pressure/continuous positive airway p. (PEEP/CPAP)
positive expiratory p.
positive inspiratory p.
posterior-anterior p.
postmembrane p.
premembrane p.
premicturition p.
proximal p.
pullback p.
pulmonary artery p. (PAP)
pulmonary artery occlusion p. (PAOP)
pulmonary artery occlusive wedge p.
pulmonary capillary wedge p.
pulmonary hypertension p.
pulmonary vascular p.
pulp p.
pulse p.
p. rate quotient
p. receptor
p. recovery
rectal resting p.
p. regulated electrohydraulic lithotripsy
resting anal sphincter p.
p. reversal
right atrial p.
right ventricular end-diastolic p.
right ventricular systolic p.
p. ring
p. rise
screen filtration p.
selection p.
shock wave p.
sinusoidal capillary p.
p. sore
sphincter of Oddi p.
spinal cord perfusion p. (SCPP)
splanchnic capillary p.
squeeze p.
static closure p.
p. study
stump p.
subglottic p.
p. support ventilation (PSV)
systolic arterial p. (SAP)
systolic blood p. (SBP)
systolic left ventricular p.
p. technique filling
tentorial p.
time p.
tissue p.
p. tolerance
tongue p.
torr p.
tourniquet p.
transglomerular hydrostatic filtration p.
transmembrane hydraulic p.
p. transmission
p. transmission ratio
transmural p.
transmyocardial perfusion p.
ureteral p.
urethral p.
p. value
vapor p.
variable positive airway p.
variceal p.
vascular p.
venous p.
venous dialysis p. (VPd)
ventilation peak p.
ventricular diastolic p.
ventricular filling p.
p. wave
p. waveform
wedge p.
wedged hepatic vein p. (WHVP)
wedged hepatic venous p.
p. welding
white without p.
zero end-expiratory p. (ZEEP)
zero end-inspiratory p.
z-point p.

pressure-controlled inverse ratio ventilation

pressure-flow

p.-f. electromyography study
p.-f. plot
p.-f. relation
p.-f. relationship

pressure-natriuresis curve

pressure-point tension ring

pressure-regulated volume control ventilation

NOTES

P

pressure-sensitive
p.-s. area
p.-s. tissue
pressure-tolerant tissue
pressure-volume
p.-v. analysis
p.-v. curve
p.-v. index
p.-v. relation
pressurized reservoir
prestandardization
prestenotic dilatation
presternal
p. notch
p. region
p. space
presternalis
presternally
presternum
presulcal
presumptive diagnosis
presurgical
p. medical evaluation
p. psychological screening (PPS)
p. state
presynaptic membrane
presystolic pressure and volume
pretarsal space
pretecta
pretemporal space
prethyroid
pretracheal
p. fascia
p. layer
p. node
p. space
pretracheales
pretrachealis
pretransplant evaluation
pretreatment
p. evaluation
p. level
pretympanic
prevention
DVT p.
extension for p.
heterotopic ossification p.
infection p.
injury p.
rod rotation p.
preventive
p. intravesical therapy
p. mastectomy
p. measure
prevertebral
p. fascia
p. ganglion
p. layer
p. soft tissue
p. space
p. space abscess
prevertebrales
prevertebralis
prevesical
prevesiculares
prewarming
Preziosi operation
prezonular space
priapus
prick
needle p.
p. puncture test
prickle cell carcinoma
prick-test
p.-t. concentration
p.-t. method
Pridie incision
Pridie-Koutsogiannis procedure
primam
primarily vascularized organ transplant
primarium
primary
p. adenocarcinoma
p. adhesion
p. amputation
p. anesthetic
p. antecubital jump bypass (PAJB)
p. arteriovenous fistula
p. bile duct carcinoma
p. biliary cirrhosis
p. cancer
p. cesarean section
p. closure
colorectal p.
p. diagnostic endoscopy
p. endpoint
p. end-to-end anastomosis
p. fibrinolysis
p. fungal infection
p. gangrene
p. gastric lymphoma (PGL)
p. gastric lymphoma staging
p. gastric non-Hodgkin lymphoma (PGL)
p. graft nonfunction
p. healing
p. hemorrhage
p. hepatic
p. herpes simplex infection
p. hyperparathyroidism
p. indirect inguinal hernia
p. inguinal herniorrhaphy
p. intraosseous carcinoma
p. lesion
p. malignancy
p. movement plane

p. myofascial trigger point
noncolorectal p.
p. origin
p. panendoscopy
p. parathyroid hyperplastic tumor
p. pathogen
p. perineal hypospadias surgery
p. position
p. procedure
p. proctocolectomy
p. prophylaxis
p. pulmonary hypertension (PPH)
p. radiation
p. rejection
p. renal calculus
p. repair
p. resection
p. rhabdomyosarcoma
p. rotation movement
p. sclerosing cholangitis
p. shock
p. sodium phosphate
p. stenting
p. surgeon
p. suture technique
p. tumor site
p. union
p. untreated HPT
p. yolk sac

primer
Bowen cavity p.
cavity p.

priming dose

primitive
p. dislocation
p. knot
p. yolk sac

primordial cyst

primum

primus

princeps, pl. **principes**
p. cervicis artery
p. pollicis artery

Princeteau tubercle

principal
p. fiber bundle
p. line
p. plane
p. point
p. visual direction

principes (*pl. of* princeps)

principle
anatomic fracture reduction p.
axial compression p.
clinical p.
closure p.
Fick p.
Goodwin cup-patch p.
image formation p.
Le Chatelier p.
line focus p.
Mitrofanoff p.
Pauli exclusion p.

Pringle
P. maneuver
P. vascular control
P. vascular control method
P. vascular control procedure
P. vascular control technique

prior drug exposure

priority
ICU care p.

prism
p. adaptation test
p. method

PRK
photorefractive keratectomy

proactive hemostasis

proatlas

probability
bone cyst fracture p.
postoperative survival p. (PSP)

proband

probing lacrimonasal duct operation

probiotic bacteria

problem
biliary p.
clinical p.
colon p.
comorbid medical p.
Coping with Health, Injuries, and P.'s (CHIP)
cosmetic p.
dermatologic p.
functional p.
gastrointestinal p.
inflammatory p.
innervation p.
medical p.
orthopedic p.
physical p.
psychological p.
rectal p.

NOTES

problem *(continued)*
surgical p.
wound p.
procallus formation
procedure
Abbe-McIndoe p.
Abbe-McIndoe-Williams p.
Abbe-Wharton-McIndoe p.
abdominal p.
ablative p.
Adams p.
advancement p.
aesthetic p.
Akin p.
Akiyama p.
Albee-Delbert p.
Aldridge sling p.
Al-Ghorab p.
Alliston p.
anchovy p.
Anderson p.
Anderson-Fowler p.
anecdotal p.
antegrade continence enema p.
antenna p.
anterior Pólya p.
anterior stabilization p.
antiincontinence p.
antireflux p.
AO p.
arterial reconstructive p.
arterial switch p.
articulatory p.
Axer-Clark p.
Badgley combination p.
Baldy-Webster p.
balloon fenestration p.
Bandi p.
Bankart p.
Barsky p.
Bartlett p.
Bassini p.
Batista p.
Baxter-D'Astous p.
Bell-Tawse p.
Belsey fundoplication p.
Bentall p.
Berman-Gartland p.
Bernard lip reconstruction p.
B.H. Moore p.
Bickel-Moe p.
bilateral inguinal hernia repair p.
Bilhaut-Cloquet p.
Billroth I, II p.
Bing-Taussig heart p.
Björk method of Fontan p.
bladder chimney p.
Blair-Brown p.
Blalock-Hanlon p.
Blalock-Taussig p.
Blatt p.
Blatt-Ashworth p.
blocking p.
Boari bladder flap p.
bone block p.
bony p.
Bose p.
bowel refashioning p.
Boyce-Vest p.
Boyd-Bosworth p.
Boyd-McLeod p.
Boytchev p.
Brahms p.
Brantigan p.
Brantigan-Voshell p.
Braun p.
breast-conserving p.
Bricker p.
Bridle p.
Bristow-Helfet p.
Bristow-May p.
Brock p.
Broström p.
Broström-Gould foot p.
Bryan p.
Bunnell-Williams p.
Burch bladder suspension p.
burn-out p.
bypass p.
Calandriello p.
Caldwell-Luc window p.
Camey p.
Campbell-Akbarnia p.
Campbell-Goldthwait p.
canalith repositioning p.
capsular shift p.
Carolinas Laparoscopic Advanced Surgery Program p.
carotid ablative p.
Castaneda p.
Castle p.
cataract p.
catheter-directed interventional p.
Cawthorne-Day p.
cecal imbrication p.
Cecil p.
Celestin p.
cervical spine stabilization p.
Chamberlain p.
Chambers p.
Charles p.
Chassar Moir-Sims p.
Chassar Moir sling p.
checkrein p.
Cherry-Crandall p.
cherry-picking p.

Chester-Winter p.
Chrisman-Snook p.
Cibis liquid silicone p.
ciliary p.
circulatory arrest p.
CLASP p.
Clayton p.
Cleveland p.
Cloward p.
Cockett p.
Cohen antireflux p.
Cole intubation p.
Collis gastroplasty p.
Collis-Nissen esophageal lengthening p.
Collis-Nissen fundoplication p.
colon p.
coloplasty p.
commando p.
compartment p.
composite pelvic resection p.
concentration p.
Connolly p.
conventional p.
core drilling p.
coronary artery revascularization p.
coronary bypass p.
corporeal rotation p.
corridor p.
Cox Maze III p.
Cracchiolo p.
curative p.
curative-intent p.
Custodis nondraining p.
cyclodestructive p.
cyclops p.
Damian graft p.
Damus-Kaye-Stansel p.
Damus-Stansel-Kaye p.
Danus-Fontan p.
Darrach p.
dartos pouch p.
Das Gupta p.
Datta p.
Davis-Kitlowski p.
Davydov p.
DAWG p.
de-airing p.
debubbling p.
debulking p.
degloving p.
dental prosthetic laboratory p.
Devine-Devine p.
Dewar posterior cervical fixation p.
diagnostic p.
Dickson-Diveley p.
DKS p.
domino p.
Donald p.
Donders p.
Dor fundoplication p.
Dorrance p.
dorsal root entry zone p.
dot-blot p.
double-stapled ileoanal reservoir p.
Douglas p.
Downey-McGlamery p.
DREZ p.
Duckett p.
Duhamel p.
Dukes p.
Duval p.
Dwyer p.
Ebbehoj p.
Eden-Hybbinette p.
Eden-Lange p.
Edwards p.
Effler-Groves mode of Allison p.
elective surgical p.
elimination p.
Elmslie p.
Elmslie-Trillat patellar p.
emergency p.
endolacrimal p.
endorectal ileoanal pull-through p.
endoscopic mucosal resection p.
endoscopy p.
end-to-end reconstruction p.
enucleation p.
esophageal sling p.
Estes p.
evacuation p.
Evans p.
Evans-Steptoe p.
Everard Williams p.
excisional biopsy p.
ex situ in vivo p.
extended Ross p.
extraanatomic bypass p.
extraarticular p.
extracorporeal p.
Faden p.
failed p.
Fairbanks-Sever p.

NOTES

procedure *(continued)*
Fasanella-Servat p.
fascial sling p.
fiberoptic intubation p.
Ficat p.
filtering p.
Fired-Hendel p.
five-incision p.
flip-flap p.
floppy Nissen fundoplication p.
Fontan-Baudet p.
Fontan-Kreutzer p.
Fontan modification of Norwood p.
forage p.
four-incision p.
four-port p.
Fowler-Stephens p.
Fox-Blazina p.
Frank p.
Fredet-Ramstedt p.
Fried-Green foot p.
Froimson p.
Frost p.
Fulford p.
Gallie p.
Gartland p.
gaseous laparoscopy p.
gasless laparoscopy p.
gastric bypass p. (GBP)
gastric emptying p. (GEP)
gastric pull-through p.
gastric pull-up p.
gastric valve tightening p.
Gelman p.
general laparoscopic surgical p.
Gilchrist p.
Gill p.
Gill-Jonas modification of Norwood p.
Gillquist p.
Gil-Vernet p.
Girard p.
Girdlestone hip p.
Girdlestone-Taylor p.
Gittes p.
Gittes-Loughlin p.
Glenn p.
Goebel p.
Goebel-Stoeckel-Frangenheim p.
Goldner-Hayes p.
Goldthwait-Hauser p.
Gould p.
Goulding p.
gracilis p.
Green p.
Gregoir-Lich p.
Gurd p.
Halban p.
hallux valgus p.
Hambly p.
Hammon p.
hamular p.
Hancock p.
Hanley rectal bladder p.
Harada-Ito p.
Harewood suspension p.
Hark p.
Harmon p.
Hartmann p.
Hass p.
Hauser patellar tendon p.
Hawkins p.
Hedley p.
Heifetz p.
hemi-Fontan p.
hemi-Koch p.
heparinization p.
Hepp-Couinaud biliary tract p.
hex p.
Heyman-Herndon clubfoot p.
Hibbs p.
Hill p.
Hinman p.
Hodor-Dobbs p.
Hoffmann-Clayton p.
Hofmeister p.
Hohmann p.
Hoke p.
Hoke-Miller p.
Hood p.
Hovanian p.
Howorth p.
Howorth-Keillor p.
Hughston p.
Hughston-Hauser p.
Hui-Linscheid p.
Hummelsheim p.
hypoglossal facial transfer p.
ileoanal pouch p.
ileoanal pull-through p.
iliac buttressing p.
infrarenal template p.
Ingelman-Sundberg gracilis muscle p.
initial screening p.
inner ear tack p.
Insall p.
installation p.
intercalary allograft p.
interventional p.
intestinal bypass p.
intraarticular p.
intraoperative p.
intraparavariceal p.
intraperitoneal p.
invasive p.

island-flap p.
isolated p.
Ito p.
Jacobaeus p.
Jaeger-Hamby p.
Jaffe p.
Jahss p.
Jannetta microvascular decompression p.
Jansey p.
Jatene arterial switch p.
jejunoileal bypass reversal p.
Jensen transposition p.
Jobe-Glousman capsular shift p.
Johnson p.
Johnson-Spiegl p.
Johnston buttonhole p.
Jonas modification of Norwood p.
Jones tube p.
J. R. Moore p.
Junod p.
Juvara p.
Kaliscinski ureteral p.
Karakousis-Vezeridis p.
Karhunen-Loeve p.
Karlsson p.
Kasai p.
Kawaii-Yamamoto p.
Kelikian p.
Kelikian-McFarland p.
Keller p.
Kelling-Madlener p.
Kelly plication p.
Kendrick p.
Kennedy p.
Kessel-Bonney p.
Kestenbaum p.
keyhole coronary bypass p.
Kidner foot p.
Kiehn-Earle-DesPrez p.
Killian frontoethmoidectomy p.
Knapp p.
Knobby-Clark p.
Ko-Airan bleeding control p.
Kocher ureterosigmoidostomy p.
Koch pouch modified p.
Kolmogorov-Smirnov p.
Kondoleon-Sistrunk elephantiasis p.
Konno p.
Koutsogiannis p.
Kraske p.
Krönlein p.
Kropp p.
Krukenberg p.
Kuhnt-Szymanowski p.
Ladd p.
Lane p.
Langenskiöld p.
Langevin updating p.
laparoscopically assisted endorectal pull-through p.
laparoscopic-assisted p.
laparoscopic bladder neck suture suspension p.
laparoscopic Burch p.
laparoscopic bypass p.
laparoscopic lymph node dissection p.
laparoscopic Nissen fundoplication p.
laparoscopic paraaortic lymph node sampling p.
laparoscopic surgical p.
laparoscopic tubal banding p.
Larmon forefoot p.
laser coagulation vaporization p. (LCVP)
Lash p.
LAST coronary bypass p.
Latarget p.
lathing p.
latissimus dorsi p.
Lauenstein p.
Leadbetter p.
Leadbetter-Politano p.
Lee p.
Le Fort p.
left atrial isolation p.
Lepird p.
L'Episcopo-Zachary p.
Lewis-Tanner p.
Lich p.
limb-lengthening p.
limb-salvage p.
limb-saving p.
limb-sparing p.
Lindeman p.
Linton p.
Lipscomb p.
Lipscomb-Anderson p.
Localio p.
loop electrocautery excision p. (LEEP)

NOTES

procedure *(continued)*
loop electrosurgical excision p. (LEEP)
loop gastric bypass p.
Lorenz p.
Lothrop frontoethmoidectomy p.
lower cervical spine p.
lower lid sling p.
Luke p.
LVR p.
Lynch frontoethmoidectomy p.
Lyon-Horgan p.
MacAusland p.
MacCarthy p.
Magnuson-Stack p.
Mahan p.
Mallory-Weiss p.
Malone ACE p.
Malone antegrade continence enema p.
Manktelow transfer p.
Mann p.
Mann-Coughlin p.
Maquet p.
Marshall-Marchetti p.
Marshall-Marchetti-Krantz p.
Martius p.
Mathieu p.
Matsen p.
Mauck p.
Maydl p.
Mayo-Fueth inversion p.
Maze III p.
McBride p.
McCall-Schumann p.
McCarroll-Baker p.
McCormick-Blount p.
McDonald p.
McElvenny-Caldwell p.
McGlamry-Downey p.
McIndoe p.
McIndoe-Hayes p.
McLaughlin p.
McVay p.
medial rotation p.
Meigs-Okabayashi p.
Michal I, II p.
microoperative p.
microsurgery p.
microsurgical epididymal sperm aspiration p.
Miller p.
minimal-access p.
minimally invasive p.
Minkoff-Nicholas p.
Mitrofanoff p.
MMK p.
Moberg key-pinch p.
modified Belsey fundoplication p.
modified Hoke-Miller flatfoot p.
modified Konno p.
modified Norfolk p.
modified Seldinger p.
modified Sugiura p.
modified Toupe p.
modified Weber-Fergusson p.
modified Wies p.
Mogensen p.
Moschcowitz p.
motion-preserving p.
multiple-port incision p.
Mumford p.
muscle-balancing p.
Mustardé otoplasty p.
Mustard intraatrial p.
needle suspension p.
needle thoracentesis p.
Neer capsular shift p.
Nesbit tuck p.
Neugebauer-LeFort p.
neurostimulating p.
neurosurgical p.
Newman p.
Nichols p.
Nicks p.
Nicola shoulder p.
Nicoll fracture repair p.
Nissen fundoplication p.
Nissen-Rosseti fundoplication p.
noncircumferential antireflux p.
nonfenestrated Fontan p.
noninvasive p.
non-rib-spreading thoracotomy incision p.
Norwood univentricular heart p.
notchplasty p.
O'Brien capsular shift p.
O'Donoghue p.
Olshausen p.
omentum majus flap p.
one-stage p.
open reconstructive p.
operant p.
operative p.
orthodontic p.
orthodox p.
orthopedic surgical p.
Orticochea p.
Osborne-Cotterill p.
osteoplastic frontal sinus p.
otic periotic shunt p.
Oudard p.
Overholt p.
palatal lengthening p.
palliative cerebrospinal shunt p.
palliative surgical p.

Palomo p.
Parrish p.
Paterson p.
Pauchet p.
pediatric laparoscopic surgical p.
pelvic pouch p.
percutaneous transhepatic biliary p.
Pereyra p.
Pereyra-Lebhertz modification of Frangenheim-Stoeckel p.
peri-vaterian therapeutic endoscopic p.
Perthes p.
Pichlmayer p.
PLIF p.
Pólya p.
portmanteau p.
posterior lumbar interbody fusion p.
posterior Pólya p.
potentially curative p.
Potts p.
Pozzi p.
Pridie-Koutsogiannis p.
primary p.
Pringle vascular control p.
psoas hitch p.
Puestow-Gillesby p.
pull-through p.
push-back p.
Putti-Platt shoulder p.
Quaegebeur p.
Quickert p.
Ramstedt p.
Ransley p.
Rastan-Konno p.
Rastelli p.
Raz p.
Raz-Leach p.
realignment p.
Récamier p.
reconstruction p.
reconstructive surgical p.
reefing p.
Rehbein p.
Reichel-Pólya p.
Reichenheim-King p.
repeat p.
restorative p.
resurfacing p.
retrogasserian p.
revascularization p.
reverse filling p.
reverse Mauck p.
reverse Putti-Platt p.
revision p.
Richardson p.
Richter and Albrich p.
Ridlon p.
Riedel frontoethmoidectomy p.
Righini p.
Ripstein p.
Rockwood p.
Rockwood-Matsen capsular shift p.
Rose p.
Ross p.
Roux-en-Y p.
Roux-Goldthwait p.
Ruiz p.
Ruiz-Mora p.
Ryerson p.
sacroiliac buttressing p.
Sade modification of Norwood p.
Salle p.
salting-out p.
salvage p.
Samilson p.
sartorial slide p.
Sato p.
Sauve-Kapandji p.
Savin p.
Sayoc p.
Schauffler p.
Schenk-Eichelter vena cava plastic filter p.
Schoemaker p.
Schonander p.
Schrock p.
scleral buckling p.
screening p.
Scudder p.
Scuderi p.
secondary p.
segment-oriented p.
Selakovich p.
Seldinger p.
semitendinosus p.
Senning transposition p.
septation p.
Shauta-Aumreich p.
Shea p.
Shirodkar p.
short lever specific contact p.
Silfverskiöld p.

NOTES

P

procedure *(continued)*
Silver p.
Simplate p.
single-stage p.
Sistrunk p.
in situ p.
sling p.
Smith-Robinson p.
Snow p.
Somerville p.
Sondergaard p.
Southwick slide p.
spatial localization p.
Spence p.
sphincter-saving p.
sphincter-sparing p.
spinal-locking p.
Spira p.
Spittler p.
SPLATT p.
split anterior tibial tendon p.
Stack shoulder p.
Staheli shelf p.
Stamey-Martius p.
Stamey modification of Pereyra p.
Stamm p.
standard gastric resection Whipple p.
standard stripping p.
standard surgical p.
Stanley Way p.
Stansel p.
stapled reconstruction p.
Steindler p.
stereotactic needle core biopsy p.
Steytler-Van Der Walt p.
Stone p.
Stoppa p.
Strayer p.
strip p.
Studer pouch p.
suburethral rectus fascial sling p.
Sugiura p.
supramesocolic surgical p.
surgical enucleation p.
Swenson pull-through p.
switch p.
Syme p.
Tachdjian p.
takedown p.
tarsal strip p.
Taylor p.
terminal Syme p.
Thal fundoplication p.
Thiersch p.
Thiersch-Duplay proximal tube p.
ThinPrep p.
Thomas p.
Thompson p.
three-stage p.
Tikhoff-Linberg p.
p. time
TIPS p.
total fundoplication p.
Toti p.
touch-up p.
Toupe p.
TRAM flap p.
transendoscopic p.
transhepatic antegrade biliary drainage p.
transvaginal Burch p.
transverse rectus abdominis muscle flap p.
Trillat p.
triple-wire p.
Tsai-Stillwell p.
tuck p.
tumbling p.
two-stage p.
two-step p.
uncinate p.
uncut Collis-Nissen fundoplication p.
unilateral inguinal hernia repair p.
untethering p.
up-and-down staircases p.
upper cervical spine p.
ureteral patch p.
urethral vesicle suspension p.
urologic laparoscopic surgical p.
urologic surgical p.
vaginal needle suspension p.
vaginal wall sling p.
valvulotomy p.
Van de Kramer fecal fat p.
Van Ness p.
vascular p.
VATS p.
ventriculoperitoneal shunting p.
video-assisted thoracic surgical p.
Vineberg p.
Vulpius p.
Vulpius-Stoffel p.
V-Y p.
W p.
Waldhausen p.
Wardill-Kilner p.
Waterhouse transpubic p.
Waterston-Cooley p.
Watson-Cheyne-Burghard p.
Watson-Jones p.
Weaver-Dunn p.
Weber p.
Weber-Fergusson p.
Wheeler p.

Whipple p.
White slide p.
Whitman talectomy p.
Whitman-Thompson p.
Wies p.
Williams p.
Wilson p.
Winograd p.
Winter p.
Womack p.
Woodward p.
yoke transposition p.
York-Mason p.
Young p.
Young-Dees p.
Yount p.
Z p.
Zancolli-Lasso p.
Zancolli static lock p.
Zarins-Rowe p.
Zoellner-Clancy p.
Z-plasty p.

procelia
procephalic
procerus muscle
process
accessory p.
acromial p.
alveolar p.
anterior clinoid p.
articular p.
basilar p.
benign p.
calcaneal p.
caudate p.
ciliary p.
Civinini p.
clinoid p.
cochleariform p.
condylar p.
condyloid p.
conoid p.
coracoid p.
corniculate p.
coronoid p.
costal p.
ensiform p.
epileptogenic p.
exocrinopathic p.
falciform p.
frontosphenoidal p.
funicular p.
healing p.
inferior articular p.
intrajugular p.
jugular p.
lateral p.
lenticular p.
malignant p.
mallear p.
mamillary p.
medial p.
mental p.
olecranon p.
papillary p.
paroccipital p.
posterior clinoid p.
pterygoid p.
pterygospinous p.
resuscitation p.
space-occupying p.
sphenoid p.
spinous p.
Stieda p.
supracondylar p.
supraepicondylar p.
temporal p.
thrombotic p.
transverse p.
trochlear p.
vaginal p.
vermiform p.
vocal p.
xiphoid p.

processus
procheilon
prochordal
Prochownik method
procidentia
procoagulant
procreate
procreation
assisted medical p.

procreative
proctagra
proctalgia
proctectasia
proctectomy
abdominoperineal p.
intersphincteric p.
Kraske transsacral p.
laparoscopic p.
mucosal p.
partial p.

NOTES

proctectomy *(continued)*
perineal p.
permanent p.
radical p.
restorative p.
sphincter-preserving p.
stapled ileal pouch-anal anastomosis without proctomucosal p.
subtotal p.
total p.
proctencleisis
procteurynter
proctitis
radiation p.
radiation-induced p.
proctocele
proctoclysis
proctococcypexy
proctocolectomy
abdominal p.
laparoscopic total p.
primary p.
restorative p.
secondary stage p.
single-stage total p.
subtotal p.
total p.
totally stapled restorative p.
total p. with ileoanal anastomosis and J pouch
proctocolitis
radiation p.
proctocolonoscopy
proctocolpoplasty
proctocystocele
proctocystoplasty
proctocystotomy
proctodynia
proctoelytroplasty
proctography
evacuation p.
proctologic
proctologist
proctology
proctoperineoplasty
proctoperineorrhaphy
proctopexy
Orr-Loygue transabdominal p.
proctoplasty
proctoptosia
proctorrhagia
proctorrhaphy
proctorrhea
proctoscopic examination
proctoscopy
rigid p.
proctosigmoidectomy
proctosigmoidoscopy
rigid p.
proctospasm
proctostasis
proctostat
proctostenosis
proctostomy
proctotomy
posterior p.
proctotresia
proctovalvotomy
procumbent
procurement
in situ split-liver p.
procurvation
product
altered gene p.
blood p.
contact activation p.
degradation p.
fibrin degradation p.
fibrinogen degradation p.
fibrinogen-fibrin degradation p.
lipid peroxidation p.
oxygen reduction p.
pyrolysis p.
rate pressure p.
tumor-cell p.
vector p.
production
biofilm p.
collagen p.
ectopic parathormone p.
excessive heat p.
metabolic heat p.
paraneoplastic ectopic ACTH p.
productive inflammation
PROEF
postoperative regimen for oral early feeding
Proetz
P. displacement technique
P. maneuver
P. position
profile
aortic valve velocity p.
coagulation p.
extraoral radiographic examination p.
facial p.
pain perception p.
Premature Infant Pain P. (PIPP)
projection p.
resting urethral pressure p.
sickness impact p.
stress urethral pressure p.
thrombogenic p.

urethral closure pressure p.
vector p.

profound hypothermia

profoundly hypothermic circulatory arrest (PHCA)

profunda
- p. brachii artery
- p. cervicalis artery

profundae

profundi

profundum

profundus
- p. artery fracture

progenitalis

progestational
- p. protection
- p. therapy

prognosis, pl. **prognoses**

prognostic
- p. block
- p. determinant
- p. factor
- p. finding
- p. indicator
- p. information
- p. marker
- p. value

prognosticator

progonoma

prograde technique

program
- aquatic stabilization p.
- back-propagation neural network p.
- Cancer Surveillance P.
- CAPRI p.
- Carolinas Laparoscopic Advanced Surgery P. (CLASP)
- conditioning p.
- diagnostic p.
- four-star exercise p.
- independent exercise p.
- Linde Walker Oxygen P.
- Muma Assessment P.
- National Marrow Donor P.
- object p.
- Organ Procurement P.
- Rothman Institute total hip p.
- safety p.
- SEER P.
- Solid Tumor Autologous Marrow Transplant P. (STAMP)
- source p.
- standard bone algorithm p.
- Starkey matrix p.
- stripping p.
- Surgical Education and Self-Assessment P. (SESAP)
- surveillance p.
- survey p.
- walking p.
- Westcott Pyramid P.
- work hardening p.

programmed
- p. electrical stimulation
- p. therapy

progression
- tumor p.

progressive
- p. abdominal distention
- P. Ambulation Scale
- p. ascites
- p. bacterial synergistic gangrene
- p. compression
- p. dilation
- p. disease
- p. extraction
- p. liver failure
- p. parenchymal destruction
- p. respiratory failure
- p. spin saturation

proinflammatory mediator

project
- Breast Cancer Detection Demonstration P.
- National Surgical Adjuvant Breast and Bowel P. (NSABP)

projection
- afferent p.
- anterior oblique p.
- anteroposterior p.
- A&P p.
- apical lordotic p.
- ascending pathway of pain p.
- axial calcaneal p.
- axial sesamoid p.
- back p.
- base p.
- bony p.
- bregma-mentum p.
- bursal p.
- Caldwell p.
- convergence p.
- coronal oblique p.
- cross-sectional p.

NOTES

P

projection *(continued)*
cross-table lateral p.
Didiee p.
divergent ray p.
dorsoplantar p.
enamel p.
erroneous p.
extradental p.
false p.
fan beam p.
p. fiber
p. fiber damage
filtered-back p.
Fischer p.
frogleg lateral p.
frontal p.
Granger p.
half-axial p.
Harris-Beath p.
Hermodsson tangential p.
horizontal p.
Isherwood p.
lateral jaw p.
left anterior oblique p.
left lateral p.
light p.
maximum-intensity p.
mental p.
Mercator p.
oblique p.
occipitomental p.
occlusal p.
orthogonal p.
PA p.
panoramic surface p.
papillary p.
parasympathetic p.
perimeter p.
posterior-superior oblique p.
posteroanterior p.
p. profile
reverse topographic p.
Rhese p.
Rungstrom p.
sagittal p.
Schüller p.
spider p.
Stenvers p.
stress dorsiflexion p.
submental vertex p.
submentovertical p.
surface p.
sympathetic p.
tangential p.
topographic p.
Towne p.
p. tract imaging
transmandibular p.
transorbital p.
transverse p.
visual p.
Waters p.

projection-reconstruction
p.-r. imaging
p.-r. technique

projective technique

prolabial

prolabium

prolactin inducible protein (PIP)

prolapse
Altemeier repair of rectal p.
anorectal mucosal p.
stomal p.

prolapsed
p. hemorrhoid
p. mitral valve syndrome
p. stoma

prolapsus

proliferating cell nuclear antigen (PCNA)

proliferation
p. area
ductal p.
fibroblast p.
follicular p.
p. zone

proliferative
p. factor
p. inflammation
p. lesion

prolongation
expiratory p.
P2 p.
pulse repetition time p.

prolonged
p. expiratory phase
p. postoperative ventilation
p. prothrombin time
p. rupture

prominence
hypothenar p.
laryngeal p.
mallear p.
osteochondral p.
pedicle screw hardware p.
styloid p.
thenar p.

prominens

prominentia, pl. **prominentiae**

prominent indentation

promontorii

promontory
pelvic p.
sacral p.
p. stimulation test

promoter
tumor p.
pronate
pronation
p. control
p. injury
pronation-abduction
p.-a. fracture
p.-a. injury
pronation-eversion
p.-e. fracture
p.-e. injury
pronation-eversion-external
p.-e.-e. rotation
p.-e.-e. rotation injury
pronation-supination
pronator
p. quadratus muscle
p. reflex
p. teres muscle
p. teres release
p. teres syndrome
p. teres tendon
prone
p. extension test
p. reduction
p. split-leg position
proneal island flap
pronephric duct
pronephros
pronglike excementosis
pronograde
pronuclear stage transfer (PROST)
prootic
propagate
propagating clustered contraction (PCC)
propagation
clot p.
propagative
propendens
proper
p. hepatic artery
p. palmar digital artery
p. plantar digital artery
properitoneal
p. fat
p. fat line
p. flank stripe
p. inguinal hernia
p. space
transabdominal p. (TAPP)
property
chemotactic p.
vasodilatory p.
prophylactic
p. angiographic intervention
p. antibiotic (PA)
p. antibiotic therapy
p. anticoagulation
p. antifungal treatment
p. bone graft
p. cholecystectomy
p. colectomy
p. fasciotomy
p. gastroenterostomy
p. gastrojejunostomy
p. intravenous antibiotic
p. irradiation
p. lymphadenectomy
p. mastectomy
p. medication
p. membrane
p. odontotomy
p. oophorectomy
p. operative stabilization
p. orchiectomy
p. resection
p. skeletal fixation
p. surgery
p. thyroidectomy
prophylaxis, pl. **prophylaxes**
antibiotic p.
antifungal p.
antithromboembolic p.
aspiration p.
CMV p.
cytomegalovirus p.
deep venous thrombosis p.
DVT p.
perioperative antibiotic p.
primary p.
stricture p.
propofol
p. infusion
p. rescue
proportional
p. assist ventilation
p. assist ventilator (PAV)
propria, pl. **propriae**
proprioceptive
p. head-turning reflex
p. neuromuscular facilitation

NOTES

proprioceptive *(continued)*
p. neuromuscular facilitation approach
proprium
proprius
proptosis
prosection
prosector tubercle
prosopalgia
prospective study
prospermia
PROST
pronuclear stage transfer
laparoscopic PROST
prostacyclin
prostaglandin
renal vasodilator p.
prostanoid
prostata
prostatae
prostatalgia
prostate
p. cancer
contact laser ablation of p. (CLAP)
female p.
p. gland
transurethral resection of p. (TURP)
transurethral resection of p. (TURP)
visual laser ablation of p.
prostatectomy
anatomical radical retropubic p.
cavernous nerve-sparing p.
laparoscopic radical p.
Madigan p.
nerve-sparing radical retropubic p.
perineal p.
radical perineal p.
radical retropubic p.
radical transcoccygeal p.
salvage p.
Stanford radical retropubic p.
suprapubic p.
total perineal p.
transurethral ablative p.
transurethral ultrasound-guided laser-induced p.
visual laser-assisted p.
Walsh radical retropubic p.
prostatic
p. adenocarcinoma
p. adenoma
p. calculus
p. carcinoma
p. duct
p. ductule
p. fluid
p. massage
p. sheath
p. sinus
p. urethra
p. urethroplasty
p. utricle
p. venous plexus
prostatica
prostatici
prostaticovesicalis
prostaticovesical plexus
prostaticus
prostatism
prostatitis
prostatocystitis
prostatocystotomy
prostatodynia
prostatolith
prostatolithotomy
prostatomegaly
prostatomy
prostatorrhea
prostatoseminal vesiculectomy
prostatotomy
prostatovesiculectomy
prostatovesiculitis
prosthesis, pl. **prostheses**
p. interface
prosthesis-cement interface
prosthetic
p. arterial graft
p. arthroplasty
p. hemiarthroplasty
p. incisional hernioplasty
p. mesh repair
p. patch
p. restoration
p. ring annuloplasty
p. valve endocarditis (PVE)
prosthetist
prosthokeratoplasty
protamine correction
protection
airway p.
automated boundary p.
barrier p.
Baxter venous/arterial management p.
cerebral p.
digital artery p.
endogenous p.
gastroduodenal mucosal p.
myocardial p.
progestational p.
radiation p.
spinal cord p.
p. test

venous/arterial management p. (VAMP)
protective antireflux operation
protein
p. content
p. C, S plasma level
p. degradation
heparin-binding p.
plasma atrial natriuretic p.
prolactin inducible p. (PIP)
p. shock therapy
p. truncation
p. truncation test
tumor necrosis factor-binding p. (TNF-bp)
proteinaceous aqueous exudation
proteinase
protein-C deficiency
proteinuria
steroid-resistant p.
proteolysis
burn-induced muscle p.
muscle p.
sepsis-induced muscle p.
proteolytic pathway
prothrombin
p. time
p. time coagulation panel
prothrombogenic agent
protocol
chemotherapy p.
evaluation p.
exsanguination p.
flashback p.
fractionation p.
perioperative standardized p.
reinjection p.
resuscitation p.
standardized p.
protoduodenum
proton
p. beam therapy
p. pump inhibition therapy
p. pump inhibitor (PPI)
protopianoma
protoplasmolysis
protozoal infection
protrude
protruded disk
protrusio
p. deformity
p. ring
protrusion
corneal p.
protrusive
p. excursion
p. jaw relation
p. line
p. occlusal position
protuberance
protuberant abdomen
protuberantia
proud graft
Proust space
provesicalis
provisional
p. fixation
p. restoration
p. stabilization
provocation test
provocative
p. chelation test
p. diskography
p. food thyroidectomy
Prowazek-Greeff body
proximad
proximal
p. aorta
p. bowel distention
p. bowel tenderness
p. bow position
p. cavity
p. centriole
p. clot
p. diverting stoma
p. end
p. endoleak
p. esophagus
p. femoral epiphysiolysis
p. femoral fracture
p. femoral resection
p. gastrectomy
p. gastric cancer
p. gastric resection
p. gastric vagotomy
p. humeral fracture
p. incision
p. interphalangeal joint approach
p. jejunum
p. limb
p. loop syndrome
p. myofascial dysfunction
p. nail matrix
p. phalanx

NOTES

proximal *(continued)*
p. portion
p. pressure
p. radioulnar articulation
p. space
p. subclavian injury
p. subtotal pancreatectomy
p. tendon rupture
p. tibial metaphysial fracture
p. tibiofibular joint dislocation
p. tumor
p. urethral sphincter
p. vascular control
p. vein
proximalis
proximal-row carpectomy
proximal-to-distal ring
proximate space
proximity
close p.
prune-belly
p.-b. abdomen
p.-b. syndrome
prune-juice
p.-j. expectoration
p.-j. peritoneal fluid
pruritic
p. erythematous patch
p. lesion
Prussak
P. pouch
P. space
PS
postcardiotomy shock
psammocarcinoma
psammoma body
psammomatous
psammosarcoma
psauoscopy
PSD
percutaneous stricture dilatation
PSE
portal-systemic encephalopathy
PSE index
pseudarthrosis repair
pseudesthesia
pseudinoma
pseudoagglutination
pseudoaneurysm
p. formation
mycotic p.
pseudoangiosarcoma
pseudoankylosis
pseudoarthritis
pseudoarthrosis repair
pseudoarticulation
pseudobiopsy technique
pseudo-blind loop syndrome
pseudoboutonnière deformity
pseudocalcification
pseudocancerous lesion
pseudocarcinoma
pseudocavitation
pseudocele
pseudocephalocele
pseudocholesteatoma
pseudochylous ascites
pseudoclaudication
pseudocoarctation of aorta
pseudocoloboma
pseudocoma
pseudocryptorchism
pseudocyst
p. drainage
pancreatic p.
pseudocystobiliary fistula
pseudocystogastrostomy
pancreatic p.
pseudodefecation
pseudodislocation
pseudoepiphysis
pseudoepithelioma
pseudoexfoliation syndrome
pseudofacilitation
pseudoganglion
Cloquet p.
pseudogestational sac
pseudoglioma
pseudohernia
pseudohydrocephaly
pseudoinfection
pseudolipoma
pseudolymphoma syndrome
pseudomasturbation
pseudomedial longitudinal fasciculus lesion
pseudomelanoma
pseudomembranous acute inflammation
pseudomeningocele
posttraumatic intradiploic p.
traumatic p.
pseudomigration
***Pseudomonas* infection**
pseudomucinous cystadenocarcinoma
pseudomyxoma
pseudoneurogenic bladder
pseudoneuroma
pseudoomphalocele
pseudoosteomalacia
pseudoosteomalacic pelvis
pseudopod formation
pseudoprolactinoma
pseudoretinoblastoma
pseudosacculation
pseudosarcoma
pseudoserous membrane

pseudostoma
pseudostratified epithelium
pseudosubluxation
pseudotabes
diabetic p.
pseudotrachoma
pseudotumor cerebrimeningeal biopsy
pseudoureterocele
pseudoxanthoma elasticum syndrome
psoas
p. fascia
p. hitch procedure
p. line
p. major muscle
p. margin
p. minor muscle
p. minor tendon
p. sheath block
psoralens, ultraviolet A (PUVA)
psoriatic arthritis
PSP
postoperative survival probability
PSS
Peritonitis Severity Score
PSV
pressure support ventilation
psychoactive
psychogenic
p. colic
p. symptom
psychologic
p. consequence
p. implication
psychological problem
psychomotor retardation
psychopharmacologic medication
psychorelaxation
psychosedation
dental p.
psychosis
psychosurgery
psychotropic medication
psychrophore
PTA
pancreatic transplantation alone
PTBD
percutaneous transhepatic biliary drainage
PTC
percutaneous transhepatic cholangiography
PTCA
percutaneous transluminal coronary angioplasty
multivessel PTCA
PTCSL
percutaneous transhepatic cholangioscopic lithotomy
PTE
pulmonary thromboendarterectomy
pterional
p. approach
p. craniotomy
pterygial tissue
pterygoid
p. artery
p. branch
p. canal
p. fissure
p. fossa
p. fovea
p. hamulus
p. lamina
p. nerve
p. notch
p. pit
p. plate
p. plexus
p. position
p. process
p. tubercle
p. tuberosity
pterygoidea
pterygoidei
pterygoideus
pterygomandibular
p. ligament
p. raphe
p. space
p. space abscess
pterygomandibularis
pterygomaxillare
pterygomaxillaris
pterygomaxillary
p. fissure
p. fossa
p. space
pterygopalatina
pterygopalatine
p. canal
p. fossa
p. fossa syndrome
p. ganglion

NOTES

pterygopalatine *(continued)*
p. groove
p. nerve
p. space
pterygopalatinum
pterygopharyngeal space
pterygopharyngeus
pterygospinale
pterygospinal ligament
pterygospinosus
pterygospinous
p. ligament
p. process
PTGDS
patellar tendon graft donor site
PTH
parathyroid hormone
PTH chemiluminescent assay
PTH level
PTLD
posttransplant lymphoproliferative disease
posttransplant lymphoproliferative disorder
ptosed
ptosis, pl. **ptoses**
ptotic organ
PTS
pediatric trauma scale
PTV
percutaneous transtracheal jet ventilation
PTX
pancreas transplant
ptyalocele
pubes (*pl. of* pubis)
pubic
p. angle
p. arch
p. arcuate ligament
p. artery
p. body
p. bone
p. branch
p. crest
p. diastasis
p. fixation
p. hair line
p. pad
p. ramus
p. region
p. spine
p. symphysis
p. tubercle
pubica
pubicum
pubiotomy
pubis, pl. **pubes**
mons p.
pubocapsular
pubocapsulare
pubococcygeal
p. line
p. muscle
pubococcygeus
pubofemoral
pubofemorale
puboprostatic
p. ligament
p. muscle
puboprostaticum
puboprostaticus
puborectalis loop
puborectal muscle
pubourethral triangle
pubovaginal
p. muscle
p. operation
pubovaginalis
pubovesicale
pubovesicalis
pubovesical muscle
Puchtler
P. alkaline Congo red method
P. Sirius red method
Puddu tendon technique
pudenda (*pl. of* pudendum)
pudendal
p. anesthesia
p. canal
p. cleft
p. hematocele
p. hernia
p. nerve
p. sac
p. slit
p. vein
pudendalis
pudendi
pudendum, pl. **pudenda**
pudic nerve
puerile respiration
puerperal
p. hematoma
p. infection
Puestow-Gillesby
P.-G. operation
P.-G. procedure
Puestow pancreaticojejunostomy
Pugh
P. classification
modified method of P.
Pugh-Child bleeding esophageal varices grading scale classification
Pulec and Freedman classification

pullback
- p. pressure
- p. pressure gradient

pulled-down colon

pull-enteroscopy

pulley
- muscular p.
- peroneal p.
- p. reconstruction
- p. suture technique

pull maneuver

pull-out wire suture technique

pull-through
- abdominal p.-t.
- Duhamel laparoscopic p.-t.
- endorectal ileal p.-t.
- endorectal ileoanal p.-t.
- ileoanal endorectal p.-t.
- p.-t. operation
- p.-t. procedure
- rapid p.-t. (RPT)
- sacroabdominoperineal p.-t.
- Soave endorectal p.-t.
- station p.-t. (SPT)
- p.-t. technique

pull-up
- gastric p.-u.
- total gastric p.-u.

pulmo, pl. **pulmones**

pulmoaortic canal

pulmona

pulmonale

pulmonales

pulmonalis

pulmonary
- p. acid aspiration syndrome
- p. angioma
- p. arborization
- p. arterial malformation
- p. arterial web
- p. arteriovenous fistula (PAF)
- p. arteriovenous malformation
- p. artery (PA)
- p. artery catheterization
- p. artery catheterization anesthetic technique
- p. artery hypertension (PAH)
- p. artery occlusion pressure (PAOP)
- p. artery occlusive wedge pressure
- p. artery pressure (PAP)
- p. artery wedge
- p. aspiration
- p. atresia
- p. autograft (PA)
- p. bacterial infection
- p. blastoma
- p. capillary wedge pressure
- p. cavitation
- p. cavity
- p. circulation
- p. collateral
- p. compliance
- p. complication
- p. contusion
- p. dysfunction
- p. effect
- p. embolectomy
- p. embolism (PE)
- p. embolization
- p. epithelial cell
- p. fibrosis
- p. function
- p. fungal infection
- p. glomangiosis
- p. homograft
- p. hypertension pressure
- p. hypoplasia
- p. hypostasis
- p. involvement
- p. ligament
- p. lobectomy
- p. lymphangioleiomyomatosis
- p. lymphangiomyomatosis
- p. manifestation
- p. mass
- p. metastasectomy
- p. metastasis
- p. orifice
- p. outflow tract
- p. overcirculation
- p. parenchymal infection
- p. pleura
- p. plexus
- p. position
- p. resection
- p. sinus
- p. stenosis repair
- p. sulcus
- p. sulcus syndrome
- p. support
- p. suppuration
- p. sympathetic blockade
- p. thromboendarterectomy (PTE)

NOTES

P

pulmonary *(continued)*
p. tissue
p. toilet
p. transplantation
p. trunk
p. tuberous sclerosis
p. tumor
p. valve anomaly
p. valve area
p. valve disease
p. valve gradient
p. valve insufficiency
p. valve replacement
p. valve restenosis
p. valve stenosis
p. valvuloplasty
p. vascular abnormality
p. vascular pressure
p. vascular resistance (PVR)
p. vascular resistance index (PVRI)
p. vein
p. venous connection anomaly
p. venous return
p. venous return anomaly
p. ventilation
p. ventilation scan
pulmonary-gas exchange
pulmones (*pl. of* pulmo)
pulmonic valve stenosis
pulmonis
pulp
p. amputation
p. approach
p. canal
p. canal therapy
p. cavity
p. devitalization
digital p.
exposed p.
p. extirpation
p. flap
p. microcirculation
p. mummification
p. pressure
red p.
splenic p.
white p.
pulpa
pulpal wall
pulpation
pulpectomy
complete p.
partial p.
pulpifaction
pulpiform
pulpify
pulpodentinal membrane
pulpoma
pulpoperiapical lesion
pulposus
pulpotomy
complete p.
formocresol p.
partial p.
total p.
pulsatile
p. hematoma
p. mass
p. pressure lavage
pulsation
pulse
abdominal p.
p. lavage irrigation
p. oximetry
peripheral p.
p. pressure
p. repetition time prolongation
p. trisection
p. value recording (PVR)
p. width
pulsed
p. electromagnetic field (PEMF)
p. irrigation
p. laser ablation
pulsed-mode operation
pulse-echo distance measurement
pulsing current for nonunion of fracture
pulsion
p. diverticulum
p. hernia
pultaceous
pulverization
Pulvertaft
P. fishmouth incision
P. weave technique
pump
p. lung
p. oxygenation
punch
p. biopsy
p. graft
p. resection
punched-out lesion
punctate
p. epithelial keratoplasty
p. hemorrhage
punctation
punctoplasty
punctum, pl. **puncta**
inferior lacrimal p.
lacrimal p.
superior lacrimal p.
puncture
antegrade p.

anterior p.
apical left ventricular p.
Bernard p.
bone marrow p.
brain p.
calix p.
cecal ligation and p. (CLP)
cisternal p.
cystic p.
dental p.
diabetic p.
diathermy p.
direct cardiac p.
direct cautery p.
direct needle p.
dural p.
endoscopic fine-needle p.
exploratory p.
femoral p.
p. incision
jejunal p.
left ventricular p.
lumbar p.
needle tracheoesophageal p.
nephrostomy p.
percutaneous needle p.
percutaneous renal p.
pericardial p.
Quincke p.
retrograde nephrostomy p.
self-sealing scleral p.
skin p.
spinal p.
splenic p.
stereotactic p.
sternal p.
subdural p.
suprapubic p.
tracheoesophageal p.
transseptal p.
ultrasound-guided nephrostomy p.
venous p.
ventricular p.
p. wound
Ziegler p.

pupil
p. dilation
exit p.

pupilla, pl. **pupillae**
pupillae sphincter muscle

pupillaris

pupillary
p. dilatation
p. line
p. margin
p. membrane
p. membrane remnant
p. muscle
p. zone

pupillodilator fiber

pupilloscopy

pupil-to-root iridectomy

puppet technique

purchase point

pure
p. cutting cautery
p. fungal infection
p. fungal organism
p. insular carcinoma
p. refractive surgery
p. rotation
p. translation

purgation

purging
immunologic method of p.
tumor cell p.

puriform
p. aspect

Purkinje network

Purmann method

purpura fulminans

purpuric lesion

purpurogenous membrane

pursestring
p. atriotomy
p. mastopexy
p. suture technique

purulence

purulent
p. exudate
p. exudation
p. inflammation
p. peritonitis

pus
p. collection
frank p.

push
p. enteroscopy
hemodynamic p.
p. maneuver
p. plus refraction technique

NOTES

P

push-back
p.-b. procedure
p.-b. technique
push-pull T technique
push-type enteroscopy
pustular
p. inflammation
p. lesion
p. patch-test reaction
pustulation
pustule
Putenney operation
Putti-Platt
P.-P. arthroplasty
P.-P. shoulder procedure
Putti posterior approach
putty kidney
PUVA
psoralens, ultraviolet A
PUVA radiation
Puzo method
PVE
prosthetic valve endocarditis
PVR
pulmonary vascular resistance
pulse value recording
pVR
perspective volume rendering
PVRI
pulmonary vascular resistance index
PVTT
portal vein tumor thrombus
pyelectasis
pyelitic
pyelitis
pyelocaliceal
pyelocaliectasis
pyelocalyceal
pyelocalycotomy
pyelocystitis
pyeloileocutaneous
pyelolithotomy
coagulum p.
open p.
pyelolymphatic
pyelolysis
pyelonephritic kidney
pyelonephritis
xanthogranulomatous p. (XCP)
pyelonephrosis
pyeloplasty
Anderson-Hynes p.
capsular flap p.
Culp spiral flap p.
disjoined p.
dismembered p.
Foley Y-plasty p.
laparoscopic dismembered p.
Scardino vertical flap p.
Thompson capsule flap p.
pyeloplication
pyeloscopy
pyelostomy
pyelotomy
extended p.
open p.
pyeloureterectasis
pyeloureterography
pyeloureterostomy
pyelovenous backflow
pyelovesicostomy
pyencephalus
pyesis
pygal
pyknic
pyknotic body
pylemphraxis
pylephlebectasis
pylethrombosis
pylorectomy
Kocher p.
pylori (*pl. of* pylorus)
pyloric
p. antrum
p. artery
p. autotransplantation
p. canal
p. constriction
p. dilation
p. gland
p. intubation
p. orifice
p. part of stomach
p. ring
p. sphincter
p. vein
pyloricae
pylorici
pyloricum
pyloricus
pyloristenosis
pylorodiosis
pylorogastrectomy
pyloromyotomy
circumumbilical p.
extramucosal p.
Fredet-Ramstedt p.
Kocher p.
laparoscopic p.
Ramstedt p.
Ramstedt-Fredet p.
pyloroplasty
double p.
Finney p.
Heineke-Mikulicz p.
Jaboulay p.

Mikulicz p.
Ramstedt p.
reconstructive p.
transhiatal p.
truncal vagotomy and p.
vagotomy and p.
Weinberg modification of p.
Yu p.
pyloroptosis
pylorostenosis
pylorostomy
pylorotomy
pylorus, pl. **pylori**
pylorus-preserving
p.-p. gastrectomy (PPG)
p.-p. pancreaticoduodenectomy
p.-p. pancreatoduodenectomy (PPPD)
p.-p. surgery
pylorus-sparing pancreaticoduodenectomy
pyocele
pyocelia
pyocephalus
pyocolpocele
pyocystis
pyodermatous
p. infection
p. skin lesion
pyogen
pyogenesis
pyogenic
p. arthritis
p. hepatic abscess
p. membrane
p. spinal infection
pyomyoma
pyonephritis
pyonephrolithiasis
pyonephrosis
pyoperitoneum
pyoperitonitis
pyopneumothorax
pyopoiesis
pyopyelectasis
pyorrhea
pyosemia
pyosis
pyospermia
pyothorax
pyoureter ectopic ureterocele
pyramid
Ferrein p.
Lallouette p.
malpighian p.
medullary p.
p. method
nasal p.
orbital p.
petrous p.
renal p.
pyramidal
p. auricular muscle
p. bone
p. decussation
p. eminence
p. epithelium
p. fracture
p. process of thyroid
p. radiation
p. tip
p. tract
p. tractotomy
pyramidale
pyramidalis
pyramidotomy
medullary p.
spinal p.
pyramis
pyretic therapy
pyriform
pyriformis
pyrogen
endogenous p.
pyrolysis product
pyruvate
p. dehydrogenase inhibition
p. metabolism
pyuria

NOTES

QOL
quality of life
QST
Quantitative Sensory Testing
Q-tip test
quadrangular
q. cartilage
q. membrane
q. space
q. therapy
quadrangularis
quadrangulation of Frouin
quadrant
circumareolar q.
left upper q.
lower lateral q.
lower medial q.
right upper q.
q. sampling technique
upper lateral q.
upper medial q.
quadrantectomy
q., axillary dissection, radiation therapy (QUART)
q. mastectomy
quadrate
q. femoral tubercle
q. muscle
quadratum
quadratus
quadriceps
q. femoris tendon
quadricepsplasty
Judet q.
Thompson q.
V-Y q.
quadrigeminal cistern
quadrilateral
q. space
q. space syndrome
quadripedal extensor reflex
quadripolar
quadruple
q. amputation
q. therapy
Quaegebeur procedure
Quaglino operation
quality
q. of life (QOL)
Q. of Well-Being Scale Self-Administered (QWB-SA)
quantification
acoustic q.
shunt q.
quantitative
q. evaluation
Q. Sensory Testing (QST)
q. stool collection
quantity
sound q.
vector q.
QUART
quadrantectomy, axillary dissection, radiation therapy
QUART procedure for breast cancer
Quartey technique
quasistatic stressed position
Quatrefages angle
quatro therapy
Quénu
Q. hemorrhoidal plexus
Q. nail plate removal technique
Quénu-Küss tarsometatarsal injury classification
questionable mass
questionnaire
Acute Low Back Pain Screening Q. (ALBPSQ)
Barriers Pain Q.
Cognitive Errors Q.
Coping Strategies Q. (CSQ)
malingering q.
McGill Pain Q. (MPQ)
MCV Pain Q.
Menstrual Distress Management Q. (MDMQ)
Owestry Disability Q. (ODQ)
Pain Coping Q. (PCQ)
SF-McGill Pain Q.
The Modified Somatic Pain Q.
quick
q. angulation technique
Q. method
Quickert
Q. procedure
Q. three-suture technique
quilt suture technique
Quinby pelvic fracture classification
Quincke puncture
Quinones
method of Q.
quinti
extensor digiti q.
quintus
quotient
pressure rate q.
ventilation/perfusion q.

QWB-SA
Quality of Well-Being Scale Self-Administered

QWB-SA form

RA
regional anesthesia
racemate
racemic
r. mixture
r. modification
racemization
rachial
rachidial
rachidian
rachiotomy
rachis, pl. **rachides, rachises**
rachitic metaphysis
rachitomy
racket nail
racket-shaped flap
Rackley method
racquet incision
racquet-shaped incision
radectomy
Radford nomogram
radiad
radial
r. bursa
r. collateral artery
r. dilator muscle
r. forearm flap
r. fracture reduction
r. head
r. head dislocation
r. head fracture
r. index artery
r. iridotomy
r. keratotomy (RK)
r. laminectomy
r. neck fracture
r. recurrent artery
r. scar
r. sclerosing lesion
r. skin incision
r. styloid fracture
r. suture track
r. wedge osteotomy
r. wrist extensor
radial-based flap
radiale
radialis
radiata
radiate sternocostal ligament
radiation
r. angiopathy
braking r.
r. burn
r. cataract
characteristic r.
r. chimera
r. damage
diagnostic r.
r. enteritis
r. enteropathy
r. exposure
general r.
geniculocalcarine r.
Goldmann coherent r.
Gratiolet r.
r. hepatitis
r. hepatopathy
homogenous r.
r. injury
intraoperative r.
involved-field r.
r. lung disease
r. monitoring
r. mucositis
r. myelopathy
r. necrosis
occipitothalamic r.
r. oncologist
optic r.
r. output
r. pneumonitis
r. poisoning
postoperative pelvic r.
r. precaution
primary r.
r. proctitis
r. proctocolitis
r. protection
PUVA r.
pyramidal r.
rectosigmoid r.
r. response
r. risk
single fraction r.
Sr-90 beta r.
superficial r.
r. survey
temporal lobe r.
r. therapy
r. treatment
Wernicke r.
whole abdominal r.
whole body r.
radiation-induced
r.-i. carcinoma
r.-i. colitis
r.-i. disease
r.-i. ischemia
r.-i. leukoencephalopathy

radiation-induced *(continued)*
r.-i. proctitis
r.-i. pulmonary toxicity
r.-i. ulceration
radiatum
radical
r. abdominal hysterectomy
r. axillary dissection
r. compartmental excision
r. curative surgery
r. cystectomy
r. en bloc removal
r. gastrectomy
r. gastric resection
r. hemorrhoidectomy
r. inguinal orchiectomy
r. lymph node dissection
r. mastectomy
r. mastoidectomy
r. mediastinal dissection
r. neck dissection
r. nephrectomy
r. nephroureterectomy
r. orchidectomy
r. palmar fasciectomy
r. pancreatoduodenectomy
r. parametrectomy
r. perineal prostatectomy
r. prefrontal lobotomy
r. proctectomy
r. retropubic prostatectomy
r. subtotal resection
r. therapy
r. total gastrectomy
r. transcoccygeal prostatectomy
r. vaginal hysterectomy
r. vulvectomy
radices (*pl. of* radix)
radicle
radicotomy
radicula
radicular
r. artery
r. canal
radicularia
radiculectomy
radiculomedullary fistula
radiculomeningeal spinal vascular malformation
radiculopathy
thoracic r.
radiectomy
radii (*pl. of* radius)
radioactive
r. concentration
r. microsphere
r. scan
r. seed implantation
radioactivity
radiobicipital
radiocapitate ligament
radiocapitellar
r. articulation
r. line
radiocarpal
r. arthroscopy
r. articulation
r. dislocation
radiocarpea
radiocolloid
radiodense lesion
radiodigital
radiofluoroscopy
televised r.
radiofrequency
r. catheter ablation (RFCA)
r. electrophrenic respiration
r. lesion
r. rhizotomy
r. thermal ablation (RFTA)
radiofrequency-generated thermal lesion
radiograph
sequential r.'s
serial r.'s
specimen r.
radiographic
r. evaluation
r. image
r. obliteration
r. technique
r. tooth repair
radiography
plain abdominal r.
postfixation r.
radioguided
r. parathyroidectomy
r. technique
radiohumeral
radioimmunoglobulin therapy
radioimmunoguided surgery
radioimmunoscintimetry
radioiodination
lactoperoxidase r.
radioiodine
r. ablation
r. ablation therapy
low-dose r.
r. treatment
radioisotope
filtered r.
r. localization
unfiltered r.
r. uptake
radiolabeled
r. sentinel node
r. serum albumin

radiolocalization
gamma-probe r.
SLN r.
radiologic
r. biliary stent placement
r. evaluation
r. evidence
r. study
r. technique
radiological
r. examination
r. sphincter
radiologist
interventional r.
vascular r.
radiology
interventional r.
radiolucent
r. crescent line
r. lesion
r. operating room table extension
radiolunate fusion
radiolus
radiolysis
radiomuscular
radiomutation
radionecrosis
radionuclide
r. scan
r. technique
radiopalmar
radiopaque
r. foreign body
r. lesion
radiopharmaceutical therapy
radiopotentiation
radioprotector
radioscaphoid fusion
radiosensitization
radio signal line
radiosurgery
LINAC-based r.
linear accelerator-based r.
stereotactic r.
radiotherapy
adjuvant r.
radiotriquetral ligament
radioulnar
r. articulation
r. dissociation
r. ligament
radisectomy
radius, pl. **radii**
r. of angulation
scaphoid r.
radix, pl. **radices**
r. point
Radley-Liebig-Brown resection
radon seed implantation
Raeder syndrome
Raff-Glantz derivative method
rag-wheel method
Rai classification
Rainville technique
raise
single heel r.
straight-leg r. (SLR)
raising
straight leg r.
rale
Ralston-Thompson pseudoarthrosis technique
Raman spectroscopy
Rambo musculoplasty
ramex
ram horn nail
rami (*pl. of* ramus)
ramicotomy
ramification
apical r.
ramisection
Ramond point
Ramon flocculation
ramotomy
superior pubic r.
Ramsay Hunt syndrome
Ramstedt
R. operation
R. procedure
R. pyloromyotomy
R. pyloroplasty
Ramstedt-Fredet pyloromyotomy
ramus, pl. **rami**
Ranawat
R. classification
R. triangle method
Ranawat-DeFiore-Straub
R.-D.-S. osteotomy
R.-D.-S. technique
Ranawat-Dorr-Inglis method
Randall plaque
random
r. bladder biopsy

NOTES

random *(continued)*
r. cutaneous flap
r. pattern flap
randomization
range
r. of excursion
r. of motion (ROM)
pain sensitivity r.
Ransley-Cantwell repair
Ransley procedure
Ransohoff operation
Ranson
R. acute pancreatitis classification
R. pancreatitis criteria
R. prognostic scoring index
Ranvier node
RAO
right anterior oblique
RAO angulation
RAO position
raphe
anogenital r.
median longitudinal r.
penile r.
perineal r.
pharyngeal r.
pterygomandibular r.
scrotal r.
rapid
r. acquisition radiofrequency-echo-steady state imaging
r. bedside imaging
r. intraoperative parathormone immunoradiometric assay
r. maxillary expansion
r. occlusion
r. pull-through (RPT)
r. pull-through esophageal manometry technique
r. recompression-high pressure oxygen
r. scan fluoroscopy
r. scan technique
r. sequence induction intubation
r. tumor lysis syndrome
r. volume resuscitation
rapid-sequence
r.-s. induction (RSI)
r.-s. induction of anesthesia
r.-s. induction anesthetic technique
rapid-volume approach
Raplon anesthesia
Rapoport test
Rappaport
R. classification
R. osteotomy
RAPS
recurrent abdominal pain syndrome
rare system reaction
rasceta
rash
acneiform r.
Rashkind
R. balloon technique
R. operation
raspberry-like density
Rastan-Konno procedure
Rastan operation
Rastelli
R. conduit
R. graft
R. operation
R. procedure
R. repair
R. type A, B, C classification of atrioventricular septal defect
rate
anastomotic complication r.
anastomotic stricture r.
average flow r.
beat-to-beat variation of fetal heart r.
blood flow r.
cerebral metabolic r. (CMR)
circulation r.
complication r.
dipole-dipole relaxation r.
disease recurrence r.
disintegration r.
early infection r.
ejection r.
expiratory flow r.
flotation r.
r. of fluid filtration
fusion nonunion r.
gallbladder ejection r.
glomerular filtration r. (GFR)
heart r. (HR)
implant survival r.
infusion r.
in-hospital mortality r.
late infection r.
leakage r.
load-deflection r.
low dose r. (LDR)
maximal expiratory flow r.
maximal ventilation r.
mean normalized systolic ejection r.
metabolic r.
mortality r.
operative mortality r.
ovulation r.
oxygen extraction r.
pacemaker adaptive r.
peak expiratory flow r.

perfusion flow r.
plasma separation r.
pressure increment r.
r. pressure product
recurrence r.
relapse r.
relaxation r.
resectability r.
Solomon-Bloembergen theory of dipole-dipole relaxation r.
stricture r.
stroke ejection r.
success r.
systolic ejection r.
transverse relaxation r.
T2 relaxation r.
vertebral osteosynthesis fusion r.
voiding flow r.

rated perceived exertion

Rathke

R. bundle
R. pouch cyst

rating of perceived exertion

ratio

adenoma-hyperplastic polyp r.
adenoma-nonadenoma r.
ankle-brachial blood pressure r.
body hematocrit-venous hematocrit r.
common mode rejection r.
cough-pressure transmission r.
cup-to-disc r.
dead space:tidal volume r.
external/internal rotation r.
fetal head:abdominal circumference r.
hand r.
head:body r.
head circumference:abdominal circumference r.
inspiratory-to-expiratory r.
international normalized r. (INR)
intrapulmonary shunt r.
MAC r.
MAC-awake r.
MAC-intubation r.
MAC-skin incision r.
MAC-Surgical incision r.
mean UV/MV r.
midexpiratory/midinspiratory flow r.
optic cup-to-disc r.
pressure transmission r.
right-to-left shunt r.
sentinel node-to-background r. (SNBR)
shunt r.
tumor:cerebellum r.
UV/MV r.
ventilation/perfusion r.

rationalization

rat-tail deformity

Rauwolfia extract

rave

fracture en r.

Raverdino operation

raw hepatic surface

ray

r. amputation
medullary r.
r. resection

Ray-Brunswick-Mack operation

Ray-Clancy-Lemon technique

Rayhack technique

Ray-McLean operation

Raynaud syndrome

Raz

R. bladder neck suspension
R. four-quadrant suspension
R. modification
R. needle suspension
R. procedure
R. urethral suspension

Raz-Leach procedure

rCABG

reoperative coronary artery bypass graft

rCBF

regional cerebral blood flow

RDS

respiratory distress syndrome

reabsorb

reaction

anaphylactoid-type r.
compensation r.
cutaneous graft-versus-host r.
eczematous r.
elimination r.
exergonic r.
extrapyramidal r.
foreign body r.
r. formation
general adaptation r.
graft-versus-host disease r.
homograft r.
immediate asthmatic r. (IAR)

NOTES

reaction *(continued)*
implant r.
inflammation r.
irritant patch-test r.
lid closure r.
litigation r.
local anesthetic r.
midazolam-induced excitatory r.
needle r.
paradoxical r.
pustular patch-test r.
rare system r.
reverse transcriptase-polymerase chain r. (RT-PCR)
scar tissue r.
whitegraft r.
reactivation tuberculosis
reactive
r. arthritis
r. dilation
r. lymphoid lesion
reactivity
airway r.
reading
benign r.
malignant r.
Read rebreathing method
real
r. adaptive relaxation
r. reconstruction
realignment procedure
real-time
r.-t. colonoscopy
r.-t. 3-D biplanar transperineal prostate implantation
r.-t. echo-planar image
r.-t. endoscopic ultrasound-guided fine-needle aspiration
r.-t. multiplanar image
r.-t. sector scanning
reamed
r. femoral nailing
r. nail
reamputation
reanastomosed
reanastomosis
laparoscopic ureteral r.
reanimation
facial r.
reanneal
reapproximation
reattachment
four-wire trochanter r.
Harris four-wire trochanter r.
reattribution technique
reauditorization
rebleeding
rebound
r. headache
r. tenderness
rebreathing
r. anesthesia
intentional r.
r. technique
Rebuck skin window technique
recalcification time
recall
memory r.
Récamier
R. operation
R. procedure
recanalization
balloon occlusive intravascular lysis enhanced r.
excimer vascular r.
laser r.
TCD r.
r. technique
umbilical vein r.
r. versus recannulization
recanalize
recannulization
recanalization versus r.
receiver saturation
recent dislocation
recently healed surgical incision
receptaculum
receptoma
receptor
acetylcholine r.
alpha-adrenergic r.
alpha-2-adrenergic r.
beta-adrenergic r.
beta-2-adrenergic r.
calcium-sensing r.
DA r.
dopamine r.
endogenous opiate r.
endometrial r.
endothelin A, B r.
high-affinity progestin r.
high threshold r.
intensity-encoded r.
mu r.
muscarinic r.
nerve growth factor r.
nicotinic r.
opioid r.
pressure r.
silent r.
up-regulation of the r.
receptor-mediated endocytosis pathway
recess
azygoesophageal r.
cecal r.

costodiaphragmatic r.
costomediastinal r.
duodenojejunal r.
elliptical r.
epitympanic r.
frontal r.
hepatorenal r.
inferior duodenal r.
inferior ileocecal r.
inferior omental r.
intersigmoid r.
Jacquemet r.
mesentericoparietal r.
paracolic r.
paraduodenal r.
parotid r.
pharyngeal r.
phrenicomediastinal r.
pineal r.
piriform r.
pleural r.
retrocecal r.
retroduodenal r.
Rosenmüller r.
sacciform r.
sphenoethmoidal r.
spherical r.
splenic r.
subhepatic r.
subphrenic r.
subpopliteal r.
superior duodenal r.
superior ileocecal r.
superior omental r.
suprabullar r.
suprapineal r.
supratonsillar r.

recession
clitoral r.
lateral rectus r.

recessional line

recession-resection

recessive
autosomal r.

recidivation

recipient
adult r.
r. hepatectomy
naive r.
OLT r.
orthotopic liver transplant r.

reciprocal relaxation

reciprocation
active r.
passive r.

recirculation
instrument r.

Recklinghausen disease type I

reclamping

reclination

reclining position

Reclus I syndrome

recoarctation of aorta

recognition
pattern r.
within-list r. (WLR)

recoil
elastic r.

recombinant
r. DNA technique
r. tissue-type plasminogen activator (RTPA, rtPA)

recommendation
FDA Anesthesia Apparatus Checkout R.'s
screening r.

reconciliation

reconditioning
mucosal r.

reconstruction
Abbe-McIndoe vaginal r.
ACL r.
alar r.
anal sphincter r.
analytic r.
Andrews iliotibial band r.
anterior capsulolabral r.
anterior cruciate ligament r.
aortic root r.
aortorenal r.
artery r.
arthroscopic anterior cruciate ligament r. (AACLR)
Bankart r.
biliary r.
Billroth I, II r.
bladder outlet r.
breast r.
Brown knee joint r.
Cabral coronary r.
Cho anterior cruciate ligament r.
Chrisman-Snook r.
circumferential esophageal r.
Clancy cruciate ligament r.

NOTES

reconstruction *(continued)*
columellar r.
constrained r.
coronal r.
corporeal r.
craniofacial r.
cruciate ligament r.
d'Aubigne femoral r.
d'Aubigne resection r.
3-D computer r.
dermal pouch r.
Dibbell cleft lip-nasal r.
distal vertebral artery r.
dural patch r.
Eaton-Littler ligament r.
Ellison lateral knee r.
endoscopic anterior cruciate ligament r.
end-to-end r.
epiglottic r.
Evans r.
exogenous r.
extraarticular r.
five-one r.
genital r.
Goldner r.
hand r.
Harmon hip r.
hemimandible r.
House r.
Hughston-Degenhardt r.
Hughston-Jacobson lateral compartment r.
immediate breast r.
index metacarpophalangeal joint r.
inferior vena cava r.
infrarenal aortic r.
innominate artery r.
Insall anterior cruciate ligament r.
intraarticular r.
iterative r.
IVC r.
joint r.
juxtacubital r.
Krukenberg hand r.
Kugelberg r.
Larson ligament r.
lateral compartment r.
Lee r.
L'Episcopo hip r.
Lewis-Tanner subtotal esophagectomy and r.
ligament r.
Longmire-Gutgeman gastric r.
lower extremity r.
MacIntosh over-the-top ACL r.
mandibular r.
r. method
Millard advancement rotation flap r.
nasal r.
Nathan-Trung modification of Krukenberg hand r.
Neer posterior shoulder r.
neoglottic r.
nipple r.
nipple-areolar r.
r. occlusal surface (RecOS)
O'Donoghue ACL r.
open r.
operative r.
oral r.
orbital rim r.
oromandibular r.
oropharyngeal r.
ossicular chain r.
osteoplastic r.
palate r.
pancreaticogastrostomy r.
papillary r.
pedicled jejunal r.
peritoneal r.
pharyngoesophageal r.
plastic r.
portal vein r.
pouch r.
r. procedure
pulley r.
real r.
renal artery r.
Rosenberg endoscopic anterior cruciate ligament r.
Roux-en-Y r.
Roux gastric r.
sagittal r.
secondary r.
septal r.
Sheen airway r.
in situ r.
socket r.
sphincter r.
S-pouch r.
staged r.
stapled r.
sternoclavicular joint r.
Swanson r.
synchronous bladder r.
Tanagho bladder neck r.
r. technique
tenoplastic r.
three-dimensional r.
thumb r.
Torg knee r.
tracheal r.
tubular r.
tubularized bladder neck r.

Turbinger gastric r.
two-stage tendon graft r.
urinary tract r.
vascular r.
Verdan osteoplastic thumb r.
vertebral artery r.
Watson-Jones r.
Whitman femoral neck r.
Wookey r.
Young-Dees bladder neck r.
Young-Dees-Leadbetter bladder neck r.
Zancolli r.

reconstructive
r. mammaplasty
r. operation
r. preprosthetic surgery
r. pyloroplasty
r. surgical procedure
r. technique

record
anesthesia r.
anesthetic r.
automated anesthesia r.
centric occluding relation r.
eccentric interocclusal r.
eccentric maxillomandibular r.
jaw relation r.
medical r.
occluding centric relation r.
terminal jaw relation r.

recording
continuous on-line r.
duodenojejunal motor r.
fasting r.
macroelectrode r.
microelectrode r.
motor r.
pulse value r. (PVR)
segmental limb pressure r.
r. session
venous outflow r.
whole-cell patch clamp r.

RecOS
reconstruction occlusal surface

recovery
anesthetic immediate r.
fluid-attenuated inversion r. (FLAIR)
neurologic r.
postoperative r.
pressure r.
r. and reorganization
r. room
r. room time
saturation r.
selective saturation r.
short tau inversion r. (STIR)
time to r.
r. time

recruitment maneuver

recta (*pl. of* rectum)

rectae

rectal
r. alimentation
r. ampulla
r. anesthesia
r. anesthetic
r. anesthetic technique
r. blind pouch
r. cancer
r. carcinoma
r. column
r. diameter
r. dilation
r. distention
r. evacuation
r. examination
r. excision
r. fascia
r. fissure
r. fistula
r. floor
r. floor line
r. fold
r. foreign body
r. hernia
r. laceration
r. mass
r. mobilization
r. mucosectomy
r. muscle cuff
r. myectomy
r. probe electroejaculation
r. problem
r. pulsed irrigation
r. resting pressure
r. sheath hematoma
r. shelf
r. sinus
r. stump
r. suction biopsy
r. surgery
r. tip

NOTES

rectal *(continued)*
r. ulceration
r. valvotomy
r. venous plexus
rectalgia
rectalis
rectangular amputation
rectectomy
recti
recticulum
endoplasmic r.
rectification
anomalous r.
inward-going r.
rectify
recto
hernia in r.
rectoanal angulation
rectocele repair
rectoclysis
rectococcygeal muscle
rectococcygeus
rectococcypexy
rectolabial fistula
rectoperineal
rectoperineorrhaphy
rectopexy
abdominal r.
anterior r.
Ekehorn r.
posterior r.
presacral r.
Ripstein anterior sling r.
Wells posterior r.
rectoplasty
rectorrhaphy
rectoscopic endometrial ablation
rectoscopy
rectosigmoid
r. anastomosis
r. carcinoma
r. junction
r. radiation
r. sphincter
r. stump
r. vein
rectosigmoidoscopy
rectosphincteric reflex
rectostenosis
rectostomy
rectotomy
rectourethral
r. fistula
r. muscle
rectourethralis
rectourinary fistula
rectouterina
rectouterine
r. cul-de-sac
r. fold
r. muscle
r. pouch
rectouterinus
rectovaginal
r. examination
r. fistula
r. pouch
r. septum
r. surgery
r. surgical treatment
rectovaginale
rectovaginalis
rectovaginouterine pouch
rectovesical
r. fascia
r. fistula
r. fold
r. muscle
r. pouch
r. septum
rectovesicale
rectovesicalis
rectovestibular fistula
rectovulvar fistula
rectum, pl. **recta**
aganglionic r.
r. cancer
colonoscopy per r.
r. irrigation
rectus
r. abdominis free flap
r. abdominis muscle
r. abdominis muscle flap
r. abdominis musculocutaneous flap
r. abdominis myocutaneous flap
r. diastasis
r. fascial wrap
r. femoris flap
r. femoris tendon
r. muscle-splitting incision
r. position
r. sheath
r. sheath hematoma
r. sheath incision
recumbent
r. incision
r. position
recurrence
distant r.
goiter r.
intraperitoneal r.
invasive r.
local r.
locoregional r.
nodal r.

noninvasive r.
peritoneal r.
port-site wound r.
r. rate
resectable extrahepatic r.
suprapubic midline r.
tumor r.
wound r.

recurrence-free survival

recurrens

recurrent

r. abdominal pain syndrome (RAPS)
r. arthralgia
r. ascites
r. aspiration
r. attack
r. corneal erosion
r. dysphagia
r. exophthalmos
r. hypercalcemia
r. incisional hernia
r. inflammation
r. interosseous artery
r. leiomyosarcoma
r. meningeal branch
r. meningeal nerve
r. nerve injury
r. nerve lesion
r. nerve lymphatic chain
r. nerve paralysis
r. patellar dislocation
r. pyogenic cholangiohepatitis (RPC)
r. pyogenic cholangitis
r. radial artery
r. thromboembolic complication
r. thromboembolic disease
r. thromboembolism
r. thrombophlebitis
r. thrombosis
r. tumor
r. ulnar artery
r. upper respiratory tract infection
r. vermian oligoastrocytoma

recurrentis

recurvation

recurvatum angulation deformity

red

r. blood cell mass
r. desaturation
r. ear syndrome
r. granulation
r. hepatization
r. induration
r. muscle
r. pulp

Reddick-Saye method

redebridement

red-eyed shunt syndrome

red-filter therapy

redilation

redintegration

redistribution hypothermia

Redman approach

Redmond-Smith operation

redo

r. CABG
r. fundoplication

redox indicator

redressement forcé

reduced liver transplant (RLT)

reduced-size

r.-s. graft
r.-s. transplant

reducible hernia

reduction

afterload r.
Agee force-couple splint r.
alar base r.
Allen r.
Aries-Pitanguy breast r.
axillary endoscopic r.
Barsky macrodactyly r.
Becton open r.
r. before resection
Boitzy open r.
calcaneal fracture r.
central cone technique r.
closed r.
cluster r.
concentric r.
Cooper r.
Cotton r.
Crosby r.
Cubbins open r.
delayed open r.
Dias-Giegerich open r.
r. division
Eaton closed r.
Eaton-Malerich r.
embryo r.
r. en masse
Essex-Lopresti open r.

NOTES

reduction *(continued)*
femoral neck fracture r.
fetal r.
Flynn femoral neck fracture r.
force-couple splint r.
Fowles open r.
fracture r.
fracture-dislocation r.
funic r.
Hankin r.
Hastings open r.
hip r.
Houghton-Akroyd open r.
incomplete r.
indirect r.
internal fixation, closed r.
interproximal r.
Kaplan open r.
Kinast indirect r.
King open r.
Lavine r.
Lejour-type breast r.
limb r.
Lowell r.
lung volume r. (LVR)
r. mammaplasty
r. mastopexy
McKeever open r.
r. method
Meyn r.
Moberg-Gedda open r.
multifetal pregnancy r.
Neer open r.
nonoperative r.
open r.
r. osteotomy
pain threshold r.
Pare r.
Parvin r.
percutaneous r.
perioperative r.
pneumatic r.
postural r.
r. potential
Pratt open r.
preload r.
prone r.
radial fracture r.
r. ring
risk r.
short-scar technique breast r.
shoulder r.
side posture r.
sigmoid loop r.
Speed-Boyd open r.
Speed open r.
spondylolisthesis r.
stable r.
stapled lung r.
sternoclavicular joint r.
stress r.
surgical r.
swan-neck deformity r.
r. syndactyly
r. technique
trial r.
tuberosity r.
r. tuberosity
tumescent technique breast r.
r. ventriculoplasty
vertical pedicle technique breast r.
volvulus r.
Wayne County r.
Weber-Brunner-Freuler open r.
weight r.
wet technique with liposuction breast r.

reduction-stabilization

redundant
r. sac tissue
r. triangular-shaped skin

reduplication
r. cataract
r. murmur

redux
chancre r.

reedy nail

reefing
r. procedure
stomach r.

reendothelialization

reentry
bundle-branch r.

reepithelialization

Rees-Ecker
R.-E. fluid
R.-E. method

Reese-Cleasby operation

Reese-Jones-Cooper operation

Reese ptosis operation

reexcision

reexpansion maneuver

reexploration
operative r.

reexplore

refashioning

reference method

referred
r. point
r. trigger-point pain
r. trigger-point phenomenon

refired

refixation

reflectance
endoscopic r.

reflected inguinal ligament

reflection
angle of r.
Campbell triceps r.
corneal r.
diaphragmatic r.
diffuse r.
guidewire r.
hepatoduodenal r.
hepatoduodenal-peritoneal r.
mirror-image r.
mucobuccal r.
pericardial r.
peritoneal r.
pleural r.
shiny cellophane r.
specular r.
total internal r.
reflectometry
acoustic r.
reflex
abdominal cardiac r.
absent gag r.
accommodation r.
Bezold-Jarisch r.
body righting r.
Breuer-Hering inflation r.
cardiopressor r.
celiac plexus r.
copper-wire r.
corneal light r.
cremasteric r.
crossed extension r.
crossed extensor r.
Cushing r.
r. erection
erector-spinal r.
r. examination
extensor thrust r.
external oblique r.
eyeball compression r.
eye-closure r.
eyelash r.
eyelid-closure r.
fixation r.
flexion-extension r.
fusion r.
gastropancreatic vagovagal r.
grasp r.
Head paradoxical r.
head-turning r.
Hering-Breuer r.
r. incontinence
inflation r.
lacrimation r.
r. ligament
mass r.
milk-ejection r.
myenteric r.
r. neurogenic bladder
oculocardiac r. (OCR)
paradoxical extensor r.
pericardial r.
pronator r.
proprioceptive head-turning r.
quadripedal extensor r.
rectosphincteric r.
renal r.
silver-wire r.
supination r.
supinator longus r.
r. sympathetic dystrophy
sympathoexcitation r.
r. therapy
vagovagal r.
r. venoconstriction
vertical suspension r.
visceral traction r.
reflexa
reflexive saccade
reflexogenic erection
reflexum
reflux
abdominal r.
abdominojugular r.
acid r.
alkaline r.
r. esophagitis
gastric r.
r. menstruation
upright r.
vesicoureteral r.
reformation
fornix r.
inferior fornix r.
reformulation
refractile body
refractive
r. keratoplasty
r. keratotomy
r. operative technique
r. surgery
refractory
r. encephalopathy
r. variceal hemorrhage

NOTES

refrigeration anesthesia
regainer space
regenerate
regenerated esophageal epithelium
regeneration
aberrant r.
r. aberration
atypical r.
axonal r.
carbon tetrachloride-induced liver r.
compensatory r.
epimorphic r.
hepatic r.
incomplete r.
liver r.
morphallactic r.
r. motor unit potential
nerve r.
neuronal r.
osteoblastic bone r.
peripheral nerve r.
squamous r.
tibial bone defect r.
tissue r.
tubular r.
regimen
adjuvant r.
antifungal r.
antiplatelet r.
treatment r.
regio, pl. **regiones**
region
abdominal r.
anal r.
ankle r.
anterior antebrachial r.
anterior brachial r.
anterior knee r.
argyrophilic nucleolar organizer r.
axillary r.
brain r.
calcaneal r.
carpal r.
choledochal r.
epigastric r.
femoral r.
gastric pacemaker r.
gluteal r.
hilar r.
hypochondriac r.
hypogastric r.
ileocecal r.
iliac r.
inframammary r.
infraorbital r.
infrascapular r.
inguinal r.
left hypochondriac r.
left lateral r.
lumbar r.
mammary r.
mental r.
nuchal r.
oral r.
orbital r.
PAG/PVG r.
paraaortic r.
parietal r.
penumbral r.
periaqueductal-periventricular r.
perineal r.
pharyngeal r.
pineal r.
popliteal r.
posterior antebrachial r.
posterior brachial r.
posterior knee r.
posterior neck r.
presternal r.
pubic r.
retroperitoneal r.
right hypochondriac r.
right iliac r.
right lateral r.
sacral r.
scapular r.
sternocleidomastoid r.
suboccipital r.
subphrenic r.
supraomental r.
suprapubic r.
sural r.
thoracoabdominal r.
umbilical r.
urogenital r.
vertebral r.
zygomatic r.
regional
r. anesthesia (RA)
r. anesthetic
r. anesthetic technique
r. block
r. cerebral blood flow (rCBF)
r. flap
r. hepatectomy
r. hypoperfusion
r. hypothermia
r. lymphadenectomy
r. lymph node basin
r. metastasis
r. node
r. wall motion abnormality (RWMA)
regiones (*pl. of* regio)
registration
image r.

registry
- Acoustic Neuroma R.
- Autologous Bone Marrow Transplant R. (ABMTR)
- Balloon Valvuloplasty R.
- Brain Tumor R.
- Kiel Pediatric Tumor R.
- Mansfield Valvuloplasty R.
- National Football Head and Neck Injury R.
- National Pediatric Trauma R. (NPTR)
- Ovarian Tumor R.
- population-based r.
- Renal Allograft Disease R.
- St. Mark polyposis r.
- tumor r.
- United Kingdom Heart Valve R.

Regnault type B mastopexy
regression
- clot r.
- r. of thrombus
- tumor r.

regressive-reconstructive approach
regurgitant lesion
regurgitation
- r. jaundice
- r. test

rehabilitation stage
rehalation
Rehbein procedure
Rehfuss method
Rehne-Delorme plication
rehydrating solution
rehydration therapy
Reichel-Pólya
- R.-P. method
- R.-P. procedure
- R.-P. stomach resection
- R.-P. technique

Reichenheim-King procedure
Reichenheim technique
Reichert
- R. cartilage
- R. membrane

Reid base line
Reifenstein syndrome
Reilly body
reimplantation
- aortorenal r.
- Cohen cross-trigonal r.
- end-to-side r.
- intentional tooth r.
- Politano-Leadbetter r.
- ureteral r.

Reinert acetabular extensile approach
reinfection tuberculosis
reinforce
- giant prosthetic r.

reinforcement
- omental r.
- pericardial r.
- peritoneal r.
- pleural patch r.

reinjection protocol
Reinke
- R. crystalloid
- R. space

reinnervation
reinoculation
reinsemination
reintegrate
reintegration
reintubation
reinversion
reirrigation
Reisseisen muscle
Reissner membrane
Reis-Wertheim vaginal hysterectomy
Reiter
- R. disease
- R. syndrome

rejection
- accelerated transplant r.
- acute allograft r.
- acute cellular r.
- acute lung r.
- acute vascular r.
- allograft corneal r.
- r. cardiomyopathy transplant
- cellular xenograft r.
- chronic allograft r.
- chronic transplant r.
- delayed hyperacute transplant r.
- ductopenic r.
- fetal r.
- fierce cellular r.
- first-set graft r.
- graft r.
- homograft r.
- hyperacute r.
- interstitial r.
- r. line
- marrow graft r.

NOTES

rejection *(continued)*
maternal r.
no r.
no infection-no r.
primary r.
renal allograft r.
second-set graft r.
total graft area r.
transplant r.
vascular r.
rejuvenation
relapse
locoregional r.
lymphoma r.
r. rate
relapsing polychondritis
relation
acentric r.
acquired centric r.
acquired eccentric jaw r.
buccolingual r.
centric jaw r.
centric occluding r.
concentration-effect r.
convenience jaw r.
cusp-fossa r.
diastolic pressure-volume r.
Duane-Hunt r.
dynamic r.
eccentric jaw r.
end-systolic pressure-volume r.
end-systolic stress-dimension r.
equivalence r.
force-frequency r.
force-length r.
force-velocity r.
force-velocity-length r.
force-velocity-volume r.
Frank-Starling r.
intermaxillary r.
interval-strength r.
jaw r.
jaw-to-jaw r.
length-resting tension r.
length-tension r.
mandibular centric r.
maxillomandibular r.
median jaw r.
occluding r.
occlusal r.
posterior border jaw r.
pressure-flow r.
pressure-volume r.
protrusive jaw r.
resting length-tension r.
rest jaw r.
retruded jaw r.
ridge r.
static r.
tension-length r.
unstrained jaw r.
ventilation/perfusion r.
ventricular end-systolic pressure-volume r.
vertical r.
working bite r.
relationship
cause-effect r.
endoscope-body position r.
end-systolic pressure-length r. (ESPLR)
intraluminal pH-pressure r.
pressure-flow r.
tissue-base r.
tumor cell-host bone r.
ventilation/perfusion r.
relative
r. curative resection
r. humidity
near-point r.
r. noncurative resection
r. response attributable to the maneuver
r. spectacle magnification
relaxant
depolarizing r.
muscle r.
neuromuscular r.
nondepolarizing r.
nondepolarizing muscle r.
r. reversal
smooth muscle r.
relaxation
adaptive r.
cardioesophageal r.
complete sphincter r.
diastolic r.
differential r.
dipole-dipole r.
dynamic r.
endothelial-dependent r.
endothelium-mediated r.
esophageal sphincter r.
incomplete r.
intraoperative stress r.
isovolumetric r.
isovolumic r.
longitudinal r.
r. method
nitric oxide blocked sphincter r.
paramagnetic shift r.
pelvic r.
r. phenomenon
r. rate
real adaptive r.
reciprocal r.

r. response
sinusoidal r.
smooth muscle r.
sphincter r.
stress r.
r. technique
r. time
r. time index
transverse r.
upper esophageal sphincter r.
uterine r.
ventricular r.
relaxing
r. incision
r. solution
release
de Quervain stenosing tenosynovitis r.
endoscopic carpal tunnel r. (ECTR)
flexor-pronator origin r.
lateral extensor r.
modified two-portal endoscopic carpal tunnel r.
physiologic pattern r.
plantar plate r.
pronator teres r.
soft-tissue r.
sustained r. (SR)
relief
r. incision
r. space
symptomatic r.
relieving incision
remain
necrotic r.
Remak
R. ganglion
R. plexus
remargination
remedial
r. inguinal exploration
r. surgery
remifentanil
remission induction
remnant
cirrhotic liver r.
Cloquet canal r.
devascularized parathyroid r.
distal r.
esophageal r.
gastric r.
r. gland
r. liver volume
mucosal r.
parathyroid r.
pupillary membrane r.
remobilization
remodeling
extracellular matrix r.
tissue r.
r. of wound
remote
r. pedicle flap
r. tier
remotivation
removable maintainer space
removal
Cameron femoral component r.
cast r.
cement r.
Collis-Dubrul femoral stem r.
colonoscopic r.
en bloc r.
endoscopic r.
excisional r.
extracorporeal CO_2 r. (ECOR)
forceps r.
foreign body r.
r. of foreign body
gastric coin r.
gland r.
Harris femoral component r.
hump r.
implant r.
laparoscopic gallbladder r.
lens r.
macroscopic tumor r.
mesh r.
metastatic tumor r.
Moreland-Marder-Anspach femoral stem r.
nail-fold r.
nail-plate r.
one-session r.
path of r.
percutaneous endoscopic r.
percutaneous stone r.
radical en bloc r.
rib r.
small polyp r.
stem r.
through-the-scope balloon r.
total surgical r.
transsphenoidal r.

NOTES

removal *(continued)*
tube r.
tumor r.
ureteral stoma r.
Winograd nail plate r.
remyelination
remyelinization
ren, pl. **renes**
renal
r. abnormality
r. adenocarcinoma
r. adenoma
r. allograft
R. Allograft Disease Registry
r. allograft rejection
r. allograft rupture
r. angiomyolipoma
r. angioplasty
r. anomaly
r. arterial embolization
r. artery
r. artery occlusive disease
r. artery orifice
r. artery reconstruction
r. artery response
r. artery stenosis
r. artery stenotic disease
r. artery stenting
r. artery thrombosis
r. autotransplantation
r. biopsy
r. branch
r. calculus
r. capsulotomy
r. cell carcinoma
r. colic
r. column
r. complication
r. compromise
r. cortex
r. cortical lobule
r. crush syndrome
r. cyst
r. cyst ablation
r. cyst decortication
r. cyst hemorrhage
r. cyst infection
r. cyst marsupialization
r. duplication
r. dysfunction
r. ectopia
r. failure
r. fascia
r. fistula
r. function
r. fungal infection
r. ganglion
r. hematoma
r. hyperfiltration
r. hypertension
r. impression
r. infarction
r. infusion therapy
r. injury repair
r. insufficiency
r. labyrinth
r. lobe
r. malrotation
r. management
r. manifestation
r. mass
r. mechanism
r. medulla
r. papilla
r. pelvis
r. pelvis carcinoma
r. plexus
r. pouch
r. preservation
r. proximal tubule preparation
r. pyramid
r. reflex
r. replacement therapy
r. revascularization
r. scintography
r. segment
r. sinus
r. sonography
r. sparring surgery
r. stone
r. surface
r. thromboendarterectomy
r. transplantation
r. tubular acidosis
r. tumor
r. vascular disease
r. vasodilator prostaglandin
r. vein
r. vein renin concentration
r. vessel
renales
renalia
renalis
renal-splanchnic steal
renaturation
renculus
rendering
perspective volume r. (pVR)
renes (*pl. of* ren)
renewal
tissue r.
renicapsule
renicardiac
reniculus, pl. **reniculi**
reniform pelvis
reninoma

reniportal
renis
renocutaneous
renogastric fistula
renointestinal
renomegaly
renopathy
renoprival
renopulmonary
renorrhaphy
renovascular hypertension
Rentrop classification
renunculus
reoperation
  planned r.
reoperative
  r. aesthetic surgery
  r. bariatric surgery
  r. blepharoplasty
  r. carotid surgery
  r. coronary artery bypass graft (rCABG)
  r. necrosectomy
  r. parathyroidectomy
  r. pelvic surgery
  r. ureteroneocystostomy
reorganization
  recovery and r.
reoxygenation
repair
  Abraham-Pankovich tendo calcaneus r.
  ACL r.
  acromioclavicular joint r.
  all-inside r.
  Allison gastroesophageal reflux r.
  Allison hiatal hernia r.
  anal sphincter r.
  anatomic r.
  aneurysm r.
  Anson-McVay hernia r.
  anterior and posterior r.
  aortic valve r.
  A&P r.
  Arlt epicanthus r.
  Arlt eyelid r.
  Atasoy-type r.
  Bankart shoulder r.
  Barnhart r.
  Bassini inguinal hernia r.
  Bassini-Stetten hernia r.
  Belsey Mark IV r.
  Belt-Fuqua hypospadias r.
  bilateral inguinal hernia r.
  bilayer patch hernia r.
  Black r.
  Blair epicanthus r.
  blepharochalasis r.
  blepharoptosis r.
  Boari ureteral flap r.
  Boerema hernia r.
  bone graft r.
  Bosworth tendo calcaneus r.
  Boyd-Anderson biceps tendon r.
  brachial plexus r.
  Brom r.
  Bunnell tendon r.
  Cantwell-Ransley epispadias r.
  Caspari r.
  cemental r.
  coarctation r.
  Collis r.
  columellar r.
  cross-trigonal r.
  crural r.
  cystocele r.
  Danus-Stanzel r.
  DeBakey-Creech aneurysm r.
  delayed primary r.
  density-dependent r.
  Devine hypospadias r.
  diaphragmatic crural r.
  dog-ear r.
  dural r.
  DuVries hammertoe r.
  dynamic r.
  early thoracoscopic r.
  Ecker-Lotke-Glazer patellar tendon r.
  Effler hiatal hernia r.
  elective hernia r.
  endoluminal r.
  endoscopic mitral valve r.
  endovascular r.
  end-to-end tendon r.
  end-to-side r.
  epineural r.
  episiotomy r.
  extensor tendon r.
  exteriorized uterine r.
  extracorporeal r.
  extraperitoneal endoscopic hernia r.
  fascicular r.
  fibrous r.

NOTES

repair *(continued)*
first-stage r.
five-one knee ligament r.
flexor tendon r.
Fontan r.
fracture r.
Froimson-Oh r.
functional r.
Gardner meningocele r.
glenohumeral dislocation r.
group fascicular r.
Halsted-Bassini hernia r.
Harrington-Allison r.
Harrington hernia r.
Hatafuku fundus onlay patch esophageal r.
Hill hiatus hernia r.
Hill median arcuate r.
histologic tooth r.
Hoguet pantaloon hernia r.
hypoplastic left heart r.
Jones first-toe r.
Kelikian-Riashi-Gleason patellar tendon r.
Kessler r.
Kleinert r.
Konno r.
Kugel hernia r.
Kuhnt-Junius r.
lacrimal gland r.
Lange tendon lengthening and r.
laparoscopic IPOM r.
laparoscopic paraesophageal hernia r. (LPHR)
laparoscopic prosthetic mesh r.
laparoscopic varicocele r.
laparoscopic ventral hernia r.
laryngeal r.
Latzko vesicovaginal fistula r.
Le Fort-Wehrbein-Duplay hypospadias r.
levator aponeurosis r.
Lich-Gregoir r.
Lichtenstein hernial r.
Lichtenstein mesh r.
Lindholm tendo calcaneus r.
Lotheissen hernia r.
MacIntosh over-the-top r.
MacNab shoulder r.
Madden r.
MAGPI hypospadius r.
Ma-Griffith tendo calcaneus r.
Mandelbaum-Nartolozzi-Carney patellar tendon r.
Marcy hernia r.
Marlex hernial r.
McVay-Cooper ligament r.
McVay inguinal hernial r.
medial r.
meniscal r.
mesh r.
Millard rotation-advancement lip r.
minimally invasive mitral valve r.
mitral valve r.
Moloney hernia r.
myelomeningocele r.
Nissen r.
Noble-Mengert perineal r.
one-stage hypospadias r.
open r.
Orr rectal prolapse r.
Palmer-Dobyns-Linscheid ligament r.
pants-over-vest hernial r.
paravaginal defect r.
patellar tendon r.
periapical tooth r.
pericardioplasty in pectus excavatum r.
perineal r.
Phaneuf-Graves r.
plastic r.
plug prosthetic mesh r.
postanal r.
posterior r.
postoperative r.
potentially lethal x-ray damage r.
premuscular prosthetic r.
primary r.
prosthetic mesh r.
pseudarthrosis r.
pseudoarthrosis r.
pulmonary stenosis r.
radiographic tooth r.
Ransley-Cantwell r.
Rastelli r.
rectocele r.
renal injury r.
reverse sigma penoscrotal transposition r.
rod fracture r.
Rodney Smith biliary stricture r.
rotator cuff r.
Scuderi r.
secondary r.
Senning r.
Sever-L'Episcopo r.
shoulder r.
Shouldice-Bassini hernia r.
in situ uterine r.
slipped Nissen r.
Speed sternoclavicular r.
sphincter r.
staged abdominal r. (STAR)
Staples r.
Staples-Black-Broström ligament r.
Stoppa hernia r.

Stoppa-type laparoscopic r.
Strickland tendon r.
sublethal x-ray damage r.
surgical r.
suture r.
Talesnick scapholunate r.
tendon r.
tension-free mesh r.
tension-free prosthetic mesh r.
TEP r.
Teuffer tendo calcaneus r.
Thal esophageal stricture r.
Theirsch-Duplay r.
thoracic aortic aneurysm r.
thoracoabdominal aortic aneurysm r.
thoracoscopic r.
tight Nissen r.
tissue r.
total extraperitoneal r.
tracheal r.
transabdominal preperitoneal r.
triad knee r.
trichiasis r.
tricuspid valve r.
triple ligamentous r.
Turco-Spinella tendo calcaneus r.
two-stage r.
ultrasound-guided compression r. (UGCR)
unilateral inguinal hernia r.
in utero r.
vaginal wall r.
vascular laceration r.
Veirs canaliculus r.
vesicovaginal r.
vest-over-pants hernia r.
videoscopic r.
volar plate r.
Watson-Jones fracture r.
Wheeler halving r.
y mesh hernia r.
York-Mason r.
Young type epispadias r.
Zancolli clawhand deformity r.

repairable parietal defect

reparative cardiac surgery

repeat

r. balloon mitral valvotomy
r. cesarean section
r. operation
r. procedure
r. revascularization

repeated

r. exposure
r. respiratory infection
r. tissue expansion

reperfusion

r. injury
ischemia and r. (I/R)

reperfusion-induced hemorrhage

reperitonealization

repetitive

r. cluster
r. nerve stimulation

rephasing

echo r.
even-echo r.

replacement

aortic valve r.
Cosgrove mitral valve r.
fluid r.
heart valve r.
homograft aortic valve r.
laparoscopic feeding tube r.
mitral valve r.
mucosal patch r.
Mueller-type femoral head r.
pulmonary valve r.
supraannular mitral valve r.
tile plate facet r.
total hip r.
total joint r.
total knee r.
tube r.
valve r.

replant

replantation

intentional r.
limb r.

repolarization

reposit

particle r.

reposition

repositioning

muscle r.

repreparation

reproductive

r. tract
r. tract abnormality

requirement

anticoagulation monitoring r.

re-resected

re-resecting

re-resection

NOTES

rerouting insertion
rerupture
rescue
r. analgesia
r. angioplasty
r. antiemetic
propofol r.
r. technique
r. therapy
resect
resectability
r. rate
surgical r.
tumor r.
resectable
r. carcinoma
r. extrahepatic recurrence
r. hepatic disease
r. liver metastasis
r. periampullary cancer
r. tumor
resection
abdominal-perineal r.
abdominoperineal r. (APR)
abdominosacral r.
absolute curative r.
absolute noncurative r.
activation map-guided surgical r.
anterior r.
r. arthrodesis
r. arthroplasty
atrial septal r.
Badgley iliac wing r.
bar r.
bilateral r.
bilobar r.
bleb r.
bone r.
bony bridge r.
bowel r.
breast r.
bronchial sleeve r.
calcaneonavicular bar r.
Carrell r.
caudal lamina r.
cesarean r.
classical subtotal r.
Clayton procedure with panmetatarsal head r.
cold-cup r.
coloanal r.
colon r.
colonic r.
colorectal cancer r.
colosigmoid r.
combined gastrointestinal r.
combined organ r.
complete r.
composite pelvic r.
condyle r.
conservative r.
craniofacial r.
CRC r.
cricotracheal r.
cryo-assisted r.
cuff r.
curative r.
D2 r.
Darrach r.
definitive r.
r. dermodesis
diathermic r.
Dillwyn-Evans r.
Dwar-Barrington r.
elective sigmoid r.
electrocautery r.
en bloc r.
endocardial r.
endometrial r.
endoscopic mucosal r. (EMR)
endoscopic snare r.
end-to-end ileo-anal anastomosis without mucosal r.
epidermoid r.
epiphysial bar r.
esophageal r.
esophagogastric r.
ex situ-in situ liver r.
extended r.
extraarticular r.
femoral r.
formal hepatic r.
gastric leiomyoma r.
gastrointestinal r.
Girdlestone r.
Guller r.
gum r.
Gurd r.
Hartmann r.
Henry r.
hepatic r.
Hoffmann panmetatarsal head r.
hyoid bone r.
ileal r.
ileocolic r.
ileocolonic r.
iliac crest r.
iliac wing r.
incomplete tumor r.
infundibular wedge r.
Ingram bony bridge r.
initial r.
innominate bone r.
intercalary r.
interdental r.
intestinal r.

Ivor-Lewis r.
Janecki-Nelson shoulder girdle r.
Karakousis-Vezeridis r.
kyphos r.
Langenskiöld bony bridge r.
laparoscopic-assisted small bowel r.
laparoscopic bowel r.
Lartat-Jacob hepatic r.
lateral rectus r.
LCVP-aided hepatic r.
LCVP-assisted major liver r.
lesser r.
levator r.
Lewis-Chekofsky r.
Lewis intercalary r.
limited r.
liver r.
lobar r.
lobe r.
Localio-Francis-Rossano r.
local radical r.
low anterior r. (LAR)
major liver r. (MLR)
Mankin r.
Marcove-Lewis-Huvos shoulder girdle r.
margin r.
r. margin
marginal r.
Mason abdominotranssphincteric r.
massive bowel r.
medial malleolus r.
metatarsal head r.
microscopic r.
Miles abdominoperineal r.
Miltner-Wan calcaneus r.
minimal transurethral r.
Mohs microsurgical r.
multiple-punch r.
multisegmental r.
Mumford r.
muscle r.
myotomy-myectomy-septal r.
nipple-flat duct r.
nonanatomic wedge r.
ovarian wedge r.
palliative r.
pancreatic tail r.
panmetatarsal head r.
parotid r.
partial cricotracheal r.
partial gastric r.
Paul-Mikulicz r.
Peet splanchnic r.
Peyman full-thickness eyewall r.
Phelps partial r.
portal vein r.
presacral r.
primary r.
prophylactic r.
proximal femoral r.
proximal gastric r.
pulmonary r.
punch r.
radical gastric r.
radical subtotal r.
Radley-Liebig-Brown r.
ray r.
reduction before r.
Reichel-Pólya stomach r.
relative curative r.
relative noncurative r.
rim r.
Rockwood r.
root end r.
R0, R1, R2 r.
scleral r.
sectoral r.
sectorial r.
segmental colonic r.
segmental lung r.
segmental pulmonary r.
segment-oriented r.
segment-oriented hepatic r.
segment-oriented liver r.
septal r.
sleeve r.
small bowel r.
sphincter-sparing r.
spleen-preserving pancreatic r.
standard gastric r.
Stener-Gunterberg r.
strip r.
subcomplete r.
submucous r.
subperiosteal r.
subtotal gastric r.
surgical r.
synchronous r.
terminal ileal r.
Thompson r.
thyroid r.
Tikhoff-Linberg shoulder girdle r.
Torek r.

NOTES

resection *(continued)*
Torpin cul-de-sac r.
transanal endoscopic microsurgical r.
transcervical r.
transoral odontoid r.
transsphenoidal microsurgical r.
transsphenoidal pituitary r. (TPR)
transthoracic vertebral body r.
transurethral r.
transverse r.
tumor r.
ultralow anterior r.
unilateral r.
VATS wedge r.
vertebral r.
Weaver-Dunn r.
wedge r.
Whipple r.

resectional
r. phase
r. phase of operation
r. technique

resection-arthrodesis
Enneking r.-a.

resection-realignment

resective
r. colostomy
r. surgery

resectoscopy

resedation

reserve
hepatic function r.
life-sustaining hepatic r.

reservoir
r. host
r. of infection
r. mucosal absorption
r. phase
pressurized r.

residual
r. abscess
r. body
r. cleft
r. cyst
r. cystic cavity
r. DCIS
r. disease
r. ductal tissue
r. focus
r. fragment
r. lesion
r. mesorectum
r. neck

residue
pharyngeal r.

resin
r. condensation
r. restoration

resistance
activated protein-C r.
alkylation r.
aortic valve r.
drug r.
extreme drug r. (EDR)
increased systemic vascular r.
insulin r.
mean airway r.
peripheral insulin r.
pulmonary vascular r. (PVR)
systemic vascular r.
tissue r.

resolution
spontaneous r.

resolvent

resonance
r. line
magnetic r. (MR)
nuclear magnetic r. (NMR)

resonant abdomen

resorption

respirable aerosol

respiration
abdominal r.
absent r.
accelerated r.
aerobic r.
agonal r.
amphoric r.
anaerobic r.
apneustic r.
artificial r.
assisted r.
asthmoid r.
Austin Flint r.
Biot r.
Bouchut r.
bronchial r.
bronchocavernous r.
bronchovesicular r.
cavernous r.
central r.
cerebral r.
Cheyne-Stokes r.
cogwheel r.
collateral r.
controlled diaphragmatic r.
Corrigan r.
cortical r.
costal r.
cyclic r.
decreased r.
diaphragmatic r.
diaphragmatic-abdominal r.

diffusion r.
direct r.
divided r.
electrophrenic r.
external r.
forced r.
granular r.
grunting r.
harsh r.
internal r.
interrupted r.
intrauterine r.
jerky r.
Kussmaul r.
Kussmaul-Kien r.
labored r.
laryngeal r.
meningitic r.
metamorphosing r.
mouth-to-mouth r.
nasal r.
nervous r.
opposition r.
oral r.
paradoxical r.
periodic r.
placental r.
puerile r.
radiofrequency electrophrenic r.
rude r.
Seitz metamorphosing r.
shallow r.
sighing r.
slow r.
sonorous r.
stertorous r.
stridulous r.
supplementary r.
suppressed r.
temperature, pulse, and r.
thoracic r.
tissue r.
transitional r.
tubular r.
ventilator-assisted r.
vesiculocavernous r.
vicarious r.
wavy r.

respirator
r. brain
r. lung

respiratoria

respiratorii

respiratorium

respiratory
r. ataxia
r. bronchiole
r. care
r. complication
r. compromise
r. depression
r. distress syndrome (RDS)
r. exchange
r. excursion
r. failure
r. insufficiency
r. inversion point
r. kinetic therapy
r. minute volume
r. syncytial virus conduit
r. syncytial virus infection
r. tract
r. tract fluid
r. tract infection

respiratory-esophageal fistula

response
anabolic r.
auditory middle-latency r. (AMLR)
baroreflex r.
biobehavioral r.
brainstem evoked r.
canal resonance r.
carbon dioxide r.
central carbon dioxide ventilatory r.
clinical r.
Cushing pressure r.
deconditioned exercise r.
detector r.
foreign body r.
hemodynamic r.
hepatic arterial buffer r.
hypercapnic ventilatory r.
hypercontractile external sphincter r.
hypermetabolic r.
hypnotic r.
hypoxic ventilatory r.
immune r.
implantation r.
inflammatory r.
irritant patch-test r.
lactation letdown r.
local twitch r. (LTR)
metabolic r.
motor r.

NOTES

response *(continued)*
motor-evoked r. (MER)
paired vasomotor r.
postburn hypermetabolic r.
radiation r.
relaxation r.
renal artery r.
senior-level trauma-team r.
sensitization r.
skin potential r.
snout r.
steady-state auditory evoked r. (SSAER)
steady-state ventilatory r.
stress r.
sympathoadrenal r.
sympathoexcitatory r.
transient auditory evoked r. (TAER)
twitch r.
ventilatory r.
white line r.

responsiveness
airway r.
baroreflex r.

rest
r. jaw relation
r. position

restenosis
aortic valve r.
r. lesion
postangioplasty r.
postballoon angioplasty r.
pulmonary valve r.

restiform body

resting
r. anal sphincter pressure
r. energy expenditure
r. length-tension relation
r. line
r. membrane potential
r. urethral pressure profile

restoration
acid-etched r.
adhesive resin-bonded cast r.
afterroot amputation r.
alloy r.
amalgam r.
Berens-Smith cul-de-sac r.
bonded cast r.
buccal r.
ceramic r.
ceramometal r.
combination r.
composite resin r.
compound r.
contour r.
r. contour
crown r.
cusp r.
dental r.
direct acrylic r.
direct composite resin r.
direct gold r.
direct resin r.
distal extension r.
esthetic r.
facial r.
facilitating r.
faulty r.
foreskin r.
full cast r.
implant r.
IMZ type r.
inlay r.
intermediate r.
intrinsic r.
large r.
maxillary r.
metal-ceramic r.
metallic r.
overhanging r.
overlay r.
permanent r.
physical r.
pinch r.
pin-supported r.
r. point
porcelain-bonded r.
porcelain-fused-to-metal r.
porcelain jacket r.
postcore r.
prosthetic r.
provisional r.
resin r.
root canal r.
silicate r.
silver amalgam r.
temporary r.
voice r.

restorative
r. colectomy
r. fixation
r. procedure
r. proctectomy
r. proctocolectomy
r. proctocolectomy technique

restriction
r. endonuclease analysis
extension r.
r. fragment length
soft-tissue r.

result
angiographic r.
cosmetic r.
cytologic r.

false-negative r.
false-positive r.
histologic r.
indocyanine green clearance r.
operative r.
postoperative r.
postprandial motor r.
short-term r.
surveillance, epidemiology, and end r. (SEER)
true-negative r.
true-positive r.

resurfacing
r. operation
r. procedure

resurgence

resuscitate

resuscitated by volume

resuscitation
blood-substitute r.
cardiac r.
cardiopulmonary r. (CPR)
delayed r.
emergency-department r.
r. endpoint
fluid r.
heart-lung r.
hypertonic-hyperoncotic fluid r.
hypotensive r.
inotrope r.
intrauterine r.
mouth-to-mouth r.
neonatal r.
newborn r.
r. period
prehospital r.
r. process
r. protocol
rapid volume r.
supranormal r.
supraphysiologic r.

resuscitation-induced pulmonary apoptosis

resuscitative
r. endpoint
r. fluid
r. thoracotomy

retained
r. foreign body
r. papilla technique
r. placental fragment

retainer closure

retard
expiratory r.

retardation
developmental r.
fetal growth r.
growth r.
healing r.
intrauterine growth r.
psychomotor r.

retching

rete, pl. **retia**
r. cord
Haller r.

retention
r. cyst
extracoronal r.
intracoronal-extracoronal r.
r. mucocele
pin r.
r. point
surgical r.
r. suture bridge
r. suture technique
urinary r.
viscera r.

retentive fulcrum line

Rethi incision

retia (*pl. of* rete)

retial

reticula (*pl. of* reticulum)

reticular
r. formation
r. lesion
r. membrane

reticularis

reticulate pigmented anomaly

reticulation

reticuloendothelioma

reticulogranuloma

reticulohistiocytoma

reticulospinal tract

reticulotomy

reticulum, pl. **reticula**
Ebner r.
extraconal fat r.

retina, pl. **retinae**

retinaculum, pl. **retinacula**
antebrachial flexor r.
caudal r.
extensor r.
Morgagni r.
patellar r.

NOTES

retinaculum *(continued)*
peroneal r.
superior peroneal r.
retinal
r. arteriovenous malformation
r. circulation
r. examination
r. excavation
r. exudate
r. flap
r. fold
r. hemorrhage
r. imbrication
r. involvement
r. macula
r. migraine
r. phacoma
r. pigment epithelial cell
r. quadrant neovascularization
r. scatter photocoagulation
r. surgeon
r. surgery
r. treatment
retinectomy
retinitis
retinoblastoma
retinoblastoma-mental retardation syndrome
retinochoroidectomy
retinocytoma
retinoic acid
retinopathy
diabetic r.
r. hemorrhage
retinopexy
pneumatic r.
retinophotoscopy
retinoscopy
Copeland r.
cylinder r.
fogging r.
streak r.
retinotomy
retothelioma
retract
retracted stoma
retractile testis
retraction
r. of clot
downward r.
lateral r.
nipple r.
panniculus r.
scar r.
soft-palate r.
r. space
stomal r.
wound r.
retractor
r. plication
retraining
computerized diaphragmatic breathing r. (CDBR)
retransplantation
cardiac r.
retreat
stabilization on r.
retreatment
lithotripsy r.
retrenchment
retrieval
intravascular foreign body r.
transvaginal ultrasonically guided oocyte r.
retroacetabular lesion
retroadductor space
retroauricular
r. free flap
r. incision
r. node
retrobulbar
r. anesthesia
r. anesthetic technique
r. hemorrhage
r. injection
r. mass
r. nerve block
r. orbital metastasis
r. space
retrocalcaneal bursa
retrocardiac
r. mass
r. space
retrocaval ureter
retrocecal
r. abscess
r. hernia
r. recess
retrocecales
retrocecalis
retrocervical
retrochiasmal
r. lesion
r. optic tract
retroclavicular injury
retroclination
retroclival structure
retroclusion
retrocolic
r. end-to-end pancreatojejunostomy
r. end-to-side choledochojejunostomy
r. end-to-side gastrojejunostomy
r. hernia
r. position
retrocollic
retrocorneal membrane

retrocrural
r. celiac plexus block
r. space
retrocuspid papilla
retrodeviation
retrodiskal
r. pad
r. temporomandibular joint pad inflammation
retrodisplacement
retroduodenal
r. artery
r. fossa
r. perforation
r. recess
retroduodenalis
retroesophageal
r. artery
r. space
retrofilling method
retroflected
retroflection
retroflexed
retroflexion
endoscopic r.
retrogasserian
r. neurectomy
r. neurotomy
r. procedure
retrogastric space
retrogeniculate lesion
retrograde
r. atrial activation mapping
r. balloon rupture
r. cannulation
r. catheter insertion
r. catheterization
r. cholangiogram
r. cholecystectomy
r. direction
r. duodenogastroscopy
r. endoscopic approach
r. femoral approach
r. hernia
r. incarceration
r. insertion point
r. intrarenal surgery
myocardium r.
r. nailing
r. nephrostomy puncture
r. obturation
r. root canal filling method
r. sphincterotomy
r. tracheal intubation anesthetic technique
r. transurethral prostatic urethroplasty
r. vascularization of superior mesenteric artery
retrohepatic
r. inferior vena cava
r. IVC
r. vein
retrohyoid bursa
retrohyoidea
retroiliac ureter
retroillumination
retroinguinale
retroinguinal space
retrojection
retrojector
retrolabyrinthine
r. presigmoid approach
r. vestibular neurectomy
retrolabyrinthine-retrosigmoid vestibular neurectomy
retrolental space
retrolingual
retrolisthesis positional dyskinesia
retromammary space
retromandibular
r. fossa
r. point
r. vein
retromandibularis
retromastoid suboccipital craniectomy
retromolar
r. fossa
r. pad
r. papilla
r. triangle
retromuscular
r. position
r. prosthetic technique
r. space
retromylohyoid space
retroocular space
retropancreatic
r. lymph node basin
retropatellar fat pad
retroperitoneal
r. adenopathy
r. approach
r. bleeding

NOTES

retroperitoneal *(continued)*
- r. cavity
- r. cutaneous ureterostomy
- r. decompression
- r. fistula
- r. gas insufflation
- r. hematoma
- r. hemorrhage
- r. hernia
- r. infection
- r. lymphadenectomy
- r. node
- r. pancreas
- r. pelvic lymph node dissection (RPLND)
- r. perforation
- r. pneumography
- r. primary rhabdomyosarcoma
- r. region
- r. soft tissue
- r. space
- r. structure
- r. viscus

retroperitoneale
retroperitoneal-iliopsoas abscess
retroperitoneoscopic nephrectomy
retroperitoneoscopy
retroperitoneum
retroperitonitis
retropharyngeal
- r. approach
- r. hematoma
- r. hemorrhage
- r. node
- r. soft tissue
- r. space

retropharyngeales
retropharyngeum
retropharynx
retroplacental hematoma
retroposed
retroposition
retropubic
- r. colpourethrocystopexy
- r. hernia
- r. Lapides-Ball bladder neck suspension
- r. space
- r. urethrolysis
- r. urethropexy
- r. urethroscopy
- r. vesiculoprostatectomy

retropubicum
retropulsed bone excision
retropulsion
retropyloric
- r. node

retropylorici
retrorectal abscess
retrosacral fascia
retrosellar structure
retrosigmoid approach
retrospection
retrospective analysis
retrosphenoidal syndrome
retrosternal
- r. air space
- r. dislocation
- r. gland
- r. hernia
- r. mass
- r. route

retrotracheal space
retrouterine
retroversioflexion
retroversion
retroverted
retrovesical space
retrovirus infection
retrovisceral
- r. fascia
- r. space

retrozygomatic space
retruded
- r. jaw relation
- r. position

retrusive excursion
return
- pulmonary venous r.
- total anomalous pulmonary venous r.
- venous r.

retzii
Retzius
- R. cavity
- line of R.
- R. space

reuniens duct
reunient
reuptake-inhibitor
- monoamine r.-i.

revaccination
revascularization
- arrested-heart r.
- arterial r.
- brain r.
- cerebral r.
- coronary r.
- heart laser r.
- lower extremity r.
- myocardial r.
- penile r.
- percutaneous transluminal coronary r.
- r. procedure
- renal r.

repeat r.
transmyocardial carbon dioxide laser r.
transmyocardial laser r. (TMLR, TMR)
revascularized tissue
reverberation
echo r.
r. room
Reverdin
R. bunionectomy
R. epidermal free graft
R. method
R. osteotomy
Reverdin-Laird
R.-L. bunionectomy
R.-L. osteotomy
Reverdin-McBride bunionectomy
reversal
ileostomy r.
r. jejunoileal bypass surgery
JIB r.
r. line
narcotic r.
r. pedicle flap
pressure r.
relaxant r.
sex r.
unfractionated heparin r.
vasectomy r.
reverse
r. augmentation
r. Barton fracture
r. bevel incision
r. Bigelow maneuver
r. Colles fracture
r. crossfinger flap
r. Dillwyn-Evans calcaneal osteotomy
r. Eck fistula
r. filling procedure
r. forearm island flap
r. gastric tube esophagoplasty
r. Hill-Sachs lesion
r. Mauck procedure
r. Monteggia fracture
r. phonation
r. Putti-Platt procedure
r. sigma penoscrotal transposition repair
r. topographic projection
r. transcriptase-polymerase chain reaction (RT-PCR)
r. Trendelenburg position
r. wedge osteotomy
r. wedge technique
reversed
r. left saphenous vein bypass graft
r. reimplanted appendicocystostomy
reverse-Y incision
reversible
r. decortication
r. shock
revision
r. hip arthroplasty
r. laparoscopy
r. procedure
shunt r.
revivification
revulsion
rewarming
Rex-Cantli-Serege line
RFCA
radiofrequency catheter ablation
RFTA
radiofrequency thermal ablation
rhabdomyolysis
acute recurrent r.
exertional r.
familial paroxysmal r.
hypoxia-induced r.
idiopathic paroxysmal r.
rhabdomyoma
cardiac r.
clinically silent r.
rhabdomyosarcoma
abdominal wall r.
advanced retroperitoneal r.
alveolar r.
primary r.
retroperitoneal primary r.
vaginal r.
rhabdosarcoma
rhabdosphincter
rhachotomy
Capener lateral r.
decompression r.
lateral r.
rhegma
rhegmatogenous
rheologic therapy

NOTES

Rhese
R. position
R. projection
rheumatica
polymyalgia r.
rheumatoid arthritis
rheumatoid-related ulceration
rhexis
hemorrhage per r.
rhinitis
rhinocanthectomy
rhinocerebral infection
rhinocheiloplasty
rhinocleisis
rhinodymia
rhinokyphectomy
rhinology
rhinopharyngeal
rhinopharynx
rhinoplasty
English r.
esthetic r.
Indian r.
Italian r.
Joseph r.
rhinoscleroma
rhinoscopy
rhinoseptal approach
rhinotomy
rhizolysis
percutaneous glycerol r.
percutaneous radiofrequency r.
percutaneous retrogasserian glycerol r.
***Rhizopus* infection**
rhizotomy
anterior r.
bilateral ventral r.
cranial nerve r.
Dana posterior r.
dorsal r.
facet r.
Frazier-Spiller r.
glycerol r.
intracranial r.
intradural dorsal spinal root r.
percutaneous radiofrequency r.
percutaneous radiofrequency dorsal r.
posterior r.
radiofrequency r.
selective posterior r.
selective sacral r.
thermal r.
trigeminal r.
rhombic
rhomboatloideus
rhombocele
rhomboid
r. ligament
r. major muscle
r. minor muscle
r. transposition flap
rhomboidal sinus
rhonchus, pl. **rhonchi**
expiratory rhonchi
rhoton suction
rhythm
ectopic r.
fibrillation r.
r. method
rhythmic
r. initiation technique
r. stabilization
rhytid
rhytidectomy
rhytidoplasty
rib
bicipital r.
bifid r.
cervical r.
costochondral r.
double-exposed r.
false r.
floating r.
r. fracture
lumbar r.
r. notching
pillar r.
r. removal
slipping r.
r. tip syndrome
true r.
vertebral r.
vertebrochondral r.
vertebrosternal r.
ribbon
r. arch technique
r. muscle
rib-cage volume
Ribes ganglion
rice body
Richard fringe
Richardson
R. procedure
R. suture technique
Riche-Cannieu anastomosis
Richet operation
Richter
R. and Albrich procedure
R. hernia
R. suture technique
Richter-Monro line
rickets
celiac r.
Ricketts-Abrams technique

rickettsial infection
Rideal-Walker method
Rideau technique
ridge
bicipital r.
epidermal r.
r. extension
external oblique r.
mesonephric r.
mylohyoid r.
osteochondral r.
Passavant r.
petrous r.
pharyngeal r.
r. relation
sphenoidal r.
supraorbital r.
temporal r.
trapezoid r.
urogenital r.
Ridley sinus
Ridlon procedure
Riedel
R. frontoethmoidectomy procedure
R. lobe
Rieger syndrome
Rieux hernia
Righini procedure
right
r. acromiodorsoposterior position
r. anterior oblique (RAO)
r. anterior oblique angulation
r. anterior occipital
r. anterior pararenal space
r. atrial pressure
r. branch
r. bundle-branch block
r. caudate lobe
r. colic artery
r. common iliac nerve
r. coronary valve
r. crural area
deviation to the r.
r. femoral artery
r. fibrous trigone
r. heart catheterization
r. hemidiaphragm
r. hypochondriac region
r. iliac region
r. inguinal hernia (RIH)
r. lateral region
r. lobe hepatectomy
r. lower extremity
r. lymphatic duct
r. main bronchus
r. middle suprarenal artery
r. midinguinal line
r. obturator artery
r. ovary
r. prostatic ligament
r. replaced hepatic artery
r. rotation
r. sagittal fissure
r. septal valve
r. sigmoid sinus
r. subclavian artery
r. subclavian vessel
r. temporoparietal craniotomy
r. testicular artery
r. thorax
r. triangular ligament
r. umbilical fold
r. upper extremity
r. upper quadrant
r. upper quadrant peritonectomy
r. ventricle
r. ventricle-pulmonary artery conduit surgery
r. ventricular end-diastolic pressure
r. ventricular outflow tract (RVOT)
r. ventricular outflow tract tachycardia
R. Ventricular Stroke Work Index (RVSWI)
r. ventricular systolic pressure
right-angled end-to-side anastomosis
right-angle technique
right-sided
r.-s. injury
r.-s. lesion
r.-s. submandibular transverse incision
r.-s. thoracotomy
right-side-down position
right-to-left shunt ratio
rigid
r. body
r. bronchoscopy
r. cervical immobilization
r. endofluoroscopy
r. endoscopic surgery
r. graft
r. grafting
r. internal fixation

NOTES

rigid *(continued)*
r. plate fixation
r. proctoscopy
r. proctosigmoidoscopy
r. ureteroscopy
rigidity
abdominal r.
boardlike r.
spinal fixation r.
rigors
frank r.
RIH
right inguinal hernia
Riley-Day syndrome
Riley-Smith syndrome
rim
r. incision
palpebral r.
r. resection
surgical occlusion r.
rima, pl. **rimae**
rim-enhancing lesion
ring
abdominal r.
abscess r.
r. abscess
amnion r.
anorectal r.
anterior limiting r.
aortic r.
r. apophysis
arterial r.
atrial r.
atrioventricular r.
B r.
r. block digital anesthetic
cardiac lymphatic r.
cataract mask r.
choroidal r.
ciliary r.
Coats white r.
collagenous trabecular r.
common annular r.
common tendinous r.
congenital r.
conjunctival r.
constriction r.
contractile r.
coronary r.
corrin r.
cricoid r.
crural r.
deep inguinal r.
distal esophageal r.
double r.
doughnut r.
drop-lock r.
dural r.
enhancing r.
epiphysial r.
r. epiphysis
esophageal A, B r.
esophageal contractile r.
esophageal contraction r.
esophageal mucosal r.
esophageal muscular r.
external inguinal r.
extracapsular arterial r.
femoral r.
fibrous r.
r. finger
r. fracture
glaucomatous r.
glial r.
gold r.
greater r.
head r.
hymenal r.
ilioinguinal r.
iliopsoas r.
inguinal r.
internal abdominal r.
internal inguinal r.
iris r.
ischial weightbearing r.
lenticular r.
r. lesion
lesser r.
lymphoid r.
mucosal esophageal r.
muscular esophageal r.
narrow internal r.
neonatal r.
orthosis drop-lock r.
osseoligamentous r.
palatopharyngeal r.
pathologic retraction r.
pelvic r.
perichondral r.
periureteric venous r.
physiologic retraction r.
Placido r.
posterior limiting r.
pressure r.
pressure-point tension r.
protrusio r.
proximal-to-distal r.
pyloric r.
reduction r.
rust r.
Schatzki esophageal r.
Schwalbe anterior border r.
scotoma r.
Soemmerring r.
r. structure
subcutaneous r.

r. sublimis apponensplasty
symblepharon r.
tentorial r.
tracheal r.
trigonal r.
T-shaped constriction r.
tympanic r.
r. ulcer
umbilical r.
vascular r.
Vieussens r.
Waldeyer r.
white r.
wide internal inguinal r.

ring-disrupting fracture

Ringer arthroscopy

ring-form congenital cataract

ring-shaped cataract

ring-wall lesion

ringworm

Rinkel serial endpoint titration

Riolan
R. anastomosis
R. arc
R. arcade
R. bone
R. muscle

Riordan
R. pollicization
R. tendon transfer technique

Ripstein
R. anterior sling rectopexy
R. procedure
R. rectal prolapse operation

Risdon approach

rise
pressure r.

Riseborough-Radin intercondylar fracture classification

risk
r. of anesthesia
anesthetic r.
bleeding r.
breast cancer r.
r. factor
Goldman classification operative r.
inherent r.
r. management of anesthesia
perforation r.
radiation r.
r. reduction
surgical r.

risorius
r. muscle

Risser
R. method
R. technique

Ritgen maneuver

Ritter-Oleson technique

Riva-Rocci method

Rives splenectomy

Rivinus
R. canal
R. duct
R. gland

Rizzoli operation

RK
radial keratotomy

RLT
reduced liver transplant

Roaf syndrome

Robert pelvis

Roberts
R. approach
R. syndrome
R. technique

robertsonian fusion

Robertson incision

Robinson
R. anterior cervical diskectomy
R. cervical spine fusion
R. morcellation

Robinson-Chung-Farahvar clavicular morcellation

Robinson-Southwick fusion technique

robotic surgery

Robson
R. point
R. position

Rochester method

Rockwood
R. acromioclavicular injury classification
R. clavicular fracture classification
R. posterior capsulorrhaphy
R. procedure
R. resection

Rockwood-Green technique

Rockwood-Matsen capsular shift procedure

rod
r. cell
r. contour preparation
r. fiber

NOTES

rod *(continued)*
r. fracture repair
r. granule
r. migration
r. placement
r. rotation prevention
r. sleeve fixation
r. spherule
Rodeck method
rod-hook construct
rodless end-loop stoma
Rodman incision
Rodney Smith biliary stricture repair
Roeder loop knot
roentgenographic evaluation
Rogers cervical fusion technique
Röhrer index
Rokitansky hernia
rolandic
r. artery
r. line
r. vein
Rolando
R. fissure
R. fracture
R. vein
role
r. fixation
inhibitory r.
roll
iliac r.
scleral r.
r. stitch
rolled shoulder lesion
rollerball
r. endometrial ablation
r. technique
Rollet incision
rolling
r. hiatal hernia
r. membrane
roll-tube technique
ROM
range of motion
rongeured
Rood technique
roof fracture
roof-patch graft
room
emergency r. (ER)
operating r. (OR)
recovery r.
reverberation r.
surgical dressing r.
trauma r.
Roos approach
root
accessory nerve r.
r. amputation
anatomical r.
r. anomaly
ansa cervicalis r.
anterior r.
bifurcation of r.
r. canal
r. canal access
r. canal débridement
r. canal disinfection
r. canal electrosterilization
r. canal filling
r. canal filling technique obturation
r. canal ionization
r. canal orifice
r. canal point
r. canal restoration
r. canal shaping
r. canal sterilization
r. canal therapy
r. canal treatment
ciliary ganglion r.
r. compression
dorsal r.
dural nerve r.
r. end resection
facial r.
facial nerve r.
r. formation
r. fracture
r. furcation
r. fusion
glossopharyngeal nerve r.
r. infiltration
r. injection
lateral r.
nail r.
nerve r.
r. perforation
posterior r.
spinal r.
trigeminal nerve r.
vagus nerve r.
ventral r.
Root-Siegal varus derotational osteotomy
rope flap
Rorabeck fasciotomy
Rosalki technique
Rosch modification
Rose
R. position
R. procedure
rosebud stoma
Rosenberg endoscopic anterior cruciate ligament reconstruction
Rosenburg operation
Rosengren operation
Rosen incision

Rosenmüller
R. body
R. fossa
R. gland
R. node
organ of R.
R. recess
valve of R.
Rosenthal
basal vein of R.
R. fiber
R. nail injury classification
R. vein
Roser-Nélaton line
Ross
R. body
R. procedure
R. technique
Rossetti modification of Nissen fundoplication
Ross-Jones test
rostra (*pl. of* rostrum)
rostrad
rostral
r. cingulotomy
r. transtentorial herniation
r. ventrolateral medulla
r. ventrolateral medulla oblongata
rostralis
rostrate
rostriform
rostrocaudal extent signal abnormality
rostrum, pl. **rostra**
rotary
r. joint
r. mounted point
r. shadowing electron microscopy
r. subluxation
rotated
externally r.
rotating
r. aspiration thromboembolectomy
r. disk oxygenation
r. frame imaging
rotating-frame zeugmatography
rotation
abduction-external r.
anisotropic r.
anterior innominate r.
axial r.
axis of r.
Borggreve limb r.
cervical general r.
clockwise r.
counterclockwise r.
r. drawer test
external r.
external-internal r.
eye r.
r. flap
flexion in abduction and external r.
flexion in adduction and internal r.
foot r.
forceps r.
r. fracture
gantry r.
hip r.
horizontal external r.
intentional r.
internal r.
internal-external r.
intersegmental r.
intestinal r.
inversion-eversion r.
inward r.
r. joint
knee r.
left r.
lumbar r.
manual r.
medial r.
r. mobility
neutral r.
opioid r.
optical r.
organoaxial r.
outward r.
pelvic r.
r. plasty
polycentric r.
posterior innominate r.
pronation-eversion-external r.
pure r.
r. recurvatum test
right r.
sagittal r.
shoulder r.
specific r.
spine r.
sternal r.
supination-external r.
synchronous scapuloclavicular r.
r. testing

NOTES

rotation *(continued)*
r. therapy
timed intermittent r.
twin bracket tooth r.
vertebral r.
visceral r.
wheel r.
rotational
r. ablation
r. burst fracture
r. contact lithotripsy
r. coronary atherectomy
r. correction
r. deformity
r. dislocation
r. flap
r. osteotomy
r. thrombectomy
rotationally induced shear-strain lesion
rotation-compression maneuver
rotationplasty
Kotz-Salzer r.
Van Ness r.
Winkelmann r.
rotator
r. cuff
r. cuff arthropathy
r. cuff lesion
r. cuff muscle
r. cuff repair
r. cuff tear
r. cuff tear arthroplasty
external r.
r. flap
internal r.
medial r.
nucleus r.
rotatores
rotatory luxation
rotavirus infection
Rothman Institute total hip program
Rotterdam Symptom Checklist
rotunda
rotundum
Rouget bulb
rough tissue handling
rouleaux formation
round
r. back deformity
r. body
r. foramen
r. hemorrhage
r. pelvis
r. shoulder deformity
r. spermatid
r. uterine ligament
rounded contour
round-robin classification
route
r. of administration
endoscopic r.
external r.
r. of injection
r. of insertion
retrosternal r.
subcutaneous r.
transthoracic r.
routine
r. bilateral neck exploration
r. laparotomy
r. unilateral exploration
Rouviere
node of R.
Roux
R. gastric reconstruction
R. gastroenterostomy
R. limb
R. limb stump
R. limb stump dehiscence
R. limb stump leak
R. stasis syndrome
Roux-duToit staple capsulorrhaphy
Roux-en-Y
R.-e.-Y. biliary bypass
R.-e.-Y. biliary bypass with antrectomy
R.-e.-Y. choledochojejunostomy
R.-e.-Y. cystojejunostomy
R.-e.-Y. distal jejunoileostomy
R.-e.-Y. esophagojejunostomy
R.-e.-Y. gastric bypass
R.-e.-Y. gastroenterostomy
R.-e.-Y. gastrojejunostomy
R.-e.-Y. hepaticojejunal anastomosis
R.-e.-Y. hepaticojejunostomy
R.-e.-Y. hepatojejunostomy
R.-e.-Y. jejunal loop incision
R.-e.-Y. limb
R.-e.-Y. limb enteroscopy
R.-e.-Y. loop
R.-e.-Y. operation
R.-e.-Y. pancreaticojejunostomy
R.-e.-Y. procedure
R.-e.-Y. procedure with vagotomy
R.-e.-Y. reconstruction
Roux-Goldthwait
R.-G. dislocation operation
R.-G. procedure
Roveda operation
Rovsing operation
Rowbotham
R. operation
R. orbital decompression
Rowe
R. calcaneal fracture classification
R. posterior shoulder approach

Rowe-Lowell
R.-L. hip dislocation classification
R.-L. system for fracture-dislocation classification
Rowe-Zarins shoulder immobilization
Rowinski
R. dacryostomy
R. operation
Royle-Thompson transfer technique
RPC
recurrent pyogenic cholangiohepatitis
RPLND
retroperitoneal pelvic lymph node dissection
RPT
rapid pull-through
RPT technique
R0, R1, R2 resection
RSI
rapid-sequence induction
RSI orotracheal intubation
RTPA, rtPA
recombinant tissue-type plasminogen activator
RT-PCR
reverse transcriptase-polymerase chain reaction
rub
peritoneal friction r.
textured fabric r.
rubber
r. band hemorrhoidectomy
r. tissue
rubber-band
r.-b. extraction
r.-b. ligation
r.-b. ligation of hemorrhoid
rubbery
r. mass
r. texture
rubbing
desensitization with towel r.
Rubbrecht
R. extirpation
R. operation
Rubens breast flap
Rubin
R. maneuver
R. tubal insufflation
rubra
rubrobulbar tract
rubroreticular tract
rubrospinal
r. decussation
r. tract
Rucker body
Ruddy incision
rude respiration
Ruedemann operation
Ruedi-Allgower classification
ruffed canal
ruga, pl. **rugae**
rugal column
rugine
rugose
rugosity
rugous
Ruiz
R. procedure
R. trapezoidal keratotomy
Ruiz-Mora
R.-M. correction
R.-M. procedure
rule
Fletcher r. of irradiation tolerance
Meyer-Overton r.
Simpson r.
Steel r. of thirds
Rungstrom projection
running
r. continuous suture technique
r. vascular technique
r. vascular technique without tension
runoff
Runyon classification
rupture
Achilles tendon r.
acute hepatic r.
adductor longus muscle r.
amnion r.
aneurysmal r.
anterior talofibular ligament r.
aortic r.
balloon r.
cardiac r.
chamber r.
chordae tendineae r.
chordal r.
choroidal r.
collateral ligament r.
complete r.
crescentic r.
diaphragmatic r.

NOTES

rupture *(continued)*
distal biceps brachii tendon r.
ERCP-induced splenic r.
esophageal r.
flexor tendon r.
Frank intrabiliary r.
gastric r.
hemidiaphragm r.
hepatic r.
hernia r.
hydatid cyst intrahepatic r.
incidental r.
inflammatory r.
infrapatellar tendon r.
interventricular septal r.
intramural esophageal r.
intraoperative r.
intraperitoneal viscus r.
intrapleural r.
longitudinal ligament r.
Mallory-Weiss mucosal r.
marginal sinus r.
membrane r.
mesenteric r.
myocardial r.
neglected r.
nonpenetrating r.
papillary muscle r.
penetrating r.
penile r.
plaque r.
postmembrane r.
prelabor membrane r.
premature amnion r.
premature membrane r.
premembrane r.
prolonged r.
proximal tendon r.
renal allograft r.
retrograde balloon r.
scar r.
scleral r.
splenic r.
spontaneous r.
stress r.
tendon r.
testicular r.
total perineal r.
transverse ligament r.
traumatic aortic r.
traumatic choroidal r.
tubal r.
ulnar collateral ligament r.
umbilical hernia r.
urinary bladder r.
uterine r.
valve r.
ventricular septal r.

ruptured
r. abdominal aortic aneurysm
r. disk
r. disk excision
r. episiotomy
r. peliotic lesion

rupture-delivery interval

Russe
R. classification
R. technique

Russe-Gerhardt method

Russell
R. fibular head autograft
hooked bundle of R.
R. percutaneous endoscopic gastrostomy
R. technique
uncinate bundle of R.

Russell-Taylor classification

rust ring

Rüter classification

Rutkow-Robbins-Gilbert classification

Rutledge extended hysterectomy classification

ruyschian membrane

Ruysch membrane

RVOT
right ventricular outflow tract

RVSWI
Right Ventricular Stroke Work Index

RWMA
regional wall motion abnormality

Rycroft operation

Rye Hodgkin disease classification

Ryerson
R. bone graft
R. procedure
R. technique

SA
septal apical
spinal anesthesia
splenic artery
SA segment
S-A
sinoatrial
SAAST
Self-Administered Alcoholism Screening test
saber-cut
s.-c. approach
s.-c. incision
sabre-shin deformity
sac
abdominal s.
air s.
allantoic s.
alveolar s.
amniotic s.
aneurysmal s.
aortic s.
bursal s.
caudal s.
chorionic s.
common dural s.
conjunctival s.
cupular blind s.
dental s.
double decidual s.
embryonic s.
empty gestational s.
enamel s.
endolymphatic s.
enterocele s.
s. extirpation
fluid-filled s.
s. formation
gestational s.
giant prosthetic reinforcement of the visceral s. (GPRVS)
greater peritoneal s.
heart s.
hernia s.
hydrocele s.
indirect hernial s.
lacrimal s.
lateral s.
lesser peritoneal s.
Mikulicz s.
nasolacrimal s.
omental s.
pericardial s.
peritoneal s.
Pleatman s.
pleural s.
preputial s.
primary yolk s.
primitive yolk s.
pseudogestational s.
pudendal s.
secondary yolk s.
serous s.
Stoppa giant prosthetic reinforcement of the visceral s.
tear s.
thecal s.
tooth s.
vestibular blind s.
vitelline s.
wide-mouth s.
yolk s.
saccade
intentional s.
reflexive s.
volitional s.
saccadic
s. eccentric target
s. eye movement
saccate
sacci (*pl. of* saccus)
sacciformis
sacciform recess
saccular
s. aneurysm
s. collection
s. spot
sacculated
sacculation
saccule
sacculotomy
sacculus, pl. **sacculi**
saccus, pl. **sacci**
saclike cavity
sacra (*pl. of* sacrum)
sacrad
sacral
s. ala
s. anesthesia
s. arcuate line
s. bar technique
s. bone tumor
s. brim target point
s. canal
s. cornua
s. crest
s. foramen
s. fracture
s. ganglion
s. hiatus

S

sacral *(continued)*
- s. horizontal plane line
- s. horn
- s. index
- s. pedicle screw fixation
- s. promontory
- s. region
- s. screw placement
- s. spine fixation
- s. spine fusion
- s. spine stabilization
- s. splanchnic nerve
- s. triangle
- s. venous plexus
- s. vertebra

sacrale
sacrales
sacral-foraminal approach
sacralia
sacralis
sacralium
sacralization
sacrectomy
sacred bone
sacri
sacroabdominoperineal pull-through
sacroanterior position
sacrococcygea
sacrococcygeal
- s. cyst
- s. disk
- s. joint
- s. junction
- s. tumor

sacrococcygeus
sacrocolpopexy
sacrodurale
sacrodural ligament
sacrofixation operation
sacrogenital fold
sacroiliac (SI)
- s. articulation
- s. buttressing procedure
- s. disarticulation
- s. dislocation
- s. extension fixation
- s. flexion fixation
- s. fracture

sacroiliaca
sacrolisthesis
sacrolumbalis
sacrolumbar
sacropelvic
sacroperineal approach
sacropexy
- abdominal s.

sacroposterior position
sacrosciatic
sacrospinal
sacrospinale
sacrospinalis
sacrospinosum
sacrospinous
- s. ligament
- s. ligament suspension
- s. ligament vaginal fixation

sacrotomy
sacrotransverse position
sacrotuberale
sacrotuberosum
sacrotuberous ligament
sacrouterine fold
sacrovaginal fold
sacrovertebral
sacrovesical fold
sacrum, pl. **sacra**
- assimilation s.
- s. fracture
- s. fusion screw fixation

saddle
- s. block anesthesia
- s. connector base
- s. lesion
- Turkish s.

saddle-nose deformity
Sade modification of Norwood procedure
Saeed technique
Saemisch
- S. operation
- S. section

Saenger
- S. operation
- S. suture technique

Safar operation
safety
- s. program

Sage-Clark
- S.-C. cheilectomy
- S.-C. technique

Sage-Salvatore acromioclavicular joint injury classification
sagittal
- s. deformity
- s. fissure
- s. plane
- s. plane instability
- s. projection
- s. reconstruction
- s. rotation
- s. section
- s. slice fracture
- s. spin-echo image
- s. suture line
- s. venous sinus

sagittalis

sagittalization
sagittal-plane imaging
sagittal-split mandibular osteotomy
Saha
S. shoulder muscle classification
S. transfer technique
Sahli method
Sakati-Nyhan syndrome
Sakellarides calcaneal fracture classification
Sakellarides-DeWeese technique
Sakoff osteotomy
saline
hypertonic lactated s.
ice-cold s.
s. injection
s. injection therapy
intravenous s.
s. lavage
s. manometer
normal s.
phosphate buffered s. (PBS)
s. solution
s. technique
saline-epinephrine
hypertonic s.-e.
Salinem infection
saliva
salivaris
salivary
s. duct
s. duct carcinoma
s. EGF
s. epithelium
s. fistula
s. gland
s. gland carcinoma
s. gland infection
s. gland tumor
s. mass
salivation
Salle procedure
salmon
s. backcut incision
s. patch
salmon-patch
s.-p. hemorrhage
s.-p. hue
salmon-pink epithelium
salpingectomy
salpinges (*pl. of* salpinx)
salpingian
salpingioma
salpingitis
salpingocele
salpingolysis
salpingoneostomy
salpingo-oophorectomy
abdominal s.-o.
bilateral s.-o.
total abdominal hysterectomy and bilateral s.-o.
unilateral s.-o.
salpingo-oophorocele
salpingo-ovariectomy
salpingo-ovariolysis
salpingopalatine
s. fold
s. membrane
salpingopexy
salpingopharyngeal
s. fascia
s. fold
s. membrane
s. muscle
salpingopharyngeus
salpingoplasty
salpingorrhaphy
salpingoscopy
salpingostomatomy
salpingostomy
linear s.
salpingotomy
abdominal s.
salpinx, pl. **salpinges**
Salter
S. epiphysial fracture classification
S. incremental line
S. innominate osteotomy
S. I-VI fracture
S. pelvic osteotomy
S. technique
Salter-Harris epiphysial fracture classification
salting-out procedure
saltwater solution
salvage
s. balloon angioplasty
s. cystectomy
s. cytology
limb s.
s. procedure
s. prostatectomy

NOTES

S

salvage *(continued)*
s. surgery
s. therapy
Salzman method
SAMBA
simultaneous areolar mastopexy and breast augmentation
same-day discharge
Samilson
S. crescentic calcaneal osteotomy
S. procedure
Sammarco-DiRaimondo modification of Elmslie technique
sample
bile s.
biopsy s.
cytology s.
FNA s.
intraoperative bile s.
peritoneal cytology s.
population s.
wire-guided biopsy s.
sampling
endocervical s.
endometrial s.
fetal tissue s.
incremental blood s.
laparoscopic paraaortic lymph node s.
lymph node s.
percutaneous fetal tissue s.
selective venous s.
tissue s.
venous s.
Sampoelesi line
Sampson cyst
Samuel position
sand
s. body
urinary s.
Sanders
S. incision
S. operation
Sandler-Dodge area-length method
Sandström body
sandwich
s. patch
s. staghorn calculus therapy
sandwiched iliac bone graft
Sanger incision
sanguification
sanguineous
s. exudate
s. infiltration
s. inflammation
s. perfusion
sanitation
sanitization
Santiani-Stone classification
Santorini
S. canal
S. cartilage
S. duct
S. fissure
S. labyrinth
S. major caruncle
S. minor caruncle
S. plexus
S. vein
SaO_2
arterial oxygen saturation
SAP
systolic arterial pressure
saphena
saphenectomy
sapheni
saphenofemoral
saphenous
s. branch
s. flap
s. hiatus
s. ICA bypass
s. opening
s. vein
s. vein bypass
s. vein bypass graft
s. vein patch graft
saphenus
Sappey
S. fiber
S. plexus
saprophyte
SAPS
simplified acute physiology score
sarcocele
sarcoid
sarcoidosis
sarcolemmal membrane
sarcology
sarcoma
Abernethy s.
spindle cell s.
undifferentiated embryonal s.
sarcomatosis
sarcomatosum
glioma s.
myxoma s.
sarcotripsy
Sargenti method
Sarmiento
S. intertrochanteric osteotomy
S. trochanteric fracture technique
sartorial slide procedure
sartorii
sartorius
Sassouni classification

satellite
s. abscess
s. lesion
s. metastasis
s. myofascial trigger point
satellitosis
Sato
S. operation
S. procedure
Satterthwaite method
saturated solution
saturation
s. analysis
arterial oxygen s. (SaO_2)
arterial oxyhemoglobin s. (SpO_2)
color s.
s. current
s. index
jugular bulb venous oxygen s.
jugular venous oxygen s. ($SjVO_2$)
mixed venous oxygen s.
s. output
oxygen s.
partial s.
progressive spin s.
receiver s.
s. recovery
secondary s.
selective s.
s. sound pressure level
step-up in oxygen s.
s. time
s. transfer
venous s.
saturnine colic
saucerization
saucerized biopsy
sausage-shaped appearance
Sauve-Kapandji procedure
Savage perineal body
Savary-Mille grading scale classification
Savin
S. operation
S. procedure
Sawyer operation
Saxtorph maneuver
Sayoc
S. operation
S. procedure
SB
septal basal
SB segment
SBP
systolic blood pressure
SC
subtotal colectomy
supracondylar
SC suspension
Scaglietti
S. closed reduction technique
S. procedure scale
scala, pl. **scalae**
scalar classification
scale
Abbreviated Injury S. (AIS)
addiction acknowledgment s.
addiction potential s.
alcohol dependence s.
Borg treadmill exertion s.
Bromage s.
Charrière s.
children's coma s.
CHIP s.
Cleveland Clinic weighted s. of endoscopic procedure
Colored Visual Analogue S. (CVAS)
coma s.
Coping with Health, Injuries, and Problems s.
dissociation, analgesia, immobility, and tension s.
ECoG performance status s.
Edinburgh 2 Coma S.
EVM grading of Glasgow Coma S.
French s.
Glasgow Coma S. (GCS)
Glasgow Outcome S.
Hospital Anxiety and Depression S.
Karnofsky s.
keratin s.
Lysholm Knee S.
MacAndrew Alcoholism S.
McMaster Quality of Life S.
Medication Quantification S.
Modified Zung Depression S.
Neonatal Infant Pain S. (NIPS)
Objective Pain S.
pain anxiety symptoms s.
pain catastrophizing s.
pediatric trauma s. (PTS)
Progressive Ambulation S.
Scaglietti procedure s.

NOTES

scale *(continued)*
Sessing pressure ulcer assessment s.
Shea pressure ulcer assessment s.
sound pressure level s.
Symptom Distress S.
verbal-rank s.
visual analog s. (VAS)
Volpicelli functional ambulation s.
Zung Depression S.
scalene
s. fascia
s. fat pad biopsy
s. hiatus
s. lymph node biopsy
s. maneuver
s. node biopsy (SNB)
s. tubercle
scalenectomy
scalenotomy
Adson-Coffey s.
scalenus
s. anterior muscle
s. anticus syndrome
s. medius muscle
s. minimus muscle
s. posterior muscle
scaling skin-colored lesion
scalloped closure
scalp
s. closure
s. incision
s. infection
s. laceration
s. muscle
s. sickle flap
subcutaneous s.
scalping
s. flap
s. flap of Converse
scan
biplane s.
computed tomography s.
contrast-enhanced CT s.
cross-vector A s.
CT s.
EMI s.
high-dose s.
iodine-131 whole-body s.
magnetic resonance imaging s.
Meckel s.
omniplane s.
peritoneovenous shunt patency s.
s. plane
postoperative CT s.
pulmonary ventilation s.
radioactive s.
radionuclide s.
scintillation s.
sector s.
serial transverse s.
sestamibi nuclear s.
stimulation s.
time position s.
transesophageal echocardiography s.
transverse s.
ventilation lung s.
ventilation/perfusion lung s.
scan-directed biopsy
Scanlon early neonatal neurobehavioral score
scanning
body s.
contrast-enhanced CT s.
CT s.
s. electron microscopy
external s.
fluorodeoxyglucose-positron emission tomography s.
s. force microscopy
functional activation PET s.
s. laser Doppler flowmetry
longitudinal s.
point s.
positron emission tomography s.
real-time sector s.
scintillation s.
sector s.
sestamibi s.
s. technique
thallium-technetium s.
total-body s.
transverse s.
whole-body s.
Scanzoni maneuver
Scanzoni-Smellie maneuver
scapha
scaphae
scaphocapitate fusion
scaphocephaly
scaphohydrocephalus
scaphoid
s. abdomen
s. bone
s. fossa
s. fracture
s. radius
scaphoidea
scaphoidei
scaphoideum
scapholunate
s. dislocation
s. dissociation
scaphotrapezial trapezoid arthritis
scapi (*pl. of* scapus)
scapula, pl. **scapulae**

scapular
s. approximation test
s. elevation
s. flap
s. line
s. muscle
s. notch
s. peroneal atrophy
s. region
scapularis
scapulectomy
Das Gupta s.
Phelps s.
scapuloanterior position
scapuloclavicular articulation
scapulohumeral
scapuloperoneal syndrome
scapulopexy
scapuloposterior position
scapulothoracic
s. dissociation
s. fusion
scapus, pl. **scapi**
scar
s. carcinoma
s. dehiscence
episiotomy s.
facetted corneal s.
s. formation
gray-white corneal s.
hypertrophic s. (HS)
incisional s.
iridectomy s.
nonpathologic s.
osteopetrotic s.
perineal s.
radial s.
s. retraction
s. rupture
sternotomy s.
thoracotomy s.
s. tissue
s. tissue reaction
Scardino
S. flap
S. vertical flap pyeloplasty
scarf
s. maneuver
s. osteotomy
s. osteotomy-bunionectomy
s. Z-osteotomy
s. Z-osteotomy-bunionectomy
s. Z-plasty
scarification test
scarify
scarless endoscopic thyroidectomy
Scarpa
S. fascia
S. foramen
S. ganglion
S. hiatus
S. liquor
S. method
S. operation
S. sheath
S. triangle
scarred skin
scarring
corneal s.
duodenal s.
gastrostomy s.
hypertrophic s.
obliterative s.
patch test s.
pathology s.
scatoma
scatoscopy
scatter
s. correction
s. photocoagulation
scavenger
superoxide s.
Schaberg-Harper-Allen technique
Schacher ganglion
Schäfer method
Schanz
S. angulation osteotomy
S. femoral osteotomy
Schatzker tibial plateau fracture classification
Schatzki esophageal ring
Schatz maneuver
Schauffler procedure
Schaumann body
Schauta vaginal operation
Schauwecker patellar wiring technique
Schede
S. clot
S. method
S. thoracoplasty
schedule
Edmonton Symptom Assessment S.

NOTES

schedule *(continued)*
Support Team Assessment S. (STAS)
Scheibe malformation
Scheie
S. classification
S. operation
S. syndrome
S. technique
S. thermal sclerostomy
schema
body s.
schematic
scheme
chemotherapeutic s.
Schenk-Eichelter vena cava plastic filter procedure
Schepens
S. operation
S. technique
Schepsis-Leach technique
Scher nail biopsy
scheroma
Schick method
Schiller-Duvall body
Schiller method
Schimek operation
schindylesis
Schirmer operation
schistocystis
schistorrhachis
schistosomal
s. bladder carcinoma
s. cystitis
schistosomiasis
ectopic cutaneous s.
schistothorax
Schlatter
S. gastrectomy technique
S. operation
Schlein elbow arthroplasty
Schlemm canal
Schmalz operation
Schmidel anastomosis
Schneider fixation
schneiderian
s. carcinoma
s. respiratory membrane
Schnute wedge resection technique
Schober
S. method
S. technique
Schobinger incision
Schoemaker
S. anastomosis
S. gastroenterostomy
S. modification
S. procedure
Schonander
S. procedure
S. technique
Schönbein operation
Schoonmaker-King single-catheter technique
Schreger line
Schreiber maneuver
Schrock procedure
Schroeder operation
Schuchardt
S. operation
S. relaxing incision
Schuknecht classification
Schüller
S. duct
S. method
S. projection
Schuller position
Schütz
S. bundle
tract of S.
Schwalbe
S. anterior border ring
S. line
S. space
Schwann cell
schwannoma
Schwartz
S. dorsiflexory osteotomy
S. method
S. tractotomy
Schwartz-Pregenzer urethropexy
Schwarz classification
sciatic
s. hernia
s. nerve block
s. nerve palsy hematoma
s. plexus
s. spine
scientific method
scimitar syndrome
scintigraphy
hepatic s.
sestamibi s.
somatostatin receptor s. (SRS)
scintillation
s. scan
s. scanning
s. vial
scintography
renal s.
scirrhous lesion
scissor-leg position
scissors dissection
scissors-excision hemorrhoidectomy
scissura
sclera, pl. **sclerae**

scleral
s. buckling operation
s. buckling procedure
s. canal
s. ectasia
s. exoplant
s. fistula
s. fistulectomy operation
s. flap
s. hemorrhage
s. resection
s. roll
s. rupture
s. search coil technique
s. shortening operation
s. sulcus
sclerectoiridectomy
sclerectomy
Holth s.
thermal s.
scleriritomy
scleroatrophic cholecystitis
sclerocorneal
s. junction
s. sulcus
sclerodermoid graft-versus-host disease
sclerokeratectomy
scleroma
scleroplasty operation
sclerosant
sclerosing
s. adenosis
s. inflammation
s. lesion
s. osteomyelitis of Garré
s. solution
s. therapy
sclerosis, pl. **scleroses**
pulmonary tuberous s.
tuberous s.
sclerostomy
posterior thermal s.
Scheie thermal s.
sclerotherapy
s. complication
emergent endoscopic s.
endoscopic injection s. (EIS)
endoscopic retrograde s.
endoscopic variceal s.
esophageal variceal s.
s. failure
fiberoptic injection s.
injection s.
intravariceal s.
paravariceal s.
variceal s.
sclerotic
s. bone lesion
s. calvarial patch
s. cemental mass
s. kidney
s. line
s. stomach
scleroticectomy
scleroticotomy
sclerotomy
anterior s.
DeWecker anterior s.
foreign body s.
Lindner s.
s. operation
posterior s.
s. with drainage
s. with exploration
scolicidal fluid
scoliosis
s. correction
s. surgery
scoliotic curve fixation
Scopinaro pancreaticobiliary bypass
score
airway s.
Aldrete s.
American Society of Anesthesiology s.
APACHE-II s.
Apgar s.
BIRADS s.
cosmetic s.
cumulative s.
cumulative pain s. (CPS)
defecation s.
discrimination s.
Dripps-American Surgical Association s.
echo s.
evacuation s.
GIQLI s.
Glasgow Coma s.'s
Glasgow Outcome S. (GOS)
Gleason s.
Injury Severity S. (ISS)

NOTES

score *(continued)*
International Classification of Diseases-9 Version of Injury Severity S. (ICISS)
Lysholm s.
MACIS s.
mangled extremity severity s.
Neurologic and Adaptive Capacity S. (NACS)
Optimal Observation S.
pancreatic necrosis prognostic s.
Parsonnet s.
Peritonitis Severity S. (PSS)
Scanlon early neonatal neurobehavioral s.
simplified acute physiology s. (SAPS)
Steward Recovery S.
symptom s.
Trauma Score and Injury Severity S. (TRISS)
visual analog pain s. (VAPS)
Yale Optimal Observation S.

scoring
s. incision
preoperative s.
s. system

scotoma, pl. **scotomata**
s. junction
s. ring

scotomization

scotoscopy

Scott
S. glenoplasty technique
S. jejunoileal bypass
S. operation
S. posterior glenoplasty

scotty-dog
s.-d. fracture
s.-d. graft

SCPP
spinal cord perfusion pressure

scratch-pad memory

scratch-type incision

screen
coagulation s.
s. filtration pressure
intravascular coagulation s.
s. oxygenation

screening
colonoscopy s.
endocrine s.
s. mammography
presurgical psychological s. (PPS)
s. procedure
s. recommendation
s. test

screw
s. angulation
s. epiphysiodesis
s. fixation
s. implantation
s. insertion
s. insertion technique
s. joint
s. loosening
s. placement
s. position perioperative monitoring
s. stabilization
s. stripout

screw-and-plate fixation

screw-and-wire fixation

screw-home mechanism

screw-in

screw-plate approach

screw-to-screw compression construct

screw-type abutment

scrota (*pl. of* scrotum)

scrotal
s. artery
s. hematocele
s. hernia
s. mass
s. pouch operation
s. pouch orchiopexy
s. raphe
s. septum
s. skin
s. skin ulcer
s. swelling
s. vein

scrotectomy
total s.

scroti

scrotiform

scrotitis

scrotocele

scrotoplasty

scrotoscopy

scrotum, pl. **scrota**

SCS
spinal cord stimulation

Scudder
S. method
S. operation
S. procedure
S. technique

Scuderi
S. procedure
S. repair
S. technique

Scultetus position

scurvy line

scyphiform

scyphoid

SEA
spinal epidural abscess
seal
cavity s.
sealed envelope technique
sealer extrusion
sealing perforation
Sealy-Laragh technique
seamless graft
seatbelt fracture
Seattle classification
sebaceae
sebaceous
s. adenocarcinoma
s. cyst
sebaceum, pl. **sebacea**
adenoma s.
Sebileau
S. hollow
S. muscle
seborrhea
second
s. cranial nerve
s. cuneiform bone
s. degree radiation injury
forced expiratory volume in 1 s. (FEV_1)
s. gas effect
s. intention
s. lumbar artery
s. pain wind-up
s. parallel pelvic plane
s. tibial muscle
secondary
s. adhesion
s. amputation
s. anesthetic
s. arrest
s. arrest of dilatation
s. articulation
s. closure
s. diagnostic biopsy
s. expansion
s. fixation
s. focal point
s. fracture
s. fungal infection
s. gangrene
s. hemorrhage
s. hernia
s. HPT
s. intention
s. lesion
s. membrane
s. myofascial trigger point
s. neuralgia
s. procedure
s. ptosis correction
s. pulmonary lobule
s. reconstruction
s. renal calculus
s. repair
s. retroperitoneal organ
s. saturation
s. stage proctocolectomy
s. surgery
s. suture technique
s. union
s. yolk sac
second-degree
s.-d. burn
s.-d. hemorrhoid
second-echo image
second-generation
second-grade fusion
second-line
s.-l. chemotherapy
s.-l. drug
second-look
s.-l. laparoscopy
s.-l. laparotomy
s.-l. operation
s.-l. surgery
second-set graft rejection
secretin stimulation
secretion
biliary s.
cholecystokinin s.
gastrin s.
insulin s.
pancreatic enzyme s.
tracheal s.
secretory
s. adenocarcinoma
s. duct
s. nerve
sectile
sectio, pl. **sectiones**
section
abdominal s.
attached cranial s.
axial s.
bar s.

NOTES

section *(continued)*
- cesarean s. (C-section)
- classical cesarean s.
- coronal s.
- cross s.
- cryostat s.
- s. cutting
- detached cranial s.
- diagonal s.
- distal shave s.
- extraperitoneal cesarean s.
- s. freeze substitution technique
- frontal s.
- frozen s. (FS)
- Giemsa-stained s.
- horizontal s.
- intraoperative frozen s.
- Kerr cesarean s.
- Latzko cesarean s.
- longitudinal s.
- low cervical cesarean s.
- lower uterine segment transverse cesarean s.
- low transverse cesarean s.
- median s.
- midfrontal plane coronal s.
- midsagittal s.
- nerve cross s.
- oblique s.
- orbital s.
- parasagittal s.
- perineal s.
- permanent s.
- pituitary stalk s.
- plastic s.
- Porro cesarean s.
- primary cesarean s.
- repeat cesarean s.
- Saemisch s.
- sagittal s.
- tangential s.
- thin s.
- transperitoneal cesarean s.
- transverse s.
- vaginal birth after cesarean s.
- vertical s.
- vestibular nerve s.

sectional
- s. root canal filling method
- s. technique

sectiones (*pl. of* sectio)

sectioning
- surgical s.

sector
- s. cut
- end-viewing s.
- s. iridectomy
- s. iridectomy operation
- lateral s.
- medial s.
- s. scan
- s. scanning

sectoral
- s. pedicle
- s. resection

sectorial
- s. branch
- s. resection

secundarium

secundus

secure intracorporeal knot

sedation
- chemical s.
- conscious s.
- ICU s.
- intravenous s.
- IV s.

sedation-induced hypoventilation

sedative
- s. effect
- s. therapy

Seddon
- S. classification
- S. dorsal spine costotransversectomy
- S. modification
- S. nerve graft
- S. technique

sedimentation
- s. equilibrium
- s. index

seeding
- instrument-tract s.
- intraluminal s.
- intraperitoneal s.
- needle tract tumor s.
- peritoneal s.
- surgical s.
- tumor s.

SEER

surveillance, epidemiology, and end result
- SEER Program

SEF

spectral edge frequency

segment
- AA s.
- AB s.
- AM s.
- anterior basal s.
- anterior inferior s.
- anterior superior s.
- apical s.
- apicoposterior s.
- bronchopulmonary s.
- cardiac s.
- cervical s.

colorectal s.
demucosalized augmentation with gastric s. (DAWG)
extramedullary s.
hepatic s.
IA s.
IB s.
inferior lingular s.
intracutaneous s.
LA s.
LB s.
lower uterine s. (LUS)
lumbar s.
medial basal s.
motion s.
occluded s.
posterior basal s.
posterosuperior s.
renal s.
SA s.
SB s.
subapical s.
subsuperior s.
superior lingular s.
venous s.

segmenta (*pl. of* segmentum)

segmental
s. alveolar osteotomy
s. bronchus
s. colonic resection
s. dilatation
s. duct
s. epidural anesthesia
s. explant
s. fixation
s. fracture
s. gastrectomy
s. hepatectomy
s. involvement
s. limb pressure recording
s. lung resection
s. mandibulectomy
s. mastectomy
s. pressure index
s. pulmonary resection
s. sphincter
s. surgery
s. tendon graft
s. vessel
s. wall motion abnormality (SWMA)

segmentalis

segmentation
s. anomaly
k space s.
s. movement
s. root canal filling method
s. sphere
volume s.

segmentectomy

segmented flap

segment-oriented
s.-o. hepatic resection
s.-o. liver resection
s.-o. procedure
s.-o. resection
s.-o. technique

segmentorum

segmentum, pl. **segmenta**

Segond fracture

segregation

Seidelin body

Seiler cartilage

Seinsheimer femoral fracture classification

Seitz metamorphosing respiration

seizure
posttraumatic s.

Selakovich procedure

Seldinger
S. cystic duct catheterization
S. method
S. percutaneous technique
S. procedure
S. retrograde wire/intubation technique

selection pressure

selective
s. anesthesia
s. angiography
s. arterial embolization
s. bowel decontamination
s. bronchial catheterization anesthetic technique
s. catheterization
s. ductal cannulation
s. excitation projection reconstruction imaging
s. inguinal node dissection
s. injection
s. intracoronary thrombolysis
s. irradiation
s. lectin-triggered apoptosis
s. lymphadenectomy

NOTES

selective *(continued)*
s. microadenomectomy
s. nonoperative management
s. photothermolysis
s. portal decompression
s. posterior rhizotomy
s. proximal vagotomy
s. sacral rhizotomy
s. saturation
s. saturation recovery
s. serotonin reuptake inhibitor (SSRI)
s. shunting
s. thoracic spine fusion
s. vascular clamping (SVC)
s. venous sampling
selenoid body
Self-Administered
S.-A. Alcoholism Screening test (SAAST)
Quality of Well-Being Scale S.-A. (QWB-SA)
self-breast examination
self-catheterization
clean intermittent s.-c.
self-expandable
self-expanding
self-help
self-infection
self-mutilation
self-obturation
intermittent s.-o.
self-reduction
self-sealing scleral puncture
self-seal pouch
self-tightening slip knot
Selinger operation
sella
empty s.
s. structure
sellae
sellaris
sellar tumor
Sell-Frank-Johnson extensor shift technique
Sellheim incision
Sellick maneuver
Selye
adaptation syndrome of S.
semantic conditioning
Semb
S. apicolysis
S. nephrectomy technique
semenuria
semicanal
semicanalis
semicartilaginous
semicircular
s. canal
s. duct
s. line of Douglas
semicircularis
semiclosed
s. anesthesia
s. circle
semicoma
semiconductor
extrinsic s.
semiconstrained total elbow arthroplasty
semielective
s. operation
s. status
semiflexed incision
semi-Fowler position
semihyalinization
semiimpermeable membrane
semilateral position
semilinear canonical correlation
semilunar
s. bone
s. cartilage
s. fibrocartilage
s. flap
s. ganglion
s. hiatus
s. incision
s. line
s. valvular septum
semilunaris
semilunate cut
semimembranosi
semimembranosus
s. muscle
s. tendon
semimembranous
seminal
s. colliculus
s. duct
s. fluid
s. gland
s. granule
s. hillock
s. tract
s. tract washout
s. vesicle
s. vesicle aspiration
seminalis
semination
seminiferous
seminis
seminoma
seminomatous
seminuria
semioblique position

semiopen
s. anesthesia
s. hemorrhoidectomy
s. sliding tenotomy
semipedunculated lesion
semipermeable membrane
semipronation
semiprone position
semireclining position
semirecumbent position
semispinalis
s. capitis muscle
s. cervicis muscle
semispinal muscle
semisulcus
semisupination
semisupine
semitendinosus
s. muscle
s. procedure
s. technique
s. tendon
semitendinous
semiupright position
Semm Z technique
Sengstaken-Blakemore method
senile
s. ectasia
s. plaque
senior-level trauma-team response
Senning
S. operation
S. repair
S. transposition procedure
Senn operation
sensate
sensation
s. level
s. time
sense of defecation
sensitive
s. plane
s. plane projection reconstruction imaging
s. point
s. visceral postsurgical disturbance
sensitivity
sensitization
central s.
s. response
sensitizing injection
sensor
calcium s.
multiparameter s.
s. operation
sensoria (*pl. of* sensorium)
sensorimotor stimulation approach
sensorineural acuity level technique
sensorium, pl. **sensoria, sensoriums**
sensory
s. block
s. blockade
s. examination
s. extinction
s. fusion
s. nerve
s. nerve fiber bundle
s. stimulation
s. tract
sentence classification
sentinel
s. blood clot
s. lymphadenectomy
s. lymph node (SLN)
s. lymph node biopsy
s. node
s. node biopsy (SNB)
s. node excision
s. node localization
s. node-to-background ratio (SNBR)
s. spinous process fracture
s. staging
SEP
somatosensory evoked potential
separation
cotton-wool s.
s. point
sepsis, pl. **sepses**
catheter s.
gram-negative s.
gram-positive s.
intraabdominal s.
peritoneal s.
postsplenectomy s.
severe human s.
systemic s.
sepsis-induced
s.-i. disseminated intravascular coagulation
s.-i. metabolic change
s.-i. muscle breakdown
s.-i. muscle proteolysis
septa (*pl. of* septum)

S

NOTES

septal
s. apical (SA)
s. basal (SB)
s. defect
s. hematoma
s. line
s. myectomy
s. myotomy
s. perforation
s. reconstruction
s. resection
s. space
septales
septate
septation
s. procedure
septectomy
atrial s.
balloon s.
Blalock-Hanlon atrial s.
Edwards s.
septi
septic
s. arthritis
s. complication
s. focus
s. shock (SS)
septicemia
septodermoplasty
septomarginal tract
septoplasty
frontal sinus s.
septorhinoplasty
esthetic s.
septostomy
atrial balloon s.
balloon atrial s.
blade atrial s.
septulum, pl. **septula**
septum, pl. **septa**
anorectal s.
anterior intermuscular s.
Bigelow s.
bridge-like s.
cartilaginous s.
Cloquet s.
colorectal s.
comblike s.
crural s.
deviated s.
endovenous s.
femoral s.
interatrial s.
intercavernosus s.
intermuscular s.
interpulmonary s.
interradicular s.
interventricular s.
membranous s.
nasal s.
orbital s.
pectiniform s.
posterior intermuscular s.
rectovaginal s.
rectovesical s.
scrotal s.
semilunar valvular s.
urogenital s.
urorectal s.
ventricular s.
Sequeira-Khanuja modification
sequela, pl. **sequelae**
sequence
caudal dysplasia s.
fast spin echo s.
FLAIR s.
turbo spin-echo s.
sequential
s. administration
s. line imaging
s. plane imaging
s. point imaging
s. radiographs
sequestration bronchopneumonia
sequestrectomy
sequestrotomy
sera (*pl. of* serum)
Serafini hernia
Serafin technique
Sergent white line
serial
s. blood gas
s. dilation
s. extraction
s. hematocrit measurement
s. imaging
s. operation
s. percutaneous liver biopsy
s. radiographic evaluation
s. radiographs
s. sonography
s. transverse scan
series
diagnostic small bowel s.
nonlaparoscopic s.
small bowel s.
upper gastrointestinal s.
series-II humeral head
serioscopy
seriscission
SER-IV fracture
serofibrinous inflammation
serofibrous
serologic
s. adhesion
s. examination

serological test
seroma cavity
seromembranous
seromucosa
seromucous gland
seromuscular
s. coat
s. colocystoplasty
s. enterocystoplasty
s. layer
s. stitch
s. suture technique
seromyectomy
duodenal s.
seromyotomy
anterior s.
laparoscopic s.
seroprotection
serosa
cecal s.
gastric s.
intact gastric s.
s. invasion
jejunal s.
serosal
s. breach
s. fluid
s. involvement
s. metastasis
s. penetration
s. tear
serosal-peritoneal metastasis
serosanguineous
seroserous
s. suture technique
serosum
serotonergic
s. system
s. tract
serous
s. acute inflammation
s. adenocarcinoma
s. cystadenocarcinoma
s. exudate
s. gland
s. layer
s. ligament
s. membrane
s. sac
serovaccination
serpentine
s. aneurysm
s. incision
serpent infection
serpiginous ulceration
serrata
serration
serratus
s. anterior muscle
s. anterior muscle flap
s. posterior inferior muscle
s. posterior superior muscle
Serres angle
Sertoli-cell-only syndrome
serum, pl. **sera**
s. alanine amino transaminase
s. alkaline phosphatase
s. ALT
s. bactericidal concentration
s. bilirubin
s. bilirubin concentration
s. calcium concentration
s. carcinoembryonic antigen
s. CEA
s. EGF
fetal bovine s. (FBS)
s. lidocaine level (SLL)
s. lithium concentration
s. neutralization
s. total bilirubin level
service
trauma s.
sesamoid
s. bone
s. cartilage
sesamoidectomy
fibular s.
sesamoideum
SESAP
Surgical Education and Self-Assessment Program
sessile
s. adenoma
s. lesion
Sessing pressure ulcer assessment scale
session
manometric recording s.
recording s.
sestamibi
s. nuclear scan
s. scanning
s. scintigraphy

NOTES

SET
signal extraction technology
set
insufflation test s.
s. point
seton
s. operation
s. wound
setpoint
setting
s. expansion
outpatient s.
outpatient surgical s.
setup
ambulatory s.
seventh cranial nerve
severe
s. deforming osteogenesis imperfecta
s. human sepsis
s. traumatic brain injury
Severin classification
Sever-L'Episcopo
S.-L. repair
S.-L. repair of shoulder
Sever modification of Fairbank technique
Sewall technique
sex
s. change operation
s. reversal
s. steroid modulation
sextant technique
sexual
s. aberration
s. evaluation
s. gland
sexualization
S-flap incision
SF-McGill Pain Questionnaire
SGO
Surgeon General's Office
SGPA
supragenicular popliteal artery
shadowing
acoustic s.
s. method
Shaffer-Hartmann method
Shaffer operation
Shaffer-Weiss classification
shaft
femoral s.
s. fracture
shagreen
s. lesion
s. patch
Shaher-Puddu classification
shallow
s. inspiration
s. respiration
sham
s. injection
s. surgery
Shambaugh incision
shank bone
shaping
root canal s.
sharing
United Network for Organ S. (UNOS)
sharp
s. angle
s. and blunt dissection
s. dilaceration
s. dissection technique
Sharpey fiber
Sharrard transfer technique
Sharrard-type kyphectomy
Shauta-Aumreich procedure
shave
s. biopsy
s. excision technique
Shea
S. pressure ulcer assessment scale
S. procedure
shear fracture
sheath
anterior s.
anterior rectus s.
axillary s.
carotid s.
common flexor s.
crural s.
femoral s.
fenestrated s.
fibrous tendon s.
flexor s.
glissonian s.
infundibuliform s.
intertubercular s.
intravenous s.
mucous s.
neurovascular s.
optic s.
paramedian s.
parotid s.
perichondral s.
plantar tendon s.
posterior rectus s.
prostatic s.
rectus s.
Scarpa s.
synovial tendon s.
vascular s.
Waldeyer s.

sheathed artery
shedding
endometrial s.
Sheehan and Dodge technique
Sheen
S. airway reconstruction
S. tip graft
sheet mesh excision
shelf
s. acetabuloplasty
Blumer s.
rectal s.
vocal s.
shell
s. nail
total hip arthroplasty with internal eccentric s.'s (THARIES)
Shelton femoral fracture classification
shelving
s. edge
s. incision
Shenton line
Shepherd fracture
shepherd's crook deformity
Sherk-Probst
S.-P. percutaneous pinning
S.-P. technique
shift
fluid s.
***Shigella* infection**
Shimazaki area-length method
shin bone
shiny cellophane reflection
ship
Fabricius s.
Shirodkar
S. operation
S. procedure
S. suture technique
shish-kebab technique
shock
allergic s.
anesthetic s.
cardiogenic s.
declamping s.
deferred s.
defibrillation s.
early unequivocal s.
endotoxic s.
endotoxin s.
heat s.
hemorrhagic s.
hyperdynamic s.
hypovolemic s.
irreversible s.
s. lung
perioperative s.
s. position
postcardiotomy s. (PS)
primary s.
reversible s.
septic s. (SS)
s. wave lithotripsy (SWL)
s. wave pressure
shoe-and-stocking position
shoelace
s. fasciotomy closure
s. stitch
shoeshine maneuver
Shone anomaly
short
s. bone
s. central artery
s. duration, unilateral, neuralgic, conjunctival injection and tearing (SUNCT)
s. esophagus type hiatal hernia
s. gastric artery
s. gastric vein
s. gastric vessel
s. head
s. hepatic vein
s. incubation hepatitis
s. lever accessory movement technique
s. lever specific contact procedure
s. oblique fracture
s. saphenous vein
s. segment spinal fusion
s. tau inversion recovery (STIR)
s. wave diathermy
short-axis plane
short-bowel syndrome
short-cone technique
shortcut sciatic pain
shortening
chordal s.
esophageal s.
short-inversion recovery imaging
short-limb Roux-en-Y gastroenterostomy
short-pulse repetition time/echo time image

NOTES

short-scar
s.-s. technique breast reduction
s.-s. technique of mastopexy
short-segment
s.-s. disease
s.-s. lesion
short-term
s.-t. convalescence
s.-t. immunosuppression
s.-t. outcome
s.-t. result
s.-t. total continence
shotgun wound
shoulder
s. amputation
s. arthroplasty
s. blade
s. disarticulation
s. dislocation
s. dislocation bone bank
s. girdle
ipsilateral s.
S. Pain and Disability Index
s. reduction
s. repair
s. rotation
Sever-L'Episcopo repair of s.
s. with bevel preparation
shoulder-strap incision
Shouldice
S. hernioplasty
S. herniorrhaphy
Shouldice-Bassini hernia repair
Shrapnell membrane
shrinkage
tumor s.
Shugrue operation
shunt
atriocaval s.
s. blockage
cavoatrial s.
central systemic-to-pulmonary s.
s. cyanosis
distal splenorenal s. (DSRS)
end-to-side portocaval s.
end-to-side splenorenal s.
s. index
s. infection
interposition mesocaval s.
intrahepatic portosystemic s.
s. manipulation
mesoatrial s.
s. muscle
s. obstruction
s. patency
s. pathway
s. placement
portacaval s.
portal-systemic s.
portosystemic s.
s. quantification
s. ratio
s. revision
side-to-side portacaval s. (SSPCS)
s. surgery
s. tap
transjugular intrahepatic portosystemic s. (TIPS)
shunting
airway s.
distal splenoadrenal s.
lumbar-peritoneal s.
pleuroperitoneal s.
portal mesenteric s.
portosystemic s.
selective s.
splenoadrenal s.
surgical portosystemic s.
ventricular peritoneal s.
ventriculoperitoneal s.
SHVC
suprahepatic inferior vena cava
SI
sacroiliac
SI joint
sialadenitis
sialoadenectomy
sialoadenotomy
sialocarcinoma
sialocele
sialolithotomy
Sibson
S. fascia
S. groove
S. muscle
Sichi operation
sickle flap
sickle-shaped canal
sickness impact profile
side
antimesenteric s.
contralateral s.
depressed s.
ipsilateral s.
luminal s.
s. port
posterior s.
s. posture reduction
side-bending barrier
side-entry access
side-lying iliac compression test
sideration
sideswipe elbow fracture
side-to-side
s.-t.-s. anastomosis
s.-t.-s. gastroenterostomy

s.-t.-s. hepatojejunostomy
s.-t.-s. portacaval shunt (SSPCS)
sidewall
pelvic s.
s. structure
SIDS
sudden infant death syndrome
sieve
s. bone
s. graft
molecular s.
Siffert intraepiphysial osteotomy
Siffert-Storen intraepiphysial osteotomy
sighing respiration
sigma
s. method
s. rectum pouch
sigmoid
s. artery
s. colon
s. colon carcinoma
s. cutaneous fistula
s. cystoplasty
s. end colostomy
s. enterocystoplasty
s. flexure
s. fold
s. fossa
s. kidney
s. loop reduction
s. mesocolon
s. rectum pouch
s. sinus ligation
s. sulcus
s. venous sinus
s. volvulus
sigmoidea
sigmoideae
sigmoidectomy
sigmoidei
sigmoideus
sigmoid-loop rod colostomy
sigmoidocystoplasty
sigmoidopexy
band s.
endoscopic s.
sigmoidoproctostomy
sigmoidorectostomy
sigmoidoscopy
fiberoptic s.
flexible s.
sigmoidostomy
sigmoidotomy
sigmoidovesical fistula
sigmoid-rectal intussusception
sign
accordion s.
Battle s.
chain-of-lakes s.
coiled spring s.
Cole s.
fabere s.
localized abdominal s.
loss-of-waist s.
s. mechanism for ventilator breathing
stacked coin s.
target s.
Thomas s.
signal
abnormal preoperative localization s.
s. attenuation
Doppler s.
electromagnetic s.
s. extraction technology (SET)
s. hemorrhage
localization s.
preoperative localization s.
signaling
downstream s.
nitric oxide s.
signature
surgical s.
signet-ring
s.-r. adenocarcinoma
s.-r. appearance
s.-r. cell carcinoma
SIH
spontaneous intracranial hypotension
SIL/ASCUS
squamous intraepithelial lesion/atypical squamous cell of undetermined significance
SIL/ASCUS lesion
Silastic
S. collar-reinforced stoma
S. lunate arthroplasty
S. ring vertical-banded gastric bypass (SRVGB)
Silber technique
silence
electrocerebral s. (ECS)

NOTES

S

silent
s. aspiration
s. autonephrectomy
s. gallstone
s. receptor
Silfverskiöld
S. lengthening technique
S. procedure
silhouette sign of Felson
silicate restoration
silicone
s. elastomer medialization
s. elastomer ring vertical gastroplasty
s. implant arthroplasty
s. implant leakage
s. intubation
s. rubber arthroplasty
s. wrist arthroplasty
siliconoma
Sillence type II-IV osteogenesis imperfecta
Silva-Costa operation
silver
s. amalgam restoration
S. bunionectomy
s. cone method
s. dollar technique
s. point root canal filling method
S. procedure
silver-fork deformity
Silver-Hildreth operation
silver-wire
s.-w. arteriole
s.-w. reflex
Silvester method
simian line
Simmonds-Menelaus
S.-M. metatarsal osteotomy
S.-M. proximal phalangeal osteotomy
Simmons
S. cervical spine fusion
S. osteotomy
Simon
S. expansion arch
S. incision
S. position
S. suture technique
Simonart band
Simonton technique
Simplate procedure
simple
s. bypass
s. cold storage preservation
s. diversion
s. external drainage
s. hepatojejunostomy
s. joint
s. mastectomy
s. mastoidectomy
s. mastopexy
s. periodontal flap
s. shoulder test (SST)
s. skull fracture
s. sound source
s. suture technique
s. transfusion
s. vulvectomy
simplex
simplification
simplified acute physiology score (SAPS)
Simpson
S. atherectomy
S. rule
Sims
S. position
S. suture technique
simultaneous
s. areolar mastopexy and breast augmentation (SAMBA)
s. bilateral percutaneous nephrolithotomy
s. compression-ventilation CPR
s. kidney-pancreas transplantation
s. method
s. pancreas and kidney (SPK)
s. pancreas-kidney transplantation
s. pancreatic-renal (SPR)
s. segmental hepatectomy
SIMV
spontaneous intermittent mandatory ventilation
synchronized intermittent mandatory ventilation
sincipital
sinciput
S incision
Sinding-Larsen-Johansson lesion
sinew
Singer-Blom endoscopic tracheoesophageal puncture technique
Singh
S. osteoporosis classification
S. osteoporosis index
single
s. adenoma
s. biopsy
s. cone root canal filling method
s. denture construction
s. fraction radiation
s. fracture
s. GSW
s. heel raise
s. hydatid disease

s. lung ventilation
s. mechanism inhaled anesthetic
s. midline extraperitoneal incision
s. pedicle TRAM flap
s. photon emission computer-aided tomography
s. proximal portal technique
s. site
s. site inhaled anesthetic
s. space technique
s. strand conformation polymorphism analysis
single-armed suture technique
single-balloon
s.-b. valvotomy
s.-b. valvuloplasty
single-breath
s.-b. diffusing capacity
s.-b. induction of anesthesia
single-echo diffusion imaging
single-fraction total body irradiation
single-incision fasciotomy
single-layer continuous closure
single-level spinal fusion
single-photon emission computed tomography
single-port
s.-p. laparoscopy
s.-p. technique
single-pour technique
single-puncture laparoscopy
single-rod construct
single-shot imaging technique
single-slice gradient-echo image
single-stage
s.-s. operation
s.-s. procedure
s.-s. tissue transfer
s.-s. total proctocolectomy
single-step esophagoplasty
single-stick method
Singleton incision
single-trocar access thoracoscopy
singulare
sinister
sinistra
sinistrae
sinistri
sinistrogyration
sinistrorotation
sinistrorse
sinistrotorsion
sinistrum
sink-trap malformation
sinoaortic denervation
sinoatrial (S-A)
s. exit block
s. nodal branch
s. nodal function
s. nodal parasympathectomy
s. node
sinocarotid nerve
sinonasal
s. carcinoma
s. cavity
s. disease
s. lesion
s. tumor
sinoscopy
sinus, pl. **sinus, sinuses**
air s.
anal s.
basilar venous s.
branchial s.
carotid s.
cavernous venous s.
s. cavity
cerebral s.
cervical s.
circular venous s.
s. closure
costomediastinal s.
cranial venous s.
dural venous s.
endodermal s.
s. endoscopy
Englisch s.
s. exit block
frontal s.
Guérin s.
Huguier s.
inferior longitudinal s.
inferior petrosal s.
inferior sagittal s.
intercavernous venous s.
s. irrigation
jugular s.
lactiferous s.
laryngeal s.
lateral s.
s. line
longitudinal vertebral venous s.
Luschka s.
Maier s.

NOTES

sinus *(continued)*
Morgagni s.
s. mucocele
oblique pericardial s.
occipital s.
osteomyelitic s.
Palfyn s.
paranasal s.
perineal s.
petrosal venous s.
petrosquamous venous s.
s. petrosus superior
phrenicocostal s.
piriform s.
pleural s.
prostatic s.
pulmonary s.
rectal s.
renal s.
rhomboidal s.
Ridley s.
right sigmoid s.
sagittal venous s.
sigmoid venous s.
sphenoidal s.
sphenoparietal venous s.
splenic s.
straight s.
s. surgery
s. tarsi syndrome
tentorial s.
s. tract
transverse pericardial s.
transverse venous s.
tympani s.
urogenital s.
venous s.

sinuscopy
maxillary s.

sinusitis
allergic fungal s.
chronic s.
fungal s.

sinusoid
hepatic s.

sinusoidal
s. capillary pressure
s. congestion
s. endothelium
s. endothelium cornucopia
s. lesion
s. relaxation

sinusotomy
Killian frontal s.

sinuvertebral nerve

siphon
carotid s.

siphonage

SIRS
systemic inflammatory response syndrome

SIS
small intestinal submucosa

Sistrunk procedure

site
alternative introduction s.
anatomic s.
anatomical s.
arterial bleeding s.
arterial entry s.
biopsy s.
bleeding s.
carcinoma of uncertain primary s.
catheter s.
coaptation s.
contralateral s.
endoscopic biopsy s.
entry s.
excisional biopsy s.
exit s.
extraabdominal s.
extraction s.
extrahepatic tumor s.
extranodal s.
extrapulmonary s.
fracture s.
graft s.
implantation s.
injection s.
introduction s.
multiple s.
s. of obstruction
osteotomy s.
patellar tendon graft donor s. (PTGDS)
peritumoral s.
pin s.
port s.
primary tumor s.
single s.
stoma s.
suprapubic extraction s.
tumor s.
wound s.

site-specific surgery

sitting position

situ
carcinoma in s. (CIS)
ductal carcinoma in s. (DCIS)
ex s.
fusion in s.
in s.
tumor in s.

situation
anatomical s.

situs

Siurala classification
six-portal synovectomy
sixth
s. cranial nerve
s. venereal disease
size
aerodynamic s.
age, distant metastases, extent of local s. (AMES)
breast s.
clot s.
crosslink plate s.
gland s.
heterogeneous gland s.
in-between s.
lesion s.
metastasis, age, completeness of resection, local invasion, and tumor s., pl. metastases (MACIS)
true s.
tumor s.
Sjöqvist intramedullary tractotomy
$SjVO_2$
jugular venous oxygen saturation
skeletal
s. abnormality
s. biopsy
s. correction
s. deformity
s. lesion
s. metastasis
s. muscle
s. muscle atrophy
s. muscle hypotonia
s. tissue
skeletale
skeletal-extraskeletal angiomatosis
skeletalis
skeleti
skeletology
skeleton
appendicular s.
axial s.
cardiac fibrous s.
fibrous s.
laryngeal s.
pelvic s.
spine s.
skeletonization
Skene
external genitalia, Bartholin, urethral, and S. (EG/BUS)
S. gland
skewer technique
skew flap
skiaporescopy
skier fracture
Skillern fracture
skin
alligator s.
s. approximation
atrophic s.
s. biopsy
s. closure
combination s.
s. conductance
s. crease
s. deficit wound
s. expansion technique
s. flap
s. flap necrosis
s. folding
s. graft neovagina
s. groove
hidden nail s.
s. incision
s. infection
s. lubrication
s. lubrication therapy
s. measurement
s. nick
ostomy s.
s. plasty
s. potential response
s. preparation
s. puncture
redundant triangular-shaped s.
scarred s.
scrotal s.
surplus s.
s. temperature
thin glossy s.
triangular-shaped s.
s. ulcer
s. window technique
s. wound
skin-colored lesion
skin-crease incision
skin-knife incision
skinned muscle fiber
Skinner classification

NOTES

skinning
s. colpectomy
s. vulvectomy
skinny-needle biopsy
skin-puncture test
skin-sparing mastectomy
skin-surfacing technique
skin-temperature gradient measurement
skin-to-tumor distance
skip
s. area
s. graft
s. lesion
s. metastasis
ski position
skived incision
Skoog
S. fasciotomy
S. technique
skull
s. base approach
s. base tumor
s. block
cloverleaf s.
s. fracture
maplike s.
steeple s.
skullcap
slack
tissue s.
slant
s. muscle operation
s. of occlusal plane
SLAP
superior labrum anterior and posterior
SLAP lesion
slaved programmed electrical stimulation
Slavianski membrane
sleep
s. dissociation
twilight s.
sleeve
s. fracture
s. graft
s. lobectomy
s. resection
s. technique
slice
s. fracture
s. preparation
sliding
s. abdominal hernia
s. esophageal hiatal hernia
s. flap
s. inlay bone graft
s. nail
s. oblique osteotomy
s. plasty
s. scale method
s. tenotomy
sling
s. and blanket technique
s. immobilization
s. ligation
s. procedure
s. and reef technique
s. suture technique
sling-ring complex
sling/wrapping technique
slippage
stomach s.
slipped
s. capital femoral epiphysis
s. hernia
s. Nissen fundoplication
s. Nissen repair
s. rib cartilage syndrome
s. vertebral apophysis
slipping
s. rib
s. rib syndrome
slit
s. catheter technique
Cheatle s.
s. hemorrhage
s. illumination
lengthwise s.
pudendal s.
s. valve
s. ventricle syndrome
vulvar s.
slit-lamp ophthalmoscopy
slitlike defect
SLL
serum lidocaine level
SLN
sentinel lymph node
SLN biopsy
SLN localization
SLN mapping
SLN radiolocalization
Sloan incision
Sloan-Kettering thyroid cancer staging
Slocum
S. amputation technique
S. fusion technique
S. maneuver
slope-shouldered lesion
slot
s. fracture
s. preparation
slot-blot
s.-b. hybridization analysis
s.-b. technique
slotted acetabular augmentation

slot-type preparation
sloughing of epithelial cell
slow
s. exchange soft tissue
s. maxillary expansion
s. respiration
slow-pathway ablation
SLR
straight-leg raise
SLR with external rotation test
Sluder
S. guillotine tonsillectomy
S. neuralgia
sludging of circulation
slush
ice s.
SMA
superior mesenteric artery
small
s. bowel biopsy
s. bowel congenital abnormality
s. bowel contrast study
s. bowel diverticular disease
s. bowel enema
s. bowel enteroscopy
s. bowel enterotomy
s. bowel followthrough examination
s. bowel idiopathic intussusception
s. bowel lesion
s. bowel lymphoma
s. bowel manometry
s. bowel resection
s. bowel series
s. bowel strangulation
s. bowel surgery
s. bowel transplant
s. bowel tumor
s. cell lung carcinoma
s. fenestra stapedotomy
s. intestinal endoscopy
s. intestinal membrane
s. intestinal submucosa (SIS)
s. intestine
s. pancreas
s. pelvis
s. polyp removal
s. round cell carcinoma
s. trochanter
Smead-Jones closure
smear
buccal s.
smegma
smegmalith
Smellie method
Smellie-Veit method
smile
endogenous s.
exogenous s.
smiley-face knotting technique
smiling incision
Smith
S. dislocation
S. eyelid operation
S. flexor pollicis longus abductorplasty
S. fracture
S. Indian technique
S. modification
S. physical capacities evaluation
S. trabeculectomy
Smith-Boyce operation
Smith-Gibson operation
Smith-Indian operation
Smith-Kuhnt-Szymanowski operation
Smith-Lemli-Opitz syndrome
Smith-Petersen
S.-P. approach
S.-P. cup arthroplasty
S.-P. hemiarthroplasty
S.-P. osteotomy
S.-P. sacroiliac joint fusion
S.-P. synovectomy
S.-P. technique
Smith-Petersen-Cave-Van Gorder anterolateral approach
Smith-Robinson
S.-R. anterior cervical diskectomy
S.-R. anterior fusion
S.-R. cervical disk approach
S.-R. cervical fusion
S.-R. interbody fusion
S.-R. operation
S.-R. procedure
S.-R. technique
Smithwick sympathectomy
SMN
surgical microscope navigation
smooth
s. muscle
s. muscle relaxant
s. muscle relaxation
s. muscular sphincter
s. skin-colored lesion

NOTES

smooth *(continued)*
s. surface cavity
s. wrap
SMP
sympathetically maintained pain
SNA
sympathetic nerve activity
snap-frozen biopsy
snapping iliopsoas tendon
snapshot GRASS technique
snare
s. cautery
s. electrocoagulation
s. excision biopsy
s. loop biopsy
s. technique
SNB
scalene node biopsy
sentinel node biopsy
SNBR
sentinel node-to-background ratio
Snellen
S. line
S. ptosis operation
S. suture technique
sniffing position
sniff method
snout response
Snow procedure
snuffbox
anatomical s.
Snyder classification
soaking solution
soak therapy
Soave
S. endorectal pull-through
S. operation
social
s. consequence
s. interaction therapy
socket
hard s.
s. joint
s. reconstruction
suspension-type s.
Soemmerring
S. muscle
S. ring
S. ring cataract
Sofield
S. femoral deficiency technique
S. osteotomy
S. pinning
soft
s. abdomen
s. callus stage
s. cataract
s. chancre
s. corn
s. event
s. exudate
s. lesion
s. palate
s. pigment stone
s. sore
s. stool
s. tissue
s. tubercle
s. wall
s. x-ray examination
s. x-ray investigation
soft-palate
s.-p. cancer
s.-p. cleft
s.-p. paralysis
s.-p. retraction
soft-tissue
s.-t. abnormality
s.-t. abscess
s.-t. curettage
s.-t. damage
s.-t. dissection
s.-t. envelope
s.-t. extremity injury
s.-t. flap
s.-t. healing
s.-t. hinge
s.-t. integrity
s.-t. interface
s.-t. interposition
s.-t. irritability
s.-t. lesion
s.-t. mass
s.-t. massage
s.-t. metastasis
s.-t. mobilization
s.-t. necrosis
s.-t. plication
s.-t. release
s.-t. restriction
s.-t. stranding
s.-t. stretching
s.-t. structure
s.-t. swelling
s.-t. thickness
s.-t. undercut
s.-t. window
soilage
peritoneal s.
soiling
colostomy s.
fecal s.
solar
s. ganglion
s. plexus
Solcia classification

soldier patch
soleal line
solei
sole laser therapy
solid
s. hidradenoma
s. hyperplasia
s. organ
s. phase extraction
s. subtype
s. tumor
S. Tumor Autologous Marrow Transplant Program (STAMP)
s. visceral hematoma
solitaire
cholesterol s.
solitarii
solitary
s. bundle
s. foramen
s. gland
s. pulmonary arteriovenous fistula
s. pulmonary mass
s. rectal ulcer
s. rectal ulcer syndrome
s. tract
solitus
Solomon-Bloembergen theory of dipole-dipole relaxation rate
solubility
solubilization
soluble
s. gas technique
solute
total body s.
solution
activating s.
aqueous s.
azeotropic s.
cardioplegic s.
cleaning s.
cold soak s.
colloid s.
colonic lavage s.
s. of contiguity
s. of continuity
crystalloid cardioplegic s.
disclosing s.
disinfecting s.
electrolyte flush s.
electrolytic s.
extracellular-like, calcium-free s.
extravasation irrigation s.
eye irrigating s.
hardening s.
hydrolysis of s.
hypotonic s.
ideal s.
intracellular-like, calcium-bearing crystalloid s.
irrigating s.
irrigation s.
lacmoid staining s.
lavage s.
nonideal s.
normal saline s.
ophthalmic ctivating s.
oxidation of s.
physiologic saline s.
physiologic salt s.
pickling s.
precipitate in s.
preservative s.
rehydrating s.
relaxing s.
saline s.
saltwater s.
saturated s.
sclerosing s.
soaking s.
solvent s.
standard s.
sterility of s.
surgical marking s.
volumetric s.
wetting s.
whole-gut lavage activating s.
solvation
solvent
s. extraction
s. solution
solvolysis
soma
somatectomy
subtotal s.
somatic
s. gene-transfer approach
s. hypoalgesia
s. mutation
s. nerve
s. pain
s. therapy
somaticosplanchnic
somaticovisceral

NOTES

somatization disorder
somatoprosthetics
somatosensory
s. evoked potential (SEP, SSEP)
s. pathway
somatostatin
s. analogue
s. receptor scintigraphy (SRS)
somatostatinoma syndrome
somatotropinoma
Somerville
S. anterior approach
S. procedure
S. technique
somite formation
somnolence
Somogyi method
Sondergaard procedure
Sondermann canal
Sones technique
sonication technique
sonic thrombolysis
sonification
Sonnenberg
S. classification
S. neurectomy
sonographic evidence
sonography
focused abdominal s.
renal s.
serial s.
sonography-guided aspiration
sonoguided biopsy
sonohysterography
sonolucent tissue
sonomicrometry
sonomicroscopy
sonorous respiration
Soper modification
Sorbie calcaneal fracture classification
sore
fungating s.
hard s.
pressure s.
soft s.
venereal s.
Soren ankle fusion
soreness
delayed onset muscle s. (DOMS)
Soriano operation
Soria operation
Sorondo-Ferré hindquarter amputation
Sorrin operation
Soto-Hall bone graft
sound
absent bowel s.'s
s. analysis
bowel s.'s
hypoactive bowel s.'s
s. pressure level
s. pressure level scale
s. quantity
sound-stimulated fetal movement
source
discrete bleeding s.
endoscopic light s.
point s.
s. program
simple sound s.
Sourdille
S. keratoplasty
S. keratoplasty operation
S. ptosis operation
Southern blot technique
Southwick
S. biplane trochanteric osteotomy
S. slide procedure
Southwick-Robinson anterior cervical approach
space
abdominal s.
acromioclavicular s.
air s.
alveolar dead s.
anatomic dead s.
anorectal s.
antecubital s.
anterior clear s.
apical s.
arachnoid s.
axillary s.
Berger s.
Bogros s.
Böttcher s.
Bowman s.
buccal s.
buccinator s.
buccopharyngeal s.
Burns s.
capsular s.
carotid s.
central palmar s.
Chassaignac s.
circumlental s.
Colles s.
coracoclavicular s.
costoclavicular s.
Cotunnius s.
cranial epidural s.
craniospinal s.
danger s.
dead s.
deep perineal s.
deep postanal anorectal s.
denture s.
digastric s.

disk s.
Disse s.
s. of Donders
echo-free s.
edentulous s.
embrasure s.
endolymphatic s.
epidural s.
episcleral s.
extracellular s.
extraction s.
extradural s.
extraperitoneal s.
extrapleural s.
extravascular s.
fascial s.
fat cell s.
first web s.
fixed maintainer s.
Fontana s.
s. of Fontana
freeway s.
geniohyoid s.
gingival s.
H s.
Henke s.
His perivascular s.
Holzknecht s.
incisural s.
increased lateral joint s.
infraglottic s.
inframesocolic s.
infraorbital s.
infratemporal s.
interalveolar s.
intercellular s.
intercondylar s.
intercostal s.
intercristal s.
interdental s.
interfascial s.
interlamellar s.
interocclusal rest s.
interprismatic s.
interproximal s.
interradicular s.
intersheath s.
intersphincteric anorectal s.
interstitial s.
intervaginal s.
intracristal s.
intrafascial s.
intramembranous s.
intrapharyngeal s.
intravaginal s.
ischiorectal anorectal s.
joint s.
k s.
Kiernan s.
lateral central palmar s.
lateral joint s.
lattice s.
leeway s.
leptomeningeal s.
Lesgaft s.
life s.
lymph s.
Magendie s.
maintainer cast s.
Malacarne s.
mandibular s.
marrow s.
masseteric s.
masseter-mandibular-pterygoid s.
masticator s.
masticatory s.
Meckel s.
medial clear s.
mediastinal s.
medullary s.
midpalmar s.
Mohrenheim s.
s. myopia
Nance leeway s.
object s.
obtainer s.
palm s.
paraglottic s.
paralaryngeal s.
parapharyngeal s.
pararenal s.
Parona s.
parotid s.
perforated s.
perianal anorectal s.
perichoroidal s.
peridental s.
peridentinoblastic s.
perihepatic s.
periimplant s.
perilenticular s.
perilymphatic s.
perineal s.
perinuclear s.

NOTES

space *(continued)*
perioptic subarachnoid s.
periotic s.
peripharyngeal s.
perirenal s.
periscleral s.
perisinusoidal s.
peritoneal s.
peritonsillar s.
perivitelline s.
pharyngeal s.
pharyngomaxillary s.
physiological dead s.
plantar s.
pleural s.
pleuroperitoneal s.
pneumatic s.
s. of Poirier
Poiseuille s.
popliteal s.
portal s.
position in s.
posterior cervical s.
postpharyngeal s.
postzygomatic s.
potassium s.
predental s.
preepiglottic s.
premasseteric s.
preperitoneal s.
presacral s.
preseptal s.
presternal s.
pretarsal s.
pretemporal s.
pretracheal s.
prevertebral s.
prezonular s.
properitoneal s.
Proust s.
proximal s.
proximate s.
Prussak s.
pterygomandibular s.
pterygomaxillary s.
pterygopalatine s.
pterygopharyngeal s.
quadrangular s.
quadrilateral s.
regainer s.
Reinke s.
relief s.
removable maintainer s.
retraction s.
retroadductor s.
retrobulbar s.
retrocardiac s.
retrocrural s.
retroesophageal s.
retrogastric s.
retroinguinal s.
retrolental s.
retromammary s.
retromuscular s.
retromylohyoid s.
retroocular s.
retroperitoneal s.
retropharyngeal s.
retropubic s.
retrosternal air s.
retrotracheal s.
retrovesical s.
retrovisceral s.
retrozygomatic s.
Retzius s.
s. of Retzius abscess
right anterior pararenal s.
Schwalbe s.
septal s.
sphenomaxillary s.
sphenopalatine s.
subacromial s.
subaponeurotic s.
subarachnoid s.
subchorial s.
subcoracoid s.
subdiaphragmatic s.
subdural s.
subgingival s.
subhepatic s.
sublingual s.
submandibular s.
submasseteric s.
submaxillary s.
submental s.
submucosal s.
subperitoneal s.
subphrenic s.
subpulmonic pleural s.
subretinal s.
subumbilical s.
superficial perineal s.
superior joint s.
supracolic s.
suprahepatic s.
suprahyoid s.
supralevator anorectal s.
supraomental s.
suprasternal s.
supratentorial s.
Tarin s.
temporal s.
Tenon s.
thenar s.
tibiofibular clear s.
tissue s.

Traube semilunar s.
Trautmann triangular s.
triangular s.
vascular s.
vertebral epidural s.
vesicocervical s.
Virchow-Robin s.
visceral s.
Waldeyer s.
web s.
Westberg s.
widened retrogastric s.
yolk s.
Zang s.
zonular s.
zygomaticotemporal s.

space-occupying
s.-o. brain lesion
s.-o. disease
s.-o. process

spacing
excessive s.

Spaeth
S. cystic bleb operation
S. ptosis operation

spall

spallation

Spälteholz preparation

span
levator s.

sparganoma

sparing therapy

Sparks
S. mandrel graft
S. mandrel technique

spasm
diffuse esophageal s. (DES)
esophageal s.
nocturnal painful tonic s. (NPTS)

spasmodic colic

spasmolysis

spastic
s. colon
s. thumb-in-palm deformity

spatial
s. localization procedure
S. Orientation Memory Test

spatium, pl. **spatia**

spatulate

spatulated

spatulation
s. condensation
graft s.
ureteral s.

Spaulding classification

Speas operation

special
s. lesion
s. reference method

specialized intralobular connective tissue

specialty
nonophthalmologic surgical s.
surgical s.

species
fungal s.

specific
s. ionization
s. modulation
s. rotation
s. survival
s. thrust manipulation

specimen
biopsy s.
catheter s.
colorectal s.
cytologic s.
cytology s.
excised s.
gastrectomy s.
mastectomy s.
operative s.
pathologic s.
preoperative FNA s.
s. radiograph
s. volume

speckled appearance

spectacle
s. correction
s. plane

spectometry
time-of-flight mass s.

spectral
s. edge
s. edge frequency (SEF)
s. edge frequency capnography
s. line

spectrometer
liquid scintillation s.
mass s.

spectrometry
gas chromatography-mass s.
gas isotope ratio mass s.
isotope dilution-mass s.
mass s.

NOTES

spectrophotometry
endoscopic reflectance s.
near-infrared s.
spectroscopic
spectroscopy
clinical s.
image-selected in vivo s.
infrared s.
magnetic resonance s.
MR s.
near-infrared s.
NMR s.
Raman s.
in vivo optical s.
specular
s. microscopy
s. reflection
speculum examination
speech
s. correction
s. detection threshold
Speed
S. arthroplasty
S. open reduction
S. osteotomy graft
S. radial head fracture classification
S. sternoclavicular repair
S. V-Y muscle-plasty
Speed-Boyd
S.-B. open reduction
S.-B. radial-ulnar technique
Spemann induction
Spence
S. and Duckett marsupialization
S. procedure
Spencer plication of vena cava
Spencer-Watson
S.-W. Z-plasty
S.-W. Z-plasty operation
sperm
s. aspiration
epididymal s.
s. immobilization test
s. microaspiration retrieval technique
s. washing insemination method
spermagglutination
spermatic
s. cord
s. duct
s. fistula
s. plexus
s. vein
s. vein ligation
spermatica
spermatici
spermaticus
spermatid
round s.
spermatocele
spermatocelectomy
spermatocyst
spermatogram
spermatolysis
spermatorrhea
spermaturia
spermiduct
spermolith
spermolysis
Spetzler anterior transoral approach
Spetzler-Martin classification
sphacelation
sphenethmoid
sphenion
sphenobasilar
sphenoccipital
sphenocephaly
sphenoethmoid
sphenoethmoidal
s. recess
sphenoethmoidalis
sphenoethmoidectomy
sphenofrontalis
sphenofrontal suture
sphenoid
s. angle
s. bone
s. emissary foramen
s. emissary vein
s. mucocele
s. process
s. sinus metastasis
sphenoidal
s. angle
s. concha
s. fissure
s. herniation
s. ridge
s. sinus
s. spine
s. turbinated bone
sphenoidale
sphenoidales
sphenoidalis
sphenoidalium
sphenoidectomy
sphenoidostomy
sphenoidotomy
sphenomalar
sphenomandibulare
sphenomandibular ligament
sphenomaxillaris
sphenomaxillary
s. fissure
s. fossa

s. space
s. suture
sphenooccipital
s. joint
s. suture
spheno-occipitalis
spheno-orbitalis
sphenoorbital suture
sphenopalatina
sphenopalatine
s. artery
s. canal
s. foramen
s. ganglion
s. ganglionectomy
s. nerve
s. space
sphenopalatinum
sphenoparietal
s. suture
s. venous sinus
sphenoparietalis
sphenopetrosa
sphenopetrosal
s. fissure
sphenorbital
sphenosalpingostaphylinus
sphenosquamosa
sphenosquamosal
sphenosquamous suture
sphenotemporal
sphenotic foramen
sphenoturbinal
sphenovomeriana
sphenovomerine suture
sphenozygomatica
sphenozygomatic suture
sphere
segmentation s.
spherica
spherical
s. lens aberration
s. recess
sphericus
spheroid
s. articulation
s. joint
spheroidea
spherule
rod s.
sphincter
anatomical s.
annular s.
anorectal s.
antral s.
artificial s.
basal s.
bicanalicular s.
Boyden s.
canalicular s.
choledochal s.
colic s.
deep anal s.
duodenal s.
duodenojejunal s.
esophageal s.
external rectal s.
external urethral s.
extrinsic s.
functional s.
Glisson s.
hepatopancreatic s.
Hyrtl s.
ileal s.
ileocecocolic s.
iliopelvic s.
incompetent s.
s. injury
internal anal s. (IAS)
internal urethral s.
intrinsic s.
lower esophageal s. (LES)
macroscopic s.
marginal s.
mediocolic s.
microscopic s.
midgastric transverse s.
midsigmoid s.
s. muscle
myovascular s.
myovenous s.
Nélaton s.
O'Beirne s.
Oddi s.
s. of Oddi dysfunction
s. of Oddi pressure
ostial s.
palatopharyngeal s.
pancreatic s.
pathologic s.
pelvirectal s.
physiological s.
postpyloric s.
prepapillary s.

NOTES

sphincter *(continued)*
preprostate urethral s.
prepyloric s.
s. preservation
proximal urethral s.
pyloric s.
radiological s.
s. reconstruction
rectosigmoid s.
s. relaxation
s. repair
segmental s.
smooth muscular s.
striated muscular s.
unicanalicular s.
Varolius s.
velopharyngeal s.
sphincteral
sphincteralgia
sphincterectomy
endoscopic s.
sphincterial
sphincteric
s. construction
s. continence
s. potency
sphincterismus
sphincteroid tract
sphincterolysis
sphincteroplasty
pancreatic s.
transduodenal s.
sphincteroscopy
sphincterotomy
biliary s.
Doubilet s.
endoscopic s. (ES)
endoscopic pancreatic duct s.
Erlangen pull-type s.
external s.
Geenen s.
internal s.
Mulholland s.
needle-knife s.
pancreatic duct s.
Parks partial s.
partial lateral internal s.
precut s.
retrograde s.
transduodenal s.
transendoscopic s.
transurethral s.
urethral s.
zipper s.
sphincter-preserving proctectomy
sphincter-saving
s.-s. method
s.-s. operation
s.-s. procedure
s.-s. surgery
s.-s. technique
sphincter-sparing
s.-s. method
s.-s. procedure
s.-s. resection
s.-s. technique
sphygmopalpation
sphygmoscopy
SPI
structured pain interview
spica cast immobilization
spiculated lesion
spider
s. angioma
s. pelvis
s. projection
spider-web
s.-w. clot
s.-w. pattern
Spiegel lobe
Spieghel line
spigelian
s. hernia
s. lobe
s. vein
Spigelius
S. hernia
S. line
S. lobe
spike burst on electromyogram of colon
spill
peritoneal s.
spillage
intraabdominal s.
intraperitoneal s.
tumor s.
Spiller-Frazier technique
spiloma
spina, pl. **spinae**
s. bifida
spinal
s. accessory nerve
s. accessory nerve-facial nerve anastomosis
afferent s.
s. analgesia
s. analgesic
s. anesthesia (SA)
s. anesthetic
s. anesthetic technique
s. angioma
s. artery
s. block
s. canal
s. column
s. column stabilization

s. compression fracture
s. cord circulation
s. cord compression
s. cord concussion
s. cord injury
s. cord injury pain
s. cord perfusion pressure (SCPP)
s. cord protection
s. cord stimulation (SCS)
s. cord tumor
s. coronal plane deformity
s. decompression
s. deformity-instability
s. delivery
s. dermal sinus tract
s. dural arteriovenous fistula
s. epidural abscess (SEA)
failed s.
s. fixation
s. fixation rigidity
s. fluid drainage
s. fusion
s. fusion pathomechanics
s. fusion position
s. fusion technique
s. ganglion
s. gate
s. headache
s. hematoma
s. infection
s. infection biopsy
s. inflammation
s. injury operative stabilization
s. instability
s. joint mobilization
s. lesion
s. manipulation
s. marrow
s. metastasis
s. mobilization technique
s. muscle
s. osteotomy
s. osteotomy stabilization
s. point
s. puncture
s. pyramidotomy
s. root
s. surgery
s. tractotomy
s. trauma
s. vascular malformation
s. vein

spinale
spinales
spinalis
spinalium
spinal-locking procedure
spinally administered
spinaloscopy
spinate
spindle
s. cell carcinoma
s. cell sarcoma
s. cell thymoma
Krukenberg corneal s.
spindle-shaped incision
spine
alar s.
angular s.
anterior inferior iliac s.
anterior superior iliac s.
Chance fracture thoracolumbar s.
s. deformity
dorsal s.
s. fracture
hemal s.
iliac s.
ischiadic s.
ischial s.
mental s.
neural s.
osteoporotic s.
posterior inferior iliac s.
posterior superior iliac s.
pubic s.
s. rotation
sciatic s.
s. skeleton
sphenoidal s.
thoracic s.
spin-echo
s.-e. image
s.-e. magnetic resonance imaging
partial saturation s.-e.
Spinelli operation
spinning disk nebulizer
spinning-top deformity
spinocerebellar tract
spinocostalis
spinogalvanization
spinoglenoid
spinolamellar line
spinolaminar line
spinomuscular

NOTES

spinoneural
spinoolivary tract
spinosum
spinosus
spinotectal tract
spinothalamic
s. cordotomy
s. pathway
s. tract (STT)
s. tractotomy
spinotransversarius
spinous
s. aspect
s. interlaminar line
s. plane
s. process
s. process fracture
spiradenoma
spiral
s. CT technique
s. dissection
s. fold
s. foraminous tract
s. ganglion
s. groove
s. incision
s. joint
s. ligament
s. line
s. membrane
s. oblique fracture
s. suture technique
spiralis
Spira procedure
spirochetal infection
spirochete infection
spirochetolysis
spirogram
forced expiratory s.
spiroscopy
Spittler procedure
Spitzka marginal tract
Spivack gastrotomy technique
SPK
simultaneous pancreas and kidney
SPK transplant
SPK transplantation
splanchnapophysial
splanchnapophysis
splanchnectopia
splanchnemphraxis
splanchnic
s. anesthesia
s. A-V fistula
s. capillary pressure
s. congestion
s. ganglion
s. hypoperfusion
s. nerve
s. oxygenation
s. oxygen consumption
s. perfusion
s. venous stasis
s. vessel
s. wall
splanchnicectomy
chemical s.
splanchnici
splanchnicotomy
splanchnicum
splanchnocele
splanchnocranium
splanchnodiastasis
splanchnolith
splanchnologia
splanchnology
splanchnomicria
splanchnoptosis
splanchnoscopy
splanchnoskeletal
splanchnoskeleton
splanchnosomatic
splanchnotomy
splanchnotribe
S-plasty
SPLATT
split anterior tibial tendon
SPLATT procedure
splayfoot deformity
spleen
accessory s.
adult wandering s.
ectopic s.
enlarged s.
floating s.
movable s.
s. preservation
s. tip
wandering s.
spleen-preserving
s.-p. distal pancreatectomy
s.-p. pancreatic resection
splen
splenectomy
abdominal s.
Henry s.
incidental s.
laparoscopic s.
open s.
Rives s.
subcapsular s.
splenectopia
spleneolus
splenetic
splenia (*pl. of* splenium)
splenial

splenic
- s. artery (SA)
- s. A-V fistula
- s. branch
- s. conservation
- s. cord of Billroth
- s. cyst
- s. flexure
- s. flexure carcinoma
- s. flexure colonoscopy
- s. fossa
- s. hilum
- s. injury
- s. laceration
- s. lesion
- s. necrosis
- s. plexus
- s. pulp
- s. puncture
- s. recess
- s. rupture
- s. sequestration syndrome
- s. sinus
- s. tissue
- s. vein
- s. vein deformity
- s. vein stump

splenica
splenicae
splenici
spleniculus
splenicum
splenicus
spleniform
splenis
spleniserrate
splenium, pl. **splenia**
splenius
splenoadrenal
- s. anastomosis
- s. shunting

splenobronchial fistula
splenocele
splenocleisis
splenocolic ligament
splenogastric omentum
splenogonadal fusion
splenoid
splenolymphatic
splenoma
splenomegaly
- congenital s.

splenonephric
splenopancreatic
splenopexy
splenophrenic
splenoptosis
splenorenal
- s. angle
- s. ligament
- s. venous anastomosis

splenorenale
splenorrhagia
splenorrhaphy
splenosis
splenotomy
splenule
splenulus, pl. **splenulus**
splenunculus, pl. **splenunculi**
splintered fracture
splinter hemorrhage
splinting
- s. of abdomen
- closed reduction/chemical s.
- extracoronal s.
- Strong dorsal extension block s.

splint/stent
- kidney internal s. (KISS)

split
- s. anterior tibial tendon (SPLATT)
- s. anterior tibial tendon procedure
- s. anterior tibial tendon transfer
- s. cuff nipple technique
- s. fixation
- s. fracture
- s. ileostomy
- s. incision
- s. liver
- s. renal function test

split-and-roll technique
split-bone technique
split-cast method
split-cord malformation
split-course technique
split-hand deformity
split-heel
- s.-h. approach
- s.-h. fracture
- s.-h. incision

split-liver
- s.-l. transplant
- s.-l. transplantation

split-lung ventilation
split-nail deformity

NOTES

split-patellar approach
split-thickness
s.-t. periodontal flap
s.-t. skin graft
splitting
s. fracture
s. lacrimal papilla operation
SpO_2
arterial oxyhemoglobin saturation
spoiled gradient-echo imaging
spondylectomy
spondylitic
s. deformity
s. myelopathy
spondylitis
ankylosing s.
juvenile ankylosing s.
spondylodesis
spondylodiscitis
lumbar s.
spondylolisthesis reduction
spondylolysis
spondylophyte
spondylothoracic
spondylotomy
spondylous
sponge
s. biopsy
s. dissection
s. explant
spongioblastoma
spongioplasty
spongiosi
spongiositis
spongiosum
spongy
s. body
s. urethra
Sponsel oblique osteotomy
spontaneous
s. adenocarcinoma
s. aliquorrhea
s. amputation
s. ascites filtration
s. breathing
s. breech extraction
s. coronary artery dissection
s. dialytic ultrafiltration
s. fracture
s. hyperemic dislocation
s. intermittent mandatory ventilation (SIMV)
s. intracranial hypotension (SIH)
s. lateral ventricle hernia
s. lesion
s. pneumothorax
s. renal hemorrhage
s. resolution
s. rupture
s. ventilation
s. ventilation anesthetic technique
s. ventrolateral hernia
sporadic
s. CRC
s. islet cell tumor
s. multigland disease
s. multigland hyperplasia
s. multiple gland parathyroid hyperplasia
s. pituitary adenoma
s. primary HPT
s. primary hyperparathyroidism
s. renal cell carcinoma
spot
ash-leaf s.
cold s.
s. compression
corneal s.
hottest s.
s. magnification
milk s.
saccular s.
utricular s.
S-pouch reconstruction
spout
ileostomy s.
SPR
simultaneous pancreatic-renal
Sprague arthroscopic technique
sprain fracture
spray-wipe-spray disinfection
spread
extrathyroid s.
lymphatic s.
metastatic s.
omental s.
peritoneal s.
spreader graft
spreading
s. depression of Leao
s. fistulation
s. hypoperfusion
Sprengel
S. anomaly
S. deformity
spring fixation
sprinter fracture
sprouting
ephaptic s.
sprue
collagenous s.
SPT
station pull-through
SPT technique
spur formation
spuria

spuriae
Spurling maneuver
spurring
sputum, pl. **sputa**
s. induction
pink frothy s.
SQ
subcutaneous
squama, pl. **squamae**
frontal s.
temporal s.
squamatization
squamocolumnar junction
squamofrontal
squamomastoid suture
squamooccipital
squamoparietal
squamopetrosal
squamosa
squamosal suture
squamosomastoidea
squamosus
squamotemporal
squamotympanic fissure
squamous
s. border
s. epithelium
s. hyperplasia
s. intraepithelial lesion
s. intraepithelial lesion/atypical squamous cell of undetermined significance (SIL/ASCUS)
s. margin
s. metaplasia
s. regeneration
s. suture
squamous intraepithelial lesion/atypical squamous cell of undetermined significance (SIL/ASCUS)
squamozygomatic
squared
kilogram per meter s.
square-shouldered lesion
squarrose
squeak
bronchopleural leak s.
squeeze pressure
SR
sustained release
Sr-90 beta radiation
SRCP
superficial renal cortical perfusion
SRS
somatostatin receptor scintigraphy
SRVGB
Silastic ring vertical-banded gastric bypass
SS
septic shock
Ssabanejew-Frank gastrostomy
SSAER
steady-state auditory evoked response
SSEP
somatosensory evoked potential
S-shaped
S-s. body
S-s. deformity
S-s. ileal pouch-anal anastomosis
S-s. incision
SSI
surgical-site infection
anterior-posterior fusion with SSI
SSPCS
side-to-side portacaval shunt
direct SSPCS
emergency SSPCS
SSRI
selective serotonin reuptake inhibitor
SSRI discontinuation syndrome
SST
simple shoulder test
stab
s. wound
s. wound incision
stability
cardiovascular s.
detrusor s.
hemodynamic s.
stabilization
anterior internal s.
anterior short-segment s.
s. approach
atlantoaxial s.
atlantooccipital s.
cervical spine s.
cervicothoracic junction s.
chest wall s.
coronoradicular s.
definitive s.
distal radioulnar joint s.
dynamic lumbar s.
flexion compression spine injury s.
fracture s.
Gruca s.

NOTES

stabilization *(continued)*
iliac crest bone graft s.
lower cervical spine posterior s.
lumbar spine s.
myoplastic muscle s.
occipitocervical s.
odontoid fracture s.
s. on retreat
prophylactic operative s.
provisional s.
rhythmic s.
sacral spine s.
screw s.
spinal column s.
spinal injury operative s.
spinal osteotomy s.
subluxation s.
thoracolumbar spine s.
s. training
TSRH crosslink s.
wire s.

stabilized
operatively s.

stabilizing fulcrum line

stable
s. burst fracture
s. cavitation
hemodynamically s.
s. reduction

stacked coin sign

stacking
breath s.

Stack shoulder procedure

Stafne idiopathic bone cavity

stage
s. B, C carcinoma
disease s.
Dukes s.
hard callus s.
s. II_E tumor
implant s.
lymph node s.
s. migration
patch s.
rehabilitation s.
soft callus s.
symptom experience s.
tumor s.

staged
s. abdominal repair (STAR)
s. bilateral stereotactic thalamotomy
s. orchiopexy
s. reconstruction
s. tympanoplasty

staghorn calculus

staging
Ann Arbor classification of Hodgkin disease s.
Astwood-Coller s. system for carcinoma
Boden-Gibb tumor s.
s. celiotomy
FAB s. of carcinoma
FIGO classification s.
Jewett and Strong s.
laparoscopic s.
s. laparotomy
multiple myeloma s.
nonoperative s.
s. operation
preoperative s.
primary gastric lymphoma s.
sentinel s.
Sloan-Kettering thyroid cancer s.
surgical s.
surgical-pathologic s.
TNM system for tumor s.
tumor s.

stagnant
s. anoxia
s. hypoxia
s. loop syndrome

stagnation

Staheli
S. shelf procedure
S. technique

Stähli pigment line

STAI
State-Trait Anxiety Inventory

stain
endocardial s.
immunohistochemical s.
Paget-Eccleston s.
port-wine s.

staining
anal canal s.
argyrophilic nucleolar organizer region s.
blue s.
corneal blood s.
extrinsic environmental s.
immunohistochemical s.
pattern of s.

staircase phenomenon

stairstep fracture

stalk
body s.

Stallard
S. eyelid operation
S. flap operation

Stallard-Liegard operation

staltic

STA-MCA
superficial temporal artery to middle cerebral artery
STA-MCA anastomosis

Stamey
S. modification of Pereyra procedure
S. needle suspension
S. operation
S. urethropexy
Stamey-Martius procedure
Stamm
S. gastroplasty
S. gastrostomy
S. metatarsal osteotomy
S. procedure
S. procedure for intraarticular hip fusion
stammering of the bladder
Stammer method
Stamm-Kader gastrotomy technique
STAMP
Solid Tumor Autologous Marrow Transplant Program
STAMP therapy
standard
s. biopsy technique
s. bone algorithm program
s. clavicular incision
s. D1 gastrectomy
s. electrode potential
s. fashion
s. formalin fixation
s. gastric resection
s. gastric resection Whipple procedure
s. Kocher incision
s. mastectomy
s. midline laparotomy
s. neck exploration
s. open approach
s. organ failure criteria
s. patient monitoring
s. radioenzymatic method
s. reduction potential
s. retroperitoneal flank incision
s. right hemicolectomy
s. solution
s. stripping procedure
s. surgical procedure
s. technique
s. thoracotomy
standardization
standardized
s. curative radical total gastrectomy
s. hepatectomy
s. protocol
stand-off weapon
Stanford
S. biopsy method
S. radical retropubic prostatectomy
S. type A, B aortic dissection
Stanford-type aortic dissection
Stanisavljevic technique
Stanley Way procedure
Stanmore shoulder arthroplasty
Stansel procedure
stapedectomy
House s.
stapedius
s. muscle
s. tendon
stapedotomy
small fenestra s.
stapes mobilization
staphylectomy
staphylococcal
s. infection
s. scalded skin syndrome
Staphylococcus epidermidis
staphylopharyngorrhaphy
staphyloplasty
staphylorrhaphy
staphylotomy
staple
s. capsulorraphy bone bank
s. capsulorrhaphy
s. fixation
s. ligated
s. line dehiscence
stapled
s. blind end
s. coloanal anastomosis
s. esophagojejunostomy
s. hemorrhoidectomy
s. ileal pouch-anal anastomosis without proctomucosal proctectomy
s. ileoanal anastomosis
s. lung reduction
s. reconstruction
s. reconstruction method
s. reconstruction procedure
s. reconstruction technique
s. stricturoplasty
Staples
S. repair
S. technique

NOTES

S

Staples-Black-Broström ligament repair
stapling
gastric s.
surgical s.
s. technique
STAR
staged abdominal repair
STAR technique
star
s. construction test
s. formation
Stark
S. classification
S. graft
Starkey matrix program
Stark-Moore-Ashworth-Boyes technique
Starlite point
startle technique
Starzl technique
STAS
Support Team Assessment Schedule
stasis
s. edema
s. gallbladder
s. liver
splanchnic venous s.
s. syndrome
s. ulceration
venous s.
state
central excitatory s.
chronic hyperparathyroid s.
dysphoric mood s.
S. end-to-end anastomosis
exhaustion s.
hypercoagulable s.
inotropic s.
local excitatory s.
mood s.
S. operation
oxidation s.
presurgical s.
thrombin-mediated consumptive s.
State-Trait Anxiety Inventory (STAI)
static
s. closure pressure
s. compliance of the total respiratory system
s. compression
s. dilation technique
s. evaluation
s. fixation
s. gangrene
s. image
s. method
s. position
s. relation
s. storage allocation
station
lymph nodal s.
node s.
perigastric node s.
perihepatic lymph nodal s.
s. pull-through (SPT)
s. pull-through esophageal manometry technique
s. test
stationary manometry
statoacoustic nerve
statoconia
statoconic membrane
status
acid-base s.
ASA physical s.
cancer s.
carrier s.
s. cribriform
s. epilepticus
s. evaluation
hepatic intracellular energy s.
hydration s.
lymph node s.
mutation carrier s.
nutritional s.
performance s.
premorbid performance s.
semielective s.
Stauffer
S. modification
S. syndrome
staurion
stay
hospital s.
length of s. (LOS)
s. suture technique
steady-state
s.-s. auditory evoked response (SSAER)
s.-s. gradient-echo imaging
s.-s. ventilatory response
steal
iliac s.
s. phenomenon
portal s.
renal-splanchnic s.
subclavian s.
steam autoclave sterilization
steamy appearance
steatocystoma
steatoma
steatotic liver
Steel
S. correction
S. maneuver
S. rule of thirds
S. triple innominate osteotomy

steep
s. head-down tilt
s. Trendelenburg position
steeple skull
steerable cystoscopy
Steffee
S. instrumentation technique
S. thumb arthroplasty
Stegemann-Stalder method
stegnosis
Steichen neurovascular free flap
Steinberg infiltration block
Steinbrocker classification
Steindler
S. flexorplasty
S. matrixectomy
S. procedure
Steinert disease
Steinmann pin fixation
stellatae
stellate
s. border breast lesion
s. configuration
s. ganglion
s. ganglion block
s. ganglion blockade
s. ganglion block anesthesia
s. ganglion block anesthetic technique
s. incision
s. laceration
s. ligament
s. mass
s. skull fracture
stellatum
stellectomy
stem
s. bronchus
s. cell
s. cell gene therapy
s. cell mobilization
s. removal
stem-loop structure
Stener-Gunterberg resection
Stener lesion
stenion
stenobregmatic
stenocephalia
stenocephalous
stenocephaly
stenocrotaphy
stenopeic iridectomy
stenosal
stenosed
stenosis, pl. **stenoses**
arterial s.
artery s.
atherosclerotic renal artery s.
calcific aortic s.
carotid artery atherosclerotic s.
cervical s.
choledochoduodenal junctional s.
congenital pyloric s.
cular subvalvular aortic s.
discrete s.
esophageal s.
granulation s.
idiopathic hypertrophic subaortic s.
ileostomy s.
pulmonary valve s.
pulmonic valve s.
renal artery s.
subglottic tracheal s.
subvalvular aortic s.
supracarinal s.
supravalvular aortic s.
tracheal s.
vessel s.
stenothorax
stenotic
s. cricoid
s. disease
s. esophagogastric anastomosis
s. lesion
s. stoma
Stensen
S. canal
S. duct
stent
s. apposition
s. construction
s. deployment
s. evaluation
s. expansion
s. graft
s. implantation
s. incrustation
s. patency
s. placement
stent-induced
s.-i. intimal hyperplasia
s.-i. pneumoperitoneum
stenting
accessory duct s.

NOTES

S

stenting *(continued)*
antral s.
biliary s.
carotid s.
carotid angioplasty with s.
endoluminal s.
endoscopic ampullary s.
endoscopic pancreatic s.
endoscopic papillotomy and s.
endoscopic retrograde biliary s.
endovascular s.
primary s.
renal artery s.
s. technique
tumor s.
stent-mounted
stent-through-wire mesh technique
Stenvers projection
step
corneal graft s.
diagnostic s.
s. graft operation
s. osteotomy
s. preparation
therapeutic s.
step-by-step technique
step-cut
s.-c. osteotomy
s.-c. transection
stepdown
s. osteotomy
s. therapy
stephanial
stephanion
stepladder incision technique
step-up in oxygen saturation
stercolith
stercoral
s. abscess
s. fecaloma
s. fistula
s. ulceration
stercoroma
stereoauscultation
stereochemistry
stereocolpogram
stereoencephalotomy
stereography
three-dimensional s.
StereoGuide stereotactic needle core biopsy
stereo-identical point
stereomagnification
stereoscopic interrogation
stereoscopy
stereoselective
stereospecific action
stereotactic
s. aspiration
s. aspiration biopsy
s. automated technique
s. brain biopsy
s. catheter drainage
s. cordotomy
s. core biopsy method
s. core biopsy technique
s. core breast biopsy
s. craniotomy
s. guidance
s. needle core biopsy
s. needle core biopsy procedure
s. neurosurgery
s. operation
s. pallidotomy
s. percutaneous needle biopsy
s. puncture
s. radiation therapy
s. radiofrequency lesioning
s. radiosurgery
s. surgery
s. surgical ablation
s. trigeminal tractotomy
s. Vim thalamotomy
s. VL thalamotomy
stereotactic
s. lesion
stereotactic-assisted radiation therapy
stereotactic-focused radiation therapy
stereotactic-guided biopsy
stereotaxic
s. surgery
s. technique
stereotaxis
volumetric s.
stereotaxy
frameless s.
sterile
s. abscess
s. field barrier
s. granuloma
s. matrix
s. technique
s. vaginal examination
sterility of solution
sterilization
chemical vapor s.
cold gas s.
defined s.
discontinuous s.
dry heat oven s.
ethylene oxide s.
ETO s.
fractional s.
gas s.
glutaraldehyde s.

intermittent s.
involuntary s.
root canal s.
steam autoclave s.
tubal s.
unsaturated chemical vapor s.
voluntary s.

sterilized
cold gas s.

steri-stripped incision

sterna (*pl. of* sternum)

sternad

sternal
s. angle
s. artery
s. branch
s. cartilage
s. development
s. fragment
s. joint
s. lifting
s. line
s. muscle
s. notch
s. part of diaphragm
s. plane
s. position
s. puncture
s. rotation

sternale

sternales

sternalgia

sternalis

sternal-occipital-mandibular immobilization

sternal-splitting incision

Sternberger antibody sandwich technique

sternen

sterni

sternochondroscapularis

sternochondroscapular muscle

sternoclavicular
s. angle
s. disk
s. joint
s. joint dislocation
s. joint reconstruction
s. joint reduction
s. junction
s. ligament
s. muscle

sternoclaviculare

sternoclavicularis

sternocleidal

sternocleidomastoid
s. artery
s. hemorrhage
s. muscle
s. muscle origin
s. region
s. vein

sternocleidomastoidea

sternocleidomastoideus

sternocostal
s. articulation
s. head
s. joint
s. triangle

sternocostale

sternocostales

sternodynia

sternofascialis

sternoglossal

sternohyoideus

sternohyoid muscle

sternoid

sternomanubrial junction

sternomastoid
s. artery
s. muscle

sternopericardiaca

sternopericardial ligament

sternoschisis

sternothyroid
s. muscle
s. muscle flap laryngoplasty

sternothyroideus

sternotomy
concomitant median s.
s. incision
median s.
s. scar

sternotracheal

sternotrypesis

sternovertebral

sternoxiphoid plane

sternum, pl. **sterna**
s. cartilage
mobile s.

sternum-splitting approach

steroid
s. concentration
endogenous s.

NOTES

steroid *(continued)*
- s. hormone
- s. injection

steroid-dependent asthmatic
steroid-resistant proteinuria
stertorous respiration
stethalgia
stetharteritis
stethoscopy
Stetta operation
Steward Recovery Score
Stewart
- S. distal clavicular excision
- S. incision
- S. styloidectomy
- S. test

Stewart-Hamilton cardiac output technique
Steytler-Van Der Walt procedure
stick-tie suture technique
Stieda
- S. fracture
- S. process

Stiegmann-Goff technique
stiff abdomen
stiffness
- fusion s.

stigma, pl. **stigmata**
- malpighian s.
- stigmata of recent hemorrhage

stigmatization
stigmatoscopy
Stiles-Bunnell transfer technique
Stilling
- canal of S.

Stillman
- S. method
- S. technique

still radiography technique
stilus
Stimson
- S. anterior shoulder reduction technique
- gravity method of S.
- S. gravity method
- S. maneuver

stimulated gracilis neosphincter technique
stimulating effect
stimulation
- anal electrical s.
- anocutaneous s.
- antidromic s.
- brain s.
- calibrated electrical s.
- cervical carcinoma s.
- cortical s.
- direct brain s.
- direct electrical nerve s.
- direct neural s.
- dorsal column s. (DCS)
- dorsal cord s.
- double-burst s.
- double simultaneous s.
- electric s.
- electrical nerve s.
- electrical surface s.
- electrogalvanic s.
- electronic bone s.
- electrophysiological s.
- external-coil electrical s.
- follicle maturation s.
- functional electrical s.
- functional neuromuscular s.
- galvanic s.
- Ganzfeld s.
- gastric electrical s.
- gingival s.
- high-voltage pulsed galvanic s.
- hilum s.
- intracranial s.
- intraoperative cavernous nerve s.
- intravaginal electrical s.
- juxtacrine s.
- magnetic s.
- magnetoelectric s.
- mechanical s.
- microamperage electrical nerve s.
- microamperage neural s.
- motor-evoked response to transcranial s. (tc-MER)
- neuromuscular electrical s.
- nociceptive s.
- noninvasive programmed s.
- ovarian s.
- ovulation s.
- paired electrical s.
- pelvic s.
- percutaneous s.
- periaqueductal gray matter s.
- periaqueductal-periventricular s.
- photic s.
- precentral cortical s.
- programmed electrical s.
- repetitive nerve s.
- s. scan
- secretin s.
- sensory s.
- slaved programmed electrical s.
- spinal cord s. (SCS)
- subthreshold s.
- supramaximal tetanic s.
- tactile s.
- s. test
- tetanic s.
- thermal s.

s. threshold
train-of-four s.
transcranial s. (TCS)
transcranial electrical s.
transcutaneous acupoint electrical s. (TAES)
transcutaneous cranial electrical s. (TCES)
transcutaneous electric s. (TES)
transcutaneous electrical nerve s.
transcutaneous electrode nerve s.
transesophageal atrial s.
transurethral electrical bladder s.
ultrarapid subthreshold s.
vagal nerve s.
vaginal electrical s.
ventricular-programmed s.
vibroacoustic s.
visual s.

stimulus, pl. **stimuli**
double extra s.
external s.
flicker-fusion s.
noxious s.
train-of-four s.
transcutaneous tetanic s.

stippled epiphysis

stippling
geographic s.

STIR
short tau inversion recovery
STIR technique

stitch
s. abscess
Allgöwer s.
baseball s.
bow-tie s.
Bunnell s.
Connell s.
cuticular s.
extramucosal s.
figure-eight s.
Fothergill s.
Frost s.
funnel s.
intracuticular s.
marker s.
mattress s.
McCall s.
roll s.
seromuscular s.
shoelace s.
tagging s.
tilt s.
tracheal safety s.
triple-throw square knot s.

St. Mark polyposis registry

Stocker
S. line
S. operation

Stockholm technique for radium therapy

stocking anesthesia

stocking-glove
s.-g. anesthesia
s.-g. pain distribution

stocking-seam incision

Stock operation

Stoffel operation

Stoll dilution egg count technique

stoma, pl. **stomas, stomata**
abdominal s.
anastomotic s.
Benchekroun s.
bowel s.
s. button
catheterizable s.
s. closure
colonoscopy per s.
concealed umbilical s.
diverting s.
dusky s.
end s.
end-loop s.
gastroenterostomy s.
gastrointestinal s.
s. hernia
ileostomy s.
loop s.
maturing the s.
Mitrofanoff s.
nippled s.
permanent s.
prolapsed s.
proximal diverting s.
retracted s.
rodless end-loop s.
rosebud s.
Silastic collar-reinforced s.
s. site
stenotic s.
s. therapist
tracheostomy s.
ureteral s.

NOTES

stoma *(continued)*
ureteric s.
Wang pleural s.
stomach
aberrant umbilical s.
s. acid
s. adenocarcinoma
bilocular s.
s. cancer metastasis
s. cardiomyotomy
Dieulafoy vascular malformation of the s.
drain-trap s.
dumping s.
hourglass s.
insufflation of s.
intrathoracic s.
leather-bottle s.
posterior s.
pyloric part of s.
s. reefing
sclerotic s.
s. slippage
thoracic s.
totally intrathoracic s.
trifid s.
upside-down s.
wallet s.
water-trap s.
stomachal
stomachic
stomal
s. colonoscopy
s. complication
s. intussusception
s. invagination
s. prolapse
s. retraction
s. ulceration
stomas (*pl. of* stoma)
stomata (*pl. of* stoma)
stomatal
stomatic
stomatomy
stomatonoma
stomatoplastic
stomatoplasty
stomatoscopy
diagnostic fiberoptic s.
stomatotomy
stomocephalus
stomodeum
stone
biliary tract s.
bladder s.
cholesterol s.
common bile duct s. (CBDS)
duct s.
endoscopic extraction pancreatic duct s.
s. extraction
extraction bile duct s.
extraction pancreatic s.
extrahepatic s.
s. fragmentation
s. granuloma formation
mounted point s.
S. procedure
renal s.
soft pigment s.
s. surgery
vein s.
stony-hard eye
Stookey-Scarff operation
stool
abdominal s.
s. evacuation
guaiac-negative s.
guaiac-positive s.
hard s.
heme-negative s.
heme-positive s.
s. impaction
soft s.
Stoppa
S. giant prosthetic reinforcement of the visceral sac
S. GPRVS
S. hernia repair
S. procedure
Stoppa-type laparoscopic repair
stop-valve airway obstruction
storage allocation
storm
thyroid s.
Stovall-Black method
stove-in chest
strabismus
paralytic s.
s. surgery
strabotomy
straddle fracture
straight
s. canal
s. catheter test
s. incision
s. leg raising
s. seminiferous tubule
s. sinus
straightening maneuver
straight-in ventriculostomy
straight-leg raise (SLR)
strain
compression s.
lysogenic s.
strain/counterstrain technique

straining
excessive s.
Straith eyelid operation
Strampelli-Valvo operation
stranding
fascial s.
soft-tissue s.
strangulated
s. hemorrhoid
s. incisional hernia
s. paraesophageal hernia
strangulation
s. necrosis
small bowel s.
strangury
strap muscle
Strassman
S. metroplasty
S. technique
transverse fundal incision of S.
strata (*pl. of* stratum)
strategy
imaging s.
injury-prevention s.
management s.
surgical s.
treatment s.
stratification
stratified
s. clot
s. epithelium
stratiform fibrocartilage
stratum, pl. **strata**
Straub technique
Strauss method
strawberry angioma
straw-colored ascites
Strayer
S. procedure
S. tendon technique
streak retinoscopy
stream
fecal s.
Streatfield-Fox operation
Streatfield operation
Streatfield-Snellen operation
strength
bone-screw interface s.
cervical extension s.
extensor hallucis longus s.
extrinsic muscle s.
graft s.
isometric cervical extension s.
wound-breaking s.
strength-duration curve
Stren intraepiphysial osteotomy
streptococcal infection
***Streptococcus* infection**
stress
cold restraint s.
s. dorsiflexion projection
s. fracture
s. lesion
operative s.
s. reduction
s. relaxation
s. response
s. rupture
surgical s.
s. ulceration
s. ulcer hemorrhage
s. urethral pressure profile
s. urinary incontinence
stress-induced gastric ulceration
stress-redistribution-reinjection thallium-201 imaging
stretch
anal s.
s. injury
stretch-and-spray technique
stretcher
stretching
soft-tissue s.
stria, pl. **striae**
corneal s.
striae of Zahn
striate
s. artery
s. body
striated
s. duct
s. muscle
s. muscle innervation
s. muscular sphincter
striation
tabby-cat s.
tigroid s.
Strickland
S. modification
S. technique
S. tendon repair
stricture
anastomotic s.
benign s.

S

NOTES

stricture *(continued)*
biliary s.
bismuth type IV s.
Caroli type I distal bile duct s.
cicatricial s.
clip-induced bile duct s.
esophageal s.
s. formation
peptic s.
s. prophylaxis
s. rate
strictureplasty
Finney s.
Heineke-Mikulicz s.
stricturoplasty
Finney s.
stapled s.
Thal s.
stricturotomy
endoscopic s.
stridor
nonorganic s.
postextubation s.
stridulous respiration
string
s. cell carcinoma
s. test
string-of-beads appearance
strip
autogenous s.
s. biopsy
s. biopsy resection technique
circumferential s.
s. perforation
s. procedure
s. resection
stripe
paratracheal tissue s.
properitoneal flank s.
stripout
screw s.
stripping
s. membrane
s. program
Stroganoff method
stroke
acute ischemic s.
s. ejection rate
exploratory s.
hemorrhagic s.
ischemic s.
nonfatal s.
perioperative s.
s. volume (SV)
stroma
stromal
s. line
s. neovascularization
stromatolysis
stromatosis
Strombeck nipple transposition
Strong dorsal extension block splinting
strongyloma
strophocephaly
Stroud pectinated area
structural
s. abnormality
s. anomaly
s. lesion
structure
abdominal s.
anatomic s.
bony s.
cord s.
cystic s.
echodense s.
endosellar s.
extraarticular s.
graft s.
helix-loop-helix s.
implant s.
infratentorial s.
major vascular s.
periesophageal s.
retroclival s.
retroperitoneal s.
retrosellar s.
ring s.
sella s.
sidewall s.
soft-tissue s.
stem-loop s.
underlying s.
vascular s.
structured pain interview (SPI)
strumectomy
median s.
strumiform
strut
s. fracture
s. fusion technique
s. graft
s. malposition
s. plate fixation
struvite
s. calculus
s. crystal formation
ST segment elevation
STT
spinothalamic tract
studding
peritoneal s.
Studebaker technique
Student-Newman-Keuls test

Studer
S. pouch procedure
S. reservoir urinary diversion
study
acoustic stimulation s.
altitude simulation s.
angiographic s.
Asymptomatic Carotid Atherosclerosis S. (ACAS)
barium swallow s.
bead chain s.
bulb-tip retrograde s.
contrast s.
coronary artery surgery s. (CASS)
cytologic s.
diagnostic s.
Doppler s.
electromyographic s.
electrophysiology s.
epidemiologic s.
exercise s.
histologic s.
imaging s.
injection s.
localization s.
manometric s.
multicentric s.
noninvasive localization s.
noninvasive venous s.
postirradiation s.
preoperative s.
pressure s.
pressure-flow electromyography s.
prospective s.
radiologic s.
small bowel contrast s.
tissue s.
T-tube s.
venographic s.
venous s.
Veterans Administration Cooperative s.
volumetric s.
stump
anastomotic s.
cervical s.
s. dehiscence
distal s.
duodenal s.
s. embolization syndrome
Hartmann s.
s. invagination
s. leak
s. ligation
s. pain
pancreatic s.
s. pressure
rectal s.
rectosigmoid s.
Roux limb s.
splenic vein s.
stunned myocardium
Sturmdorf
S. operation
S. suture technique
stuttering
exteriorized s.
urinary s.
stye, pl. **styes**
styliform
styloauricularis
styloauricular muscle
styloglossus
s. muscle
stylohyal
stylohyoid
s. branch
s. ligament
s. muscle
s. process syndrome
stylohyoideum
stylohyoideus
styloid
s. cornu
s. prominence
s. syndrome
styloidea
styloidectomy
Stewart s.
styloidei
vagina processus s.
stylolaryngeus
stylomandibular
s. ligament
s. membrane
stylomandibulare
stylomastoid
s. artery
s. foramen
s. vein
stylomastoidea
stylomastoideum
stylomaxillary ligament
stylopharyngeal muscle

NOTES

stylopharyngeus
stylostaphyline
stylosteophyte
styptic collodion
Suarez-Villafranca operation
Suave-Kapandji arthroplasty
subabdominal
subabdominoperitoneal
subacromial
- s. bursa
- s. space

subacromialis
subacute
- s. inflammation

subanal
subanesthetic concentration
subaortici
subapicale
subapical segment
subaponeurotic space
subarachnoid
- s. anesthesia
- s. block
- s. cavity
- s. cistern
- s. hemorrhage
- s. injection
- s. space

subarachnoidale
subarcuata
subarcuate fossa
subarcuatus
subareolar tenderness
subastragalar dislocation
subaural
subauricular
subaxial
subaxillary
subcapital
- s. fracture
- s. osteotomy

subcapsular
- s. hemorrhage
- s. renal hematoma
- s. splenectomy

subcartilaginous
subcaudate tractotomy
subcecal fossa
subchondral
subchorial
- s. hemorrhage
- s. space

subchorionic
- s. hematoma
- s. hemorrhage

subchoroidal approach
subciliary incision
subclassification
subclavia
subclaviae
subclavian
- s. arteriovenous fistula
- s. artery
- s. artery aneurysm
- s. artery occlusion
- s. central venous catheter insertion
- s. duct
- s. groove
- s. injury
- s. line
- s. loop
- s. lymphatic trunk
- s. muscle
- s. nerve
- s. periarterial plexus
- s. perivascular block
- s. steal
- s. steal syndrome
- s. sulcus
- s. triangle
- s. vein
- s. vein catheterization
- s. vein patch angioplasty
- s. vessel exposure

subclavian-subclavian bypass
subclavianus
subclavicular approach
subclavii
subclavius
subclinical infection
subcoma therapy
subcomplete resection
subcondylar
- s. deformity
- s. oblique osteotomy

subconjunctival
- s. hemorrhage
- s. injection

subcoracoid
- s. bursa
- s. shoulder dislocation
- s. space

subcorneal blister
subcortical hemorrhage
subcostal
- s. artery
- s. flank incision
- s. groove
- s. line
- s. muscle
- s. nerve
- s. plane
- s. port
- s. position
- s. transperitoneal incision
- s. vein

subcostale
subcostalis
subcostosternal
subcranial
subcruralis
subcrureus
subcutanea
subcutaneous (SQ)
s. acromial bursa
s. anastomosis
s. calcaneal bursa
s. dose
s. emphysema
s. fascia
s. fasciotomy
s. flap
s. fungal infection
s. hematoma
s. implantation
s. implanted injection port
s. infrapatellar bursa
s. injection
s. mastectomy
s. necrosis
s. necrotizing infection
s. olecranon bursa
s. operation
s. plane
s. portion
s. ring
s. route
s. scalp
s. tibialis posterior tenotomy
s. tissue
s. transfusion
subcutaneum
subcuticular suture technique
subcutis
subdeltoid
s. bursa
s. fat plane obliteration
subdeltoidea
subdiaphragmatic
s. abscess
s. space
subdigastric node
subdorsal
subduce
subdural
s. abscess
s. block
s. cavity
s. cleft
s. effusion
s. electrode array
s. grid implantation
s. hematoma
s. hematorrhachis
s. hemorrhage
s. hygroma
s. puncture
s. space
subdurale
subendocardial
subependymal
s. brain calcification
s. brain nodule
s. extension
s. giant cell astrocytoma
s. hemorrhage
subependymoma
subepithelial
s. hemorrhage
s. membrane
subepithelium
subfalcial herniation
subfascial
s. hematoma
s. prepatellar bursa
subfrontal approach
subfrontal-transbasal approach
subgaleal
s. abscess
s. emphysema
s. hematoma
s. hemorrhage
subgingival space
subglenoid shoulder dislocation
subglottic
s. cavity
s. edema
s. pressure
s. tracheal stenosis
subgluteal hematoma
subgrundation
subhepatic
s. abscess
s. recess
s. space
subhepaticus
subhuman primate donor
subhyaloid hemorrhage
subhyoid bursa
subiculum

NOTES

S

subiliac
subilium
subimplant membrane
subinfection
subinguinal
s. fossa
s. incision
s. microsurgical varicocelectomy
s. triangle
subintimal hemorrhage
subjacent tissue
subject
human s.
supine human s.
subjugal
sublabial
s. incision
s. midline rhinoseptal approach
s. perforation
sublaminar fixation
sublation
sublesional ulceration
sublethal x-ray damage repair
subligamentous dissection
sublimation
sublimis
sublingual
s. artery
s. bursa
s. caruncula
s. crescent
s. cyst
s. duct
s. fold
s. fossa
s. ganglion
s. gland
s. hematoma
s. papilla
s. pit
s. space
s. space abscess
s. vein
sublinguale
sublingualis
sublumbar
subluxation
rotary s.
s. stabilization
submammary incision
submandibular
s. duct
s. fossa
s. ganglion
s. node
s. space
s. space abscess
s. triangle
submandibulares
submandibularis
submandibulectomy
submasseteric
s. space
s. space abscess
submassive PE
submaxillaris
submaxillary
s. duct
s. fossa
s. ganglion
s. space
s. triangle
submembranous placental hematoma
submental
s. artery
s. fistula
s. hematoma
s. node
s. space
s. space abscess
s. triangle
s. vein
s. vertex projection
submentale
submentales
submentalis
submentovertical projection
submucosa
jejunal s.
small intestinal s. (SIS)
submucosal
s. dissection
s. gastric hemorrhage
s. invasion
s. mass
s. plexus
s. space
s. urethral augmentation
s. vascular dilation
submucosus
submucous
s. membrane
s. resection
submuscular implantation
subnarcotic
subnasal
subneural
suboccipital
s. decompression
s. muscle
s. nerve
s. region
s. triangle
s. venous plexus
suboccipitales
suboccipitalis

suboccipital-subtemporal approach
suboccipital-transmeatal approach
suboptimal
s. examination
s. surgery
subparalyzing dose
subparietal
subpatellar
subpectoral
s. implantation
s. implantation technique
s. plane
s. pocket
subpelviperitoneal
subpericardial
subperichondrial excision
subperiosteal
s. abscess
s. dissection
s. exposure
s. fracture
s. hematoma
s. hemorrhage
s. implant abutment
s. implant one-phase technique
s. infection
s. resection
subperiosteally
subperitoneal
s. fascia
s. space
subperitonealis
subperitoneoabdominal
subperitoneopelvic
subpetrosal
subpharyngeal
subphrenic
s. abscess
s. fluid
s. recess
s. region
s. space
subphrenici
subpleural
subplexal
subpopliteal recess
subpopulation
subpreputial
subpubic
s. angle
s. hernia
subpubicus
subpulmonary
subpulmonic pleural space
subpyloric
s. node
subpylorici
subretinal
s. damage
s. hemorrhage
s. neovascularization
s. neovascular membrane
s. space
s. surgery
subsarcolemma cisterna
subsartorial canal
subscale
catastrophizing s.
cognitive anxiety s.
fear s.
helplessness s.
subscapular
s. artery
s. branch
s. bursa
s. fossa
s. muscle
s. nerve
s. vein
subscapulares
subscapularis
s. muscle
s. tendon
subsector
subsegmental hepatectomy
subsegmentectomy
hepatic s.
subselective embolization
subserosa
subserous
subspinous
substance
cement s.
compact s.
s. concentration
corneal s.
cortical s.
exogenous s.
exophthalmos-producing s.
extracellular ground s.
glandular s.
medullary s.
müllerian inhibiting s.
muscular s.

S

NOTES

substance *(continued)*
s. P
tumor polysaccharide s.
vasoactive s.
substantia
substernal
s. angle
s. gland
substernomastoid
substitute
blood s.
hypooncotic plasma s.
substitutional cardiac surgery
substitution transfusion
substructure
subsuperior segment
subsuperius
subtalar
s. articulation
s. dislocation
subtemporal
s. decompression
s. dissection
subtemporal-intradural approach
subtendinous
s. iliac bursa
s. prepatellar bursa
subtentorial lesion
subthreshold stimulation
subthyroideus
subtotal
s. colectomy (SC)
s. distal pancreatectomy
s. esophagectomy
s. esophagoplasty
s. gastrectomy
s. gastric exclusion
s. gastric resection
s. glossectomy
s. hepatectomy
s. lateral meniscectomy
s. maxillectomy
s. pancreatoduodenectomy
s. parathyroidectomy
s. proctectomy
s. proctocolectomy
s. somatectomy
s. supraglottic laryngectomy
s. thyroidectomy
subtraction
image s.
s. technique
subtrochanteric
s. femoral fracture
s. incision
s. osteotomy
subtrochlear
subtype
comedo s.
cribriform s.
micropapillary s.
papillary s.
solid s.
tumor s.
subumbilical
s. incision
s. infection
s. space
subungual hematoma
suburethral rectus fascial sling procedure
subvaginal
subvalvular aortic stenosis
subvertebral
subvitrinal
subvolution
subxiphoid
s. limited pericardiotomy
s. port
subzonal insemination
subzygomatic
succenturiate
successive approximation
success rate
sucking wound
Sucquet
S. anastomosis
S. canal
Sucquet-Hoyer
S.-H. anastomosis
S.-H. canal
sucrose test
suction
airway s.
s. aspiration
s. biopsy
bulb s.
continuous NG s.
s. curettage
diastolic s.
s. dissection
s. drainage
Frazier s.
Gomco s.
s. injury
lavage and s.
low intermittent s.
s. method
nasogastric s.
nasopharyngeal s.
nasotracheal s.
NG s.
orogastric s.
perilimbal s.

rhoton s.
s. suspension
suctioning
endotracheal s.
suction-irrigation technique
sudation
Suda type I, II, III papilla classification
sudden infant death syndrome (SIDS)
Sudeck critical point
sudomotor axon reflex testing
sudoriferae
sudoriferous
s. duct
s. gland
Sugarbaker operation
sugar-icing liver
suggillation
postmortem s.
Sugioka transtrochanteric rotational osteotomy
Sugiura
S. esophageal variceal transection
S. procedure
suite
endoscopy s.
sulcal artery
sulcate
sulciform
sulcomarginal tract
sulculus
sulcus, pl. **sulci**
ampullary s.
atrioventricular s.
calcaneal s.
carotid s.
cerebral s.
chiasmatic s.
cingulate s.
coronary s.
deltopectoral s.
s. fixated position
s. fixation
implant gingival s.
inferior petrosal s.
internal spiral s.
intertubercular s.
mentolabial s.
nymphocaruncular s.
nymphohymenal s.
preauricular s.
pulmonary s.
scleral s.
sclerocorneal s.
sigmoid s.
subclavian s.
superior petrosal s.
supraacetabular s.
talar s.
terminalis s.
sulfacytine
sulfation
sulfonation
sulfur and silver point
Summerskill operation
sump syndrome
sun
s. and chemical combination damage
s. exposure
SUNCT
short duration, unilateral, neuralgic, conjunctival injection and tearing
SUNCT syndrome
Sunderland nerve injury classification
superacromial
superanal
superciliaris
superciliary arch
supercilii
supercilium
superduct
superexcitation
superfecundation
superfetation
superficial
s. angioma
s. anterior larynx
s. anterior wall
s. brachial artery
s. branch
s. burn
s. cardiac plexus
s. cervical artery
s. circumflex iliac artery
s. epigastric artery
s. excision
s. external pudendal artery
s. forearm
s. head
s. implantation
s. inguinal fascia
s. keratectomy

NOTES

superficial *(continued)*
s. lamellar keratoplasty
s. layer
s. lymphatic vessel
s. neck
s. orbit
s. palmar arch
s. palmar artery
s. parotidectomy
s. perineal artery
s. perineal pouch
s. perineal space
s. radiation
s. renal cortical perfusion (SRCP)
s. subumbilical infection
s. suture technique
s. temporal artery
s. temporal artery to middle cerebral artery (STA-MCA)
s. temporal artery-to-MCA bypass
s. temporalis artery
s. temporal plexus
s. thrombophlebitis
s. type
s. volar artery
s. wound
superficiale
superficiales
superficialis
superficialization
supergenual
superimpregnation
superinfection
fungal s.
superior
s. aberrant ductule
s. alveolar artery
s. angle
s. arcuate bundle
s. boundary
s. carotid triangle
s. cerebellar artery
s. cervical cardiac branch
s. cervical ganglion
s. cervical ganglionectomy
s. costal facet
s. costal pit
s. dislocation
s. duodenal fold
s. duodenal fossa
s. duodenal recess
s. edge
s. epigastric artery
s. face
s. fascia
s. flap
s. flexure
s. gluteal artery
s. gluteal neurovascular bundle
s. hemorrhoidal artery
s. hemorrhoidal plexus
s. horn
s. hypogastric plexus
s. hypophysial artery
s. ileocecal recess
s. intercostal artery
s. internal parietal artery
s. joint space
s. labial artery
s. labial branch
s. labrum anterior and posterior (SLAP)
s. lacrimal duct
s. lacrimal papilla
s. lacrimal punctum
s. laryngeal cavity
s. laryngeal nerve external branch
s. larynx
s. lateral genicular artery
s. leaf
s. lingular segment
s. margin
s. meatus
s. medial genicular artery
s. mediastinum
s. mesenteric arterial system
s. mesenteric artery (SMA)
s. mesenteric ganglion
s. mesenteric plexus
s. mesenterorenal bypass technique
s. oblique tendon
s. omental recess
s. orbit
s. orbital fissure
s. orbital fissure syndrome
s. pancreaticoduodenal artery
s. parathyroid
s. parietal lobe
s. pelvic aperture
s. peroneal retinaculum
s. petrosal sulcus
s. phrenic artery
s. pole
s. pubic ramotomy
s. pubic ramus
s. rectal artery
s. rectal fold
s. rectal plexus
s. sector iridectomy
sinus petrosus s.
s. suprarenal artery
s. tarsus
s. thoracic aperture
s. thoracic artery
s. thyroid artery
s. thyroid notch

s. thyroid plexus
s. thyroid tubercle
s. tibial articulation
s. ulnar collateral artery
s. vena cava
s. vena cava syndrome
s. vertebral notch
s. vesical artery

superiores
superior-intradural approach
superioris
superius
superlactation
superligamen
supernate
supernumerary
s. breast
s. gland
s. organ

superolateral
superovulation induction
superoxide-mediated endothelial cell dysfunction
superoxide scavenger
superpetrosal
superpigmentation
superselective
s. microcoil embolization
s. vagotomy

supersensitivity
superstructure
super-wet technique
supinate
supination
s. deformity
s. injury
s. reflex

supination-adduction fracture
supination-eversion
s.-e. fracture
s.-e. injury

supination-external
s.-e. rotation
s.-e. rotation IV fracture
s.-e. rotation injury

supination-inversion rotation injury
supination-plantar flexion injury
supinator
s. crest
s. longus reflex
s. muscle

supinatoris
supine
s. human subject
s. hypotensive syndrome
s. position

supine-oblique approach
supple bowel
supplementary
s. analgesia
s. canal
s. oxygen
s. respiration

supplementation
calcitriol s.
calcium carbonate s.
postoperative s.
temporary postoperative s.
vitamin D s.

supply
arterial s.
blood s.
compensatory blood s.
tumor blood s.

support
advanced trauma life s. (ATLS)
blood pressure s.
excessive lip s.
external s.
extracorporeal life s. (ECLS)
inspiratory pressure s.
mechanical ventilatory s.
parenteral nutritional s.
pulmonary s.
s. suture technique
systemic pressure s.
S. Team Assessment Schedule (STAS)
ventilator s.
ventilatory s.
volume-assured pressure s.

supporting tissue
suppository
suppressed respiration
suppression
twitch s.

suppressor
tumor s.

suppurant
suppurate
suppuration
alveodental s.
pulmonary s.

NOTES

suppurativa
hidradenitis s.
suppurative
s. acute inflammation
s. cholecystitis
s. chronic inflammation
s. exudate
s. granulomatous inflammation
s. infection
supraacetabular
s. groove
s. sulcus
supraacetabularis
supraacromial
supraanal
supraannular
s. mitral valve replacement
supraarytenoid cartilage
supraauricular point
supraaxillary
suprabuccal
suprabullar recess
supracarinal stenosis
supracerebellar approach
supracervical
s. hysterectomy
s. incision
suprachoroid
s. lamina
s. layer
suprachoroidal hemorrhage
suprachoroidea
supraciliary canal
supraclavicular
s. approach
s. block
s. brachial block anesthesia
s. compression
s. examination
s. lymph node biopsy
s. muscle
s. nerve
s. triangle
supraclaviculares
supraclavicularis
supraclinoid aneurysm
supracolic space
supracondylar (SC)
s. amputation
s. humeral fracture
s. line
s. process
s. suspension
s. varus osteotomy
s. Y-shaped fracture
supracondyloid
supracostal
supracotyloid
supracrestal
s. line
s. plane
supracricoid partial laryngectomy
supracristale
supracristalis
supracristal plane
supradiaphragmatic
supraduodenal
s. approach
s. artery
supraduodenalis
supraepicondylar process
supragenicular popliteal artery (SGPA)
supraglenoid tubercle
supraglottic laryngectomy
supraglottoplasty
suprahepatic
s. cuff
s. inferior vena cava (SHVC)
s. IVC
s. space
s. vena cava
suprahyoid
s. branch
s. gland
s. muscle
s. neck dissection
s. space
s. triangle
suprahyoidei
suprainguinal
suprainterparietal bone
supraintestinal
supralevator
s. anorectal space
s. pelvic exenteration
s. perirectal abscess
supralumbar
supramalleolar
s. flap
s. varus derotation osteotomy
supramammary
supramandibular
supramastoid fossa
supramaxillary
supramaximal tetanic stimulation
suprameatal
s. pit
s. triangle
suprameatica
supramental
supramentale
point B, s.
supramesocolic surgical procedure
supranasal
supraneural

supranormal
s. CI
s. hemodynamic therapy
s. resuscitation
s. value
supranuclear lesion
supraomental
s. region
s. space
supraomohyoid neck dissection
supraoptic
s. anastomosis
s. canal
supraopticohypophysial tract
supraorbital
s. arch
s. artery
s. canal
s. foramen
s. margin
s. nerve
s. notch
s. pericranial flap
s. point
s. ridge
s. vein
supraorbitale
supraorbitalis
supraorbital-pterional approach
supraorbitomeatal
suprapapillary Roux-en-Y duodenojejunostomy
suprapatellar
s. bursa
s. pouch
suprapatellaris
suprapelvic
supraperiosteal flap
supraphysiologic
s. fluid
s. fluid technique
s. resuscitation
suprapineal recess
suprapleuralis
suprapleural membrane
supraprostatectomy
suprapubic
s. cystotomy
s. extraction site
s. hernia
s. lithotomy
s. midline recurrence
s. needle aspiration
s. Pfannenstiel incision
s. port
s. prostatectomy
s. puncture
s. region
s. urethrovesical suspension operation
suprapyloric
s. node
suprapyloricus
suprarenal
s. body
s. capsule
s. cortex
s. filter placement
s. gland
s. impression
s. medulla
s. plexus
s. vein
suprarenalectomy
suprarenalis
suprascapular
s. artery
s. ligament
s. nerve
s. nerve compression
s. notch
s. vein
suprascapularis
suprasellar
s. low-density lesion
s. mass
s. subarachnoid cistern
suprasphincteric fistula
supraspinal
supraspinale
supraspinalis muscle
supraspinata
supraspinatus muscle
supraspinous
s. fossa
s. ligament
s. muscle
suprasternal
s. bone
s. examination
s. notch
s. plane
s. space
suprasternale

NOTES

suprasymphysary
supratemporal
supratentorial
s. approach
s. arteriovenous malformation
s. craniotomy
s. lesion
s. space
s. tumor
suprathoracic
Suprathreshold Adaptation Test
supratonsillar
s. fossa
s. recess
supratragic tubercle
supratragicum
supratrochlear
s. artery
s. nerve
s. vein
supratrochleares
supraumbilical incision
supravaginal
supravaginalis
supravalvar
supravalvular aortic stenosis
supraventricular
s. arrhythmia
s. crest
supraventricularis
supraversion
supravesical fossa
supravesicalis
suprema
supremae
supreme
s. intercostal artery
s. intercostal vein
surae
sural
s. artery
s. nerve biopsy
s. region
suralis
surface
acromial articular s.
auricular s.
s. biopsy
buccal s.
s. cooling technique
costal s.
cut s.
denture foundation s.
diaphragmatic s.
s. disinfection
dorsal s.
endosteal s.
s. epithelium
extensor s.
external s.
foundation s.
glenoid s.
hepatic s.
implant-bearing s.
inferior s.
internal s.
s. irradiation
s. landmark
s. membrane
orbital s.
ovarian s.
peritoneal s.
posterior s.
s. projection
raw hepatic s.
reconstruction occlusal s. (RecOS)
renal s.
s. replacement hip arthroplasty
temporal s.
s. tension theory of narcosis
tissue ingrowth s.
surface-projection rendering image
surfactant
hydrolysis of s.
surgeon
American College of S.'s (ACS)
American Society for Colon and Rectal S.'s (ASCRS)
colorectal s.
endocrine s.
Fellow of American College of S.'s (F.A.C.S.)
general s.
S. General's Office (SGO)
gynecologic s.
oculoplastic s.
pancreatic s.
parathyroid s.
pediatric s.
plastic s.
primary s.
retinal s.
thoracic s.
thyroid s.
trauma s.
vascular s.
surgeon-dependent technique failure
surgeon's knot
surgery
ablative cardiac s.
adjustable-suture strabismus s.
adult cardiovascular s.
adult scoliosis s.
ambulatory s.
American Board of S. (ABS)
anorectal s.

anterior cervical spine s.
anterior cervicothoracic junction s.
anterior lower cervical spine s.
antiglaucoma s.
antireflux s.
aortic reconstructive s.
apically repositioned flap in mucogingival s.
arterial reconstructive s.
arthroscopic laser s.
aseptic s.
asymmetric s.
bariatric s.
bat ear s.
beating-heart bypass s.
bench s.
breast-conserving s.
bypass s.
cardiac s.
cardiothoracic s.
cardiovascular s.
carotid s.
cataract s.
cervical decompression s.
cervical disk s.
cervicothoracic junction s.
ciliodestructive s.
clean contaminated s.
closed s.
colon and rectal s.
colorectal s.
combination s.
s. complication
computer-assisted stereotactic s.
concomitant antireflux s.
conservation s.
conservative s.
conventional s.
corneal s.
cosmetic s.
craniofacial reconstructive s.
cranio-orbital s.
curative-intent s.
cytoreductive s.
debulking s.
decompressive s.
definitive s.
dental s.
dentofacial s.
dialysis access s.
dirty s.
double jaw s.
DREZ s.
ECA-PCA bypass s.
elective s.
elective cosmetic s. (ECS)
emergency s.
emergent s.
endocrine s.
endodontic s.
endoscopic s.
endoscopic cardiac s.
endoscopic sinus s.
endoscopic video-assisted s.
endovascular s.
epilepsy s.
esthetic s.
excisional cardiac s.
exploratory s.
ex situ bench s.
extracorporeal s.
extracranial-intracranial bypass s.
eyelid s.
eye muscle s.
failed s.
featural s.
femorodistal reconstructive s.
fetal s.
filtration s.
first ray s.
fistulizing s.
flexible endoscopic s.
functional endoscopic sinus s. (FESS)
gastric bypass s.
gastric reduction s.
gastrointestinal s.
general thoracic s.
glaucoma s.
hand-assisted laparoscopic s. (HALS)
hepatic resectional s.
hepatobiliary s.
hip replacement s.
hypotensive s.
hysteroscopic s.
ileal pouch s.
image-guided s. (IGS)
inadequate s.
intestinal s.
intraabdominal s.
intradural tumor s.
intralacrimal s.
intranasal sinus s.

NOTES

surgery *(continued)*
intraorbital s.
jejunoileal bypass s.
keyhole s.
knee replacement s.
labyrinthine s.
lacrimal s.
laparoscopically assisted s.
laparoscopic-assisted aortic reconstructive s.
laparoscopic bariatric s.
laparoscopic colorectal cancer s.
laparoscopic Dorr antireflux s.
laparoscopic Toupet anti-reflux s.
laryngeal framework s.
laser s.
laser-filtering s.
Lich-Gregoir kidney transplant s.
limb-salvage s.
limb-sparing s.
local s.
lower extremity s.
lung volume reduction s.
major abdominal s.
major nonvascular abdominal s.
mandibular s.
maxillary s.
maxillofacial s.
microscopically controlled s.
minimal access general s.
minimally invasive robotic heart valve s.
minor s.
Mohs micrographic s.
mucogingival s.
nasal endoscopic s.
navigated brain tumor s.
navigational s.
nephron-sparing s.
neurologic s.
neurological s.
neuroma relocation s.
nonbench s.
noncardiac s.
nonvascular abdominal s.
oculoplastic s.
oncoplastic s.
open anti-reflux s.
open disk s.
open heart s. (OHS)
oral and maxillofacial s.
orbital s.
orthognathic s.
osseous s.
palliative s.
pancreatic s.
parathyroid s.
parenchymal sparing s.
pediatric cardiovascular s.
pediatric ophthalmic s.
pelvic colonic s.
penile venous ligation s.
periapical s.
peripheral vascular s.
plastic and reconstructive s.
port-access technique for coronary bypass s.
portal decompression s.
portal-systemic shunt s.
posterior lower cervical spine s.
posterior lumbar interbody fusion s.
posterior lumbar spine and sacrum s.
posterior upper cervical spine s.
preprosthetic s.
primary perineal hypospadias s.
prophylactic s.
pure refractive s.
pylorus-preserving s.
radical curative s.
radioimmunoguided s.
reconstructive preprosthetic s.
rectal s.
rectovaginal s.
refractive s.
remedial s.
renal sparring s.
reoperative aesthetic s.
reoperative bariatric s.
reoperative carotid s.
reoperative pelvic s.
reparative cardiac s.
resective s.
retinal s.
retrograde intrarenal s.
reversal jejunoileal bypass s.
right ventricle-pulmonary artery conduit s.
rigid endoscopic s.
robotic s.
salvage s.
scoliosis s.
secondary s.
second-look s.
segmental s.
sham s.
shunt s.
sinus s.
site-specific s.
small bowel s.
sphincter-saving s.
spinal s.
stereotactic s.
stereotaxic s.
stone s.
strabismus s.

suboptimal s.
subretinal s.
substitutional cardiac s.
symmetric s.
targeted s.
telepresence s.
telerobotic-assisted laparoscopic s.
thoracic s.
thyroglossal cyst s.
total hip replacement s.
total knee replacement s.
transperitoneal hand-assisted laparoscopic s.
transsexual s.
transsphenoidal s.
transsphincteric s.
trauma s.
tubal reconstruction s.
tumor s.
upper gastrointestinal tract s.
urologic s.
vaginal s.
valvular heart s.
vascular abdominal s.
video-assisted thoracoscopic s. (VATS)
video-assisted thorascopic s. (VATS)
videoscopic hernia s.
vitreoretinal s.
vitreous s.
volume reduction s. (VRS)
weight reduction s.

surgical

s. abdomen
s. access
s. adjunct
s. admitting unit
s. anatomy
s. anesthesia
s. approach
s. autoimmunization
s. bone impression
s. change
s. cholecystectomy
s. cholecystostomy
s. clinician
s. correction
s. crown lengthening
s. cystgastrostomy
s. débridement
s. debulking
s. defect
s. diagnosis
s. diathermy
s. drape combustion
s. dressing room
S. Education and Self-Assessment Program (SESAP)
s. emergency
s. emphysema
s. endarterectomy
s. endodontics
s. enucleation
s. enucleation method
s. enucleation procedure
s. enucleation technique
s. eruption
s. erysipelas
s. estrogen ablation
s. excision
s. excision biopsy
s. exposure
s. extirpation
s. failure
s. field
s. flap
s. incision
s. indication
s. infection
s. intervention
s. keratometry
s. ligation
s. maggot
s. maggot therapy
s. management
s. maneuver
s. margin
s. marking solution
s. microscope navigation (SMN)
s. neck
s. neck fracture
s. neonate
s. neurangiographic technique
s. neurology
s. occlusion rim
s. oncologist
s. oncology
s. orthodontia
s. orthodontics
s. outcome
s. pancreatic disease
s. patch grafting
s. pathology

surgical *(continued)*
s. perspective
s. placement
s. portal decompression
s. portosystemic shunting
s. positioning
s. preparation
s. problem
s. pulp exposure
s. reduction
s. repair
s. resectability
s. resection
s. retention
s. risk
s. sectioning
s. seeding
s. signature
s. specialty
s. staging
s. stapling
s. strategy
s. stress
s. suture technique
s. thrombectomy
s. trauma
s. treatment
s. treatment objective
s. treatment option
s. tuberculosis
s. vagotomy
s. weight loss
s. wound
surgically
s. corrected hypertension
s. treated patient
surgical-pathologic staging
surgical-radiologic minicholecystostomy
surgical-site infection (SSI)
surplus skin
surrenal
surveillance
endoscopic s.
s. endoscopy
graft s.
s. mechanism
s. program
s. technique
surveillance, epidemiology, and end result (SEER)
survey
s. line
s. program
radiation s.
survival
breast cancer-specific s. (BCSS)
s. curve
disease-free s. (DFS)
distant recurrence-free s. (DRFS)
graft s.
locoregional recurrence-free s. (LRRFS)
long-term s.
postoperative s.
recurrence-free s.
specific s.
susceptibility gene
suspended
s. animation
s. inspiration
suspended-pedicle approach
suspension
Aldridge-Studdefort urethral s.
Alexander-Adams uterine s.
Baldy-Webster uterine s.
bladder neck s.
Burch bladder s.
Burch iliopectineal ligament urethrovesical s.
Coffey s.
corporeal sacrospinous s.
corset s.
cuff s.
endoscopic bladder neck s.
extraperitoneal laparoscopic bladder neck s.
fingertrap s.
flexible hinge s.
Gilliam-Doleris uterine s.
Gittes-Loughlin bladder neck s.
s. laryngoscopy
minimal-incision pubovaginal s.
Olshausen s.
Pereyra bladder neck s.
Pereyra needle s.
Raz bladder neck s.
Raz four-quadrant s.
Raz needle s.
Raz urethral s.
retropubic Lapides-Ball bladder neck s.
sacrospinous ligament s.
SC s.
Stamey needle s.
suction s.
supracondylar s.
urethral s.
uterine s.
suspension-type socket
suspensory
s. ligament
s. muscle
s. sling operation
suspicion
clinical s.

suspicious
s. abnormality
s. finding
s. FNA
s. lesion
s. microcalcification
sustained
s. pressure technique
s. release (SR)
sustentacular tissue
sustentaculum
Sutherland-Greenfield osteotomy
Sutherland-Rowe incision
sutura, pl. **suturae**
sutural
s. bone
s. diastasis
s. ligament
suture
s. anastomosis
s. anchor technique
apical s.
basilar s.
bregmatomastoid s.
s. bridge
cervical s.
s. closure
s. closure technique
coronal s.
cranial s.
dentate s.
ethmoidolacrimal s.
ethmoidomaxillary s.
s. failure
false s.
s. fatigue
s. fixation
frontal s.
frontoethmoidal s.
frontomaxillary s.
frontonasal s.
frontoparietal s.
frontosphenoid s.
frontozygomatic s.
infraorbital s.
interendognathic s.
intermaxillary s.
internasal s.
interparietal s.
s. joint
lacrimoconchal s.
lacrimomaxillary s.
lambdoid s.
s. ligated
s. ligation
s. line
s. line cancer
s. line dehiscence
nasomaxillary s.
neurocentral s.
occipital s.
occipitomastoid s.
occipitoparietal s.
occipitosphenoid s.
palatine s.
palatoethmoidal s.
palatomaxillary s.
parietal s.
parietomastoid s.
petrobasilar s.
petrospheno-occipital s.
petrosquamous s.
petrotympanic s.
s. plication
s. repair
sphenofrontal s.
sphenomaxillary s.
sphenooccipital s.
sphenoorbital s.
sphenoparietal s.
sphenosquamous s.
sphenovomerine s.
sphenozygomatic s.
squamomastoid s.
squamosal s.
squamous s.
temporal s.
transosseous s.
tympanomastoid s.
tympanosquamosal s.
zygomaticofrontal s.
zygomaticomaxillary s.
zygomaticotemporal s.
suturectomy
sutured
doubly s.
sutureless
s. bowel anastomosis
s. colostomy closure
s. laparoscopic extraperitoneal inguinal herniorrhaphy
suturing
Bard endoscopic s.
conventional s.

NOTES

suturing *(continued)*
direct s.
intracorporeal s.
magnetic control s. (MCS)
needleless s.
suxamethonium
SV
stroke volume
SVC
selective vascular clamping
swage
swallow
barium s.
s. method
swamp carcinoma
Swan incision
swan-neck
s.-n. deformity reduction
s.-n. finger deformity
Swanson
S. classification
S. Convex condylar arthroplasty
S. radial head implant arthroplasty
S. reconstruction
S. silicone wrist arthroplasty
S. technique
sweat
s. duct
s. gland
sweat-gland
s.-g. adenocarcinoma
s.-g. adenoma
Swedish approach
Sweet method
swelling
external s.
genital s.
levator s.
lysosomal s.
scrotal s.
soft-tissue s.
Swenson pull-through procedure
Swiss roll embedding technique
switch
compression s.
s. operation
s. procedure
switched B-gradient technique
swivel dislocation
SWL
shock wave lithotripsy
SWMA
segmental wall motion abnormality
sword-fighting
sycoma
sycosiform fungous infection
Sydney
S. line
S. system gastritis classification
sylvian
s. approach
s. aqueduct
s. cistern
s. dissection
s. fissure
s. fistula
s. hematoma
s. line
s. point
s. vein
Sylvius
valve of S.
symblepharon ring
Syme
S. ankle disarticulation amputation
S. external urethrotomy
S. procedure
Symington anococcygeal body
symmetric
s. surgery
s. thumb duplication
s. vertebral fusion
symmetry
s. operation
s. plane
sympathectomy
cervical perivascular s.
cervicothoracic s.
chemical s.
Leriche s.
lumbar s.
periarterial s.
preganglionic s.
presacral s.
Smithwick s.
transdermal s.
visceral s.
sympathetic
s. blockade
s. blockade anesthetic technique
s. branch
s. ganglion block anesthetic technique
s. interruption
s. microneurography
s. nerve
s. nerve activity (SNA)
s. nerve block
s. projection
s. trunk
sympathetically
s. maintained pain (SMP)
s. mediated pain
sympathetoblastoma

sympathic
sympathicectomy
sympathicoblastoma
sympathicogonioma
sympathicotripsy
sympathicus
sympathoadrenal response
sympathoblastoma
sympathoexcitation
  s. reflex
sympathoexcitatory response
sympathogonioma
sympatholysis
sympatholytic agent
sympathomimetic agent
symperitoneal
symphyseotomy
symphyses (*pl. of* symphysis)
symphysialis
symphysic
symphysion
symphysiotomy
symphysis, pl. **symphyses**
  cardiac s.
  intervertebral s.
  mandibular s.
  manubriosternal s.
  mental s.
  pleural s.
  pubic s.
symptom
  acute s.
  chronic reflux s.
  S. Distress Scale
  s. experience stage
  s. formation
  ipsilateral hemispheric s.
  s. magnification syndrome
  myelopathic s.
  neurologic s.
  nonspecific s.
  postoperative s.
  presenting s.
  psychogenic s.
  s. score
  transient neurologic s. (TNS)
  unremitting s.
symptomatic
  s. infection
  s. patient
  s. primary HPT
  s. relief
  s. traumatic dissection
symptomatology
symptoms
symptothermal method
synadelphus
synanastomosis
synandrogenic
synapse, pl. **synapses**
  excitatory s.
synaptosome
synarthrodia
synarthrodial joint
synarthrosis, pl. **synarthroses**
syncephalus
synchondrodial joint
synchondroseotomy
synchondrosis, pl. **synchondroses**
  s. xiphosternalis
synchondrotomy
synchrocyclotron operation
synchronization
synchronized
  s. fibrillation
  s. intermittent mandatory ventilation (SIMV)
  s. intermittent mechanical ventilation
synchronous
  s. bladder reconstruction
  s. emergence
  s. hepatic metastasis
  s. intermittent mandatory ventilation
  s. lesion
  s. pathology
  s. resection
  s. scapuloclavicular rotation
  s. tumor
  s. urinary tract infection
syncope
syncretio
syncytial knot
syndactyl
syndactylia
syndactylization
syndactylous
syndactyly
  Diamond-Gould reduction s.
  Kelikian-Clayton-Loseff surgical s.
  reduction s.
syndectomy
syndesmectomy

NOTES

syndesmectopia
syndesmodial joint
syndesmopexy
syndesmophyte
bridging s.
syndesmoplasty
syndesmorrhaphy
syndesmotic
syndesmotomy
syndrome
abdominal compartment s.
abdominal muscle deficiency s.
acrofacial s.
acute coronary s.
acute disconnection s.
acute respiratory distress s. (ARDS)
adhesive s.
adrenal feminization s.
adult respiratory distress s. (ARDS)
afferent loop s.
aglossia-adactylia s.
Alport s.
amniotic infection s.
angio-osteohypertrophy s.
ankyloglossia superior s.
anomalous innominate artery compression s.
anterior cavernous sinus s.
anterior chest wall s.
anterior spinal artery s.
Apert s.
Arnold-Chiari s.
Ascher s.
Bannayan-Riley-Ruvalcaba s.
Behçet s.
bent-nail s.
bile-plug s.
billowing mitral valve s.
black patch s.
blind loop s.
blind pouch s.
Bloodgood s.
blue toe s.
body cast s.
Boerhaave s.
bowel bypass s.
brittle nail s.
Budd-Chiari s.
Burnett s.
burning feet s.
calcaneal spur s.
callosal disconnection s.
camptomelic s.
cancer susceptibility s.
capsular exfoliation s.
Caroli s.
cauda equina s.
cavernous sinus s.
celiac artery compression s. (CCS)
celiac band s.
central anticholinergic s.
central cord s.
central heel pad s.
cerebellomedullary malformation s.
cerebellopontine angle s.
cervical acceleration-deceleration s.
cervical compression s.
cervical fusion s.
Cheatle s.
Chiari II s.
chronic hyperventilation s.
classic multiple organ failure s.
clinical s.
clivus s.
cloverleaf skull s.
cluster tic s.
coarctation s.
Cogan s.
common peroneal nerve s.
compartment compression s.
compensatory antiinflammatory response s. (CARS)
complex regional pain s. (CRPS)
complex regional pain s. I, II
compression s.
congenital central hypoventilation s.
congenital ring s.
Cooper s.
cord traction s.
coronary s.
Costen s.
Cronkhite-Canada s.
Crouzon s.
crush s.
cutaneomucouveal s.
Dandy-Walker s.
D chromosome ring s.
deafferentation pain s.
Dejerine-Roussy s.
de Quervain s.
dialysis disequilibrium s.
dialysis encephalopathy s.
disconnection s.
DISH s.
dumping s.
dural shunt s.
Eagle s.
Eagle-Barrett s.
ectopic ACTH s.
embryonic fixation s.
entrapment s.
euthyroid sick s.
excited skin s.
exertional anterior compartment s.
exertional compartment s.

exertional deep posterior compartment s.
exfoliation s.
exploding head s.
extraarticular pain s.
extrapyramidal s.
failed back surgery s.
familial aortic ectasia s.
familial atypical multiple mole melanoma s.
familial cardiac myxoma s.
familial cholestasis s.
familial polyposis s.
FAM-M s.
female urethral s.
feminization s.
fetal aspiration s.
fibrofascial compartment s.
first arch s.
flapping valve s.
floppy valve s.
Fraley s.
Franceschetti s.
Fraser s.
Frey s.
functional prepubertal castration s.
G s.
gastrojejunal loop obstruction s.
glomangiomatous osseous malformation s.
glucagonoma s.
Gorlin-Chaudhry-Moss s.
Hadju-Cheney acroosteolysis s.
Hallermann-Streiff s.
Hallermann-Streiff-François s.
Hanhart s.
head-bobbing doll s.
hemangioma-thrombocytopenia s.
hemispheric disconnection s.
hemolytic uremic s.
hepatorenal s.
hereditary cancer s.
hereditary flat adenoma s.
Hinman s.
HNPCC s.
Horner s.
Hutchison s.
hyaline membrane s.
hymenal s.
hyoid s.
hypersensitive xiphoid s.
hyperventilation s.
hypoplastic left heart s.
immotile cilia s.
impaired regeneration s.
infantile choriocarcinoma s.
inherited cancer s.
innominate artery compression s.
intersection s.
iridocorneal endothelial s.
iridocorneal epithelial s.
Jacod s.
Jeune s.
jugular foramen s.
Kasabach-Merritt s.
Klippel-Trenaunay s.
Klippel-Trenaunay-Weber s.
lactic acidosis and stroke-like s.
Larsen s.
levator ani s.
levator scapulae s.
loculation s.
lower nephron s.
Luys body s.
Lynch s.
Maffucci s.
malignant external otitis s.
Mallory-Weiss s.
mandibulofacial dysotosis s.
mangled extremity s.
Marfan s.
Marin Amat s.
MASS s.
massive bowel resection s.
maternal deprivation s.
meconium aspiration s.
meconium plug s.
megacystic s.
megacystis-megaureter s.
megacystis-microcolon-intestinal hypoperistalsis s.
MEN s.
MEN-2a, -2b s.
Mendelson s.
Ménière s.
minimal-change nephrotic s.
minimal-lesion nephrotic s.
Mirizzi s.
mitochondrial myopathy, encephalopathy, lactic acidosis, and stroke-like s. (MELAS)
mitral valve prolapse s.
Mohr s.
monofixation s.

S

NOTES

syndrome *(continued)*
Morquio s.
mucocutaneous lymph node s.
mucocutaneous pigmentation of Peutz-Jeghers s.
mucosal neuroma s.
mucous plug s.
müllerian duct derivation s.
multiple endocrine neoplasia s.
multiple endocrine neoplasia type 2a, 2b s.
multiple hamartoma s.
multiple mucosal neuroma s.
multiple organ dysfunction s. (MODS)
multiple organ failure s.
multiple pterygium s.
myofascial pain s.
nail-patella s.
nail-patella-elbow s.
naviculocapitate fracture s.
nephritic s.
nerve compression-degeneration s.
neuroleptic malignant s. (NMS)
neurovascular compression s.
nevoid basal cell carcinoma s.
nonocclusive mesenteric ischemia s.
OAV s.
obesity-hypoventilation s.
occipital condyle s.
ocular-mucous membrane s.
oculobuccogenital s.
oculomandibulofacial s.
oculovertebral s.
OFD s.
Ogilvie s.
optic tract s.
orbital apex s.
organic short bowel s.
orofaciodigital s.
osteogenesis imperfecta congenita s.
osteomyelofibrotic s.
osteopathia striata s.
osteoporosis pseudoglioma s.
Ostrum-Furst s.
otomandibular s.
ovarian hyperstimulation s.
ovarian overstimulation s.
ovarian vein s.
pacemaker s.
Paget-von Schrötter s.
pain s.
Papillon-Léage and Psaume s.
parasellar s.
paratrigeminal s.
Parsonage-Turner s.
pericardiotomy s.
pericolic membrane s.
peritubal s.
peroneal compartment s.
persistent müllerian duct s.
Peutz-Jeghers s.
pharyngeal pouch s.
Phocas s.
piriformis s.
placental hemangioma s.
popliteal web s.
postadrenalectomy s.
postcardiotomy s.
postcholecystectomy s.
postcolonoscopy distention s.
postcommissurotomy s.
postembolization s.
posterior interosseous nerve compression s.
postfundoplication s.
postgastrectomy s.
postirradiation s.
postlaminectomy s.
postpericardiotomy s.
postphlebitic s.
postpolypectomy coagulation s.
posttubal ligation s.
postvagotomy s.
preexcitation s.
prolapsed mitral valve s.
pronator teres s.
proximal loop s.
prune-belly s.
pseudo-blind loop s.
pseudoexfoliation s.
pseudolymphoma s.
pseudoxanthoma elasticum s.
pterygopalatine fossa s.
pulmonary acid aspiration s.
pulmonary sulcus s.
quadrilateral space s.
Raeder s.
Ramsay Hunt s.
rapid tumor lysis s.
Raynaud s.
Reclus I s.
recurrent abdominal pain s. (RAPS)
red ear s.
red-eyed shunt s.
Reifenstein s.
Reiter s.
renal crush s.
respiratory distress s. (RDS)
retinoblastoma-mental retardation s.
retrosphenoidal s.
rib tip s.
Rieger s.
Riley-Day s.
Riley-Smith s.
Roaf s.

Roberts s.
Roux stasis s.
Sakati-Nyhan s.
scalenus anticus s.
scapuloperoneal s.
Scheie s.
scimitar s.
Sertoli-cell-only s.
short-bowel s.
sinus tarsi s.
slipped rib cartilage s.
slipping rib s.
slit ventricle s.
Smith-Lemli-Opitz s.
solitary rectal ulcer s.
somatostatinoma s.
splenic sequestration s.
SSRI discontinuation s.
stagnant loop s.
staphylococcal scalded skin s.
stasis s.
Stauffer s.
stump embolization s.
stylohyoid process s.
styloid s.
subclavian steal s.
sudden infant death s. (SIDS)
sump s.
SUNCT s.
superior orbital fissure s.
superior vena cava s.
supine hypotensive s.
symptom magnification s.
systemic inflammatory response s. (SIRS)
Takayasu s.
terminal reservoir s.
testicular feminization s.
tethered cord s.
third and fourth pharyngeal pouch s.
thoracic compression s.
thoracic endometriosis s.
thoracic outlet s. (TOS)
Thorn s.
Tillaux-Phocas s.
Tolosa-Hunt s.
tooth-and-nail s.
transient compartment s.
translocation Down s.
transplant lung s.
transurethral resection s.
Treacher Collins s.
trisomy 8 s.
trisomy C s.
Trotter s.
tumor lysis s.
Turcot s.
twin-twin transfusion s. (TTTS)
urethral s.
uterine hernia s.
uveoencephalitic s.
valgus extension overload s.
vanished testis s.
vascular ring s.
VATER association s.
Vernet s.
vertebral subluxation s.
vibration s.
vibrator hand s.
Villaret s.
visual deprivation s.
vitreoretinal traction s.
Wartenberg s.
Weyers-Thier s.
yellow nail s.

synechia, pl. **synechiae**
s. formation

synechiotomy
Paufique s.

synechotomy
synectenterotomy
synencephalocele
synergism
synergistic
s. interaction
s. muscle

synergy
drug s.

syngeneic
s. graft
s. tissue
s. transplantation

syngenesioplastic transplantation
syngenesioplasty
syngenesiotransplantation
syngnathia
syngraft
synonychia
synorchidism
synoscheos
synostectomy
synosteology
synostosis

NOTES

synotia
synovectomy
  Albright s.
  arthroscopic s.
  carpal s.
  dorsal s.
  Inglis-Ranawat-Straub elbow s.
  palmar s.
  Porter-Richardson-Vainio s.
  six-portal s.
  Smith-Petersen s.
  volar s.
  Wilkinson s.
synovia (*pl. of* synovium)
synovial
  s. biopsy
  s. bursa
  s. cavity
  s. fistula
  s. fluid
  s. fluid examination
  s. fold
  s. frenula
  s. frenum
  s. fringe
  s. gland
  s. hernia
  s. herniation
  s. joint
  s. ligament
  s. membrane
  s. tendon sheath
  s. tissue
  s. villus
synoviale
synoviales
synovialis
synovioma
  benign giant cell s.
  malignant s.
synoviparous
synovitis
synovium, pl. **synovia**
synpolydactyly
synthesis, pl. **syntheses**
  collagen s.
  first-strand cDNA s.
synthetic
  s. augmentation
  s. method
syphilid
syphilis
syphilitic fever
syphiloma of Fournier
syringadenoma
syringeal
syringectomy
syringes (*pl. of* syrinx)
syringoadenoma
syringocarcinoma
syringocele
syringocisternostomy
syringocystadenoma
syringocystoma
syringohydromyelic cavity
syringoma
syringomeningocele
syringomyeli
syringomyelia
syringomyelic
  s. dissociation
  s. hemorrhage
syringomyelocele
syringomyelus
syringotome
syringotomy
syrinx, pl. **syringes**
syssarcosic
syssarcosis
syssarcotic
system
  anesthetic s.
  APACHE-II s.
  arterial s.
  autologous melanoma s.
  behavioral inhibition s. (BIS)
  biliary s.
  Breast Imaging Reporting and Data S. (BIRADS)
  cartilaginous part of skeletal s.
  celiac arterial s.
  central nervous s.
  circle s.
  Clinical Classification S. (CCS)
  closed anesthesia s.
  coronary sinus perfusion s.
  digestive s.
  duct s.
  ductal s.
  electromagnetic s.
  endogenous opioid s.
  enteric nervous s.
  extracellular matrix s.
  Facial Action Coding S.
  Fatal Accident Reporting S.
  force feedback s.
  intracranial venous s.
  lacrimal s.
  lymphoma s.
  Maximally Discriminative Facial Coding S.
  mesenteric arterial s.
  musculoskeletal s.
  needle-free s.
  needleless intravenous administration s.

nervous s.
neuronavigational s.
neurotransmitter s.
node lymphoma s.
open anesthesia s.
opioid s.
optical s.
organ s.
Pain Relief Scoring S.
pediatric anesthesia s.
perfusion s.
peripheral access s. (PAS)
pin-index safety s.
preoperative scoring s.
scoring s.
serotonergic s.
static compliance of the total respiratory s.
superior mesenteric arterial s.
therapeutic intervention scoring s. (TISS)
TNM staging s.
trauma s.
United States Renal Data S.
vascular s.
vein s.
venous s.
vertical vein s.

systema

systematic

s. method
s. sextant biopsy

systematization

systemic

s. absorption
s. adjuvant therapy
s. antibiotic
s. anticoagulation
s. antifungal therapy
s. arteriovenous fistula
s. chemotherapy
s. condition
s. disease
s. dissection
s. endotoxemia
s. examination
s. fungal infection
s. hypoperfusion
s. hypotension
s. immunotherapy
s. inflammatory response syndrome (SIRS)
s. lesion
s. lupus
s. oxygen extraction
s. perfusion
s. pressure support
s. radioimmunoglobulin therapy
s. sepsis
s. vascular resistance
s. venodilation
s. venous circulation

systolic

s. arterial pressure (SAP)
s. blood pressure (SBP)
s. ejection murmur
s. ejection rate
s. left ventricular pressure
s. pressure time index

Szymanowski-Kuhnt operation

Szymanowski operation

NOTES

T

T fracture
T incision
T lesion
T myelotomy
T phenotypic lymphocyte
T sign

T1

first twitch height

T1-weighted spin-echo image
T2 relaxation rate
T2-weighted spin-echo image
tabby-cat striation
tabetic

t. crisis
t. dissociation

tablature
table

inner t.
vitreous t.

tabulation
TAC

total abdominal colectomy

TACC

thoracic aortic cross-clamping

Tachdjian

T. classification
T. procedure

tachistoscopy
tachycardia

atrial ectopic t.
atrioventricular reentry t.
automatic ectopic t.
bundle-branch reentrant t.
ectopic atrial t.
endless-loop t.
exercise-induced ventricular t.
junctional ectopic t.
pacemaker-mediated t.
right ventricular outflow tract t.
torsade de pointes ventricular t. (TdPVT)

tachyphylaxis
tacrolimus-based immunosuppression
tactic

thyroidectomy t.
thyroid surgical t.

Tactilaze angioplasty
tactile

t. anesthesia
t. stimulation

TAER

transient auditory evoked response

TAES

transcutaneous acupoint electrical stimulation

tagging stitch
tagliacotian operation
tail

artery of the pancreatic t.
t. bone
pancreatic t.
t. tumor
t. vertebra

tailbone
tailor bunionectomy
Tait flap
Tajima

T. method
T. suture technique

Takayasu

T. arteritis
T. disease
T. syndrome

takedown

t. abdominal approach
bilateral ureterostomy t.
colostomy t.
t. procedure

talar

t. avulsion fracture
t. canal
t. dislocation
t. neck fracture
t. osteochondral fracture
t. sulcus

talc

t. insufflation
t. operation
t. peritonitis
t. pleurodesis

talectomy

Trumble t.

Talesnick scapholunate repair
tali (*pl. of* talus)
talipes cavus deformity
talocalcaneal

t. angle
t. articulation
t. fusion

talocalcaneare
talocalcaneonavicular articulation
talocrural joint
talonaviculare
talonavicular fusion
taloscaphoid
talotibial
talus, pl. **tali**

T

tamp
tamponade
balloon tube t.
low-pressure t.
t. needle tract
tract t.
tamponage
tamponing
tamsulosin
Tanagho
T. bladder flap urethroplasty
T. bladder neck reconstruction
tandem
t. clipping technique
t. colonoscopy
t. construction
t. lesion
tangential
t. biopsy
t. colonic submucosal injection
t. débridement
t. excision
t. incision
t. projection
t. section
t. tract
t. wound
tangent screen examination
Tanner operation
Tansini operation
Tansley operation
tantalum cranioplasty
tap
abdominal t.
peritoneal t.
shunt t.
tape mark
tapered tip
taper point
tapetum
tapinocephalic
tapinocephaly
TAPP
transabdominal properitoneal
tapping
glabellar t.
target
fixation t.
t. gland
t. lesion
t. plasma
t. plasma concentration (TPC)
saccadic eccentric t.
t. sign
target-controlled infusion (TCI)
targeted
t. brain biopsy
t. lobar deflation
t. surgery
targeting
tumor t.
Tarin space
Tarkowski method
tarsal
t. amputation
t. bone fracture
t. canal
t. dislocation
t. fold
t. gland
t. joint infection
t. laceration
t. ligament
t. medullostomy
t. membrane
t. plate
t. strip procedure
t. wedge osteotomy
tarsectomy
Blaskovics t.
Kuhnt t.
tarsen
tarsi (*pl. of* tarsus)
tarsocheiloplasty
tarsoconjunctival flap
tarsometatarsal
t. amputation
t. articulation
t. dislocation
t. fracture-dislocation
t. truncated-wedge arthrodesis
tarsophalangeal
tarsoplasty
tarsorrhaphy
bilateral temporary t.
tarsotomy
transverse t.
tarsus, pl. **tarsi**
inferior t.
superior t.
tartrate
Tasia operation
taste pathway
tattooing
colonic t.
Taussig-Bing anomaly
Taussig-Morton
T.-M. node dissection
T.-M. operation
Taussig operation
Tawara
T. node
node of Aschoff and T.
Taylor
T. approach

T. procedure
T. suture technique
Taylor-Daniel-Weiland technique
Taylor-Townsend-Corlett iliac crest bone graft
TBF
tracheal blood flow
TBI
traumatic brain injury
TBSA
total body surface area
TBW
total body weight
TC
total colectomy
TCD
transcranial Doppler
TCD recanalization
T-cell
cytolytic T.-c. (CTL)
T.-c. depleted bone marrow transplantation
T.-c. line
TCES
transcutaneous cranial electrical stimulation
TCI
target-controlled infusion
TCM
thick cutaneous melanoma
Tc-99m
technetium-99m
tc-MER
motor-evoked response to transcranial stimulation
TCNB
Tru-Cut needle biopsy
T-condylar fracture
T-configuration
TCS
transcranial stimulation
TD
thermodilution
TDCO
thermodilution cardiac output
TdPVT
torsade de pointes ventricular tachycardia
TE
tracheoesophageal
TE fistula
TEA
thromboendarterectomy
teacup fracture
Teale-Knapp operation
team
trauma t.
TEAP
transesophageal atrial pacing
TEAP threshold
tear
bucket-handle t.
esophageal t.
flap meniscal t.
inadvertent serosal t.
Mallory-Weiss t.
mesenteric t.
rotator cuff t.
t. sac
serosal t.
teardrop
t. fracture
t. line
tearing
excessive t.
short duration, unilateral, neuralgic, conjunctival injection and t. (SUNCT)
technetium-99m (Tc-99m)
technic
technical
t. consideration
t. factor
t. failure
technician
OR t.
technique
abdominal pressure t.
abduction traction t.
ablative t.
Ace-Colles frame t.
acid etch bonding t.
adduction traction t.
afterloading t.
agglutination t.
airbrasive t.
air-gap t.
airway occlusion t.
Albert suture t.
Alexander t.
Allison suture t.
alternating suture t.
American laryngectomy t.
Amplatz t.
Amspacher-Messenbaugh t.

NOTES

technique *(continued)*
Anderson-Hutchins t.
Andrews t.
anesthetic t.
angiographic road-mapping t.
angle bisection t.
angle suture t.
antegrade double balloon-double wire t.
antegrade/retrograde cardioplegia t.
anterior quadriceps musculocutaneous flap t.
anterior sandwich patch t.
anterograde transseptal t.
antireflux ureteral implantation t.
AO t.
APOLT t.
Appolito suture t.
apposition suture t.
approximation suture t.
Araki-Sako t.
arcuate suture t.
Argyll-Robertson suture t.
Arlt suture t.
Armaly-Drance t.
Armistead t.
Aronson-Prager t.
arrested-heart revascularization t.
arterial cannulation anesthetic t.
arthrographic capsular distention and rupture t.
ascending t.
aseptic t.
ASIF screw fixation t.
Asnis t.
assay t.
assisted reproductive t.
Atasoy V-Y t.
Atkinson t.
atraumatic suture t.
atrial-well t.
autosuture t.
Avila t.
avulsion t.
Axenfeld suture t.
axillary block anesthetic t.
axillary perivascular t.
Ayre spatula-Zelsmyr cytobrush t.
Babcock suture t.
back-and-forth suture t.
Badgley t.
bag-of-bones t.
Bailey-Badgley t.
Bailey-Dubow t.
Baker t.
Balacescu-Golden t.
balanced anesthetic t.
balloon catheter t.
balloon-catheter and basket-retrieval t.
balloon tamponade t.
Bandi t.
Banks-Laufman t.
Barcat t.
bare scleral t.
Barkan t.
Barraquer suture t.
barrier t.
Barron hemorrhoidal banding t.
Barsky t.
baseball suture t.
basic t.
basilar suture t.
basket extraction t.
basket fragmentation t.
basketing t.
Bass t.
Bassini t.
bastard suture t.
Batch-Spittler-McFaddin t.
Bauer-Tondra-Trusler t.
Baumgard-Schwartz tennis elbow t.
Beall-Webel-Bailey t.
Beckenbaugh t.
Becker t.
Béclard suture t.
Becton t.
Begg light wire differential force t.
behavioral t.
Bell-Tawse open reduction t.
Belsey fundoplication t.
Belt t.
bench surgical t.
Bentall composite graft t.
Bentall inclusion t.
Bertrandi suture t.
Beverly-Douglas lip-tongue adhesion t.
bilateral inguinal hernia repair t.
Billroth I, II t.
bioprogressive t.
biopsy t.
biparietal suture t.
Bircher-Weber t.
bisecting angle t.
bisecting-the-angle t.
bitewing t.
Black t.
Black-Broström staple t.
Blackburn t.
bladder neck preserving t.
Blair t.
Blair-Byars hypospadias t.
blanket suture t.
Bleck recession t.

Blenderm patch t.
blind nasal intubation anesthetic t.
blind nasotracheal intubation anesthetic t.
blind-spot projection t.
Bloom-Raney modification of Smith-Robinson t.
Blount tracing t.
Blundell-Jones t.
Bohlman cervical fusion t.
Bohlman triple-wire t.
bolster suture t.
bolus intravenous anesthetic t.
bone t.
Bonfiglio-Bardenstein t.
Bonfiglio modification of Phemister t.
Bonola t.
boost t.
bootstrap two-vessel t.
Bora t.
Borggreve-Hall t.
bougienage t.
Bowers t.
Bowles t.
Box t.
Boyd-Anderson t.
Boyden chamber t.
Boyd-McLeod tennis elbow t.
Boyes brachioradialis transfer t.
Bozeman suture t.
Braasch bulb t.
brachial plexus block anesthetic t.
Brackett-Osgood-Putti-Abbott t.
Brackin t.
Brady-Jewett t.
Brand tendon transfer t.
breast-conserving t.
Brecher-Cronkite t.
Brecher new methylene blue t.
bregmatomastoid suture t.
Brenner gastrojejunostomy t.
bridle suture t.
Brockenbrough t.
Brockhurst t.
bronchoscopy anesthetic t.
Brooks t.
Brooks-Jenkins atlantoaxial fusion t.
Brooks-Seddon transfer t.
Broström injection t.
Brown t.
Brown-Beard t.
Brown-Brenn t.
Brown-Wickham t.
Bruhat t.
Bruser t.
Bryan-Morrey t.
Buck-Gramcko t.
Bugg-Boyd t.
bulk pack t.
bunching suture t.
Buncke t.
Bunnell atraumatic t.
Bunnell suture t.
Bunnell tendon transfer t.
Burch bladder suspension t.
Burgess t.
buried mass far-and-near suture t.
Burkhalter modification of Stiles-Bunnell t.
Burkhalter transfer t.
Burrows t.
buttonhole suture t.
button suture t.
Buxton bolus suture t.
bypass t.
cable wire suture t.
Caldwell-Coleman flatfoot t.
Callahan fusion t.
Camino catheter t.
Camitz t.
Campbell t.
Canale t.
canal/wall-up t.
Capello t.
Cape Town t.
capitonnage suture t.
capping t.
capsule flap t.
capsule forceps t.
cardiovascular imaging t.
Carey Ranvier t.
Carnesale t.
carotid preservation t.
Carrell fibular substitution t.
Carrel suture t.
catheterization t.
catheter-securing t.
caudal epidural anesthetic t.
cavernosal alpha blockade t.
Cave-Rowe shoulder dislocation t.
celiac plexus block anesthetic t.
cell separation t.
cement t.

NOTES

technique *(continued)*
cementless t.
central anesthetic t.
central slip sparing t.
central venous cannulation anesthetic t.
cephalotrigonal t.
cervical plexus block anesthetic t.
cervical screw insertion t.
cervical spondylotic myelopathy fusion t.
chain suture t.
channel shoulder pin t.
Charters t.
Chaves-Rapp muscle transfer t.
Cherney suture t.
chevron t.
chew-in t.
Chiari t.
Childress ankle fixation t.
chloramine-T t.
cholangiographic t.
Cho tendon t.
Chow t.
Chrisman-Snook ankle t.
Cierny-Mader t.
Cincinnati t.
circular suture t.
circulatory arrest anesthetic t.
circumcision suture t.
clamp-and-sew t.
clamshell t.
Clancy ligament t.
Clark transfer t.
classic DSRS t.
Clayton-Fowler t.
clearance t.
Cleveland-Bosworth-Thompson t.
clip t.
closed-circuit anesthetic t.
closed-gloving t.
closed tubule fixation t.
Cloward t.
Coakley suture t.
coaptation suture t.
cobalt-60 moving strip t.
cobbler's suture t.
Cobb scoliosis measuring t.
Codivilla tendon lengthening t.
Coffey t.
Coffey-Witzel jejunostomy t.
Cofield t.
Cohen cross-trigonal t.
cold saline-induced paresthesia t.
Cole t.
Coleman flatfoot t.
Collis broken femoral stem t.
Collis-Nissen fundoplication t.
Coltart fracture t.
combination of isotonics t.
combined spinal-epidural anesthetic t.
compensation t.
composite addition t.
composite pelvic resection t.
compound suture t.
compression t.
computer-assisted continuous infusion anesthetic t.
computer-controlled drug administration anesthetic t.
computer-controlled infusion anesthetic t.
Connell suture t.
Connolly t.
continuous gum t.
continuous infusion anesthetic t.
continuous pull-through t.
continuous spinal anesthetic t.
continuous suture t.
continuous-wave t.
contoured anterior spinal plate t.
contraceptive t.
contract-relax t.
controlled release anesthetic t.
controlled water-added t.
conventional t.
Conyers t.
Coomassie brilliant blue t.
Coonse-Adams t.
Cope t.
Copeland t.
coracoclavicular t.
Corbin t.
coronary flow reserve t.
costotransversectomy t.
cough CPR t.
Counsellor-Flor modification of McIndoe t.
Cozen-Brockway t.
crash t.
Crawford graft inclusion t.
Crawford-Marxen-Osterfeld t.
Creech t.
Crego tendon transfer t.
cricoid pressure anesthetic t.
cross-facial t.
cross-section t.
Crown suture t.
cruciform suture t.
crushing t.
Crutchfield reduction t.
cryosurgical t.
Cubbins shoulder dislocation t.
Culcher-Sussman t.
culturing t.

cup-patch t.
Cupper suture t.
Curtis t.
Curtis-Fisher knee t.
Cushing suture t.
cushioning suture t.
cutaneous suture t.
cutdown t.
cuticular suture t.
Czerny-Lembert suture t.
Czerny suture t.
Darrach-McLaughlin shoulder t.
Davey-Rorabeck-Fowler decompression t.
Davis drainage t.
Debeyre-Patte-Elmelik rotator cuff t.
decompression t.
decortication t.
DEFT t.
Deisting prostatic dilation t.
delayed primary suture t.
deliberate hypotension anesthetic t.
demand-adapted administration anesthetic t.
Denis Browne urethroplasty t.
Dennis t.
de novo needle-knife t.
DePalma modified patellar t.
depth pulse t.
dermal suture t.
descending t.
destructive interference t.
Devonshire t.
Dewar-Barrington clavicular dislocation t.
Dewar-Harris shoulder t.
Dewar posterior cervical fusion t.
Deyerle femoral fracture t.
diagnostic t.
Dias-Giegerich fracture t.
Dickinson calcaneal bursitis t.
Dickson transplant t.
Dieffenbach-Duplay hypospadias t.
differential force t.
differential spinal block anesthetic t.
digital subtraction t.
dilator-and-sheath t.
dilution-filtration t.
Dimon-Hughston t.
Diprivan t.
direct/indirect t.
direct insertion t.
distraction t.
Dixon t.
Dolenc t.
Doll trochanteric reattachment t.
Doppler auto-correlation t.
Dor fundoplication t.
dot-blot t.
Dotter t.
Dotter-Judkins t.
double-armed suture t.
double-balloon t.
double-button suture t.
double-dummy t.
double-folded cup-patch t.
double-freeze t.
double-looped semitendinosus t.
double-rod t.
double-sealant t.
double-staple t.
double-stapled ileoanal reservoir t.
double stapling t. (DST)
double-stick t.
double-tube t.
double-wire t.
Douglas bag t.
dowel t.
doweling spondylolisthesis t.
Drake tandem clipping t.
DREZ modification of Eriksson t.
drilling t.
driven equilibrium Fourier transform t.
Drummond spinous wiring t.
Drummond wire t.
dry field t.
dual impression t.
duct-to-mucosa t.
Dufourmentel t.
dunking t.
Dunn t.
Dunn-Brittain foot stabilization t.
Duplay I, II t.
Dupuytren suture t.
DuVries deltoid ligament reconstruction t.
Dyban t.
dye dilution t.
dynamic bolus tracking t.
Eames t.
Eastwood t.
Eaton-Littler t.

NOTES

technique *(continued)*
Eaton-Malerich fracture-dislocation t.
Eberle contracture release t.
ECG signal-averaging t.
Ecker-Lotke-Glazer tendon reconstruction t.
edge-to-edge suture t.
Eftekhar broken femoral stem t.
Eggers tendon transfer t.
Eisenberger t.
Eklund t.
elliptical excision t.
Ellis-Jones peroneal tendon t.
Ellison t.
Ellis skin traction t.
Emmet suture t.
en bloc, no-touch t.
Ender femoral fracture t.
endobronchial intubation anesthetic t.
endodontic t.
endofluoroscopic t.
endorectal ileoanal pull-through t.
endoscope-assisted t.
endoscopic-assisted t.
endoscopic-assisted microsurgical t.
endoscopic mucosal resection t.
endovascular stenting t.
end-to-end reconstruction t.
end-to-side vasoepididymostomy t.
entangling t.
enucleation t.
epiaortic imaging t.
epidural blood patch anesthetic t.
epineural suture t.
epithelialization t.
Erickson-Leider-Brown t.
Eriksson brachial block t.
Eriksson ligament t.
erysiphake t.
esophageal banding t.
Essex-Lopresti axial fixation t.
Essex-Lopresti calcaneal fracture t.
Evans ankle reconstruction t.
eversion t.
everting interrupted suture t.
evoked potential t.
exchange t.
excisional biopsy t.
excision-curettage t.
ex situ-in situ t.
extraanatomical renal revascularization t.
extraanatomic bypass t.
extraarticular t.
extracorporeal t.
extraction balloon t.
extradural anesthetic t.
extravesical ureteral reimplantation t.
extremity mobilization t.
extubation anesthetic t.
ex vivo t.
FA t.
facet excision t.
Fahey t.
Fahey-O'Brien t.
Fairbanks t.
Falk vesicovaginal fistula t.
far-and-near suture t.
Farmer t.
fast exposure t.
fat-suppression t.
feeder-frond t.
femoral 3-in-1 t.
Ferkel torticollis t.
ferning t.
fiberoptic bronchoscopy anesthetic t.
fiberoptic endoscopy anesthetic t.
fiberoptic tracheal intubation anesthetic t.
Fick t.
Ficoll-Hypaque t.
Fielding modification of Gallie t.
figure-of-eight suture t.
filling first t.
finger fracture t.
Finochietto-Billroth I gastrectomy t.
first-line screening t.
first-pass t.
first rib resection via subclavicular approach t.
Fish cuneiform osteotomy t.
fixation t.
fixation suture t.
FLAK t.
Flamm t.
flap t.
Flatt t.
flicker-fusion frequency t.
Flick-Gould t.
flip-flap t.
floppy Nissen fundoplication t.
flow detection t.
flow interruption t.
flow mapping t.
fluid loading anesthetic t.
fluorescent antibody staining t. (FAST)
fluoroscopic pushing t.
flush-and-bathe t.
flushing t.
Flynn t.
Fones t.
Forbes modification of Phemister graft t.

Ford triangulation t.
fore-and-aft suture t.
Forest-Hastings t.
forward triangle t.
Fourier-acquired steady-state t. (FAST)
four-maximal breath preoxygenation t.
four-port t.
Fowles dislocation t.
Frank permanent gastrotomy t.
Fraunfelder no-touch t.
Freebody-Bendall-Taylor fusion t.
freehand suturing t.
free ligature suture t.
free-root insertion t.
French fracture t.
Fried-Hendel tendon t.
Froimson t.
frontalis sling t.
Frost suture t.
functional t.
Furnas-Haq-Somers t.
furrier's suture t.
fusion t.
Gaenslen split-heel t.
Gallie atlantoaxial fusion t.
Gallie wiring t.
Galveston t.
Gambee suture t.
Ganley t.
Garceau tendon t.
gaseous laparoscopy t.
gasless laparoscopy t.
gastric valve tightening t.
gated t.
Gaur balloon distention t.
Gelman t.
Gély suture t.
general anesthetic t.
George Lewis t.
Ger t.
Getty decompression t.
Giannestras modification of Lapidus t.
Gibson suture t.
gift wrap suture t.
Gilbert-Tamai-Weiland t.
Gillies-Millard cocked-hat t.
Gill-Manning-White spondylolisthesis t.
Gill sliding graft t.
Gil-Vernet t.
Gittes t.
Gledhill t.
Glen Anderson t.
gliding-hole-first t.
gloved-fist t.
Glover suture t.
Glynn-Neibauer t.
Goebel-Frangenheim-Stoeckel t.
Goldberg t.
Goldmann kinetic t.
Goldmann static t.
Goldner-Clippinger t.
gold plate t.
gold seed implantation t.
Goldstein spinal fusion t.
Gomco t.
Goodwin t.
Goodwin-Hohenfellner t.
Goodwin-Scott t.
Gordon-Broström t.
Gordon joint injection t.
Gordon-Taylor t.
Gould suture t.
grabbing t.
gracilis flap t.
grasping t.
Graves t.
gravimetric t.
Green-Banks t.
Greulich-Pyle t.
Grice-Green t.
Grimelius t.
Gritti-Stokes knee amputation t.
groove suture t.
Grosse-Kempf tibial t.
Groves-Goldner t.
Gruber suture t.
Grüntzig t.
Guhl t.
guidewire exchange t.
guidewire and mini-snare t.
Gussenbauer suture t.
Guttmann t.
Guyon ankle amputation t.
guy suture t.
Guyton-Friedenwald suture t.
Hackethal stacked nailing t.
Håkanson t.
half-mouth t.
Hall t.
Halsted suture t.

NOTES

technique *(continued)*
Hamas t.
Hamou t.
Hardinge t.
harelip suture t.
Hark t.
Harmon transfer t.
Harriluque t.
Harris suture t.
Hartel t.
Hartmann reconstruction t.
Hassmann-Brunn-Neer elbow t.
Hasson t.
Hauri t.
Hauser patellar realignment t.
Hawkins inside-out nephrostomy t.
Hawkins single-stick t.
head turn t.
Heaney t.
helical suture t.
hemostat t.
hemostatic suture t.
Hendler unitunnel t.
Henning inside-to-outside t.
Henry acromioclavicular t.
hepatic vascular isolation t.
Hermodsson internal rotation t.
Hey-Groves fascia lata t.
Hey-Groves-Kirk t.
Hey-Groves ligament reconstruction t.
Heyman-Herndon-Strong t.
Higgins t.
high-amplitude sucking t.
high-heat casting t.
high-kV t.
high-tension suturing t.
Hill-Nahai-Vasconez-Mathes t.
Hitchcock tendon t.
Hodgson t.
Hofmeister t.
Hohl-Moore t.
Hoke-Kite t.
hold-relax t.
hole-in-one t.
Hood t.
Hoppenfeld-Deboer t.
Hori t.
horizontal mattress suture t.
hot biopsy t.
Hotchkiss-McManus PAS t.
hot-dog t.
Houghton-Akroyd fracture t.
House t.
Hovanian transfer t.
Howard t.
Hughes modification of Burch t.
Hughston-Jacobson t.
Hungerford t.
Hunt-Early t.
Huntington tibial t.
hybridization-subtraction t.
hybridoma t.
hydroflow t.
hydrogen inhalation t.
hygroscopic t.
hypogastric plexus block anesthetic t.
hypothermia anesthetic t.
Ilizarov limb-lengthening t.
image-related screening t.
imaging t.
imbricated suture t.
immediate extension t.
immersion t.
immunohistochemical t.
implanted suture t.
impression t.
indicator dilution t.
indirect t.
indocyanine green indicator dilution t.
induced hypotension anesthetic t.
induction anesthetic t.
infiltration anesthetic t.
Inglis-Cooper t.
Inglis-Ranawat-Straub t.
inhalation anesthetic t.
injection t.
inotrope resuscitation t.
Insall ligament reconstruction t.
insemination swim-up t.
insertion t.
inside-out t.
inside-to-outside t.
insufflation anesthetic t.
intercostal nerve block anesthetic t.
interference screw t.
interlocking suture t.
internal jugular vein cannulation anesthetic t.
internal jugular vein catheterization anesthetic t.
internal jugular vein puncture anesthetic t.
interpleural anesthetic t.
interrupted suture t.
interscalene block anesthetic t.
interspinous segmental spinal instrumentation t.
interventional t.
intraarticular anesthetic t.
intracorporeal knotting t.
intradermal mattress suture t.
intradermal tattooing t.

intramuscular preanesthetic medication anesthetic t.
intraoperative computer-assisted spinal orientation t.
intraperitoneal t.
intrathecal cannulation anesthetic t.
intrathecal morphine anesthetic t.
intravenous cannulation anesthetic t.
intravenous oxygen-15 water bolus t.
intubation anesthetic t.
invaginating suture t.
invagination t.
invasive t.
inverting knot t.
ischemic-tourniquet t.
isolation t.
isometric t.
Ivalon suture t.
Jaboulay-Doyen-Winkleman t.
Jacobs locking-hook spinal rod t.
Jansey t.
Jeffery t.
jejunoileal bypass reversal t.
Jerne t.
jet ventilation anesthetic t.
J loop t.
Jobert suture t.
Johnson pelvic fracture t.
Johnson staple t.
Johnston pursestring suture t.
Jones-Brackett t.
Jones and Jones wedge t.
Jones-Politano t.
Jorgensen t.
Judd pyloroplasty t.
Judkins t.
Judkins-Sones t.
jugular t.
Kader-Senn gastrotomy t.
Kalt suture t.
kangaroo tendon suture t.
Kapandji t.
Kapel elbow dislocation t.
Kaplan t.
Kashiwagi t.
Kates-Kessel-Kay t.
Kato thick smear t.
Kaufer tendon t.
Kaufmann t.
Kehr t.
Kelikian-Clayton-Loseff t.
Kelikian-Riashi-Gleason t.
Kellogg-Speed fusion t.
Kelly suture t.
Kendrick t.
Kendrick-Sharma-Hassler-Herndon t.
Kennedy ligament t.
Kern t.
Kessler suture t.
Kety-Schmidt inert gas saturation t.
keyhole tenodesis t.
Keystone t.
Kidde cannula t.
King t.
King-Richards dislocation t.
King-Steelquist t.
Kirk thigh amputation t.
Kirschner suture t.
kissing balloon t.
Kjolbe t.
Klein t.
Klisic-Jankovic t.
Knoll refraction t.
Knott t.
Koch t.
Krawkow-Cohn t.
Krawkow-Thomas-Jones t.
Krempen-Craig-Sotelo tibial nonunion t.
Krönig t.
Kumar-Cowell-Ramsey t.
Kumar spica cast t.
Küntscher t.
Kutler finger amputation t.
Labbé gastrotomy t.
labiolingual t.
lace suture t.
Lamaze t.
Lamb-Marks-Bayne t.
Lambrinudi t.
laparoscopic colposuspension t.
laparoscopic lymph node dissection t.
laparoscopic Nissen fundoplication t.
laparoscopic paraaortic lymph node sampling t.
laparoscopic stripping t.
Lapides t.
Lapidus hammertoe t.
large-core t.
Larson t.

NOTES

T

technique *(continued)*
laryngeal mask insertion anesthetic t.
laryngoscopy anesthetic t.
laser welding t.
lateral bending t.
lateral window t.
Laurell t.
layer t.
Lazarus-Nelson t.
LCVP-aided t.
LDN t.
Leach t.
Leadbetter modification t.
Leboyer t.
Le Dentu suture t.
Le Dran suture t.
LeDuc t.
Lee t.
Lefèvre gastrectomy t.
Le Fort suture t.
Lehman t.
Leibolt t.
Leksell t.
Lembert suture t.
Lenart-Kullman t.
lens suture t.
lesser sac t.
letterbox t.
Lewit stretch t.
Lich extravesical t.
Lich-Gregoir t.
Lichtman t.
lid-loading t.
Liebolt radioulnar t.
ligate-divide-staple t.
ligation suture t.
light-around-wire t.
Limberg t.
limb-saving t.
Lindholm t.
lingual split-bone t.
Lipscomb t.
Lister t.
Little t.
Littler t.
Littler-Cooley t.
Lloyd-Roberts fracture t.
localization t.
local standby anesthesia t.
locking suture t.
lock-stitch suture t.
Löffler suture t.
long cone t.
loop gastric bypass t.
loop-on mucosa suture t.
Losee modification of MacIntosh t.
Losee sling and reef t.
loss-of-resistance t.
lost wax pattern t.
LowDye taping t.
low-flow anesthetic t.
Lown t.
Ludloff t.
lumbar accessory movement t.
lumbar anesthetic t.
Luque instrumentation concave t.
Luque instrumentation convex t.
Luque sublaminar wiring t.
LUS scanning t.
Lyden t.
Lyden-Lehman t.
Lynn t.
MacIntosh t.
macroelectrode recording t.
Madden t.
Magerl translaminar facet screw fixation t.
Magilligan measuring t.
Magnuson t.
Ma-Griffith t.
Maitland t.
Majestro-Ruda-Frost tendon t.
Malawer excision t.
Mallory t.
Mancini t.
mandibular swing t.
Mankin t.
manometric t.
Manske t.
manual push-pull t.
Maquet t.
Marbach-Weil t.
March t.
Marcus-Balourdas-Heiple ankle fusion t.
Marks-Bayne t. for thumb duplication
Marlex plug t.
Marshall ligament repair t.
Marshall-McIntosh t.
marsupialization t.
Martin patellar wiring t.
Martin reduction t.
masking t.
masquerade t.
MAST t.
Mathieu t.
Matti-Russe t.
Mazet t.
McCauley t.
McConnell t.
McElfresh-Dobyns-O'Brien t.
McElvenny t.
McFarland-Osborne t.
McFarlane t.

McGoon t.
McKeever-Buck elbow t.
McLaughlin-Hay t.
McLean t.
McMaster t.
McReynolds open reduction t.
McVay t.
Meares-Stamey t.
mechanical ventilation anesthetic t.
Mehn-Quigley t.
Meigs suture t.
membrane catheter t.
Menghini biopsy t.
Mensor-Scheck t.
Merendino t.
Messerklinger t.
Meyerding-Van Demark t.
Michal II t.
microelectrode recording t.
microinvasive t.
micromanipulation t.
microsurgery t.
microsurgical t.
microtransducer t.
micro-tubulotomy t.
microvascular t.
midface degloving t.
Milch cuff resection of ulna t.
Milch elbow t.
Milford mallet finger t.
Millen t.
mille pattes t.
Millesi modified t.
minilaparotomy t.
minimal-access t.
minimal leak t.
minimally invasive surgical t.
Mital elbow release t.
miter t.
Mitrofanoff continent urinary diversion t.
Mizuno t.
Mizuno-Hirohata-Kashiwagi t.
modified Belsey fundoplication t.
modified brachial t.
modified Cantwell t.
modified Child t.
modified Hassan open t.
modified piggyback t.
modified Pomeroy t.
modified Sacks-Vine push-pull t.
modified Seldinger t.
modified Toupe t.
modified V-Y advancement t.
Moe scoliosis t.
Mohs fresh tissue chemosurgery t.
Mohs microsurgery t.
molecular t.
monitored anesthesia care anesthetic t.
monitoring t.
Monticelli-Spinelli distraction t.
Moore t.
morcellation t.
Morgan-Casscells meniscus suturing t.
Morrison t.
Mose t.
motor point block anesthetic t.
MPB t.
MPGR t.
MP-RAGE t.
Mubarak-Hargens decompression t.
mucosal relaxing incision t.
Mueller t.
Mullins blade t.
multiple inert gas elimination t. (MIGET)
multiple-port incision t.
muscle energy t.
muscle-splitting t.
Nalebuff-Millender lateral band mobilization t.
nasotracheal intubation anesthetic t.
nasovesicular catheter t.
Nealon t.
near-and-far suture t.
needle-knife t.
needle thoracentesis t.
needle-through-needle single interspace t.
nerve stimulator anesthetic t.
nerve suture t.
neural arch resection t.
neuroablative t.
neuroleptanalgesia anesthetic t.
Neviaser acromioclavicular t.
Neviaser-Wilson-Gardner t.
Nicholas five-in-one reconstruction t.
Nicholas ligament t.
Niebauer-King t.
Nikaidoh-Bex t.
Nirschl t.

NOTES

technique *(continued)*
Nissen fundoplication t.
Nissen-Rosseti fundoplication t.
nitrous oxide-opioid-barbiturate anesthetic t.
nitrous oxide-oxygen-opioid anesthetic t. (N_2O-O_2-opioid anesthetic technique)
no-leak t.
noninvasive t.
nonlaparoscopic t.
nonoptimal t.
non-rib-spreading thoracotomy incision t.
N_2O-O_2-opioid anesthetic t.
nitrous oxide-oxygen-opioid anesthetic technique
noose suture t.
Norfolk t.
Northern blot t.
no-touch t.
N2-Sargenti t.
Oakley-Fulthorpe t.
Ober-Barr transfer t.
Ober tendon t.
O'Brien akinesia t.
Obtura injectable t.
off-center isoperistaltic t.
Ogata t.
Okamura t.
Ollier t.
Omer-Capen t.
one-lung ventilation anesthetic t.
one-phase subperiosteal implant t.
one-pour t.
onlay t.
onlay-tube-onlay urethroplasty t.
open drop t.
open flap t.
open-gloving t.
open Hasson t.
open laparoscopic t.
open palm t.
open-sky t.
operative t.
O'Phelan t.
optimal t.
oral anesthetic t.
Orandi t.
orbital exenteration gastroscopic access t.
Orticochea scalping t.
Osborne-Cotterill elbow t.
Osgood modified t.
Osmond-Clarke t.
Ostrup harvesting t.
Ouchterlony t.
Ouchterlony gel diffusion t.
outside-to-outside arthroscopy t.
over-and-over suture t.
Overhauser t.
overlapping suture t.
over-the-wire t.
Oxford t.
Pacey t.
Pack t.
Pagenstecher suture t.
Palfyn suture t.
palliative t.
Palmer t.
Palmer-Widen shoulder t.
Palomo t.
Pancoast suture t.
pants-over-vest t.
Papineau t.
Paquin t.
paradoxical t.
parallel t.
paralleling t.
paresthesia anesthetic t.
Paré suture t.
Parker-Kerr suture t.
Parrish-Mann hammertoe t.
Parvin gravity t.
PAS t.
passive gliding t.
patch t.
Paterson t.
patient-controlled analgesia anesthetic t.
Paulos ligament t.
Pauwels t.
Peacock transposing t.
peg-and-socket t.
pelviscopic clip ligation t.
Percoll t.
percutaneous insertion t.
percutaneous interventional t.
perfusion hypothermia t.
perfusion measurement t.
peribulbar anesthetic t.
pericostal suture t.
peripheral nerve block anesthetic t.
Perry t.
Perry-Nickel t.
Perry-O'Brien-Hodgson t.
Perry-Robinson cervical t.
Petit suture t.
Pheasant elbow t.
Phemister-Bonfiglio t.
Phemister onlay bone graft t.
phrenic nerve block anesthetic t.
Pichlmayer t.
Pierrot-Murphy tendon t.
pinch-grasp injection t.
pin suture t.

plaque t.
plastic matrix t.
plastic suture t.
plicating suture t.
Pólya t.
Ponsky pull or guidewire insertion t.
porcelain cervical ditching t.
Porstmann t.
Porter-Richardson-Vainio t.
posterior flap t.
posterolateral costotransversectomy t.
postresection filling t.
Pratt t.
premuscular mesh t.
presaturation t.
preservation t.
pressure half-time t.
primary suture t.
Pringle vascular control t.
Proetz displacement t.
prograde t.
projection-reconstruction t.
projective t.
pseudobiopsy t.
Puddu tendon t.
pulley suture t.
pull-out wire suture t.
pull-through t.
pulmonary artery catheterization anesthetic t.
Pulvertaft weave t.
puppet t.
pursestring suture t.
push-back t.
push plus refraction t.
push-pull T t.
quadrant sampling t.
Quartey t.
Quénu nail plate removal t.
quick angulation t.
Quickert three-suture t.
quilt suture t.
radiographic t.
radioguided t.
radiologic t.
radionuclide t.
Rainville t.
Ralston-Thompson pseudoarthrosis t.
Ranawat-DeFiore-Straub t.
rapid pull-through esophageal manometry t.
rapid scan t.
rapid-sequence induction anesthetic t.
Rashkind balloon t.
Ray-Clancy-Lemon t.
Rayhack t.
reattribution t.
rebreathing t.
Rebuck skin window t.
recanalization t.
recombinant DNA t.
reconstruction t.
reconstructive t.
rectal anesthetic t.
reduction t.
refractive operative t.
regional anesthetic t.
Reichel-Pólya t.
Reichenheim t.
relaxation t.
rescue t.
resectional t.
restorative proctocolectomy t.
retained papilla t.
retention suture t.
retrobulbar anesthetic t.
retrograde tracheal intubation anesthetic t.
retromuscular prosthetic t.
reverse wedge t.
rhythmic initiation t.
ribbon arch t.
Richardson suture t.
Richter suture t.
Ricketts-Abrams t.
Rideau t.
right-angle t.
Riordan tendon transfer t.
Risser t.
Ritter-Oleson t.
Roberts t.
Robinson-Southwick fusion t.
Rockwood-Green t.
Rogers cervical fusion t.
rollerball t.
roll-tube t.
Rood t.
Rosalki t.
Ross t.
Royle-Thompson transfer t.
RPT t.
running continuous suture t.

NOTES

technique *(continued)*
running vascular t.
Russe t.
Russell t.
Ryerson t.
sacral bar t.
Saeed t.
Saenger suture t.
Sage-Clark t.
Saha transfer t.
Sakellarides-DeWeese t.
saline t.
Salter t.
Sammarco-DiRaimondo modification of Elmslie t.
Sarmiento trochanteric fracture t.
Scaglietti closed reduction t.
scanning t.
Schaberg-Harper-Allen t.
Schauwecker patellar wiring t.
Scheie t.
Schepens t.
Schepsis-Leach t.
Schlatter gastrectomy t.
Schnute wedge resection t.
Schober t.
Schonander t.
Schoonmaker-King single-catheter t.
scleral search coil t.
Scott glenoplasty t.
screw insertion t.
Scudder t.
Scuderi t.
sealed envelope t.
Sealy-Laragh t.
secondary suture t.
sectional t.
section freeze substitution t.
Seddon t.
segment-oriented t.
Seldinger percutaneous t.
Seldinger retrograde wire/intubation t.
selective bronchial catheterization anesthetic t.
Sell-Frank-Johnson extensor shift t.
Semb nephrectomy t.
semitendinosus t.
Semm Z t.
sensorineural acuity level t.
Serafin t.
seromuscular suture t.
seroserous suture t.
Sever modification of Fairbank t.
Sewall t.
sextant t.
sharp dissection t.
Sharrard transfer t.
shave excision t.
Sheehan and Dodge t.
Sherk-Probst t.
Shirodkar suture t.
shish-kebab t.
short-cone t.
short lever accessory movement t.
Silber t.
Silfverskiöld lengthening t.
silver dollar t.
Simon suture t.
Simonton t.
simple suture t.
Sims suture t.
Singer-Blom endoscopic tracheoesophageal puncture t.
single-armed suture t.
single-port t.
single-pour t.
single proximal portal t.
single-shot imaging t.
single space t.
skewer t.
skin expansion t.
skin-surfacing t.
skin window t.
Skoog t.
sleeve t.
sling and blanket t.
sling and reef t.
sling suture t.
sling/wrapping t.
slit catheter t.
Slocum amputation t.
Slocum fusion t.
slot-blot t.
smiley-face knotting t.
Smith Indian t.
Smith-Petersen t.
Smith-Robinson t.
snapshot GRASS t.
snare t.
Snellen suture t.
Sofield femoral deficiency t.
soluble gas t.
Somerville t.
Sones t.
sonication t.
Southern blot t.
Sparks mandrel t.
Speed-Boyd radial-ulnar t.
sperm microaspiration retrieval t.
sphincter-saving t.
sphincter-sparing t.
Spiller-Frazier t.
spinal anesthetic t.
spinal fusion t.
spinal mobilization t.

spiral CT t.
spiral suture t.
Spivack gastrotomy t.
split-and-roll t.
split-bone t.
split-course t.
split cuff nipple t.
spontaneous ventilation anesthetic t.
Sprague arthroscopic t.
SPT t.
Staheli t.
Stamm-Kader gastrotomy t.
standard t.
standard biopsy t.
Stanisavljevic t.
stapled reconstruction t.
Staples t.
stapling t.
STAR t.
Stark-Moore-Ashworth-Boyes t.
startle t.
Starzl t.
static dilation t.
station pull-through esophageal manometry t.
stay suture t.
Steffee instrumentation t.
stellate ganglion block anesthetic t.
stenting t.
stent-through-wire mesh t.
step-by-step t.
stepladder incision t.
stereotactic automated t.
stereotactic core biopsy t.
stereotaxic t.
sterile t.
Sternberger antibody sandwich t.
Stewart-Hamilton cardiac output t.
stick-tie suture t.
Stiegmann-Goff t.
Stiles-Bunnell transfer t.
Stillman t.
still radiography t.
Stimson anterior shoulder reduction t.
stimulated gracilis neosphincter t.
STIR t.
Stoll dilution egg count t.
strain/counterstrain t.
Strassman t.
Straub t.
Strayer tendon t.
stretch-and-spray t.
Strickland t.
strip biopsy resection t.
strut fusion t.
Studebaker t.
Sturmdorf suture t.
subcuticular suture t.
subpectoral implantation t.
subperiosteal implant one-phase t.
subtraction t.
suction-irrigation t.
superficial suture t.
superior mesenterorenal bypass t.
super-wet t.
support suture t.
supraphysiologic fluid t.
surface cooling t.
surgical enucleation t.
surgical neurangiographic t.
surgical suture t.
surveillance t.
sustained pressure t.
suture anchor t.
suture closure t.
Swanson t.
Swiss roll embedding t.
switched B-gradient t.
sympathetic blockade anesthetic t.
sympathetic ganglion block anesthetic t.
Tajima suture t.
tandem clipping t.
Taylor-Daniel-Weiland t.
Taylor suture t.
telescoping suture t.
tendon suture t.
tension band wiring t.
tension suture t.
Terzis t.
test dose anesthetic t.
Teuffer t.
Thal fundoplication t.
thermal expansion t.
thermocatalytic t.
thermodilution t.
Thiersch suture t.
thiopental-sufentanil-desflurane-nitrous oxide anesthetic t.
Thomas t.
Thomas-Thompson-Straub transfer t.
Thompson t.
Thompson-Henry t.

NOTES

technique *(continued)*
Thompson-Loomer t.
thoracic epidural anesthetic t.
thoracolumbar spondylosis surgical t.
threaded-hole-first t.
three-loop t.
three-portal t.
through-and-through suture t.
thyroidectomy t.
thyroid surgical t.
tissue-sparing t.
titration t.
Todd-Evans stepladder tracheal dilatation t.
Tohen tendon t.
Tom Jones suture t.
Tompkins median bivalving t.
tongue-and-groove suture t.
topical anesthetic t.
Torg t.
Torgerson-Leach modified t.
total etch t.
total fundoplication t.
total intravenous anesthetic t.
Toupe t.
tracheal extubation anesthetic t.
tracheal intubation anesthetic t.
tracheal suction anesthetic t.
traction suture t.
transanal stapling t.
transarterial anesthetic t.
transcranial electrical stimulation anesthetic t.
transdermal anesthetic t.
transfixing suture t.
transiliac bar t.
translaryngeal guided intubation anesthetic t.
transmucosal drug administration anesthetic t.
transtracheal jet ventilation anesthetic t.
trapezius stimulation anesthetic t.
Trethowan-Stamm-Simmonds-Menelaus-Haddad t.
triangulation t.
triple-wire t.
trocar t.
trocar-cannula t.
Trusler aortic valve t.
tubal ligation band t.
tube-shift t.
tube-within-tube t.
Tuffier morcellement t.
Tullos t.
tumbling t.
Turco clubfoot release t.
turn-and-suction biopsy t.
Turnbull t.
twisted suture t.
twist-off t.
two-layer open t.
two-needle t.
two-patch t.
two-portal t.
two-pour t.
two-sleeve t.
two-stage tendon grafting t.
two-step t.
ultrasonographic t.
ultrasound anesthetic t.
uncut Collis-Nissen fundoplication t.
underlay fascia t.
unilateral inguinal hernia repair t.
uninterrupted suture t.
unitunnel t.
unlocking spiral t.
upgated t.
Ussing chamber t.
Van Lint modified t.
Van Milligen eyelid repair t.
vascular isolation t.
Vastamäki t.
Veleanu-Rosianu-Ionescu t.
velocity catheter t.
venous access t.
ventral bending t.
Verdan t.
Verhoeff suture t.
vertical-cut t.
vertical mattress suture t.
Vidal-Ardrey fracture t.
video-assisted t.
videofluoroscopic t.
video transurethral resection t.
Vim-Silverman t.
volumetric t.
Volz-Turner reattachment t.
von Haberer-Finney gastrectomy t.
Vulpius-Compere tendon t.
V-Y advancement t.
Wadsworth t.
Wagner open reduction t.
Wagoner cervical t.
Waldhausen subclavian flap t.
Wallace t.
Wanger reduction t.
Warner-Farber ankle fixation t.
Warwick and Ashken t.
wash t.
washed-field t.
water-suppression t.
Watkins fusion t.
Watson t.
Watson-Cheyne t.

wax-matrix t.
wax pattern thermal expansion t.
Weaver-Dunn acromioclavicular t.
Weber-Brunner-Freuler-Boitzy t.
Weber-Vasey traction-absorption wiring t.
Weckesser t.
Weinstein-Ponseti t.
Welch t.
Wertheim-Bohlman t.
West-Soto-Hall patellar t.
whipstitch suture t.
Whitesides t.
Whitesides-Kelly cervical t.
whole blood lysis t.
Wick catheter t.
Wickham t.
Williams-Haddad t.
Willi glass crown t.
Wilson t.
Wilson-Jacobs tibial fracture fixation t.
Wilson-McKeever shoulder t.
window t.
Windson-Insall-Vince grafting t.
Winograd t.
Winter spondylolisthesis t.
wire removal t.
Wirth-Jager tendon t.
Wölfler suture t.
Woodward t.
^{133}Xe intravenous injection t.
xenon-washout t.
Young t.
Young-Dees t.
Y-suture t.
Zancolli rerouting t.
Zariczny t.
Zarins-Rowe ligament t.
Zavala t.
Zazepen-Gamidov t.
Zeier transfer t.
Zielke t.
Z-suture t.
Zuker and Manktelow t.

technocausis

technology
assisted-reproduction t.
controlled release silver t.
endoluminal t.
endoscopic t.
endovascular t.
fluorescent optode t.
laparoscopic t.
signal extraction t. (SET)

tecta

tectobulbar tract

tectocephalic

tectocephaly

tectology

tectonic
t. epikeratoplasty
t. keratoplasty

tectopontine tract

tectoria

tectorial membrane

tectospinal
t. decussation
t. tract

TEE
transesophageal echocardiography

teeth
canine t.
central incisor t.
extruded t.
t. ligation
molar t.
premolar t.

TEF
tracheoesophageal fistula

Teflon granuloma

teflurane

TEG
thromboelastography

tegmentotomy

tela, pl. **telae**

telangiectasia

telangiectatic angioma

telangioma

telecobalt therapy

telelectrocardiogram

telencephalic malformation

telencephalization

telepresence surgery

telerobotic-assisted laparoscopic surgery

telescoping
t. nail
t. suture technique

televised radiofluoroscopy

television microscopy

TeLinde operation

telomerase

TEM
transanal endoscopic microsurgery

NOTES

T

temperature
ambient t.
axilla t.
basal body t.
bladder t.
body t.
brain t.
esophagus t.
flash-point t.
t. gradient
heat production t.
hyperthermic t.
intraoperative core body t.
normal body t.
normothermic t.
t., pulse, and respiration
skin t.
t. threshold
temperature-compensated vaporizer
temple
tempora (*pl. of* tempus)
temporal
t. aponeurosis
t. apophysis
t. arteritis
t. artery
t. artery biopsy
t. bone
t. bone fracture
t. bone tumor
t. branch
t. canal
t. fascia
t. fossa
t. incision
t. line
t. lobectomy
t. lobe radiation
t. muscle
t. orientation
t. plane
t. process
t. ridge
t. space
t. space infection
t. squama
t. surface
t. suture
t. vein
t. wedge
temporal-cerebral arterial anastomosis
temporale
temporalis
t. fascia flap
t. muscle flap
t. tendon
temporary
t. cavity phenomenon
t. diverting colostomy
t. end colostomy
t. fecal diversion
t. loop ileostomy
t. nerve blockade
t. pacemaker placement
t. palsy
t. postoperative supplementation
t. restoration
temporization
temporoauricular
temporofrontal tract
temporohyoid
temporomalar
temporomandibular
t. articular disk
t. joint
t. joint articulation
t. joint dislocation
t. ligament
t. luxation
t. nerve
t. pain
temporomandibulare
temporomandibularis
temporomaxillary vein
temporooccipital
temporoparietalis
temporoparietal muscle
temporopontine tract
temporosphenoid
temporozygomatica
tempus, pl. **tempora**
tenacious adhesion
tendency
thrombotic t.
tender
t. line
t. point
tenderness
abdominal t.
diffuse abdominal t.
marked t.
proximal bowel t.
rebound t.
subareolar t.
tendinea
tendineae
tendines (*pl. of* tendo)
tendineus
tendinis
vagina fibrosa t.
tendinitis
tendinomyoplastic amputation
tendinoplasty
tendinosuture
tendinous
t. arch

t. cord
t. inscription
t. insertion
t. opening
tendinum
tendo, pl. **tendines**
t. Achillis
tendolysis
tendon
abductor pollicis longus t.
Achilles t.
adductor magnus t.
anterior tibialis t.
attenuation of t.
biceps t.
calcaneal t.
calcanean t.
central t.
t. centralization
central perineum t.
common annular t.
common extensor t.
conjoined t.
conjoint t.
cricoesophageal t.
digital extensor t.
elbow extensor t.
erector spinae t.
t. excursion
extensor carpi radialis brevis t.
extensor carpi radialis longus t.
extensor carpi ulnaris t.
extensor digiti minimi t.
extensor digiti quinti t.
extensor digitorum t.
extensor digitorum brevis t.
extensor digitorum communis t.
extensor digitorum longus t.
extensor hallucis longus t.
extensor indicis proprius t.
extensor pollicis brevis t.
extensor pollicis longus t.
extensor quinti t.
fibularis longus t.
fibularis tertius t.
flexor carpi radialis t.
flexor digitorum longus t.
flexor digitorum profundus t.
flexor digitorum superficialis t.
flexor hallucis brevis t.
flexor hallucis longus t.
flexor pollicis longus t.
gracilis t.
t. graft
hamstring t.
heel t.
iliopsoas t.
intermediate digastric t.
intermediate omohyoid t.
t. interposition arthroplasty
lateral rectus t.
latissimus dorsi t.
masseter t.
peroneal brevis t.
peroneal longus t.
plantaris t.
popliteus t.
posterior tibialis t.
pronator teres t.
psoas minor t.
quadriceps femoris t.
rectus femoris t.
t. repair
t. rupture
semimembranosus t.
semitendinosus t.
snapping iliopsoas t.
split anterior tibial t. (SPLATT)
stapedius t.
subscapularis t.
superior oblique t.
t. suture technique
temporalis t.
thumb extensor t.
toe extensor t.
t. transplantation
trefoil t.
triceps t.
vastus medialis t.
wrist extensor t.
t. of Zinn
tendoplasty
tendotomy
tendovaginal
tenectomy
tenesmus
tenia, pl. **teniae**
free t.
mesocolic t.
omental t.
tenial
teniamyotomy
tenodesis
calcaneal t.

NOTES

tenodesis *(continued)*
extensor t.
MacIntosh extraarticular t.
tenolysis
tenomyoplasty
tenomyotomy
Tenon
T. capsule
T. membrane
T. space
tenonectomy
tenontology
tenontomyoplasty
tenontomyotomy
tenontoplastic
tenontoplasty
tenontotomy
tenophyte
tenoplastic reconstruction
tenoplasty
tenorrhaphy
tenosuture
tenosynovectomy
dorsal t.
flexor t.
tenosynovitis
de Quervain t.
tenotomy
adductor t.
Arroyo t.
Arruga t.
Braun shoulder t.
curb t.
extensor t.
free t.
graduated t.
intrasheath t.
t. operation
percutaneous t.
semiopen sliding t.
sliding t.
subcutaneous tibialis posterior t.
transverse t.
Veleanu-Rosianu-Ionescu adductor t.
Z marginal t.
Z-plasty t.
tensile
tension
t. by applanation
t. band fixation
t. band wiring technique
t. endothorax
extrapolated end-tidal carbon dioxide t. ($PETCO_2$)
t. fracture
isometric venous t.
oxygen t.
t. pneumopericardium
t. pneumothorax
running vascular technique without t.
t. suture technique
tissue oxygen t.
twitch t.
tension-free
t.-f. anastomosis
t.-f. hernioplasty
t.-f. hiatoplasty
t.-f. mesh implantation
t.-f. mesh repair
t.-f. prosthetic mesh repair
tension-length relation
tensor
t. fascia femoris flap
t. fascia lata muscle
t. fascia lata muscle flap
t. insertion
t. tympani canal
tenth cranial nerve
tentoria (*pl. of* tentorium)
tentorial
t. herniation
t. laceration
t. nerve
t. notch
t. pressure
t. ring
t. sinus
tentorii
tentorium, pl. **tentoria**
tenue
tenuis
Tenzel rotational cheek flap
TEP
totally extraperitoneal
TEP repair
teratoblastoma
teratocarcinoma
pineal t.
teratogenic medication
teratogen-induced malformation
teratologic dislocation
teratoma
mature t.
teratomatous
teratoneuroma
teratospermia
terebration
teres
t. major muscle
teretis
tergal
tergum
terminad
terminal
t. bronchiole

t. cisterna
t. colostomy
t. crest
t. duct carcinoma
t. head
t. hinge position
t. ileal pouch
t. ileal resection
t. ileostomy
t. ileum
t. ileum intubation
t. infection
t. jaw relation record
t. line
t. neosalpingostomy
nociceptor afferent peripheral t.
t. plane
t. reservoir syndrome
t. Syme procedure
t. ventriculostomy
t. web

terminale

terminalis
t. sulcus

terminalization

terminolateral

terminolaterally

terminoterminal anastomosis

terminus, pl. **termini**

terrace

territory
hepatic t.

Terson operation

tertiary
t. amputation
t. care
t. healing
t. trauma center

tertius

Terzis technique

TES
transcutaneous electric stimulation

tessellation

Tessier
T. classification
T. craniofacial operation
T. osteotomy

test
abduction external rotation t.
acoustic stimulation t.
Adson t.
air t.
alcohol used disorders identification t.
Allen t.
anorectal function t.
Apley compression t.
articulation t.
artificial erection t.
Astrand 6-minute submaximal cycle ergometer t.
axial compression t.
balloon expulsion t.
baroreceptor t.
Behçet skin puncture t.
Bielschowsky-Parks head-tilt, three-step t.
Bielschowsky three-step, head-tilt t.
bladder neck elevation t.
Bonney t.
breast stimulation contraction t.
breath excretion t.
Brodie-Trendelenburg tourniquet t.
bronchial inhalation challenge t.
bronchoprovocation t.
caffeine and halothane contracture t. (CHCT)
carpal compression t.
cavity t.
chlormerodrin accumulation t.
CholesTrak t.
Cholestron PRO t.
CLO t.
closed patch t.
CO_2 inhalation t.
cold pressor t. (CPT)
compression t.
concentration performance t.
confrontation visual field t.
corneal staining t.
Cortrosyn stimulation t.
Crampton t.
deep articulation t.
diagnostic articulation t.
differential ureteral catheterization t.
Digit Symbol Substitution T.
disk space saline acceptance t.
t. dose anesthetic technique
double Maddox rod t.
DR-70 tumor marker t.
Dunnett t.
Dupuy-Dutemps dacryocystorhinostomy dye t.

NOTES

test *(continued)*
Durkan carpal compression t.
dye exclusion t.
dye reduction spot t.
ergonovine provocation t.
excitability t.
external rotation-abduction stress t.
external rotation-recurvatum t.
extrastimulus t.
extrinsic entrapment t.
fast-flush t.
Feagin shoulder dislocation t.
femoral nerve traction t.
fetal acoustic stimulation t.
Finger Oscillation T.
fistula t.
flexion-rotation-drawer knee instability t.
fluctuation t.
fluorescein instillation t.
fluorescein string t.
foramen compression t.
foraminal compression t.
forced generation t.
forearm ischemic exercise t.
forearm supination t.
forward traction t.
Friberg microsurgical agglutination t.
gastric accommodation t.
germ tube t.
Gruber t.
hair bulb incubation t.
head compression t.
head distraction t.
head-down tilt t.
head-dropping t.
head-tilt t.
head-up tilt t.
head-up tilt-table t.
hepaplastin t.
high-altitude simulation t.
Hollander t.
Howard t.
Hughston external rotation recurvatum t.
human ovum fertilization t.
hyperventilation t.
iliac compression t.
implantation t.
indocyanine green retention t.
Ingram-Withers-Speltz motor t.
t. injection
Korotkoff t.
Kruskal-Wallis t.
labyrinthine fistula t.
lacrimal irrigation t.
line t.
liver function t.
localization t.
lumbar extension t.
lumbar rotation t.
Luria-Delbruck fluctuation t.
Maddox rod t.
Maddox wing t.
Mann-Whitney t.
Marshall t.
Marshall-Marchetti t.
matchstick t.
Maudsley Mentation T.
maximum stimulation t.
memory guidance saccade t.
MHA-TP t.
Michigan Abuse Screening T. (MAST)
mobilization t.
MUGA exercise stress t.
Multistage Maximal Effort exercise stress t.
nasal provocation t.
nerve excitability t.
neutralization t.
nipple stimulation t.
nonparametric t.
Noyes flexion rotation drawer t.
Object Classification T.
obturator t.
occlusive patch t.
one-hour office pad t.
one-minute endoscopy room t.
open application t.
open patch t.
Pachon t.
parametric t.
Parks-Bielschowsky three-step, head-tilt t.
penetration t.
Peptavlon stimulation t.
percutaneous pressure ureteral perfusion t.
perimeter corneal reflex t.
perineal nerve terminal motor latency t.
peritoneal equilibration t.
Perthes t.
postcoital t.
prick puncture t.
prism adaptation t.
promontory stimulation t.
prone extension t.
protection t.
protein truncation t.
provocation t.
provocative chelation t.
Q-tip t.
Rapoport t.

regurgitation t.
Ross-Jones t.
rotation drawer t.
rotation recurvatum t.
scapular approximation t.
scarification t.
screening t.
Self-Administered Alcoholism Screening t. (SAAST)
serological t.
side-lying iliac compression t.
simple shoulder t. (SST)
skin-puncture t.
SLR with external rotation t.
Spatial Orientation Memory T.
sperm immobilization t.
split renal function t.
star construction t.
station t.
Stewart t.
stimulation t.
straight catheter t.
string t.
Student-Newman-Keuls t.
sucrose t.
Suprathreshold Adaptation T.
Thompson t.
thymol tumidity t.
tissue compression t.
tourniquet t.
traction t.
transillumination t.
Trieger t.
trunk incurvation t.
tube dilution t.
tube precipitin t.
tumor skin t.
twitch height t.
two-point discrimination t.
University of Pennsylvania Smell Identification T.
vaginal cornification t.
vaginal mucification t.
Valpar whole body range of motion t.
vertical compression t.
vibration threshold t.
Visual-Motor Integration T.
in vitro contracture t.
Von Frey t.
walking ventilation t.
washout t.
Whitaker pressure-perfusion t.
Wilcoxon signed-rank t.
wire loop t.

testalgia

testectomy

testes (*pl. of* testis)

testicle

testicular
t. adrenal-like tissue
t. appendage
t. artery
t. biopsy
t. carcinoma
t. cord
t. duct
t. ectopia
t. feminization syndrome
t. mass
t. metastasis
t. plexus
t. rupture
t. torsion
t. tumor
t. vein

testicularis

testiculus

testing
compression t.
confrontation t.
Doppler ultrasound segmental blood pressure t.
genetic t.
palpation t.
patch t.
penile injection t.
Quantitative Sensory T. (QST)
rotation t.
sudomotor axon reflex t.
tilt-table t.

testis, pl. **testes**
t. cord
cryptorchid t.
t. fracture
movable t.
retractile t.
torsion t.
undescended t.

testitis

testoid

tetanic
t. fade

NOTES

tetanic *(continued)*
t. stimulation
t. stimulation method
tetanization
tetanus
cephalic t.
extensor t.
head t.
traumatic t.
tetany
duration t.
hyperventilation t.
postoperative t.
tethered cord syndrome
tetracaine
hyperbaric t.
liposome-encapsulated t.
tetraethylammonium
tetragonus
tetralogy of Fallot
Teuffer
T. technique
T. tendo calcaneus repair
Teutleben ligament
TEVP
transesophageal ventricular pacing
Texas Scottish Rite Hospital (TSRH)
texture
echo t.
firm t.
rubbery t.
textured fabric rub
T-fastener gastropexy
TFCC
triangular fibrocartilage complex
TG
total gastrectomy
TGF
transforming growth factor
Thal
T. esophageal stricture repair
T. esophagogastroscopy
T. esophagogastrostomy
T. fundic patch operation
T. fundoplasty
T. fundoplication
T. fundoplication method
T. fundoplication procedure
T. fundoplication technique
T. stricturoplasty
thalamectomy
thalamencephalic
thalamencephalon
thalamic
t. circulation
t. pain
t. plane
thalamic-subthalamic hemorrhage
thalamocaudate arteriovenous malformation
thalamostriate vein
thalamotomy
gamma t.
staged bilateral stereotactic t.
stereotactic Vim t.
stereotactic VL t.
Vim t.
thallium-technetium scanning
Thal-Nissen fundoplasty
thanatopsy
Thane method
THARIES
total hip arthroplasty with internal eccentric shells
THE
transhiatal esophagectomy
theater
operating t.
twin operating t.
thebesian
t. circulation
t. vein
theca, pl. **thecae**
thecal
t. sac
t. sac compression
theca-lutein cyst
thecoma
luteinized t.
ovarian t.
Theden method
Theile muscle
Theirsch-Duplay repair
thele
theleplasty
thenad
thenal
thenar
t. eminence
t. flap
t. muscle
t. prominence
t. space
thenaris
thenen
theory
gate-control t.
membrane expansion t.
Pauling t.
therapeutic
t. alternative
t. anesthesia
t. angiogenesis
t. approach
t. arsenal
t. colonoscopy

t. dissection
t. effect
t. efficacy
t. endpoint
t. insemination
t. intervention scoring system (TISS)
t. iridectomy
t. irradiation
t. laparoscopy
t. lymph node dissection (TLND)
t. modality
t. nerve block
t. option
t. phlebotomy
t. step
t. upper endoscopy

therapist
stoma t.

therapy
ablation t.
ablative laser t.
active appliance t.
active assistive motion t.
adjunct t.
adjunctive suppressive medical t.
adjuvant chemoradiation t.
adjuvant drug t.
aerosol t.
alternate-day t.
alternative t.
amplitude-summation interferential current t.
anaclitic t.
angina-guided t.
antiarrhythmic t.
antibiotic t.
anticoagulant t.
anticoagulation t.
antiemetic t.
antifungal t.
antihormonal t.
antilymphoid t.
antireflux t.
antithrombotic t.
apotreptic t.
argon laser t.
around-the-clock oral maintenance bronchodilator t.
augmentation t.
balloon photodynamic t.
belly bath t.
biomagnetic t.
bite plane t.
boron neutron-capture t.
Bragg peak proton-beam t.
breast conservation t. (BCT)
breast-conserving t.
breast-preservation t.
brisement t.
bronchoscopic photodynamic t.
buprenorphine narcotic analgesic t.
Cancell t.
cerebral protective t.
chest physical t.
chronic opioid analgesic t. (COAT)
Clinitron air-fluidized t.
coagulative laser t.
cobalt t.
cognitive-behavioral t.
combined chemoradiation t.
compartmental radioimmunoglobulin t.
complementary t.
concomitant t.
conditioning t.
conformal radiation t.
conservative t.
contact dissolution t.
continuous renal replacement t.
convulsive t.
corrective t.
Crozat t.
deep chest t.
definitive local t.
device t.
diagnostic surgical t.
diathermic t.
dilation t.
diuretic t.
dressing t.
dual t.
electrical stimulation t.
electric aversion t.
electric differential t.
electroconvulsive t.
electrotherapeutic sleep t.
endocavitary radiation t.
endoluminal t.
endoscopic hemostatic t.
endoscopic injection t.
endoscopic laser t.
endoscopic pancreatic t.
endoscopic photodynamic t.

NOTES

T

therapy *(continued)*
endourological t.
endovascular t.
enterostomal t.
eradication t.
erythropoietin t.
esophageal photodynamic t.
ethanol injection t.
expansion and activator t.
extended field irradiation t.
external beam radiation t.
external vacuum t.
external x-ray t.
ex vivo gene t.
factor replacement t.
fast neutron radiation t.
fetal drug t.
focused radiation t.
fractionated radiation t.
frappage t.
frequency-difference interferential current t.
functional orthodontic t.
gene replacement t.
gene-transfer t.
grenz ray t.
HDR intracavitary radiation t.
hemofiltration t.
hepatic arterial t.
herbal t.
high-dose radioiodine t.
high-voltage t.
hydration t.
hyperbaric oxygen t.
hyperthermia t.
ImmTher t.
immunocompetent tissue t.
implosive t.
incremental t.
indirect pulpal t.
Indoklon t.
InFerno moist heat t.
infrared t.
inhalation t.
injection t.
innovative t.
instillation t.
insulin coma t.
insulin shock t.
interferential t.
interlesional t.
internal radiation t.
interstitial photodynamic t.
interstitial radiation t.
interventional t.
intraarterial t.
intracavernous injection t.
intracavitary radiation boost t.
intracorporeal injection t.
intradiscal electrothermal t. (IDET)
intralesional t.
intraperitoneal radiation t.
intraspinal t.
intrathecal t.
intravascular fluid t.
intravenous antibiotic t.
intravenous hydration t.
intravenous ozone t.
intraventricular t.
invasive t.
ischemia-guided medical t.
isolation perfusion t.
IV fluid t.
Kelsey unloading exercise t.
ketoprofen analgesic t.
laser t.
LDR intracavitary radiation t.
life-saving form of t.
Livingstone t.
local t.
long-term oxygen t.
Lymphapress compression t.
magnet t.
manipulative t.
medical t.
microcurrent t.
microwave t.
migraine abortive t.
morphine narcotic analgesic t.
MTBE t.
multimodal adjuvant t.
multimodality t.
multiple t.
myoablative t.
myofunctional t.
Nd:YAG laser t.
negative pressure t.
neoadjuvant t.
neodymium:YAG laser t.
neutron beam t.
neutron capture t.
nonspecific t.
nonsurgical t.
occlusal t.
occlusion t.
occlusive t.
occupational t.
ocular radiation t.
open surgical t.
operative t.
optimal t.
orthodontic t.
outpatient physical t.
oxygen t.
PA t.
palliative t.

pancreatic intraluminal radiation t.
parenteral t.
particle beam radiation t.
PEMF t.
penile injection t.
penile vein occlusion t.
percussion t.
percutaneous embolization t.
percutaneous ethanol injection t.
percutaneous microwave coagulation t.
percutaneous transcatheter t.
perfusion t.
periodontal t.
perioperative antibiotic t.
permanent anticoagulant t.
photodynamic t. (PDT)
photoradiation t.
physical t.
placebo t.
plasma exchange t.
pool t.
positional release t.
postnatal t.
postoperative anticoagulation t.
postradiation t.
posttransplant immunosuppression t.
postural t.
prenatal t.
preoperative t.
preventive intravesical t.
progestational t.
programmed t.
prophylactic antibiotic t.
protein shock t.
proton beam t.
proton pump inhibition t.
pulp canal t.
pyretic t.
quadrangular t.
quadrantectomy, axillary dissection, radiation t. (QUART)
quadruple t.
quatro t.
radiation t.
radical t.
radioimmunoglobulin t.
radioiodine ablation t.
radiopharmaceutical t.
red-filter t.
reflex t.
rehydration t.
renal infusion t.
renal replacement t.
rescue t.
respiratory kinetic t.
rheologic t.
root canal t.
rotation t.
saline injection t.
salvage t.
sandwich staghorn calculus t.
sclerosing t.
sedative t.
skin lubrication t.
soak t.
social interaction t.
sole laser t.
somatic t.
sparing t.
STAMP t.
stem cell gene t.
stepdown t.
stereotactic-assisted radiation t.
stereotactic-focused radiation t.
stereotactic radiation t.
Stockholm technique for radium t.
subcoma t.
supranormal hemodynamic t.
surgical maggot t.
systemic adjuvant t.
systemic antifungal t.
systemic radioimmunoglobulin t.
telecobalt t.
thermal t.
three-cornered t.
three-dimensional conformal radiation t.
thrombolytic t.
timed-sequential t.
tocolytic t.
tongue thrust t.
total push t.
transcatheter arterial embolization t.
transfusion t.
transgenic t.
transurethral collagen injection t.
transvenous t.
triadic t.
trial of conservative t.
trimodality t.
triple intrathecal t.
tumor t.
ultrasonic t.

NOTES

therapy *(continued)*
ultrasound t.
ultrasound-guided shock wave t.
unfractionated heparin t.
vocal fold fixation t.
voice t.
volume t.
whole-brain radiation t.
wide-field radiation t.
wide-range radiation t.
will t.
xenogenic cell t.
x-ray t.
therencephalous
thermal
t. ablation
t. anesthesia
t. balance
t. coefficient expansion
t. death point
t. disinfection
t. expansion technique
t. injury
t. keratoplasty
t. necrosis
t. rhizotomy
t. sclerectomy
t. stimulation
t. therapy
thermally active method
thermal/perfusion balloon angioplasty
thermic anesthesia
thermocatalytic technique
thermocauterectomy
thermocautery
thermochemotherapy
thermocoagulation
thermodilution (TD)
bolus t. (BTD)
t. cardiac output (TDCO)
t. method
t. technique
thermodynamic theory of narcosis
thermogenesis
nonshivering t.
thermogram
thermographic examination
thermography
thermokeratoplasty
thermolysis
thermometry
tympanic t.
thermopenetration
thermoregulation
perianesthetic t.
thermoregulatory vasoconstriction
thermorhizotomy
thermosclerectomy
thermosclerostomy
thermosclerotomy
thermotherapy
microwave t.
transurethral microwave t.
thick cutaneous melanoma (TCM)
thickened
t. nail
t. synovial membrane
thickening
endocardial t.
heel pad t.
postlumpectomy skin t.
thickness
Breslow t.
endometrial t.
end-systolic wall t. (ESWT)
soft-tissue t.
Thiersch
T. anal incontinence operation
T. graft operation
T. medium split free graft
T. method
T. procedure
T. suture technique
T. thin split free graft
Thiersch-Duplay
T.-D. proximal tube procedure
T.-D. tube graft
T.-D. urethral construction
T.-D. urethroplasty
thigh
t. bone
t. graft arteriovenous fistula
t. joint
posterior t.
thimble valvotomy
thin
t. basement membrane
t. basement membrane disease
t. glossy skin
t. section
thin-needle biopsy
thinning
corneal t.
ThinPrep procedure
thin-section axial image
thiol
t. augmentation
t. modification
thiopental-sufentanil-desflurane-nitrous oxide anesthetic technique
third
t. cranial nerve
t. and fourth pharyngeal pouch syndrome
t. occipital nerve
t. parallel pelvic plane

t. space fluid accumulation
Steel rule of t.'s
t. trochanter
t. ventriculostomy

third-degree
t.-d. burn
t.-d. hemorrhoid
t.-d. radiation injury

third-grade fusion
Thiry fistula
Thiry-Vella fistula
Thoma ampulla
Thomas
T. classification
T. extrapolated bar graft
T. operation
T. procedure
T. sign
T. technique

Thomas-Thompson-Straub transfer technique
Thomas-Warren incision
Thom flap laryngeal reconstruction method
Thompson
T. anterolateral approach
T. anteromedial approach
T. capsule flap pyeloplasty
T. excision
T. ligament
T. line
T. posterior radial approach
T. procedure
T. quadricepsplasty
T. resection
T. technique
T. telescoping V osteotomy
T. test

Thompson-Epstein femoral fracture classification
Thompson-Hatina method
Thompson-Henry technique
Thompson-Loomer technique
Thomson operation
thoracentesis
needle t.

thoraces (*pl. of* thorax)
thoracic
t. anesthesia
t. aneurysm
t. aorta
t. aortic aneurysm repair
t. aortic cross-clamping (TACC)
t. aortic disease
t. aortic dissection
t. aortic plexus
t. approach
t. axis
t. cage
t. cardiac branch
t. cardiac nerve
t. cavity
t. compression syndrome
t. diskectomy
t. disk herniation
t. duct
t. duct fistula
t. endometriosis syndrome
t. epidural analgesia
t. epidural anesthetic technique
t. epidural catheterization
t. esophagogastrostomy
t. esophagus
t. facet fusion
t. ganglion
t. girdle
t. great vessel
t. index
t. inlet
t. inlet soft tissue
t. inlet vascular injury
t. interspinal muscle
t. intertransverse muscle
t. kidney
t. lesion
t. limb
t. longissimus muscle
t. outlet compression
t. outlet syndrome (TOS)
t. plane
t. radiculopathy
t. respiration
t. rotator muscle
t. short esophagomyotomy
t. spinal fusion
t. spinal nerve
t. spine
t. spine biopsy
t. spine fracture
t. spine kyphotic deformity
t. spine scoliotic deformity
t. spine vertebral osteosynthesis
t. stomach
t. surgeon

NOTES

thoracic *(continued)*
t. surgery
t. vein
t. vertebra
t. vertebral body
t. wall
thoracica
thoracicae
thoracici
thoracicoabdominal
thoracicoacromial
thoracicohumeral
thoracicus
thoracis
thoracoabdominal
t. aneurysm
t. aortic aneurysm repair
t. esophagectomy
t. esophagogastrectomy
t. extrapleural approach
t. gunshot wound
t. incision
t. injury
t. intrapleural approach
t. nerve
t. region
t. retroperitoneal lymphadenectomy
t. trauma
thoracoacromial
t. artery
t. flap
t. trunk
t. vein
thoracoacromialis
thoracoceloschisis
thoracocentesis
thoracocyllosis
thoracocyrtosis
thoracodorsal
t. artery
t. nerve
thoracodorsalis
thoracoepigastric
t. flap
t. vein
thoracoepigastrica
thoracograph
thoracolaparotomy
thoracolumbalis
thoracolumbar
t. aponeurosis
t. burst fracture
t. fascia
t. junction surgical exposure
t. outflow
t. retroperitoneal approach
t. spine anterior exposure
t. spine fracture
t. spine fracture-dislocation
t. spine stabilization
t. spine vertebral osteosynthesis
t. spondylosis surgical technique
thoracolysis
thoracomelus
thoracophrenolaparotomy
thoracoplasty
conventional t.
costoversion t.
Delorme t.
Schede t.
Wilms t.
thoracopneumoplasty
thoracoschisis
thoracoscopic
t. approach
t. diskectomy
t. esophageal mobilization
t. esophagomyotomy
t. pericardiectomy
t. repair
t. talc insufflation
thoracoscopic-assisted esophagectomy
thoracoscopy
single-trocar access t.
thoracostenosis
thoracosternotomy
thoracostomy
closed chest t.
tube t.
thoracotomy
anterior t.
anterolateral t.
t. approach
axillary t.
bilateral anterior t.
book t.
clamshell t.
emergency department t. (EDT)
emergency room t.
ER t.
esophagectomy with t.
t. incision
left-sided t.
Lewis t.
limited t.
limited anterior small t. (LAST)
median t.
muscle-sparing t.
open t.
resuscitative t.
right-sided t.
t. scar
standard t.
trapdoor t.

thorascopic
t. apical pleurectomy
t. drainage
thorax, pl. **thoraces**
left t.
Peyrot t.
right t.
Thorel bundle
Thorn
T. maneuver
T. syndrome
Thornell microlaryngoscopy
threaded-hole-first technique
three-body wear
Three Color Concept of wound classification
three-cornered
t.-c. bone
t.-c. therapy
three-dimensional
t.-d. conformal radiation therapy
t.-d. contouring
t.-d. FATS method
t.-d. Fourier transform gradient-echo imaging
t.-d. projection reconstruction imaging
t.-d. reconstruction
t.-d. stereography
three-field
t.-f. dissection
t.-f. lymphadenectomy
three-in-one block
three-loop
t.-l. ileal pouch
t.-l. technique
three-part fracture
three-plane deformity
three-point
t.-p. bending moment
t.-p. touch
three-portal technique
three-quadrant hemorrhoidectomy
three-snip punctum operation
three-square flap
three-stage procedure
three-trocar technique cholecystectomy
threshold
apneic t.
atrial defibrillation t.
current perception t. (CPT)
defibrillation t.
detection t.
displacement t.
double-point t.
experimental t.
fibrillation t.
flicker-fusion t.
median detection t.
noise detection t.
pacemaker t.
pressure pain t. (PPT)
t. shift method
speech detection t.
stimulation t.
TEAP t.
temperature t.
ventilation t.
throat anesthesia
thrombase
thrombasthenia
thrombectomy
chemical t.
early t.
mechanical t.
percutaneous rotational t.
rotational t.
surgical t.
thrombi (*pl. of* thrombus)
thrombin
human t.
thrombin-mediated consumptive state
thromboangiitis obliterans
thromboasthenia
thrombocythemia
thrombocytopenia
heparin-induced t. (HIT)
immune-mediated unfractionated heparin-induced t.
unfractionated heparin-induced t.
thromboelastogram
thromboelastograph
thromboelastography (TEG)
thromboembolectomy
percutaneous aspiration t.
rotating aspiration t.
thromboembolic
t. complication
t. disease
t. event
t. fistula
t. risk factor

NOTES

thromboembolism
recurrent t.
venous t.
thromboendarterectomy (TEA)
pulmonary t. (PTE)
renal t.
thrombogenesis
thrombogenic
t. disorder
t. foreign body
t. profile
thrombolysis
coronary t.
T. in Myocardial Infarction (TIMI)
t. in myocardial infarction classification
selective intracoronary t.
sonic t.
urokinase t.
thrombolytic
t. agent
t. therapy
thrombopathy
thrombophlebitis
recurrent t.
superficial t.
thromboplastin
tissue t.
thromboprophylaxis
thrombosed
t. graft
t. internal and external hemorrhoid
thrombosin
thrombosis, pl. **thromboses**
acute mesenteric venous t.
arterial t.
chronic t.
deep vein t.
deep venous t. (DVT)
diffuse microvascular t.
early graft t.
effort t.
graft t.
intimal t.
t. of IVC
portal t.
postoperative deep venous t. (PODVT)
recurrent t.
renal artery t.
vascular access t.
venous effort t.
widespread portal system t.
thrombostasis
thrombotic
t. complication
t. disease
t. episode
t. gangrene
t. process
t. tendency
Thrombo-Wellcotest method
thrombus, pl. **thrombi**
deep venous t.
t. extension
peripheral t.
portal tumor t.
portal vein tumor t. (PVTT)
regression of t.
tumor t.
vein tumor t.
through-and-through
t.-a.-t. fracture
t.-a.-t. laceration
t.-a.-t. suture technique
t.-a.-t. V-shaped horizontal osteotomy
through-knee amputation
through-the-scope
t.-t.-s. balloon dilation
t.-t.-s. balloon removal
thrower fracture
thrust manipulation
thulium:YAG laser angioplasty
thumb
t. deformity
t. duplication
t. extensor tendon
t. metacarpophalangeal joint approach
t. reconstruction
t. web
thumb-in-palm deformity
thumbprinting
thymectomy
cervical t.
complete t.
neonatal t.
video-assisted thoracoscopic t.
thymi (*pl. of* thymus)
thymic
t. artery
t. branch
t. carcinoma
t. cyst
t. duct
t. mass
t. vein
thymicae
thymici
thymicolymphatic
thymocyte NA^+/H^+ exchanger
thymol
t. flocculation
t. tumidity test
thymolipoma

thymoma
spindle cell t.
thymus, pl. **thymi**
t. gland
t. gland excision
xenotransplantation t.
thymusectomy
thyroarytenoideus
thyroarytenoid muscle
thyrocele
thyrocervical
t. artery
t. trunk
thyrocervicalis
thyrochondrotomy
thyroepiglottic
t. ligament
t. muscle
thyroepiglotticum
thyroepiglotticus
thyroglobulin
thyroglossal
t. cyst surgery
t. duct
t. duct cyst
t. fistula
thyrohyal
thyrohyoid
t. ligament
t. membrane
t. muscle
thyrohyoidea
thyrohyoideus
thyroid
t. adenoma
t. axis
t. body
t. cancer
t. carcinoma
t. cartilage
t. cystadenoma
t. eminence
t. endocrine disorder
t. gland
goitrous t.
t. hormone serum concentration
t. hyperplasia
t. ima artery
t. lamina
t. lobe
t. lobectomy
t. muscle
t. needle biopsy
t. neoplasia
t. nodule
t. nodule ablation
t. operation
t. pathology
pyramidal process of t.
t. resection
t. storm
t. surgeon
t. surgical tactic
t. surgical technique
t. tissue
t. tumor
t. vein
thyroidal hernia
thyroidea
thyroideae
thyroidectomize
thyroidectomy
breast approach t.
complete t.
completion t.
gasless endoscopic t.
near-total t.
outpatient t.
prophylactic t.
provocative food t.
scarless endoscopic t.
subtotal t.
t. tactic
t. technique
total t.
videoendoscopic t.
thyroidei
thyrointoxication
thyrolaryngeal
thyrolingual duct
thyromental distance
thyropalatine
thyroparathyroidectomy
thyropharyngeal
thyroplasty
thyroptosis
thyrotomy
thyrotoxic coma
Ti
inspiratory time
TIA
transient ischemic attack
tibia, pl. **tibiae**
tibiad

NOTES

tibial
t. acceleration
t. augmentation block
t. bending fracture
t. bone defect regeneration
t. condyle fracture
t. crest
t. diaphysial fracture
t. epiphysis
t. intertendinous bursa
t. metaphysis
t. open fracture
t. plafond fracture
t. plateau fracture
t. plateau fracture-dislocation
t. shaft fracture
t. triplane fracture
t. tuberosity fracture
t. tuberosity osteotomy
tibialis
t. posterior dislocation
tibiocalcaneal
t. arthrodesis
t. medullary nailing
tibiocalcanean
tibiofascialis
tibiofemoral articulation
tibiofibular
t. articulation
t. clear space
t. diastasis
t. fusion
t. joint dislocation
t. line
tibionavicular
tibionaviculare
tibioperoneal
t. trunk angioplasty
t. vessel angioplasty
tibioscaphoid
tibiotalar
t. fusion
posterior t.
tibiotalocalcaneal
t. arthrodesis
t. fusion
Tibone posterior capsulorrhaphy
tic
t. douloureux
dystonic t.
tidal
t. drainage
t. volume
Tiedemann nerve
tier
remote t.
ties-over-stent
tightening
gastric valve t.
tight Nissen repair
tight-to-shaft (TTS)
tigroid
t. appearance
t. striation
tigrolysis
Tikhoff-Linberg
T.-L. procedure
T.-L. shoulder girdle resection
Tilden method
tile
T. classification
t. plate facet replacement
Tillaux
extraocular muscles of T.
Tillaux-Chaput fracture
Tillaux-Kleiger fracture
Tillaux-Phocas syndrome
Tillett operation
tilt
base-ring t.
filter t.
head-down t.
head-up t.
steep head-down t.
t. stitch
Trendelenburg t.
tilt-table testing
time
acceleration t.
activated clotting t. (ACT)
activated coagulation t.
anesthesia t.
anesthetic t.
association t.
average extubation t.
bleeding t.
blood-brain equilibration t.
carotid ejection t.
celite-activated clotting t. (CACT)
cerebral circulation t.
circulation t.
cold ischemia t.
concentration times t.
correlation t.
deceleration t. (DCT)
decimal reduction t.
Duke bleeding t.
duration t.
ejection t.
electrode response t.
evolution t.
execution t.
explosive doubling t.
followup t.
forced expiratory t.

helium equilibration t.
heparin neutralized thrombin t. (HnTT)
hepatic ischemic t.
high-dose thrombin t. (HiTT)
inspiration t.
inspiratory t. (Ti)
interhemispheric propagation t.
isovolumic relaxation t.
Ivy method of bleeding t.
kaolin-activated clotting t. (KACT)
lag t.
Lee-White clotting t.
t. of maximum concentration
mean circulation t.
Mielke bleeding t.
nucleation t.
operating t.
operative t.
plasma clotting t.
t. position scan
preoperative evolution t.
preservation t.
t. pressure
procedure t.
prolonged prothrombin t.
prothrombin t.
recalcification t.
t. to recovery
recovery t.
recovery room t.
relaxation t.
saturation t.
sensation t.
total respiratory t. (Ttot)
total tourniquet t.
tourniquet t.
tumor doubling t.
ventilator t.
ventricular activation t.
voice termination t.
warm ischemic t.

time-concentration curve
time-cycled ventilation
timed
t. forced expiratory volume
t. intermittent rotation
timed-sequential therapy
time-of-flight mass spectometry
TIMI
Thrombolysis in Myocardial Infarction
TIMI classification
Tim knot
tip
t. angle
intraabdominal t.
nasal t.
overprojecting nasal t.
papillary muscle t.
pyramidal t.
rectal t.
spleen t.
tip-of-the-tongue phenomenon
TIPS
transjugular intrahepatic portosystemic shunt
TIPS procedure
TISS
therapeutic intervention scoring system
tissue
abdominal adipose t.
aberrant t.
t. ablation
acellular pannus t.
acinar t.
adipose connective t.
ampullary granulation t.
anechoic t.
aneurysm t.
aneurysmal t.
angiomatous neoplastic t.
anisotropic t.
aortic aneurysm t.
t. approximation
t. architecture
areolar connective t.
atrioventricular conduction t.
attenuating t.
t. bank
t. blocking
border t.
breast biopsy t.
bronchial-associated lymphoid t.
brown adipose t.
bursa-equivalent t.
bursal t.
cancellous t.
capsular support t.
cartilaginous t.
caseated t.
cementoid t.
cervical soft t.
chromaffin t.
cicatricial t.

NOTES

tissue *(continued)*
t. coagulation
collagenous t.
t. compression
t. compression test
t. conductivity
t. confirmation
conjunctiva-associated lymphoid t.
connective t.
corneal t.
coronal pulp t.
crushed t.
cryostat t.
cutaneous t.
denuded connective t.
t. detritus
devitalized t.
diffuse lymphatic t.
t. dissection
donor t.
t. Doppler imaging
dorsal t.
earlobe adipose t.
echogenic t.
ectopic endometrial t.
elastic t.
enveloping scar t.
episcleral t.
t. expansion
extraarticular t.
extracapsular t.
extraperitoneal t.
exuberant granulation t.
fatty prostatic t.
fetal lymphoid t.
fibroadipose t.
fibroblastic t.
fibroelastic t.
fibrofatty breast t.
fibrotic t.
fibrous connective t.
fibrous scar t.
t. fluke
functional renal t.
t. fusion
Gamgee t.
ganglial t.
gastrointestinal-associated lymphoid t.
gingival t.
glandular t.
granulation t.
granulomatous t.
gut-associated lymphoid t. (GALT)
hard and soft t.
healthy t.
hemangiomatous t.
hematopoietic t.
hilar structure scar t.
His-Purkinje t.
histiocytic t.
t. homogeneity
hyperplastic t.
hypertrophic granulation t.
hypocellular fibrous t.
t. hypoxia
t. imprint
t. ingrowth surface
interdental t.
interfascicular fibrous t.
t. interposition
interstitial t.
intervening connective t.
intralobular connective t.
isotropic t.
keratinized t.
ligamentous support t.
t. ligand
lipoma-like t.
lipomatous t.
liver t.
t. loss
t. lymph
lymphatic t.
lymphoid t.
mammary t.
maternal t.
mesenchymal t.
mesothelial t.
mineralized t.
t. molding
mucosa-associated lymphoid t. (MALT)
muscular t.
musculoskeletal t.
myeloid t.
myocardial t.
nasion soft t.
t. necrosis
necrotic/fibrotic t.
necrotic hyalinized t.
neoplastic t.
nephrogenic t.
neural t.
nodal t.
nonviable t.
nonvital t.
normal t.
nuclear t.
t. nutrition
oral t.
orbital adipose t.
orbitonasal t.
osseous t.
t. oxygenation
t. oxygen tension

pancreatic t.
paracancerous t.
paraoral t.
parathyroid t.
paravaginal soft t.
parenchymal t.
penoid t.
t. perfusion
periadvential t.
periapical t.
periarticular t.
pericanalicular connective t.
periesophageal t.
periimplant t.
perilobular connective t.
perinephric t.
perineural t.
perinodal t.
periosteal t.
peripancreatic t.
peripheral lymphoid t.
periprostatic t.
petrotympanic t.
pharyngeal t.
t. pH monitoring
placental t.
polypoid t.
preepiglottic soft t.
t. preservation
t. pressure
t. pressure measurement
pressure-sensitive t.
pressure-tolerant t.
prevertebral soft t.
pterygial t.
pulmonary t.
redundant sac t.
t. regeneration
t. remodeling
t. renewal
t. repair
residual ductal t.
t. resistance
t. respiration
retroperitoneal soft t.
retropharyngeal soft t.
revascularized t.
rubber t.
t. sampling
scar t.
skeletal t.
t. slack
slow exchange soft t.
soft t.
sonolucent t.
t. space
specialized intralobular connective t.
splenic t.
t. study
subcutaneous t.
subjacent t.
supporting t.
sustentacular t.
syngeneic t.
synovial t.
testicular adrenal-like t.
t. texture abnormality
thoracic inlet soft t.
t. thromboplastin
thyroid t.
t. tolerance
t. tolerance dose
t. transfer
t. transplant
t. transplantation
t. trauma
t. trimming
trophoblastic t.
tuberculosis granulation t.
t. typing
vascular t.
viable t.
viscoelastic t.
vital t.
t. water content
t. welding
xenogeneic t.

tissue-base relationship
tissue-bearing area
tissue-borne
tissue-equivalent
tissue-sparing technique
tissue-supported base
tissue-tissue-supported base
titratable
titration
coulometric t.
Dean and Webb t.
potentiometric t.
Rinkel serial endpoint t.
t. technique
titubation
head t.

NOTES

TIVA
total intravenous anesthesia
TKA
total knee arthroscopy
TLND
therapeutic lymph node dissection
TME
total mesorectal excision
TMLR
transmyocardial laser revascularization
TMR
transmyocardial laser revascularization
TNF
tumor necrosis factor
TNF-alpha
tumor necrosis factor-alpha
TNF-bp
tumor necrosis factor-binding protein
TNM
tumor, node, metastasis
TNM carcinoma classification
TNM staging system
TNM system for tumor staging
TNS
transient neurologic symptom
to-and-fro anesthesia
tocolysis
tocolytic therapy
Todd-Evans stepladder tracheal dilatation technique
toddler fracture
Tod muscle
toe
Butler procedure to correct overlapping t.'s
catheter t.
t. extensor
t. extensor muscle
t. extensor tendon
great t.
toe-block anesthesia
toenail
embedded t.
ingrowing t.
toe-phalanx transplantation
TOF
train-of-four
Tohen tendon technique
toilet
cavity t.
peritoneal t.
pulmonary t.
tolazoline
Toldt
T. fascia
line of T.
T. membrane
white line of T.
tolerance
anesthetic t.
histologic t.
pressure t.
tissue t.
Tolosa-Hunt syndrome
tomentum
Tom Jones suture technique
tomography
computed t. (CT)
contrast-enhanced computed t.
expiratory computed t.
fluorodeoxyglucose-positron emission t.
positron emission t. (PET)
single-photon emission computed t.
single photon emission computer-aided t.
ultrafast CT electron beam t.
ultrafast spiral computed t.
Tompkins median bivalving technique
tongue
t. bone
t. fasciculation
t. flap
t. fracture
mandibular t.
t. plication
t. pressure
t. thrust classification
t. thrust therapy
tongue-and-groove suture technique
tongue-in-groove operation
tongue-jaw-neck dissection
tonometer
indentation t.
tonometry
applanation t.
gastric t.
indentation t.
nasogastric t.
tonsil
Gerlach t.
tonsilla, pl. **tonsillae**
tonsillar
t. branch
t. crypt
t. fold
t. hernia
t. herniation
tonsillaris
tonsillectomy
t. and adenoidectomy
Sluder guillotine t.
tonsilloadenoidectomy
tooth
anatomical t.
t. extraction

t. fracture
t. hemisection
t. immobilization
t. mass
t. migration
t. perforation
t. plane
t. position
t. sac
t. transplantation
tooth-and-nail syndrome
tooth-to-tooth position
topectomy
Topel knot
tophus
topical
t. anesthetic
t. anesthetic technique
t. antibacterial agent
t. antibiotic
t. cooling
t. hemostatic agent
t. iodine application
t. oropharyngeal anesthesia
Topinard facial angle
topistic
topographic projection
top-up
epidural t.-u.
Torek
T. operation
T. orchiopexy
T. resection
Torg
T. classification
T. knee reconstruction
T. technique
Torgerson-Leach modified technique
tori (*pl. of* torus)
toric ablation
Torkildsen ventriculocisternostomy
Tornwaldt cyst
Torode-Zieg classification
Toronto pelvic fracture classification
Torpin cul-de-sac resection
torque
light wire t.
translation of t.
unwanted screw t.
torrential hemorrhage
torr pressure
torsade de pointes ventricular tachycardia (TdPVT)
torsion
angle of femoral t.
biliary tract t.
extravaginal testicular t.
intravaginal t.
perinatal t.
testicular t.
t. testis
unilateral testicular t.
torsional fracture
torso
t. crease
t. injury
torsoclusion
tortipelvis
tortuous intercostal artery
toruloma
torulopsis infection
torus, pl. **tori**
t. fracture
TOS
thoracic outlet syndrome
total
t. abdominal colectomy (TAC)
t. abdominal evisceration
t. abdominal hysterectomy
t. abdominal hysterectomy and bilateral salpingo-oophorectomy
t. ankle arthroplasty
t. anomalous pulmonary venous return
t. articular replacement arthroplasty
t. articular resurfacing arthroplasty
t. axial node irradiation
t. bilateral vagotomy
t. bilirubin level
t. biopsy
t. body fat
t. body hypothermia
t. body irradiation
t. body solute
t. body surface area (TBSA)
t. body water
t. body weight (TBW)
t. breech extraction
t. colectomy (TC)
t. colonic aganglionosis
t. colonoscopy
t. continence
t. cystectomy

NOTES

total *(continued)*
t. dehiscence
t. ear obliteration
t. elbow arthroplasty
t. endoscopic esophagectomy
t. erythrocyte volume
t. etch technique
t. ethmoidectomy
t. exchangeable potassium measurement
t. excisional operation
t. extraperitoneal repair
t. fundoplication
t. fundoplication method
t. fundoplication procedure
t. fundoplication technique
t. gastrectomy (TG)
t. gastric pull-up
t. gastric wrap
t. glossectomy
t. graft area rejection
t. hip arthroplasty
t. hip arthroplasty with internal eccentric shells (THARIES)
t. hip replacement
t. hip replacement surgery
t. hypophysectomy
t. internal reflection
t. intravenous anesthesia (TIVA)
t. intravenous anesthetic technique
t. joint arthroplasty
t. joint replacement
t. keratoplasty
t. knee arthroplasty
t. knee arthroscopy (TKA)
t. knee replacement
t. knee replacement surgery
t. laparoscopic esophagectomy
t. laryngectomy
t. laryngopharyngectomy
t. L-chain concentration
t. left hepatectomy
t. lobectomy
t. lymphoid irradiation
t. mastectomy
t. meniscectomy
t. mesorectal excision (TME)
t. nodal irradiation
t. pancreatectomy
t. parathyroidectomy
t. parenteral alimentation
t. parenteral nutrition (TPN)
t. patellectomy
t. patellofemoral joint arthroplasty
t. pelvic exenteration
t. pericystectomy
t. perineal prostatectomy
t. perineal rupture
t. petrosectomy
t. proctectomy
t. proctocolectomy
t. proctocolectomy with ileoanal anastomosis and J pouch
t. prostatoseminal vesiculectomy
t. protein concentration
t. pulpotomy
t. push therapy
t. respiratory time (Ttot)
t. retrocolic end-to-side gastrojejunostomy
t. scrotectomy
t. shoulder arthroplasty
t. space analysis
t. spinal anesthesia
t. surgical removal
t. thoracic esophagectomy
t. thyroidectomy
t. time to intubation (TTI)
t. tourniquet time
t. transfusion
t. vascular exclusion
t. vascular isolation (TVI)
t. wrist arthroplasty

total-body scanning

totally
t. extraperitoneal (TEP)
t. extraperitoneal inguinal herniorrhaphy
t. intrathoracic stomach
t. stapled restorative proctocolectomy

Toti
T. operation
T. procedure

Toti-Mosher operation

touch
three-point t.

touch-up procedure

Toupe
T. method
T. procedure
T. technique

Toupet
T. fundoplasty
T. hemifundoplication
T. hemifundoplication fundoplication

tourniquet
t. control
t. ischemia
t. ischemic pain
t. occlusion
t. paralysis
t. pressure
t. test
t. time

tourniquet-induced pain

Tourtual
T. canal
T. membrane
Towako method
Towne projection
Townley-Paton operation
toxemia
toxic
t. epidermal necrolysis
t. granulation
toxicity
aminoglycoside t.
endocrine t.
extramedullary t.
glutamate t.
neostigmine t.
oxygen t.
radiation-induced pulmonary t.
toxin
botulinum A t.
t. exposure
extracellular t.
Toynbee muscle
TPC
target plasma concentration
TPN
total parenteral nutrition
TPR
transsphenoidal pituitary resection
trabecula, pl. **trabeculae**
trabecular
t. bone fracture
t. membrane
t. network
trabeculated
t. bladder
t. bone lesion
trabeculation
trabeculectomy
Cairns t.
t. operation
Smith t.
trabeculopexy
argon laser t.
trabeculoplasty
argon laser t.
laser t.
trabeculotomy
trace anesthetic
tracer dilution
trachea, pl. **tracheae**
tracheal
t. adenoma
t. agenesis
t. aspiration
t. bifurcation angle
t. block
t. blood flow (TBF)
t. branch
t. cartilage
t. compression
t. extubation anesthetic technique
t. fenestration
t. fracture
t. gland
t. intubation
t. intubation anesthetic technique
t. ligation
t. node
t. reconstruction
t. repair
t. ring
t. safety stitch
t. secretion
t. stenosis
t. suction anesthetic technique
t. topical analgesia
t. triangle
t. tug
t. tumor
t. ulceration
t. web
tracheales
trachealia
trachealis muscle
trachelalis
trachelectomy
trachelematoma
trachelian
tracheloclavicularis
tracheloclavicular muscle
trachelomastoid
trachelomastoideus
trachelopexy
tracheloplasty
trachelorrhaphy
trachelos
tracheloschisis
trachelotomy
tracheoaerocele
tracheobiliary fistula
tracheobronchial
t. anomaly

NOTES

T

tracheobronchial *(continued)*
t. foreign body
t. node
tracheobronchoesophageal fistula
tracheobronchoscopy
tracheocele
tracheocutaneous fistula
tracheoesophageal (TE)
t. fistula (TEF)
t. puncture
tracheolaryngeal
tracheopharyngeal
tracheoplasty
tracheostomy
definitive t.
elective dilatational t.
emergency t.
flap t.
Great Ormond Street t.
Montgomery t.
percutaneous dilational t.
t. stoma
tracheotomy
trachoma gland
track
pin t.
radial suture t.
tracking
electromagnetic t.
optical t.
Tracrium
tract
abnormal fetal urogenital t.
aerodigestive t.
alimentary t.
Arnold t.
association t.
atriodextrofascicular t.
atriofascicular t.
atrio hisian bypass t.
atrionodal bypass t.
auditory t.
bile t.
biliary t.
bronchial t.
Burdach t.
bypass t.
central tegmental t.
cerebellorubral t.
cerebellothalamic t.
cholinergic t.
Collier t.
concealed bypass t.
corticobulbar t.
corticopontine t.
corticospinal t.
crossed pyramidal t.
cuneocerebellar t.
dead t.
deep liver t.
deiterospinal t.
dental sinus t.
dentatothalamic t.
dermal sinus t.
digestive t.
t. dilation
direct pyramidal t.
dopaminergic t.
dorsolateral t.
extrapyramidal t.
fastigiobulbar t.
fetal urogenital t.
fistulous t.
Flechsig t.
frontopontine t.
frontotemporal t.
gastrointestinal t.
geniculocalcarine t.
geniculotemporal t.
genital t.
genitourinary t.
GI t.
Gowers t.
habenulointerpeduncular t.
hepatic outflow t.
Hoche t.
hypothalamohypophysial t.
ileal inflow t.
ileal outflow t.
iliopubic t.
iliotibial t.
infected t.
inflammatory sinus t.
inflow t.
intestinal t.
intramural fistulous t.
lateral corticospinal t.
left ventricular outflow t. (LVOT)
Lissauer t.
liver t.
Loewenthal t.
mamillothalamic t.
Marchi t.
mesolimbic-mesocortical t.
Monakow t.
t. of Münzer and Wiener
nasal t.
needle t.
nerve t.
nigrostriatal t.
nodo-hisian bypass t.
nodoventricular t.
occipitocollicular t.
occipitopontine t.
occipitotectal t.
olfactory t.

olivocerebellar t.
olivospinal t.
optic t.
ororespiratory t.
outflow t.
pancreaticobiliary t.
parietopontine t.
perineal sinus t.
portal t.
posterior spinocerebellar t.
prepyramidal t.
pulmonary outflow t.
pyramidal t.
reproductive t.
respiratory t.
reticulospinal t.
retrochiasmal optic t.
right ventricular outflow t. (RVOT)
rubrobulbar t.
rubroreticular t.
rubrospinal t.
t. of Schütz
seminal t.
sensory t.
septomarginal t.
serotonergic t.
sinus t.
solitary t.
sphincteroid t.
spinal dermal sinus t.
spinocerebellar t.
spinoolivary t.
spinotectal t.
spinothalamic t. (STT)
spiral foraminous t.
Spitzka marginal t.
sulcomarginal t.
supraopticohypophysial t.
t. tamponade
tamponade needle t.
tangential t.
tectobulbar t.
tectopontine t.
tectospinal t.
temporofrontal t.
temporopontine t.
tree-barking urinary t.
T-tube t.
tuberoinfundibular t.
Türck t.
UGI t.
upper aerodigestive t.
upper gastrointestinal t. (UGI)
upper respiratory t.
urinary t.
urogenital t.
uveal t.
ventral spinocerebellar t.
ventral spinothalamic t.
ventricular outflow t.
vestibulospinal t.
vocal t.
Waldeyer t.
Wolff-Parkinson-White bypass t.
wound t.

traction
t. alopecia
t. aneurysm
t. application
t. atrophy
t. detachment
t. diverticulum
t. epiphysis
t. fracture
gentle t.
t. headache
t. suture technique
t. test

tractotomy
anterolateral t.
bulbar cephalic pain t.
dorsal column t.
intramedullary t.
medullary spinothalamic t.
mesencephalic t.
pontine spinothalamic t.
pyramidal t.
Schwartz t.
Sjöqvist intramedullary t.
spinal t.
spinothalamic t.
stereotactic trigeminal t.
subcaudate t.
trigeminal t.
Walker t.

traditional method

trafficking
membrane t.

tragicus muscle

tragus, pl. **tragi**

training
joint protection t.
stabilization t.

train-of-four (TOF)

NOTES

train-of-four *(continued)*
t.-o.-f. stimulation
t.-o.-f. stimulus
t.-o.-f. transmission
Trainor-Nida operation
Trainor operation
trajector
trajectory
bullet t.
missile t.
TRALD
transfusion-related acute lung injury
TRAM
transverse rectus abdominis muscle
TRAM flap
TRAM flap procedure
tram line
trampoline fracture
trance coma
tranquilization
tranquilizer
transabdominal
t. approach
t. laparoscopic herniorrhaphy
t. mucosectomy
t. preperitoneal hernioplasty
t. preperitoneal repair
t. properitoneal (TAPP)
transacromial approach
transactivation
transaminase
alanine amino t. (ALT)
glutamic oxaloacetic t.
glutamic pyruvic t.
serum alanine amino t.
transanal
t. approach
t. endoscopic microsurgery (TEM)
t. endoscopic microsurgical resection
t. excision
t. mucosectomy
t. mucosectomy with handsewn anastomosis
t. pouch advancement
t. stapling technique
t. ultrasonography
transanimation
transantral
t. approach
t. ethmoidal approach
t. ethmoidectomy
transaortic valve gradient
transarterial
t. anesthetic technique
t. chemoembolization
transarticular wire fixation
transaxial scan plane
transaxillary
t. apical bullectomy
t. approach
transbrachioradialis approach
transbronchial
t. lung biopsy
t. needle aspiration
transcallosal transventricular approach
transcanine approach
transcaphoid fracture
transcapillary hydrostatic pressure gradient
transcapitate
t. fracture
t. fracture-dislocation
transcapitellar wire fixation
transcardiac membranotomy
transcarpal amputation
transcatheter
t. ablation
t. arterial embolization therapy
t. closure
transcavernous transpetrous apex approach
transcerebellar hemispheric approach
transcervical
t. approach
t. balloon tuboplasty
t. femoral fracture
t. intrafallopian tube transfer
t. resection
t. tubal access
transchondral fracture
transclavicular approach
transcoccygeal approach
transcochlear
t. approach
t. cochleovestibular neurectomy
t. vestibular neurectomy
transcondylar fracture
transcortical transventricular approach
transcranial
t. Doppler (TCD)
t. electrical stimulation
t. electrical stimulation anesthetic technique
t. frontal-temporal-orbital approach
t. stimulation (TCS)
transcranial-supraorbital approach
transcriptional control
transcubital approach
transcutaneous
t. access
t. acupoint electrical stimulation (TAES)
t. biopsy
t. cranial electrical stimulation (TCES)

t. electrical nerve stimulation
t. electric stimulation (TES)
t. electrode nerve stimulation
t. oxygen monitoring
t. oxygen pressure measurement
t. partial pressure of oxygen
t. tetanic stimulus
transcylindrical cholecystectomy
transcystic
t. approach
t. drain
t. drainage
transdermal
t. administration
t. analgesic
t. anesthesia
t. anesthetic technique
t. sympathectomy
transduction
complex signal t.
transduodenal
t. approach
t. endoscopic decompression
t. pancreatectomy
t. sphincteroplasty
t. sphincterotomy
transect
transected
t. ductule
t. vertical gastric bypass
transection
aortic t.
atlantooccipital t.
esophageal t.
hepatic parenchymal t.
t. incision
parenchymal t.
t. plane
step-cut t.
Sugiura esophageal variceal t.
traumatic aortic t.
transendoscopic
t. electrocoagulation
t. laser photocoagulation
t. procedure
t. sphincterotomy
transepiphyseal fracture
transesophageal
t. atrial pacing (TEAP)
t. atrial stimulation
t. echocardiography (TEE)
t. echocardiography scan
t. echocardiography with pacing
t. endoscopy
t. ligation of varix
t. varix ligation
t. ventricular pacing (TEVP)
transethmoidal
transfemoral
t. liver biopsy
t. venous catheterization
transfer
adenoviral t.
barber pole stripe t.
composite free tissue t.
dermal fat-free tissue t.
free flap t.
free tissue t.
gamete intrafallopian tube t. (GIFT)
maternal-placental-fetal drug t.
microvascular free flap t.
Ober-Barr procedure for brachioradialis t.
placental t.
pronuclear stage t. (PROST)
saturation t.
single-stage tissue t.
split anterior tibial tendon t.
tissue t.
transcervical intrafallopian tube t.
in vitro fertilization-embryo t.
wraparound neurovascular composite free tissue t.
transferrin
melanoma t.
transfibular approach
transfixation
transfixing suture technique
transfixion
transforaminal passage
transform
driven equilibrium Fourier t. (DEFT)
transformary mass
transformation
hemorrhagic t.
malignant t.
neoplastic t.
t. zone
transforming growth factor (TGF)
transfrontal approach
transfuse

NOTES

transfusion
acute blood t.
allogenic blood t.
arterial t.
blood product t.
coagulation factor t.
direct t.
double-volume exchange t.
drip t.
exchange t.
exsanguination t.
homologous blood t.
immediate t.
indirect t.
intraperitoneal blood t.
intraperitoneal fetal t.
intrauterine intraperitoneal fetal t.
mediate t.
perioperative t.
peritoneal t.
simple t.
subcutaneous t.
substitution t.
t. therapy
total t.
transfusion-related
t.-r. acute lung injury (TRALD)
t.-r. air embolism
t.-r. lung injury (TRLI)
transgastric
t. fine-needle aspiration biopsy
t. ligation
t. plication
transgastrostomic enteroscopy
transgenic therapy
transglomerular hydrostatic filtration pressure
transgluteal approach
transhamate
t. fracture
t. fracture-dislocation
transhepatic
t. antegrade biliary drainage procedure
t. approach
t. catheterization
transhiatal
t. approach
t. blunt esophagectomy
t. esophagectomy (THE)
t. esophagojejunostomy
t. pyloroplasty
transhiatally
transhyoid pharyngotomy
transient
t. auditory evoked response (TAER)
t. azotemia
t. cavitation
t. compartment syndrome
t. edema
t. hiatal hernia
t. hypocalcemia
t. ischemic attack (TIA)
t. lesion
t. neurologic deficit
t. neurologic symptom (TNS)
t. osteoporosis of hip
t. visual obscuration
transiliac
t. amputation
t. bar technique
t. fracture
t. rod fixation
transillumination test
transischiac
transition
cervicothoracic t.
transitional
t. cell carcinoma
t. epithelium
t. respiration
t. zone biopsy
transjugular
t. hepatic biopsy
t. insertion
t. intrahepatic portosystemic shunt (TIPS)
t. liver access
t. liver biopsy
translabyrinthine and suboccipital approach
translaryngeal
t. guided intubation anesthetic technique
t. tracheal intubation
translation
anterior t.
anteroposterior t.
caudal t.
cephalad t.
coronal plane deformity sagittal t.
dorsal t.
force t. (FTR)
t. injury
t. mobility
t. motion
posterior t.
pure t.
t. of torque
ulnar t.
vertical t.
translational
t. fracture
t. position

translocation
bacterial t.
t. Down syndrome
translucent
transluminal
t. coronary angioplasty
t. extraction atherectomy
transmandibular-glossopharyngeal approach
transmandibular projection
transmastoid approach
transmeatal
t. approach
t. tympanoplasty incision
transmediastinal posterior esophagoplasty
transmembrane hydraulic pressure
transmesenteric
t. hernia
t. plication
transmetatarsal amputation
transmigration
ovular t.
transmission
double-burst t.
t. electron microscopy
iatrogenic t.
t. image
neuromuscular t.
pressure t.
train-of-four t.
transmucosal
t. delivery
t. drug administration anesthetic technique
transmural
t. approach
t. closure
t. hydrostatic pressure gradient
t. inflammation
t. pressure
transmutation
transmyocardial
t. carbon dioxide laser revascularization
t. laser revascularization (TMLR, TMR)
t. perfusion pressure
transnasal
t. administration
t. bile duct catheterization
t. biopsy
t. endoscopy
transocular
transolecranon approach
transomental posterior gastroenterostomy
transoral
t. approach
t. endoscopy
t. odontoid resection
transorbital
t. leukotomy
t. lobotomy
t. projection
transosseous suture
transpalatal approach
transpapillary
t. approach
t. biopsy
t. cannulation
t. catheterization
t. endoscopic cholecystotomy
transparietal
transpedicular
t. approach
t. screw-rod fixation
transpelvic
t. amputation
t. gunshot wound
transperineal palladium 103
transperineurial passage
transperitoneal
t. approach
t. cesarean section
t. exposure
t. hand-assisted laparoscopic surgery
t. laparoscopic adrenalectomy
t. laparoscopic nephrectomy
t. laparoscopic nephroureterectomy
transplacental hemorrhage
transplant
acute rejection of liver t.
adult-to-adult living related donor living t.
autologous bone marrow t.
auxiliary t.
cadaveric hand t.
cadaveric whole organ t.
corneal t.
domino t.
fetal tissue t.
Gallie t.
heart t.
hepatic t.
lamellar corneal t.

T

transplant *(continued)*
- liver t.
- living-related small bowel t.
- lung t.
- t. lung syndrome
- t. nephrectomy
- orthotopic liver t. (OLT)
- pancreas t. (PTX)
- penetrating corneal t.
- placental tissue t.
- primarily vascularized organ t.
- reduced liver t. (RLT)
- reduced-size t.
- t. rejection
- rejection cardiomyopathy t.
- small bowel t.
- SPK t.
- split-liver t.
- tissue t.

transplantar

transplantation
- adrenal medulla t.
- allogenic t.
- allograft t.
- anhepatic stage of liver t.
- autogenous tooth t.
- autologous blood stem cell t.
- autologous bone marrow t. (ABMT)
- auxiliary partial orthotopic liver t. (APOLT)
- bone marrow t.
- Bosworth femoroischial t.
- brain t.
- bridge organ t.
- cardiac t.
- clinical intestinal t.
- composite tissue t.
- corneal t.
- Cowen-Loftus toe-phalanx t.
- cryopreserved extrapelvic ovarian t.
- femoroischial t.
- fetal liver t.
- fetal thymus t.
- fresh extrapelvic ovarian t.
- heart t.
- heart-lung t.
- hepatic t.
- hepatocyte t.
- heterotopic t.
- homogenous tooth t.
- homotopic t.
- intestinal t.
- kidney t.
- liver t.
- living-related donor t.
- living-related liver t. (LRLT)
- lung t.
- muscle-tendon t.
- neonatal pulmonary t.
- organ t.
- orthoptic t.
- orthotopic heart t.
- orthotopic liver t. (OLT)
- osteoarticular allograft t.
- pancreas t.
- pancreas-kidney t.
- pancreatic t.
- pancreaticoduodenal t.
- piggyback liver t.
- pigment cell t.
- pituitary gland t.
- pulmonary t.
- renal t.
- simultaneous kidney-pancreas t.
- simultaneous pancreas-kidney t.
- SPK t.
- split-liver t.
- syngeneic t.
- syngenesioplastic t.
- T-cell depleted bone marrow t.
- tendon t.
- tissue t.
- toe-phalanx t.
- tooth t.
- xenograft t.

transplantectomy

transplanted stamp graft

transpleural

transpleurodiaphragmatic

transport
- air critical-care t.

transportation

transposition
- carotid t.
- t. flap
- penoscrotal t.
- Strombeck nipple t.
- Z-plasty t.

transpubic incision

transpupillary cyclophotocoagulation

transpyloric plane

transpyloricum

transradial approach

transrectal
- t. approach
- t. surgical treatment
- t. ultrasound-guided sextant biopsy

transrectus incision

transsacral
- t. fracture

transscaphoid
- t. dislocation fracture
- t. perilunate dislocation

transscrotal

transsection

transseptal
t. approach
t. left heart catheterization
t. orchiopexy
t. puncture
transsexualism
transsexual surgery
transsinus approach
transsphenoidal
t. approach
t. evacuation
t. hypophysectomy
t. microsurgical resection
t. operation
t. pituitary resection (TPR)
t. removal
t. surgery
transsphincteric
t. anal fistula
t. surgery
transstenotic pressure gradient measurement
transsternal approach
transsylvian approach
transtentorial
t. approach
t. herniation
transthermia
transthoracic
t. approach
t. diskectomy
t. dissection
t. esophagectomy
t. needle aspiration
t. needle aspiration biopsy
t. Nissen fundoplication
t. percutaneous fine-needle aspiration biopsy
t. route
t. vertebral body resection
transthoracotomy
transtorcular approach
transtracheal
t. aspirate
t. aspiration
t. jet
t. jet ventilation
t. jet ventilation anesthetic technique
transtriquetral
t. fracture
t. fracture-dislocation
transtrochanteric
t. approach
t. rotational osteotomy
transtubercular plane
transtympanic neurectomy
transubstantiation
transudation
transudative
t. ascites
t. inflammation
transumbilical breast augmentation (TUBA)
transureteroureteral anastomosis
transureteroureterostomy (TUU)
transurethral
t. ablative prostatectomy
t. balloon dilatation
t. balloon dilation
t. collagen injection therapy
t. electrical bladder stimulation
t. laser incision
t. marsupialization
t. microwave thermotherapy
t. needle ablation
t. resection
t. resection of bladder tumor (TURBT)
t. resection of prostate (TURP)
t. resection of prostate (TURP)
t. resection syndrome
t. sphincterotomy
t. ultrasound-guided laser-induced prostatectomy
t. ureterorenoscopy
transvaginal
t. approach
t. Burch procedure
t. fallopian tube catheterization
t. tubal catheterization
t. ultrasonically guided oocyte retrieval
t. ultrasonographic examination
t. urethrolysis
transvector
transvenous
t. approach
t. liver biopsy
t. therapy
transventricular mitral valve commissurotomy
transversa
transversalis fascia

NOTES

transversarium
transverse
t. abdominal muscle
t. anthelicine groove
apical t. (AP-T)
t. aponeurotic arch
t. approach
t. arytenoid muscle
t. cervical artery
t. colectomy
t. colon
t. colostomy
t. comminuted fracture
t. costal facet
deep-gastric t. (DG-T)
t. duodenotomy
t. facial
t. facial artery
t. facial fracture
t. fascia
five-chamber t. (5C-T)
t. fixation
t. fixator application
t. foramen
four-chamber t. (4C-T)
t. fundal incision of Strassman
t. head
t. ligament rupture
lower uterine segment t. (LUST)
t. magnetization phase
t. mastectomy
t. mastectomy incision
t. maxillary fracture
t. mesocolon
midpapillary t. (MP-T)
mitral valve-t. (MV-T)
t. oval pelvis
t. palatine fold
t. pancreatic artery
t. pericardial sinus
t. plane
t. plane motion insufficiency
t. process
t. process fracture
t. projection
t. rectal fold
t. rectus abdominis muscle (TRAM)
t. rectus abdominis muscle flap
t. rectus abdominis muscle flap procedure
t. relaxation
t. relaxation rate
t. resection
t. scan
t. scanning
t. scapular artery
t. section
t. section of heart
t. section imaging
t. skin incision
t. suture of Krause
t. tarsotomy
t. tenotomy
t. venous sinus
t. vesical fold
transversectomy
transverse-loop rod colostomy
transversely oriented endplate compression fracture
transversi
transversocostal
transversospinalis
transversospinal muscle
transversostomy
transversourethralis
transversovertical index
transversus
t. abdominis aponeurosis
t. abdominis muscle
transxiphoid approach
Trantas operation
tranylcypromine
trapdoor
t.-d. approach
t.-d. fragment
t.-d. thoracotomy
trapezia (*pl. of* trapezium)
trapezial
trapeziform
trapezii
trapeziometacarpal fusion
trapezium, pl. **trapezia**
t. fracture
trapezius
t. flap
t. stimulation anesthetic technique
trapezoid
t. body
t. line
t. method
t. ridge
trapezoidal
t. incision
t. keratotomy
t. osteotomy
trapezoidea
trapezoideum
trap incision
Trasylol
Traube-Hering curve
Traube semilunar space
trauma, pl. **traumas, traumata**
American Association for the Surgery of T. (AAST)
avulsion t.

blunt hepatic t.
t. care
corneal t.
external t.
foreign body t.
genital tract t.
head t.
hepatic t.
inadvertent t.
intraoral t.
pancreatic t.
t. patient
penetrating t.
perineal impact t.
t. room
T. Score and Injury Severity Score (TRISS)
t. service
spinal t.
t. surgeon
t. surgery
surgical t.
t. system
t. team
thoracoabdominal t.
tissue t.
truncal t.
t. victim

trauma-related death

traumasthenia

traumata (*pl. of* trauma)

traumatic

t. amputation
t. anesthesia
t. aortic rupture
t. aortic transection
t. atlantooccipital dislocation
t. brain injury (TBI)
t. cardiac arrest
t. cervical disk herniation
t. choroidal rupture
T. Coma Data Bank
t. corneal abrasion
t. diaphragmatic hernia
t. false aneurysm
t. fistula
t. fracture
t. gangrene
t. inflammation
t. internal carotid artery dissection
t. intracranial hematoma
t. lesion
t. progressive encephalopathy
t. pseudomeningocele
t. renal mass
t. tetanus

traumatism

traumatize

traumatologist

orthopedic t.

traumatology

traumatonesis

traumatopathy

traumatopnea

traumatosepsis

traumatotherapy

Trautmann triangular space

Treacher Collins syndrome

treadmill

t. exercise
t. exercise capacity

treatment

acidification t.
acorn t.
allocation of t.
alternative t.
anoplasty t.
antifungal t.
Boyd-Ingram-Bourkhard t.
Carrel t.
chemotherapeutic t.
cholecystectomy t.
chronic anoplasty t.
cognitive behavior t. (CBT)
complementary t.
compression rod t.
computer-assisted t.
conservative surgical t.
continuous medical t.
Dakin-Carrel t.
definitive t.
diabetic retinal t.
dialysis t.
distraction/compression scoliosis t.
dual compression scoliosis t.
endoscopic t.
endovascular graft t.
esophageal dilation t.
ex vivo marrow t.
ferromagnetic microembolization t.
Gelfoam particles transarterial embolization t.
graft t.
hemodialysis t.

NOTES

treatment *(continued)*
insulin coma t.
intracavernosal injection t.
intravesical chemotherapeutic t.
iodine t.
laparoscopic t.
lipiodol transarterial embolization t.
local t.
locoregional t.
medical t.
mitomycin transarterial embolization t.
t. modality
multidisciplinary pain t. (MPT)
nonsurgical t.
open surgical t.
operative t.
t. option
percutaneous endovascular t.
photocoagulation t.
prophylactic antifungal t.
radiation t.
radioiodine t.
rectovaginal surgical t.
t. regimen
retinal t.
root canal t.
t. strategy
surgical t.
transrectal surgical t.
ureteral surgical t.

tree
biliary t.
bronchial t.
cannulation of the biliary t.
endobronchial t.
extrahepatic biliary t.
iliac arterial t.
intrahepatic biliary t.

tree-barking urinary tract

trefoil
t. deformity
t. tendon

Treitz
T. arch
T. fascia
T. fossa
T. hernia
T. ligament
T. muscle

trellis formation

trema

trematode infection

tremor
essential t.
parkinsonian t.

Trendelenburg
T. operation
T. position
T. tilt

trepanation
corneal t.
dental t.

trephination
dental t.
open-sky t.

trephine needle biopsy

Treponema
microhemagglutination *T. pallidum* (MHA-TP)
T. pallidum immobilization

Trethowan metatarsal osteotomy

Trethowan-Stamm-Simmonds-Menelaus-Haddad technique

Treves
T. fold
T. operation

triad
acute compression t.
Beck t.
Charcot t.
hepatic t.
t. knee repair
portal t.
Virchow t.
wall-echo shadow t.

triadic therapy

triage

triaging

trial
t. cementation
t. of conservative therapy
European Carotid Surgery T. (ECST)
neuraxial medication t.
neurostimulation t.
North American Symptomatic Carotid Endarterectomy T. (NASCET)
t. point
t. reduction

triangle
anal t.
anterior t.
Assézat t.
auricular t.
axillary t.
Béclard t.
Burow t.
Calot t.
carotid t.
cephalic t.
cervical t.
Charcot t.
digastric t.
Elaut t.

facial t.
Farabeuf t.
femoral t.
frontal t.
Grynfeltt t.
Henke t.
Hesselbach t.
inferior carotid t.
inferior occipital t.
infraclavicular t.
inguinal t.
interscalene t.
Labbé t.
Langenbeck t.
Lesser t.
Lesshaft t.
Lieutaud t.
lumbar t.
lumbocostoabdominal t.
Macewen t.
Malgaigne t.
Marcille t.
muscular t.
occipital t.
omoclavicular t.
omotracheal t.
Petit lumbar t.
Pirogoff t.
pubourethral t.
retromolar t.
sacral t.
Scarpa t.
sternocostal t.
subclavian t.
subinguinal t.
submandibular t.
submaxillary t.
submental t.
suboccipital t.
superior carotid t.
supraclavicular t.
suprahyoid t.
suprameatal t.
tracheal t.
umbilicomammillary t.
urogenital t.
vesical t.
Weber t.

triangular
t. advancement flap
t. aponeurosis
t. bone
t. capsulotomy
t. cartilage
t. fascia
t. fibrocartilage complex (TFCC)
t. fold
t. fossa
t. ligament of liver
t. muscle
t. space

triangulare

triangularis

triangular-shaped skin

triangulation
indirect t.
t. stapling method
t. technique

triaxial total elbow arthroplasty

tribasilare

tributary
venous t.

triceps
t. bursa
t. flap
t. tendon

tricepsplasty

trichangion

trichiasis repair

trichilemmoma
desmoplastic t.

trichion

trichodiscoma

tricholemmoma

trichoma

***Trichomonas* infection**

trichoscopy

tricipital

triclofos

tricorn

tricornute

tricorrectional bunionectomy

tricuspid
t. position
t. valve annuloplasty
t. valve anulus
t. valve area
t. valve disease
t. valve flow
t. valve repair
t. valvuloplasty

tridermoma

Trieger test

NOTES

triethiodide
gallamine t.
trifacial nerve
trifid stomach
trifurcation
t. injury
t. involvement
popliteal artery t.
trigastric
trigeminal
t. cave
t. cavity
t. decompression
t. dermatome
t. ganglion
t. impression
t. nerve
t. nerve root
t. neuralgia
t. rhizotomy
t. tractotomy
trigeminale
trigeminalis
trigemini
trigeminus
trigger
t. point
t. point injection
triggered ventilation
trigger-point inactivation
trigona (*pl. of* trigonum)
trigonal ring
trigone
habenular t.
inguinal t.
Lieutaud t.
right fibrous t.
vertebrocostal t.
trigonectomy
trigonitis
trigonocephaly
trigonum, pl. **trigona**
Trillat procedure
trilobate
trimalleolar ankle fracture
trimming
tissue t.
trimodality therapy
triophthalmos
triotus
triphalangeal thumb deformity
triphenyltetrazolium staining method
Tripier
T. operation
T. operation throw square knot
triplane
t. osteotomy
t. tibial fracture
triple
t. anastomosis
t. hemisection
t. innominate osteotomy
t. intrathecal therapy
t. ligamentous repair
t. lobe hepatectomy
t. loop pouch
t. point
triple-balloon valvuloplasty
triple-lumen infusion
triple-throw square knot stitch
triple-wire
t.-w. procedure
t.-w. technique
triplication
tripod
t. fracture
Haller t.
tripodia
tri-point
tripsinization
triquetral
t. bone
t. fracture
triquetrolunate dislocation
triquetropisiform articulation
triquetrous cartilage
triquetrum
triradial
triradiate
t. acetabular extensile approach
t. line
t. transtrochanteric approach
triradius
triscaphe fusion
trisection
pulse t.
trisectorectomy
trisegmentectomy
trisomy
t. C syndrome
t. 8 syndrome
trisplanchnic
TRISS
Trauma Score and Injury Severity Score
tristichia
triticea
triticeal cartilage
triticeum
trituration
trivalve
TRLI
transfusion-related lung injury
trocar
t. cystostomy
t. drainage method
t. gas leak

t. injury
t. site hernia
t. technique
t. wound
t. wound bleed
t. wound site complication
trocar-cannula technique
trocar-related injury
trochanter
greater t.
lesser t.
t. major
t. minor
small t.
third t.
trochanterian
trochanteric
t. bursa
t. crest
t. migration
t. osteotomy
trochanterica
trochanterplasty
trochantin
trochantinian
trochlea, pl. **trochleae**
trochlear
t. fossa
t. fovea
t. nerve
t. process
t. synovial bursa
trochleariform
trochleariformis
trochlearis
trochleiform
trochoid
t. articulation
t. joint
Trolard vein
Tronzo intertrochanteric fracture classification
trophectoderm biopsy
trophedema
trophic
t. fracture
t. lesion
trophoblastic tissue
tropism
facet t.
Trotter syndrome
trough line
Trousseau point
Troutman operation
Truc
T. flap
T. operation
Tru-Cut needle biopsy (TCNB)
true
t. aneurysm
t. diverticulum
t. exfoliation
t. hernia
t. knot
t. muscle
t. mutation
t. negative
t. pelvis
t. positive
t. rib
t. size
t. vertebra
t. vocal cord
true-negative result
true-positive result
Trumble talectomy
trumpet
nasal t.
truncal
t. lesion
t. melanoma
t. trauma
t. vagotomy
t. vagotomy and gastroenterostomy
t. vagotomy and pyloroplasty
truncated tarsometatarsal wedge arthrodesis
truncated-wedge
t.-w. arthrodesis
truncation
t. phenomenon
protein t.
truncus, pl. **trunci**
trunk
accessory nerve t.
anterior vaginal t.
brachiocephalic t.
bronchomediastinal t.
celiac t.
costocervical t.
t. duplication
hepatic venous t.
t. incurvation test
intestinal t.

NOTES

trunk *(continued)*
jugular lymphatic t.
linguofacial t.
lumbar t.
lumbosacral t.
nerve t.
posterior vaginal t.
pulmonary t.
subclavian lymphatic t.
sympathetic t.
thoracoacromial t.
thyrocervical t.
upper t.
vagal t.
venous t.
Trusler
T. aortic valve technique
T. technique of aortic valvuloplasty
trypsin
crystallized t.
trypsinization
Tsai-Stillwell procedure
Tscherne classification
Tscherne-Gotzen tibial fracture classification
T-shaped
T-s. capsulotomy
T-s. constriction ring
T-s. incision
TSRH
Texas Scottish Rite Hospital
TSRH crosslink stabilization
TSRH rod fixation
Tsuji laminaplasty
T-tack gastropexy
TTI
total time to intubation
Ttot
total respiratory time
TTS
tight-to-shaft
TTS balloon dilation
TTTS
twin-twin transfusion syndrome
T-tube
T-t. drainage
T-t. placement
T-t. study
T-t. tract
T-t. tract choledochofiberoscopy
T-t. tract choledochoscopy
TUBA
transumbilical breast augmentation
tuba, pl. **tubae**
tubage
tubal
t. branch
t. insufflation
t. ligation
t. ligation band technique
t. reconstruction surgery
t. rupture
t. sterilization
tubaria
tubariae
tubatorsion
tube
auditory t.
t. cecostomy
t. decompression
diagnostic t.
digestive t.
t. dilution test
embryonic neural t.
end t.
endothelial t.
eustachian t.
t. extrusion
fallopian t.
t. feeding
t. flap graft
t. gastrostomy
germ t.
knuckle of t.
t. leakage
medullary t.
t. migration
molar t.
neural t.
t. placement
t. precipitin test
t. removal
t. replacement
t. thoracostomy
tube-carina distance
tubectomy
tubed
t. free skin graft
t. groin flap
t. pedicle flap
t. urethroplasty
tube-fed patient
tube-patient distance
tuber, pl. **tubera**
calcaneal t.
cortical t.
frontal t.
omental t.
parietal t.
tubercle
accessory t.
anatomical t.
anterior t.
auricular t.
calcaneal t.
carotid t.

Chassaignac t.
conoid t.
corniculate t.
cuneiform t.
dental t.
dissection t.
dorsal radius t.
genial t.
genital t.
Gerdy t.
hard t.
iliac t.
inferior thyroid t.
infraglenoid t.
jugular t.
labial t.
Lisfranc t.
Lister t.
mamillary t.
marginal t.
maxillary t.
mental t.
Morgagni t.
obturator t.
t. osteotomy
pharyngeal t.
Princeteau t.
prosector t.
pterygoid t.
pubic t.
quadrate femoral t.
scalene t.
soft t.
superior thyroid t.
supraglenoid t.
supratragic t.
wedge-shaped t.
Whitnall orbital t.
Wrisberg t.
Zuckerkandl t.

tubercula (*pl. of* tuberculum)
tuberculation
tuberculization
tuberculocele
tuberculoma
tuberculosis
central nervous system t.
endobronchial t.
endometrial t.
extraarticular t.
extrapulmonary t.
extrathoracic t.
exudative t.
t. granulation tissue
inhalation t.
peritoneal t.
reactivation t.
reinfection t.
surgical t.

tuberculous
t. abscess
t. arthritis
t. caseation
t. infiltration
t. lesion

tuberculum, pl. **tubercula**
first-degree t.
Zuckerkandl t.

tuberoinfundibular tract
tuberositas
tuberosity
costal t.
t. fragment
masseteric t.
pterygoid t.
reduction t.
t. reduction

tuberous
t. sclerosis
t. sclerosis-associated renal cell carcinoma
t. sclerosis-associated tumor
t. sclerosis complex

tube-shift technique
tube-to-film distance
tube-within-tube technique
tubi (*pl. of* tubus)
tuboabdominal
tuboligamentous
tuboovarian abscess
tuboperitoneal
tuboplasty
balloon t.
transcervical balloon t.
ultrasound transcervical t.

tubotorsion
tubouterine implantation
tubovaginal
tubular
t. aneurysm
t. basement membrane
t. carcinoma
t. colonic duplication
t. excretory mass

T

NOTES

tubular *(continued)*
t. reconstruction
t. regeneration
t. respiration
t. vertical gastroplasty
tubularized
t. bladder neck reconstruction
t. cecal flap
tubulation
tubule
Albarran y Dominguez t.
convoluted seminiferous t.
Henle t.
mesonephric t.
paragenital t.
straight seminiferous t.
uriniferous t.
tubuli (*pl. of* tubulus)
tubulization
tubulovillar lesion
tubulovillous adenoma
tubulus, pl. **tubuli**
tubus, pl. **tubi**
tuck
t. position
t. procedure
Tudor-Thomas
T.-T. graft
T.-T. operation
Tuffier morcellement technique
tuft fracture
tug
tracheal t.
Tukey post-hoc correction
Tullos technique
tumbler
t. flap
t. graft
tumbling
t. procedure
t. technique
t. technique operation
tumescent technique breast reduction
tummy tuck flap
tumor
abdominal t.
t. ablation
Abrikosov t.
adenoid t.
alveolar t.
ampullary t.
t. angiogenesis
t. antigen
antral t.
aortic body t.
t. ascites
t. bed
benign bone t.
biliary tract t.
bleeding t.
blood t.
t. blood supply
blood vessel t.
t. blush
body t.
bone t.
brain t.
brown fat t.
t. bulk
t. burden
Buschke-Löwenstein t.
t. capsule
carcinoid t.
cardiac t.
carotid body t.
celiac t.
t. cell
t. cell-host bone relationship
t. cell purging
cervical t.
colon t.
colorectal primary t.
debulking of t.
deep t.
t. defect
diffuse t.
discrete t.
distal t.
t. dormancy mode
t. doubling time
dumbbell t.
duodenal t.
t. embolism
embryonal t.
t. encapsulation
endocrine t.
t. erosion
esophageal t.
extrahepatic t.
eye t.
eyelid t.
t. feature
focal t.
focus of t.
fungating t.
gastric stromal t.
genital tract t.
glial t.
t. grade
t. grading
gritty t.
t. growth
gynecologic t.
hepatic t.
hyperplastic t.
t. hypoxia

t. imaging
t. infiltration
infratentorial t.
t. initiation
intracranial t.
intraluminal t.
intramedullary t.
intramyocardial t.
t. invasion
invasive t.
islet cell t.
isolated metastatic t.
t. kinetic model
lacrimal gland t.
liver t.
t. location
lumbar t.
lung t.
t. lysis syndrome
malignant t.
t. marker
t. mass
mediastinal t.
metastatic t.
midbody t.
mixed t.
multifocal t.
musculoskeletal t.
t. necrosis
t. necrosis factor (TNF)
t. necrosis factor-alpha (TNF-alpha)
t. necrosis factor-binding protein (TNF-bp)
t. neovasculature
neuroendocrine t.
t., node, metastasis (TNM)
t., node, metastasis carcinoma classification
nonfamilial malignant endocrine t.
nonfunctional malignant t.
nonseminomatous testicular t.
ocular t.
optic nerve t.
oral cavity t.
orbital t.
t. origin
ovarian t.
t. oxygenation
Pancoast t.
pancreatic endocrine t.
parathyroid t.
phyllodes t.
pituitary t.
t. ploidy
t. plop
t. polysaccharide substance
potato t.
primary parathyroid hyperplastic t.
t. progression
t. promoter
proximal t.
pulmonary t.
t. receptor protein negative
t. recurrence
recurrent t.
t. registry
t. regression
t. removal
renal t.
t. resectability
resectable t.
t. resection
sacral bone t.
sacrococcygeal t.
salivary gland t.
t. seeding
sellar t.
t. shrinkage
sinonasal t.
t. site
t. in situ
t. size
t. skin test
skull base t.
small bowel t.
solid t.
t. spillage
spinal cord t.
sporadic islet cell t.
t. stage
t. stage grouping
stage II_E t.
t. staging
t. stenting
t. subtype
t. suppressor
t. suppressor gene
t. suppressor oncogene
supratentorial t.
t. surgery
synchronous t.
tail t.
t. targeting
temporal bone t.

NOTES

tumor *(continued)*
testicular t.
t. therapy
t. thrombus
thyroid t.
tracheal t.
transurethral resection of bladder t. (TURBT)
tuberous sclerosis-associated t.
t. ulceration
unresectable t.
t. vascularity
t. vessel
t. volume
von Hippel-Lindau t.
Wilms renal t.
tumor-bearing kidney
tumor-cell product
tumor:cerebellum ratio
tumorectomy
tumor-free margin
tumorigenesis
foreign body t.
tumor-like bone condition
tumor-related death
tumor specific
tumor-targeting ability
tunable dye laser lithotripsy
tunic
mucosal t.
muscular t.
tunica, pl. **tunicae**
tunicary hernia
tunnel
catheter t.
t. creation
t. graft
t. infection
t. and sling fixation
t. of Wertheim
tunneled ventriculostomy
tunneling
Tupper arthroplasty
turbid peritoneal fluid
turbinal
turbinate
turbinated
turbinectomy
Turbinger gastric reconstruction
turbinoplasty
turbo spin-echo sequence
TURBT
transurethral resection of bladder tumor
turcica
Türck
T. bundle
T. tract
Turco clubfoot release technique
Turco-Spinella tendo calcaneus repair
Turcot syndrome
Turkish saddle
Turk line
turn-and-suction biopsy technique
Turnbull
T. colostomy
T. end-loop ileostomy
T. multiple ostomy operation
T. technique
turned-down tendon flap
turned-up pulp deformity
Turner operation
turnover flap
TURP
transurethral resection of prostate
turunda, pl. **turundae**
tutamen, pl. **tutamina**
TUU
transureteroureterostomy
TVI
total vascular isolation
Tweed method
twelfth cranial nerve
twilight sleep
twin
t. bracket tooth rotation
t. formation
t. method
t. operating theater
Twining line
twin-twin transfusion syndrome (TTTS)
twirling method
twisted
t. fundoplication
t. suture technique
twist-off technique
twitch
t. depression
evoked t.
t. height
t. height test
t. response
t. suppression
t. tension
two-bellied muscle
two-chamber longitudinal (2C-L)
two-dimensional
t.-d. Fourier transformation imaging
t.-d. Fourier transform gradient-echo imaging
t.-d. monitoring
two-dye method
two-field dissection
two-flight exertional dyspnea
two-inclinometer method
two-layer
t.-l. anastomosis

t.-l. enteroenterostomy
t.-l. latex closure
t.-l. open technique
two-loop J-shaped ileal pouch
two-microphone acoustic reflection method
two-needle technique
two-part fracture
two-patch technique
two-piece ostomy pouch
two-plane
t.-p. deformity
t.-p. fluoroscopy
t.-p. occlusion
two-point
t.-p. discrimination test
t.-p. nerve block
two-portal technique
two-pour technique
two-quadrant hemorrhoidectomy
two-sleeve technique
two-stage
t.-s. hip fusion
t.-s. procedure
t.-s. repair
t.-s. Syme amputation
t.-s. technique mastectomy
t.-s. tendon grafting technique
t.-s. tendon graft reconstruction
two-step
t.-s. orchiopexy
t.-s. pancreatoduodenectomy
t.-s. procedure
t.-s. technique
two-team dissection
two-trocar laparoscopic cholecystectomy
Tycos pressure infusion line
tylectomy
tylion
tyloma
tympani
chorda t.
t. sinus
tympanic
t. bone
t. canal
t. canaliculus
t. cavity
t. membrane
t. membrane measurement
t. neurectomy
t. notch
t. plexus
t. ring
t. thermometry
tympanica
tympanitic abdomen
tympanohyal bone
tympanomastoid
t. fissure
t. suture
tympanomastoidea
tympanomastoidectomy
tympanomeatal flap
tympanoplasty
t. mastoidectomy
t. ossiculoplasty
staged t.
type I–V t.
tympanosquamosa
tympanosquamosal suture
tympanosquamous fissure
tympanotemporal
tyndallization
type
t. B-1, -2 lesion
t. I–IV canal
t. C pelvic ring fracture
depressed t.
histologic t.
macroscopic t.
t. I, II, III, IIIA, IIIB, IIIC open fracture
superficial t.
t. I–V tympanoplasty
ulcerated t.
typhlectasis
typhlectomy
typhlodicliditis
typhloempyema
typhlolithiasis
typhlon
typhlopexy
typhlorrhaphy
typhlostomy
typhlotomy
typhloureterostomy
typhoidal cholecystitis
typical skin lesion
typing
tissue t.
tyroma
Tyrrell fascia
Tyson gland

NOTES

NOTES

UA
umbilical arterial
UA blood
UAL
ultrasonic-assisted liposuction
ubinemia
UC
ulcerative colitis
UGCR
ultrasound-guided compression repair
UGI
upper gastrointestinal tract
UGI endoscopy
UGI tract
Uhl
U. anomaly
U. malformation
UICC
Union Internationale Contre le Cancer
UICC tumor classification
ulcer
aphthous u.
cervical u.
collar-button-like u.
Cruveilhier u.
duodenal u.
gastric u.
genital u.
ischemic u.
neuropathic u.
oral aphthous u.
penetrating u.
peptic u.
perforated peptic u.
postsclerotherapy u.
ring u.
scrotal skin u.
skin u.
solitary rectal u.
ulcerated
u. mucosa
u. type
ulceration
acute hemorrhagic u.
anal u.
anastomotic u.
aphthous u.
A.S.A.-induced gastric u.
catarrhal marginal u.
CMV-associated u.
CMV-induced esophageal u.
collar-button u.
corneal u.
diffuse u.
duodenal u.
esophageal u.
gastric u.
gastrointestinal u.
genital u.
herpes epithelial tropic u.
intertrigo with u.
intestinal u.
ischemic infected u.
labial u.
linear u.
marginal u.
mucosal u.
mucous membrane u.
nasal mucosal u.
necrotic u.
oral u.
patchy colonic u.
postbulbar u.
radiation-induced u.
rectal u.
rheumatoid-related u.
serpiginous u.
stasis u.
stercoral u.
stomal u.
stress u.
stress-induced gastric u.
sublesional u.
tracheal u.
tumor u.
ulcerative
u. colitis (UC)
u. inflammation
ulcerogenic fistula
ulcerogranuloma
ulectomy
ulegyria
uletomy
Ullmann line
Ulloa operation
ulna, pl. **ulnae**
ulnar
u. artery
u. branch
u. bursa
u. collateral ligament rupture
u. deviation deformity
u. drift deformity
u. fracture
u. head
u. head excision
u. hemiresection interposition arthroplasty
u. motor neurectomy
u. translation

ulnari
ulnaris
extensor carpi u. (ECU)
ulnocarpal
ulocarcinoma
uloid
ulotomy
ultrabrachycephalic
ultrafast
u. CT electron beam tomography
u. spiral computed tomography
ultrafiltration
continuous arteriovenous u.
dialytic u.
extracorporeal u.
glomerular u.
modified u.
spontaneous dialytic u.
ultra-high-frequency ventilation
ultra-high-magnification endoscopy
ultraligation
ultralow
u. anterior resection
u. anterior resection parastomal infection
ultramicroscopy
ultrarapid subthreshold stimulation
ultrasonic
u. aspiration
u. attenuation
u. cutting
u. dissection
u. endovaginal finding
u. fragmentation
u. lithotresis
u. lithotripsy
u. nebulizer
u. therapy
ultrasonic-assisted liposuction (UAL)
ultrasonication
ultrasonographic
u. data
u. technique
ultrasonographically-guided injection
ultrasonography
carotid duplex u.
color duplex u.
Doppler duplex u.
duplex u.
endoanal u.
endoscopic u. (EUS)
high-resolution u.
intraoperative u. (IOUS)
laparoscopic u. (LUS)
laparoscopic intracorporeal u. (LICU)
open intraoperative u.
transanal u.
ultrasonography-guided fine-needle aspiration biopsy
ultrasonosurgery
ultrasound
u. anesthetic technique
cervical u.
Doppler u.
u. examination
u. guidance
u. image
intraoperative u. (IOUS)
laparoscopic u.
preoperative u.
u. therapy
u. transcervical tuboplasty
ultrasound-assisted percutaneous endoscopic gastrostomy
ultrasound-guided
u.-g. anterior subcostal liver biopsy
u.-g. automated large-core breast biopsy
u.-g. bronchoscopy
u.-g. compression repair (UGCR)
u.-g. core breast biopsy
u.-g. core-needle biopsy (US-CNB)
u.-g. echo biopsy
u.-g. fine-needle aspiration
u.-g. fine-needle aspiration biopsy (US-FNAB)
u.-g. needle biopsy
u.-g. nephrostomy puncture
u.-g. shock wave therapy
u.-g. stereotactic biopsy
ultraterminal excementosis
ultraviolet (UV)
u. blood irradiation
psoralens, u. A (PUVA)
ultropaque method
umbilectomy
umbilical
u. arterial (UA)
u. artery
u. artery blood
u. artery catheterization
u. circulation
u. cord
u. cord anomaly
u. cord hematoma
u. fissure
u. fistula
u. fossa
u. hernia
u. hernia rupture
u. herniorrhaphy
u. mass
u. notch
u. plane
u. plate

u. port
u. prevesical fascia
u. region
u. ring
u. skin-knife incision
u. vein (UV)
u. vein blood
u. vein catheterization
u. vein to maternal vein (UV/MV)
u. vein recanalization
u. venous
umbilicalis
umbilicate
umbilication
umbilici (*pl. of* umbilicus)
umbilicomammillary triangle
umbilicovesical fascia
umbilicus, pl. **umbilici**
umbo
umbrascopy
umbrella closure
unanticipated hepatic disease
unattended laboratory operation
unavoidable hemorrhage
unbanded gastroplasty
uncal
u. herniation
unci (*pl. of* uncus)
unciform bone
unciforme
uncinate
u. bundle of Russell
u. groove
u. pancreas
u. procedure
u. process fracture
u. process mass
uncinatum
uncinectomy
uncipressure
uncommitted metaphysial lesion
uncomplicated
u. acute cholecystitis
u. angiomyolipoma
unconstrained shoulder arthroplasty
uncontrollable glaucoma
uncovertebral joint
uncus, pl. **unci**
uncut
u. Collis-Nissen fundoplication
u. Collis-Nissen fundoplication method
u. Collis-Nissen fundoplication procedure
u. Collis-Nissen fundoplication technique
underangulation
undercorrection
undercut
soft-tissue u.
underlay fascia technique
underlying
u. cardiomyopathy
u. cause
u. structure
underresuscitated
underresuscitation
undersensing
pacemaker u.
underventilation
undescended testis
undifferentiated
u. adenocarcinoma
u. connective tissue disease
u. embryonal sarcoma
u. lesion
u. squamous cell carcinoma
undifferentiation
undisplaced fracture
undiversion
Undritz anomaly
undulating membrane
unfiltered
u. preparation
u. radioisotope
unfractionated
u. heparin antibody
u. heparin-induced thrombocytopenia
u. heparin reversal
u. heparin therapy
ungual
u. fibroma
u. labia
ungualabia
unguis, pl. **ungues**
unguium
uniaxial joint
unicaliceal kidney
unicanalicular sphincter
unicompartmental knee arthroplasty
unicondylar fracture
unification
unifocal optic nerve lesion

unilateral
u. amputee
u. anesthesia
u. approach
u. diaphragmatic elevation
u. hemidysplasia cornification disorder
u. hemilaminectomy
u. hernia
u. hypophysectomy
u. inguinal hernia repair
u. inguinal hernia repair method
u. inguinal hernia repair procedure
u. inguinal hernia repair technique
u. interfacetal dislocation
u. intrafacetal dislocation
u. laryngeal paralysis
u. lobectomy
u. neck exploration
u. nephrectomy
u. pallidotomy
u. parathyroidectomy
u. pedicle cannulation
u. pneumoretroperitoneum
u. resection
u. sacroiliac approach
u. salpingo-oophorectomy
u. subcostal incision
u. testicular torsion
unilobar disease
unilocular
u. cyst
u. cystic lesion
u. joint
unimalleolar fracture
uninhibited neurogenic bladder
uninterrupted suture technique
union
delayed fracture u.
fibrous u.
U. Internationale Contre le Cancer (UICC)
osteonal bone u.
primary u.
secondary u.
vicious u.
unipedicled flap
unipennate muscle
unipennatus
unipolar cauterization
uniportal arthroscopic microdiskectomy
unique
u. NCRLM
u. noncolorectal liver metastasis
unit
autologous blood u.
autologous RBC u.
day care surgical u. (DCSU)
Hounsfield u. (HU)
inpatient dialysis u.
intensive care u. (ICU)
low-grade suction u.
u. of mass
u. membrane
neurosurgical intensive care u. (NICU)
postanesthesia care u. (PACU)
surgical admitting u.
United
U. Kingdom Heart Valve Registry
U. Network for Organ Sharing (UNOS)
U. States Renal Data System
uniting
u. canal
u. cartilage
u. duct
unitunnel technique
University of Pennsylvania Smell Identification Test
unlocking spiral technique
unmonitored local anesthesia
UNOS
United Network for Organ Sharing
unplanned valgus osteotomy
unreamed nailing
unreduced dislocation
unremitting symptom
unrepositioned flap
unresectability
unresectable
u. extrahepatic disease
u. hepatoblastoma
u. lesion
u. metastasis
u. periampullary cancer
u. tumor
unresuscitated
unroofing
unsaturated chemical vapor sterilization
unsex
unshuntable portal hypertension
unstable
u. angina
u. bladder
u. fracture
u. fracture-dislocation
unstrained jaw relation
unstriated muscle
untethering procedure
untreated
u. HPT
u. hyperparathyroidism
ununited fracture
unusual opportunistic infection
unwanted screw torque

up-and-down staircases procedure
upgated technique
UPJ
ureteropelvic junction
U pouch
U-pouch construction
upper
u. abdominal evisceration
u. adenoma
u. aerodigestive tract
u. airway obstruction
u. alimentary endoscopy
u. cervical spine anterior exposure
u. cervical spine fusion
u. cervical spine procedure
u. end
u. endoscopy and colonoscopy
u. esophageal sphincter relaxation
u. extremity
u. extremity nerve block
u. eyelid
u. gastrointestinal bleeding
u. gastrointestinal endoscopy
u. gastrointestinal panendoscopy
u. gastrointestinal series
u. gastrointestinal tract (UGI)
u. gastrointestinal tract surgery
u. genital tract infection
u. GI hemorrhage
u. GI tract foreign body
u. incisor angulation
u. intestinal endoscopy
u. jaw
u. jaw bone
u. jejunal motility
u. jejunal motor pattern
u. jejunum
u. lateral quadrant
u. lid
u. lip
u. medial quadrant
u. mediastinum
u. midline incision
u. respiratory tract
u. respiratory tract infection
u. respiratory tract mucosa
u. small bowel motor disturbance
u. subscapular nerve
u. thoracic wall
u. thorax aperture
u. tract disease
u. trapezius flap
u. trunk
up-regulation of the receptor
upright
u. position
u. reflux
upright-Y incision
upside-down stomach
upsiloid
uptake
local lymphatic u.
lymphatic u.
placental u.
radioisotope u.
urachal
u. carcinoma
u. fistula
u. fold
u. ligament
uraniscoplasty
uraniscorrhaphy
uranoplasty
Wardill-Kilner four-flap u.
uranorrhaphy
uranostaphyloplasty
uranostaphylorrhaphy
uraroma
urate
urate-associated inflammation
uratoma
urban
U. operation
u. trauma center
Urbaniak
U. neurovascular free flap
U. scapular flap
urea hydrolysis
urea-impermeable membrane
urecchysis
uredema
urelcosis
uremia
uremia-related coagulopathy
uremic
u. coma
u. gastrointestinal lesion
u. inflammation
ureter
curlicue u.
ectopic u.
extravesical infrasphincteric ectopic u.

NOTES

ureter *(continued)*
u. implantation
postcaval u.
retrocaval u.
retroiliac u.
ureteral
u. bladder augmentation
u. branch
u. carcinoma
u. catheterization
u. colic
u. duplication
u. ectopia
u. fistula
u. injury
u. meatotomy
u. meatus
u. patch procedure
u. perforation
u. pressure
u. reimplantation
u. spatulation
u. stent placement
u. stoma
u. stoma removal
u. surgical treatment
ureteralgia
ureterectasia
ureterectomy
distal u.
ureteric
u. branch
u. fold
u. pelvis
u. plexus
u. stoma
ureterica
ureterici
uretericus
ureteris
ureteritis
ureterocalicostomy
ureterocele
ectopic u.
orthotopic u.
pyoureter ectopic u.
ureterocelorraphy
ureterocolic fistula
ureterocolonic anastomosis
ureterocolostomy
ureterocutaneous fistula
ureterocystoplasty
ureterocystostomy
ureteroendoscopy
ureteroenteric
ureteroenterostomy
ureterohydronephrosis
ureteroileal anastomosis
ureteroileocecoproctostomy
ureteroileoneocystostomy
ureteroileostomy
Bricker u.
ureterolithiasis
ureterolithotomy
laparoscopic u.
ureterolysis
combined u.
extravesical u.
intravesical u.
Lich-Gregoir u.
Pacquin u.
Politano-Leadbetter u.
ureteroneocystostomy
Glen Anderson u.
u. herniation
Politano-Leadbetter u.
reoperative u.
ureteroneopyelostomy
ureteronephrectomy
ureteropelvic
u. junction (UPJ)
u. obstruction
ureteroperitoneal fistula
ureteroplasty
ileal patch u.
ureteroproctostomy
ureteropyelitis
ureteropyeloneostomy
ureteropyelonephrostomy
ureteropyeloplasty
ureteropyeloscopy
flexible u.
ureteropyelostomy
ureteropyosis
ureterorectostomy
ureterorenoscopy
transurethral u.
ureterorrhagia
ureterorrhaphy
ureteroscopy
rigid u.
ureterosigmoid anastomosis
ureterosigmoidostomy
ileocecal u.
Maydl u.
ureterostenoma
ureterostenosis
ureterostoma
ureterostomy
cutaneous loop u.
Davis intubated u.
high-loop cutaneous u.
low-loop cutaneous u.
retroperitoneal cutaneous u.

ureterotomy
Davis intubated u.
intubated u.
ureterotrigonoenterostomy
ureterotubal anastomosis
ureteroureteral anastomosis
ureteroureterostomy
ureterouterine fistula
ureterovaginal fistula
ureterovesical obstruction
ureterovesicoplasty
Leadbetter-Politano u.
ureterovesicostomy
urethra
anterior u.
female u.
fixed drain pipe u.
male u.
membranous u.
penile u.
posterior u.
prostatic u.
spongy u.
urethrae
urethral
u. artery
u. atresia
u. calculus
u. carcinoma
u. caruncle
u. closure mechanism
u. closure pressure profile
u. coaptation
u. crest of male
u. dilation
u. diverticulectomy
u. gland
u. groove
u. lacuna
u. opening
u. papilla
u. pressure
u. pressure measurement
u. sphincterotomy
u. suspension
u. syndrome
u. vesicle suspension procedure
urethralgia
urethralis
urethrectomy
urethremorrhagia
urethrism
urethritis
urethrobalanoplasty
urethrobulbar
urethrocavernous fistula
urethrocecal anastomosis
urethrocele
urethrocystometry
urethrocystopexy
urethrocystoscopy
urethrodynia
urethrohymenal fusion
urethrolysis
retropubic u.
transvaginal u.
urethropenile
urethroperineal
urethroperineoscrotal
urethropexy
Gittes u.
Lapides-Ball u.
Marshall-Marchetti-Krantz u.
retropubic u.
Schwartz-Pregenzer u.
Stamey u.
urethroplasty
Badenoch u.
Cantwell-Ransley u.
Cecil u.
modified Young u.
onlay island-flap u.
pedicle flap u.
prostatic u.
retrograde transurethral prostatic u.
Tanagho bladder flap u.
Thiersch-Duplay u.
tubed u.
urethroprostatic
urethrorectal fistula
urethrorrhagia
urethrorrhaphy
urethrorrhea
urethroscopic
urethroscopy
retropubic u.
urethrospasm
urethrostaxis
urethrostenosis
urethrostomy
perineal u.
Poncet perineal u.
urethrotomy
direct-vision internal u.

NOTES

urethrotomy *(continued)*
endoscopic optical u.
external u.
internal u.
perineal u.
Syme external u.
urethrovaginal fistula
urethrovesical
urethrovesicopexy
urge incontinence
uricosuria
urinae
urinaria
urinariae
urinarius
urinary
u. apparatus
u. bladder
u. bladder rupture
u. calcium excretion
u. calculus
u. catheterization
u. conduit
u. EGF
u. exertional incontinence
u. extraversion
u. fistula
u. organ
u. retention
u. sand
u. stuttering
u. tract
u. tract abnormality
u. tract anomaly
u. tract disease
u. tract disorder
u. tract infection
u. tract injury
u. tract obstruction
u. tract reconstruction
urinary-umbilical fistula
urinary-vaginal fistula
urination
delayed u.
urine specimen collection
uriniferous tubule
urinogenital
urinogenous
urinoma
urinoscopy
urinosexual
urocele
urocheras
urochesia
urocyst
urocystic
urocystis
urodynamics
urodynia
urogenital
u. anomaly
u. apparatus
u. canal
u. cleft
u. diaphragm
u. fistula
u. membrane
u. region
u. ridge
u. septum
u. sinus
u. tract
u. triangle
urogenitale
urogenitalis
urogenous
urokinase thrombolysis
urolith
urolithiasis
urolithic
urolithology
urologic
u. anesthesia
u. complication
u. laparoscopic surgical procedure
u. oncology
u. operation
u. surgery
u. surgical procedure
u. system cancer
urological evaluation
urologist
pediatric u.
urology
pediatric u.
Uromat dilation
uroncus
uronephrosis
uronoscopy
uropathy
obstructive u.
uropoiesis
uropoietic
uropsammus
urorectal
u. membrane
u. septum
uroscheocele
uroschesis
uroscopy
urosepsin
urosepsis
urostomy
urothelial
u. basement membrane
u. carcinoma

urothelium
urothorax
urticaria
urtication
US-CNB
ultrasound-guided core-needle biopsy
use
off-label u.
use-dependent sodium channel blocker
US-FNAB
ultrasound-guided fine-needle aspiration biopsy
U-shaped
U-s. incision
U-s. jejunal pouch
U-s. scalp flap
Ussing chamber technique
uterectomy
uteri (*pl. of* uterus)
uterina
uterinae
uterine
u. adenocarcinoma
u. anomaly
u. artery
u. aspiration
u. cavity
u. compression
u. evaluation
u. fibromyoma
u. gland
u. hernia
u. hernia syndrome
u. incision
u. infection
u. lysosome level
u. mass
u. papillary serous carcinoma
u. perforation
u. relaxation
u. rupture
u. sarcoma metastasis
u. suspension
u. vein
u. venous plexus
u. window
uterinus
uteroabdominal
uterocervical
uterocystostomy
uterofixation
uterolysis
laparoscopic u.
uteroovarian
uteroparietal
uteropelvic
uteroperitoneal fistula
uteropexy
uteroplacental circulation
uteroplasty
uterosacral
u. block
u. fold
u. ligament
uteroscopy
uterotomy
uterotubal
uterovaginal
u. canal
u. plexus
uteroventral
uterovesical
u. fold
u. ligament
u. pouch
uterovesicalis
uterus, pl. **uteri**
masculine u.
utilization
impaired oxygen u.
oxygen u.
utricle
prostatic u.
utricular spot
utriculitis
utriculosaccular duct
utriculosaccularis
U-turn maneuver
UV
ultraviolet
umbilical vein
UV blood
UV irradiation
uveal
u. metastasis
u. tract
uveitis
anterior u.
endogenous u.
posterior u.
uveoencephalitic syndrome
uveoplasty
uviofast

NOTES

uvioresistant
uviosensitive
UV/MV
- umbilical vein to maternal vein
  - UV/MV ratio

uvula, pl. **uvuli**
- Lieutaud u.

uvulae
uvular muscle
uvulectomy
uvuli (*pl. of* uvula)
uvulopalatopharyngoplasty
uvulopalatoplasty
- laser-assisted u. (LAUP)

uvulotomy
Uyemura operation

V_A
alveolar ventilation per minute
V_E
minute ventilation
V_A
VAC
vacuum-assisted closure
vaccinia
v. infection
v. melanoma oncolysate (VMO)
vaccinization
VACTERL
vertebral, anal, cardiac, tracheal, esophageal, renal, limb
VACTERL anomaly
vacuolation
vacuole
vacuolization
basket-weave v.
isometric tubular v.
vacuum
v. aspiration
constant v.
v. extraction
v. extractor delivery
vacuum-assisted closure (VAC)
VAE
venous air embolism
vagal
afferent v.
v. arrest
v. body
v. nerve stimulation
v. trunk
vagalis
vagectomy
vagi (*pl. of* vagus)
vagina, pl. **vaginae**
azygos artery of v.
v. fibrosa tendinis
v. masculina
posterior fornix of v.
v. processus styloidei
vaginae
vaginal
v. adenocarcinoma
v. anomaly
v. artery
v. birth after cesarean delivery
v. birth after cesarean section
v. carcinoma
v. celiotomy
v. column
v. condyloma
v. cone biopsy
v. construction
v. cornification test
v. cuff
v. cystourethropexy
v. ectopic anus
v. electrical stimulation
v. examination
v. fistula
v. foreign body
v. gland
v. hernia
v. hysterectomy
v. hysterotomy
v. infection
v. inflammation
v. laceration
v. lithotomy
v. mass
v. mucification test
v. myomectomy
v. needle suspension procedure
v. nerve
v. opening
v. orifice
v. perineorrhaphy
v. process
v. rhabdomyosarcoma
v. surgery
v. venous plexus
v. vesicostomy
v. wall approach
v. wall repair
v. wall sling procedure
vaginales
vaginalis
vaginapexy
vaginate
vaginectomy
vaginitis
vaginoabdominal
vaginocele
vaginofixation
Dührssen v.
vaginohysterectomy
vaginolabial hernia
vaginoperineal
vaginoperineoplasty
vaginoperineorrhaphy
vaginoperineotomy
vaginoperitoneal
vaginopexy
Norman Miller v.
vaginoplasty
cutback-type v.

vaginoplasty *(continued)*
Fenton v.
posterior flap v.
vaginoscopy
pediatric v.
vaginotomy
vaginourethroplasty
vaginovesical
vaginovulvar
vagoaccessorius
vagoglossopharyngeal
vagolysis
vagotomy
v. and antrectomy with gastroduodenostomy
bilateral v.
gastric v.
highly selective v.
laparoscopic v.
laser laparoscopic v.
medical v.
parietal cell v.
posterior truncal v.
proximal gastric v.
v. and pyloroplasty
Roux-en-Y procedure with v.
selective proximal v.
superselective v.
surgical v.
total bilateral v.
truncal v.
vagovagal reflex
vagus, pl. **vagi**
v. nerve
v. nerve root
Vaino MP arthroplasty
Valentine position
valgus
v. angulation
v. deformity
v. extension overload syndrome
v. wedge-prop osteotomy
v. Y-shaped prop osteotomy
valgus-external rotation injury
validation
histopathologic v.
vallate papilla
vallecula, pl. **valleculae**
Valleix point
Valls-Ottolenghim-Schajowicz needle biopsy
Valpar whole body range of motion test
Valsalva
V. maneuver
V. muscle
value
acid-base v.
diagnostic v.
high predictive v.
intracranial pressure v.
negative predictive v. (NPV)
positive predictive v. (PPV)
postprandial v.
predictive v.
pressure v.
prognostic v.
supranormal v.
valva, pl. **valvae**
valve
v. ablation
v. of Bauhin
v. bladder
Cabot trumpet v.
Carpentier-Edwards stented bovine pericardial v.
Carpentier-Edwards stented porcine xenograft v.
v. cinefluoroscopy
v. cusp
v. debris
expiratory v.
v. of Guérin
v. of Hasner
v. of Heister
v. of Houston
ileocecal v.
v. leaflet
left coronary v.
mitral v.
v. orifice area
v. patency
v. replacement
right coronary v.
right septal v.
v. of Rosenmüller
v. rupture
slit v.
v. of Sylvius
v. of Vieussens
v. wrapping
valvectomy
valved conduit anastomosis
valvoplasty
valvotomy
aortic v.
balloon aortic v.
balloon mitral v.
balloon pulmonary v.
balloon tricuspid v.
double-balloon v.
Inoue balloon mitral v.
Longmire v.
mitral balloon v.
mitral valve v.
percutaneous mitral balloon v.

rectal v.
repeat balloon mitral v.
single-balloon v.
thimble v.

valvula, pl. **valvulae**
Amussat v.
Gerlach v.

valvular
v. aortic disease
v. heart disease
v. heart surgery

valvule
lymphatic v.

valvulectomy

valvuloplasty
aortic v.
bailout v.
balloon aortic v.
balloon dilation v.
balloon mitral v.
balloon pulmonary v.
Carpentier tricuspid v.
catheter balloon v.
double-balloon v.
intracoronary thrombolysis balloon v.
mitral v.
multiple-balloon v.
percutaneous balloon aortic v.
percutaneous balloon mitral v.
percutaneous balloon pulmonic v.
percutaneous transluminal balloon v.
pulmonary v.
single-balloon v.
tricuspid v.
triple-balloon v.
Trusler technique of aortic v.

valvulotomy
balloon v.
v. procedure

VAMP
venous/arterial management protection
Baxter VAMP

van
v. Buren disease
v. Buren operation
V. de Kramer fecal fat procedure
V. Herick modification
V. Hoorne canal
V. Hoorn maneuver
V. Lint anesthesia
V. Lint flap
V. Lint injection
V. Lint lid block
V. Lint modified technique
V. Milligen eyelid repair technique
V. Milligen operation
V. Ness procedure
V. Ness rotationplasty

vanished testis syndrome

Vannas capsulotomy

vapor
anesthetic v.
v. density
partial pressure of water v.
v. pressure

vaporization
Contact Laser v.
laser v.

vaporize

vaporizer
draw-over v.
flow-over v.
temperature-compensated v.

VAPS
visual analog pain score

variability
heart rate v. (HRV)
index of v.
interpretation v.

variable
v. positive airway pressure
v. screw placement

variable-dose patient-controlled anesthesia (VDPCA)

variable-release compression

variation
anatomic v.
anatomical v.
biliary anatomic v.

varication

variceal
v. band ligation
v. bleeding
v. column
v. decompression
v. hemorrhage
v. pressure
v. sclerotherapy
v. wall

varicella infection

varicella-zoster virus infection

varicelliform lesion

varices (*pl. of* varix)

NOTES

varicocele
varicocelectomy
laparoscopic v.
microsurgical inguinal v.
subinguinal microsurgical v.
varicose
v. aneurysm
v. vein stripping and ligation
varicotomy
variety
diffuse v.
multifocal v.
variocele
variolation
variolization
varix, pl. **varices**
actively bleeding varix
aneurysmal v.
coil-shaped v.
ectopic v.
esophageal v.
v. ligation
Okuda transhepatic obliteration of v.
percutaneous transhepatic obliteration of esophageal v.
peristomal v.
transesophageal ligation of v.
Varolius sphincter
varus
v. hindfoot deformity
v. rotation shortening osteotomy
varus-valgus plane
VAS
visual analog scale
vas, pl. **vasa**
vascular
v. abdominal surgery
v. abnormality
v. access
v. access patient
v. access thrombosis
v. accident
v. anastomosis
v. anatomy
v. anomaly
v. bed
bifurcated v. graft
v. bundle
v. cannulation
v. circle
v. complication
v. compression
v. control
v. decompensation
v. disease
v. disease death
v. ectasia
v. endothelial growth factor (VEGF)
v. endothelium
v. exclusion
v. fold
v. injury
v. invasion
v. isolation technique
v. laceration
v. laceration repair
v. loop
v. malformation
v. manifestation
v. medicine
v. metastasis
v. neoplasm
v. nerve
v. net
v. occlusion
v. pedicle
v. perforation
v. plexus
v. pressure
v. procedure
v. radiologist
v. reconstruction
v. rejection
v. renal mass
v. ring
v. ring division
v. ring syndrome
v. sheath
v. space
v. structure
v. surgeon
v. system
v. tissue
v. watershed
v. zone
vascularis
vascularity
tumor v.
vascularization
vascularize
vascularized
v. bone graft
v. free flap
vasculature
extracranial v.
extracranial cerebral v.
vasculitic lesion
vasculitis
diffuse v.
leukocytoclastic v.
widespread v.
vasculo-Behçet disease
vasculobiliary pedicle
vasculocardiac

vasculomyelinopathy
vasculopathy
graft v.
vasculosa
vasculosi
vasculosus
vasectomy
no-scalpel v.
v. reversal
vasoactive
v. medication
v. substance
vasoconstriction
hypoxic pulmonary v. (HPV)
isoflurane-induced v.
thermoregulatory v.
vasocutaneous fistula
vasodilatation
vasodilation
vasodilator
v. administration
v. agent
arterial-selective intravenous v.
v. infusion
mesenteric v.
vasodilator-stimulated rCBF single photon emission computed tomographic measurement
vasodilatory property
vasoepididymostomy
vasoganglion
vasoligation
vasomotor nerve
vasoneuropathy
vasoneurosis
vasopressin
intravenous v.
vasopressor
vasoproliferation
vasopuncture
vasoreflex
vasorelaxation
vasorum
vasosection
vasostimulant
vasostomy
vasotomy
vasovagal
vasovasostomy
vasovesiculectomy
Vastamäki technique
vastus
v. medialis tendon
VATER
vertebral, anus, tracheoesophageal, radial, and renal
VATER association
VATER association syndrome
Vater
V. ampulla
V. fold
V. papilla
VATS
video-assisted thoracoscopic surgery
video-assisted thorascopic surgery
VATS procedure
VATS wedge resection
Vaughan Williams antiarrhythmic drug classification
vault
cranial v.
V-banded gastroplasty
VBG
vertical banded gastroplasty
VBG pouch
VCP
vocal cord paralysis
VDPCA
variable-dose patient-controlled anesthesia
Veau classification
Vecchietti
V. method
V. operation
$VECO_2$
carbon dioxide elimination
vection
vector
v. phase
v. product
v. profile
v. quantity
vecuronium neuromuscular blocking
vegetative lesion
VEGF
vascular endothelial growth factor
veil
aqueduct v.
vein
aberrant obturator v.
accessory cephalic v.
adrenal v.
anastomotic v.

NOTES

V

vein *(continued)*
angular v.
appendicular v.
aqueous v.
arcuate v.
arterial v.
ascending lumbar v.
auricular v.
autogenous v.
autologous internal jugular v.
axillary v.
azygos v.
basal v.
basilic v.
basivertebral v.
brachiocephalic v.
bronchial v.
Browning v.
buccal v.
Burow v.
canaliculus v.
capillary v.
cardiac v.
central v.
cephalic v.
cerebellar v.
cerebral v.
cervical v.
choroid v.
ciliary v.
circumflex v.
colic v.
collateral v.
comitans v.
common basal v.
common facial v.
condylar emissary v.
v. confluence
coronary v.
costoaxillary v.
cremasteric v.
v. cuff
v. decompression
deep cervical v.
descending genicular v.
digital v.
diploic v.
dorsispinal v.
emissary v.
epigastric v.
esophageal v.
ethmoidal v.
facial v.
femoral v.
fetal intrahepatic v.
frontal v.
v. of Galen malformation
gastric v.
gastroepiploic v.
gonadal v.
v. graft
great saphenous v.
hemiazygos v.
hemorrhoidal v.
hepatic portal v.
human umbilical v. (HUV)
hypogastric v.
hypophyseoportal v.
ileal v.
ileocolic v.
iliac v.
inferior alveolar v.
inferior interosseous v.
inferior lateral genicular v.
inferior medial genicular v.
infraorbital v.
innominate cardiac v.
intercapitular v.
intercostal v.
internal auditory v.
internal jugular v.
internal maxillary v.
internal pudendal v.
internal thoracic v.
intervertebral v.
intestinal v.
intraportal v.
jugular v.
juxtahepatic v.
Labbé v.
labial v.
labyrinthine v.
lacrimal v.
laryngeal v.
left brachiocephalic v.
left subclavian v. (LSV)
lingual v.
long thoracic v.
lumbar v.
Marshall oblique v.
mediastinal v.
meningeal v.
mesenteric v.
musculophrenic v.
nasofrontal v.
native portal v.
v. obstruction
occipital cerebral v.
occipital emissary v.
v. occlusion
ophthalmic v.
orbital v.
v. orifice
ovarian v.
palatal v.
pancreatic v.

pancreaticoduodenal v.
paratonsillar v.
paraumbilical v.
parietal emissary v.
parotid v.
v. patch
v. patch angioplasty
patent portal v.
pericardiacophrenic v.
pericardial v.
peripheral v.
peritoneal v.
peroneal v.
petrosal v.
pharyngeal v.
phrenic v.
popliteal v.
portal v.
portal-systemic collateral v.
posterior anterior jugular v.
posterior auricular v.
posterior facial v.
posterior intercostal v.
posterior interosseous v.
posterior labial v.
posterior parotid v.
posterior scrotal v.
prepyloric v.
proximal v.
pudendal v.
pulmonary v.
pyloric v.
rectosigmoid v.
renal v.
retrohepatic v.
retromandibular v.
rolandic v.
Rolando v.
Rosenthal v.
Santorini v.
saphenous v.
scrotal v.
short gastric v.
short hepatic v.
short saphenous v.
spermatic v.
sphenoid emissary v.
spigelian v.
spinal v.
splenic v.
sternocleidomastoid v.
v. stone
stylomastoid v.
subclavian v.
subcostal v.
sublingual v.
submental v.
subscapular v.
supraorbital v.
suprarenal v.
suprascapular v.
supratrochlear v.
supreme intercostal v.
sylvian v.
v. system
temporal v.
temporomaxillary v.
testicular v.
thalamostriate v.
thebesian v.
thoracic v.
thoracoacromial v.
thoracoepigastric v.
thymic v.
thyroid v.
Trolard v.
v. tumor thrombus
umbilical v. (UV)
umbilical vein to maternal v. (UV/MV)
uterine v.
v. valve wrapping
vertebral v.
vertical v.
Vesalius v.
vesical v.
vestibular v.
vidian v.
Vieussens v.
vorticose v.
v. wall

Veirs canaliculus repair
vela (*pl. of* velum)
velamen, pl. **velamina**
velamentous insertion
velamentum, pl. **velamenta**
velamina (*pl. of* velamen)
velar
Veleanu-Rosianu-Ionescu
V.-R.-I. adductor tenotomy
V.-R.-I. technique
veliform
Vella fistula
vellication

NOTES

vellus
velocity
v. catheter technique
migration v.
velopharyngeal
v. closure
v. port
v. sphincter
veloplasty
functional v.
Velpeau
V. canal
V. deformity
V. fossa
V. hernia
velum, pl. **vela**
corneal v.
vena, pl. **venae**
venacavaplasty
face-to-face v.
venectomy
venereal
v. condyloma
v. sore
venereology
venesection
venipuncture
Venn-Watson classification
venoablation
percutaneous v.
venobiliary fistula
venoconstriction
mesenteric v.
reflex v.
venodilation
nitrate-induced v.
systemic v.
venogram
venographic study
venography
contrast v.
wedge hepatic v.
venolysis
circumferential v.
venom extract
venoperitoneostomy
venosa
venosi
venostasis
venostomy
venosum
venosus
venotomy
venous
v. access
v. access technique
v. admixture
v. air embolism (VAE)
v. anastomosis
v. angioma
v. angle
v. blood gas
v. channel
v. circulation
v. collateral
v. compression
v. confluence
v. cutdown
v. dialysis pressure (VPd)
v. effort thrombosis
v. embolization
v. foramen
v. gangrene
v. groove
v. hemorrhage
v. hypercarbia
v. injury
v. insufficiency
v. interposition graft
v. intravasation
v. invasion
v. ligament
v. line
v. loop
v. malformation
maternal v. (MV)
v. occlusion
v. outflow
v. outflow recording
v. pathology
v. plexus
v. pressure
v. puncture
v. return
v. sampling
v. saturation
v. segment
v. sheath patch
v. sinus
v. stasis
v. stasis disease
v. study
v. system
v. thromboembolism
v. tributary
v. trunk
umbilical v.
v. web
v. web disease
venous/arterial management protection (VAMP)
venous-occlusion volume plethysmography
venous-related complication
venous-to-venous anastomosis
venovenostomy

venovenous
v. bypass (VVB)
v. extracorporeal bypass
venter
ventilation
v. agent
airway pressure release v. (APRV)
alveolar v.
artificial v.
assist-control mode v.
assisted v.
bag-and-mask v.
bagged mask v.
bag-valve-mask-assisted v.
v. circuit
v. collateralization
continuous-flow v.
continuous mandatory v.
continuous positive pressure v. (CPPV)
control of v.
controlled v.
controlled mechanical v. (CMV)
control-mode v.
cuirass v.
v. defect
difficult v.
emergency v.
v. equivalent
extended mandatory minute v. (EMMV)
forced mandatory intermittent v.
hand v.
heart synchronized v.
HFJ v.
high-frequency v. (HFV)
high-frequency jet v. (HFJV)
high-frequency oscillation v.
high-frequency oscillatory v. (HFOV)
high-frequency percussive v.
high-frequency positive-pressure v. (HFPPV)
v. index (VI)
inspired v. (VI)
intermittent demand v.
intermittent mandatory v. (IMV)
intermittent mechanical v.
intermittent positive pressure v. (IPPV)
inverse-ratio v.
jet v.
local exhaust v.
low-frequency jet v.
v. lung scan
manual v.
maximal voluntary v.
maximum voluntary v. (MVV)
mechanical v.
minute v. (V_E)
mouth-to-mouth v.
neonate v.
noninvasive positive-pressure v. (NPPV)
one-lung v. (OLV)
oscillatory v.
partial liquid v.
v. peak pressure
percutaneous transtracheal jet v. (PTV)
positive-pressure v. (PPV)
postoperative v.
pressure control v. (PCV)
pressure control inverse ratio v. (PCIRV)
pressure-controlled inverse ratio v.
pressure-regulated volume control v.
pressure support v. (PSV)
prolonged postoperative v.
proportional assist v.
pulmonary v.
single lung v.
split-lung v.
spontaneous v.
spontaneous intermittent mandatory v. (SIMV)
synchronized intermittent mandatory v. (SIMV)
synchronized intermittent mechanical v.
synchronous intermittent mandatory v.
v. threshold
time-cycled v.
transtracheal jet v.
triggered v.
ultra-high-frequency v.
volume-cycled decelerating-flow v.
ventilation/perfusion (V/Q)
v./p. abnormality
v./p. defect
v./p. distribution
v./p. imaging
v./p. inequality

NOTES

ventilation/perfusion *(continued)*
- v./p. lung scan
- v./p. mismatch
- v./p. quotient
- v./p. ratio
- v./p. relation
- v./p. relationship

ventilator
- v. dependency
- high-frequency jet v.
- high-frequency positive-pressure v.
- v. management
- proportional assist v. (PAV)
- v. support
- v. time
- v. weaning

ventilator-assisted respiration
ventilator-associated pneumonia
ventilator-induced
- v.-i. lung injury (VILI)
- v.-i. pneumopericardium
- v.-i. pneumothorax

ventilatory
- v. depression
- v. response
- v. support

venting percutaneous gastrostomy
ventral
- v. bending technique
- v. hernia
- v. herniorrhaphy
- v. root
- v. sacrococcygeal ligament
- v. sacrococcygeus muscle
- v. spinocerebellar tract
- v. spinothalamic tract
- v. tegmental decussation

ventralis
ventricle
- laryngeal v.
- lateral v.
- left v.
- Morgagni v.
- right v.

ventricular
- v. aberration
- v. access
- v. activation time
- v. canal
- v. depolarization abnormality
- v. diastolic pressure
- v. dilation
- v. endoaneurysmorrhaphy
- v. endomyocardial biopsy
- v. end-systolic pressure-volume relation
- v. filling pressure
- v. fold
- v. inflow anomaly
- v. inflow tract obstruction
- v. ligament
- v. outflow tract
- v. outflow tract obstruction
- v. perforation
- v. peritoneal (VP)
- v. peritoneal shunting
- v. phonation
- v. preexcitation
- v. puncture
- v. relaxation
- v. septal defect closure
- v. septal rupture
- v. septal wound defect
- v. septum
- v. tachycardia/ventricular fibrillation

ventriculare
ventricularis
ventricularization
ventricular-programmed stimulation
ventriculectomy
- partial left v.

ventriculi (*pl. of* ventriculus)
ventriculocisternostomy
- Torkildsen v.

ventriculocordectomy
ventriculomastoidostomy
ventriculomegaly
ventriculoperitoneal
- v. shunting
- v. shunting procedure
- v. shunt placement

ventriculoplasty
- reduction v.

ventriculopuncture
ventriculorum
ventriculoscopy
ventriculostomy
- straight-in v.
- terminal v.
- third v.
- tunneled v.

ventriculotomy
- encircling endocardial v.
- partial encircling endocardial v.

ventriculus, pl. **ventriculi**
ventrocystorrhaphy
ventroinguinal
ventrolateral hernia
ventroposterolateral (VPL)
ventroptosis
ventroscopy
ventrotomy
ventrum penis flap
venula, pl. **venulae**
venular lesion

venule
high endothelial v.
vera
verae
verapamil
veratridine
veratrin
verbal-rank scale
verbotonal method
Verdan
V. osteoplastic thumb reconstruction
V. technique
Verga
accessory venous sinus of V.
verge
anal v.
Verhoeff
V. operation
V. suture technique
Verhoeff-Chandler
V.-C. capsulotomy
V.-C. operation
verification
intraoperative v.
Vermale operation
Verman needle biopsy
vermian fossa
vermicular colic
vermiculation
vermiform
v. appendage
v. appendix
v. body
v. process
vermiformis
mesenteriolum processus v.
vermilion border
vermilionectomy
Vermont spinal fixator articulation
Vernet syndrome
Verneuil
V. canal
V. operation
vernix membrane
verrucous lesion
vertebra, pl. **vertebrae**
basilar v.
caudal v.
cervical v.
coccygeal v.
dorsal v.
false v.
lumbar v.
picture frame v.
v. plana fracture
sacral v.
tail v.
thoracic v.
true v.
wedge-shaped v.
vertebral
v., anal, cardiac, tracheal, esophageal, renal, limb (VACTERL)
v., anus, tracheoesophageal, radial, and renal (VATER)
v., anus, tracheoesophageal, radial, and renal anomaly
v. arch
v. artery
v. artery disease
v. artery reconstruction
v. body
v. body anterior cortex
v. body corpectomy
v. body decompression
v. body fracture
v. bone mass
v. canal
v. column
v. compression
v. dissection
v. epidural space
v. exposure
v. foramen
v. fusion
v. ganglion
v. groove
v. nerve
v. notch
v. osteosynthesis
v. osteosynthesis fusion rate
v. region
v. resection
v. rib
v. ring apophysis
v. rotation
v. stable burst fracture
v. subluxation complex
v. subluxation syndrome
v. vein
v. venous plexus
v. wedge compression fracture
vertebrale

NOTES

vertebralis
vertebrarium
vertebrated
vertebrectomy
Bohlman anterior cervical v.
cervical spondylotic myelopathy v.
vertebroarterial foramen
vertebroarterialis
vertebrochondral rib
vertebrocostal trigone
vertebrofemoral
vertebroiliac
vertebropelvic ligament
vertebrosacral
vertebrosternal rib
vertex, pl. **vertices**
v. position
vertical
v. angulation
v. banded gastroplasty (VBG)
v. banded gastroplasty pouch
v. compression
v. compression test
v. condensation root canal filling method
v. divergence position
v. flap
v. gastric bypass
v. illumination
v. index
V. lip biopsy
v. mastopexy
v. mattress suture technique
v. maxillary excess
v. midline incision
v. osteotomy
v. partial laryngectomy
v. pedicle technique breast reduction
v. plane
v. relation
v. ring gastroplasty (VRG)
v. section
v. shear fracture
v. Silastic ring gastroplasty
v. suspension reflex
v. tooth fracture
v. translation
v. uterine incision
v. vein
v. vein system
v. versus horizontal preparation
vertical-cut
v.-c. method
v.-c. technique
verticalis
vertically acquired infection
vertices (*pl. of* vertex)
verticomental
vertiginous migraine
vertigo
benign paroxysmal positional v. (BPPV)
cyclic v.
positional v.
verumontanitis
verumontanum
Verwey eyelid operation
very
v. large scale integration
v. late activation
v. low density lipoprotein (VLDL)
Vesalius
V. bone
canal of V.
V. foramen
V. vein
vesica, pl. **vesicae**
vesical
v. calculus
v. diverticulectomy
v. fistula
v. gland
v. lithotomy
v. plexus
v. triangle
v. vein
vesicalis
vesication
vesicle
air v.
brush-border membrane v.
v. hernia
optic v.
otic v.
seminal v.
vesicoabdominal
vesicoacetabular fistula
vesicobullous lesion
vesicocele
vesicocervical space
vesicoclysis
vesicocolic fistula
vesicocutaneous fistula
vesicoenteric fistula
vesicofixation
vesicointestinal fistula
vesicolithiasis
vesicomyectomy
vesicomyotomy
vesicoovarian fistula
vesicoprostatic
vesicopubic
vesicorectal fistula
vesicorectostomy
vesicosalpingovaginal fistula

vesicosigmoid
vesicosigmoidostomy
vesicospinal
vesicostomy
cutaneous v.
preputial continent v.
vaginal v.
vesicotomy
vesicoumbilical ligament
vesicoureteral reflux
vesicourethral
v. anastomosis
v. canal
vesicouterina
vesicouterine
v. fistula
v. ligament
v. pouch
vesicouterinum
vesicouterovaginal
vesicovaginal
v. fistula
v. repair
vesicovaginorectal fistula
vesicovaginostomy
vesicovisceral
vesicula, pl. **vesiculae**
vesicular
v. acute inflammation
v. appendage
v. granulomatous inflammation
v. venous plexus
v. viral infection
vesiculation
vesiculectomy
prostatoseminal v.
total prostatoseminal v.
vesiculitis
vesiculocavernous respiration
vesiculoprostatectomy
retropubic v.
vesiculoprostatitis
vesiculosa
vesiculotomy
Vesling line
vessel
aberrant v.
abnormally feeding blood v.
absorbent v.
afferent lymphatic v.
anterior great v.
bleeding v.
blood v.
celiac v.
chyle v.
collateral v.
deep lymphatic v.
v. distention
ectatic v.
endosteal v.
v. exposure
gastric v.
inflow v.
infrapopliteal v.
innominate v.
intercostal v.
lacteal v.
v. ligation
lumbar v.
lymph v.
lymphatic v.
nutrient v.
pancreaticoduodenal arcade v.
parent v.
periesophageal blood v.
portal v.
posterior great v.
renal v.
right subclavian v.
segmental v.
short gastric v.
splanchnic v.
v. stenosis
superficial lymphatic v.
thoracic great v.
tumor v.
v. wall
vessel-containing plate
vest
vestibula (*pl. of* vestibulum)
vestibular
v. blind sac
v. canal
v. canaliculus
v. crest
v. fissure
v. fold
v. ganglion
v. gland
v. labyrinth
v. ligament
v. membrane
v. nerve
v. nerve section

NOTES

vestibular *(continued)*
v. neurectomy
v. vein
v. window
vestibulare
vestibularis
vestibule
esophagogastric v.
gastroesophageal v.
labial v.
nasal v.
vestibuli
vestibulitis
vestibulocochlear nerve
vestibuloplasty
vestibulospinal tract
vestibulourethral
vestibulum, pl. **vestibula**
vestige
vestigialis
vestigial muscle
vest-over-pants
v.-o.-p. hernia repair
v.-o.-p. herniorrhaphy
Veterans Administration Cooperative study
V-flap meatoplasty
VI
inspired ventilation
ventilation index
viability
flap v.
viable tissue
vial
multidose v.
scintillation v.
vibrating line
vibration
v. condensation
v. disease
v. neuritis
v. syndrome
v. threshold test
vibrational angioplasty
vibrator hand syndrome
***Vibrio fetus* infection**
vibrissa, pl. **vibrissae**
vibroacoustic stimulation
vicarious respiration
vicious union
Vicq d'Azyr bundle
victim
trauma v.
Victor Gomel method
Vidal-Ardrey fracture technique
video
v. endoscopy
v. esophagoscopy
v. fluoroscopy
v. image
v. mediastinoscopy
v. small-bowel enteroscopy
v. thoracoscopic drainage
v. transurethral resection technique
video-assisted
v.-a. excisional biopsy
v.-a. gastrectomy
v.-a. technique
v.-a. thoracic surgical procedure
v.-a. thoracoscopic surgery (VATS)
v.-a. thoracoscopic thymectomy
v.-a. thorascopic surgery (VATS)
v.-a. transsternal radical esophagectomy
videoendoscopic-assisted microsurgery
videoendoscopic thyroidectomy
videoendoscopy
videoesophagogoscopy
videofluoroscopic technique
videofluoroscopy
videolaparoscopic cardiomyotomy
video-laparoscopic guidance
videomicroscopy
videoscopic
v. evaluation
v. fundoplication
v. hernia surgery
v. repair
videostroboscopy
videothoracoscopy
videourodynamic evaluation
vidian
v. canal
v. nerve
v. neuralgia
v. vein
Viers operation
Vieussens
V. ansa
V. ganglion
V. limbus
V. ring
valve of V.
V. vein
view
abdominal v.
anterior v.
apical lordotic v.
Boehler calcaneal v.
Boehler lumbosacral v.
Breuerton v.
cine v.
coned-down v.
decubitus v.
frontal x-ray v.
laparoscopic transhiatal v.

lateral x-ray v.
one-plane v.
vigil
coma v.
vigilance monitoring
vigorous hydration
VILI
ventilator-induced lung injury
Villaret syndrome
villoma
villosa
villous
v. atrophy
v. epithelium
villus, pl. **villi**
arachnoid v.
intestinal v.
peritoneal v.
pleural v.
synovial v.
villusectomy
Vim-Silverman
V.-S. technique
V.-S. technique for liver biopsy
Vim thalamotomy
Vincent infection
vinculum, pl. **vincula**
Vindelov method flow cytometry analysis
Vineberg procedure
vinyl chloride exposure
violaceous lesion
violation
peritoneal v.
pleural v.
vipoma
Virag operation
viral
v. marker
v. respiratory infection
Virchow
V. metastasis
V. triad
Virchow-Robin
V.-R. space
V.-R. space dilatation
virga
virginal membrane
virginity
virgin neck
virilia
virilis
virilization
virtual
v. colonoscopy
v. cystoscopy
v. point
virus
adenoidal-pharyngeal-conjunctival v.
coxsackievirus A, B v.
Epstein-Barr v. (EBV)
hepatitis C v. (HCV)
human immunodeficiency v. (HIV)
viscera (*pl. of* viscus)
viscerad
visceral
v. anesthesia
v. angiomyolipoma
v. edema
v. hamartoma
v. herniation
v. hyperalgesia
v. injury
v. layer
v. lesion
v. muscle
v. nerve
v. node
v. pain
v. pelvic fascia
v. perfusion
v. pericardiectomy
v. pericardium
v. peritoneum
v. pleura
v. postsurgical disturbance
v. pouch
v. rotation
v. space
v. sympathectomy
v. traction reflex
viscerale
viscerales
visceralgia
visceralis
viscerobronchial cardiovascular anomaly
viscerocranium
visceroinhibitory
visceroparietal
visceroperitoneal
visceropleural
visceroptosis
viscerosensory

NOTES

visceroskeletal
visceroskeleton
viscerosomatic
viscerotomy
viscerum
viscoelastic tissue
viscosity
viscus, pl. **viscera**
abdominal v.
abdominopelvic v.
herniated v.
hollow v.
v. injury
intraperitoneal v.
viscera retention
retroperitoneal v.
Visick dysphagia classification
vision
central v.
direct laparoscopic v.
laparoscopic v.
presbyopic v.
visiting nurse
visor flap
visual
v. analog pain score (VAPS)
v. analog scale (VAS)
v. analysis
v. association area
v. closure
v. compromise
v. deprivation syndrome
v. direction
v. extinction
v. fixation
v. function evaluation
v. laser ablation
v. laser ablation of prostate
v. laser-assisted prostatectomy
v. line
v. method
v. orientation
v. pathway
v. plane
v. point
v. preservation
v. projection
v. stimulation
visualization
contrast v.
direct fluoroscopic v.
double-contrast v.
endoscopic v.
fluoroscopic v.
inadequate v.
visually triggered headache
Visual-Motor Integration Test
vital
v. capacity
v. knot
v. tissue
vitamin D supplementation
vitelline
v. duct anomaly
v. fistula
v. membrane
v. sac
vitellointestinal cyst
vitiation
vitreal
v. hemorrhage
v. membrane
vitrectomy
anterior v.
closed-system pars plana v.
core v.
open-sky v.
port v.
posterior v.
Weck-cel v.
vitreolysis
vitreoretinal
v. surgery
v. traction syndrome
vitreoretinopathy
exudative v.
familial exudative v.
vitreous
v. aspiration
v. breakthrough hemorrhage
v. cavity
v. foreign body
v. hernia
v. herniation
v. humor
v. membrane
v. neovascularization
v. surgery
v. table
vitreum
vitrification
vividialysis
vividiffusion
vivification
vivo
ex v.
in v.
VLDL
very low density lipoprotein
VMO
vaccinia melanoma oncolysate
polyvalent VMO
vocal
v. cord
v. cord atrophy

v. cord injection
v. cord movement
v. cord palsy
v. cord paralysis (VCP)
v. dysfunction
v. fold
v. fold approximation
v. fold fixation therapy
v. ligament
v. muscle
v. process
v. shelf
v. tract

vocale

vocalis muscle

Vogel method

Vogt operation

voice

v. disorder of phonation
eye, motor, v. (EVM)
v. restoration
v. termination time
v. therapy

voiding

v. flow rate
v. urethral pressure measurement

Voigt line

vola

volar

v. angulation
v. angulation deformity
v. aspect
v. epineurolysis
v. finger approach
v. interosseous artery
v. midline approach
v. midline oblique incision
v. plate arthroplasty
v. plate arthroplasty technique fracture-dislocation
v. plate repair
v. radial approach
v. semilunar wrist dislocation
v. synovectomy
v. ulnar approach
v. zig-zag finger incision

volaris

volarward approach

volatile

v. anesthesia
v. anesthetic
v. anesthetic agent

volatilization

volitional saccade

Volkmann

V. canal
V. clawhand deformity
V. fracture
V. ischemic contracture

volotrauma

Volpicelli functional ambulation scale

volsella

volume

abdominal v.
biopsy v.
blood transfusion v.
circulation v.
compartmental v.
drain v.
end-expiratory lung v. (EELV)
end-inspiratory v.
v. expansion
expiratory reserve v.
expiratory residual v.
extracellular fluid v. (ECFV)
fiber bundle v.
forced expiratory v.
gland v.
injection v.
intraperitoneal v.
intravascular v.
liver v.
maximal expiratory flow v.
median biopsy v.
minute v.
v. plethysmography
presystolic pressure and v.
v. reduction surgery (VRS)
remnant liver v.
respiratory minute v.
resuscitated by v.
rib-cage v.
v. segmentation
specimen v.
stroke v. (SV)
v. therapy
tidal v.
timed forced expiratory v.
total erythrocyte v.
tumor v.
weight-based peritoneal exchange v.

volume-assured pressure support

volume-cycled decelerating-flow ventilation

NOTES

V

volumetric
v. analysis
v. capnometry
v. method
v. solution
v. stereotaxis
v. study
v. technique
volumetry
CT v.
voluntary
v. area
v. guarding
v. sterilization
volvulus
cecal v.
gastric v.
midgut v.
v. reduction
sigmoid v.
Volz arthroplasty
Volz-Turner reattachment technique
vomer
vomerine canal
vomerobasilar canal
vomeronasal
v. cartilage
v. nerve
vomerorostral canal
vomerorostralis
vomerovaginal
v. canal
v. groove
vomerovaginalis
vomicose
vomit
bilious v.
vomiting
postoperative nausea and v. (PONV)
vomitus
coffee-grounds v.
von
V. Ammon operation
V. Bergman hernia
v. Blaskovics-Doyen operation
v. Claus chronometric method
V. Ebner gland
v. Ebner line
v. Economo disease
V. Frey test
v. Graefe operation
V. Haberer-Finney anastomosis
v. Haberer-Finney gastrectomy technique
V. Haberer gastroenterostomy
v. Hippel-Lindau disease
v. Hippel-Lindau tumor
v. Hippel operation
v. Kossa method
v. Langenbeck bipedicle mucoperiosteal flap
V. Langenbeck palatal closure
v. Langenbeck pedicle flap
v. Noorden incision
v. Willebrand factor
vortex, pl. **vortices**
vorticose vein
Vostal radial fracture classification
V-osteotomy
Japas V-o.
off-set V-o.
VP
ventricular peritoneal
VPd
venous dialysis pressure
VPL
ventroposterolateral
VPL pallidotomy
V/Q
ventilation/perfusion
VRG
vertical ring gastroplasty
VRS
volume reduction surgery
V-shaped
V-s. incision
V-s. osteotomy
V-sign of Naclerio
V-slope method
V-to-Y closure
Vulpius-Compere tendon technique
Vulpius procedure
Vulpius-Stoffel procedure
vulsella
vulva, pl. **vulvae**
vulvar
v. adenoid cystic adenocarcinoma
v. biopsy
v. carcinoma
v. infection
v. pigmented lesion
v. slit
vulvectomy
Basset radical v.
Parry-Jones v.
radical v.
simple v.
skinning v.
vulvitis
vulvocrural
vulvoplasty
vulvouterine
vulvovaginal
v. carcinoma
v. cystectomy

v. gland
v. lesion
v. premenarchal infection

vulvovaginoplasty
Williams v.

VVB
venovenous bypass

V-Y
V-Y advancement
V-Y advancement flap
V-Y advancement technique
V-Y gastroplasty
V-Y Kutler flap
V-Y plasty
V-Y procedure
V-Y quadricepsplasty

NOTES

V

W
W hernia
W procedure
Wachendorf membrane
Wackenheim clivus canal line
Wadsworth
W. elbow approach
W. posterolateral approach
W. technique
Wagener-Clay-Gipner classification
Wagner
W. classification
W. closed pinning
W. modification of Syme amputation
W. open reduction technique
W. skin incision
W. two-stage Syme amputation
Wagoner
W. cervical technique
W. posterior approach
wagon-wheel fracture
Wagstaffe fracture
wake-up evaluation
Walcher position
Waldeyer
W. fossa
W. gland
W. ring
W. ring lesion
W. sheath
W. space
W. tract
Waldhauer operation
Waldhausen
W. procedure
W. subclavian flap technique
Walker tractotomy
walking
w. epidural anesthetic
w. program
w. ventilation test
wall
anterior abdominal w.
anterior aortic w.
anterior rectus sheath w.
anterior thoracic w.
aortic w.
bile duct w.
w. of body
bowel w.
cavity w.
chest w.
cyst w.
deep anterior w.
duct w.
edematous bowel w.
fibrotic w.
gastric w.
gingival cavity w.
intermediate anterior w.
w. invasion
lateral w.
nail w.
nasal w.
nontumoral gastric w.
orbital w.
parietal w.
peripheral cavity w.
posterior oropharyngeal w.
posterior rectus sheath w.
pulpal w.
w. push maneuver
soft w.
splanchnic w.
superficial anterior w.
thoracic w.
upper thoracic w.
variceal w.
vein w.
vessel w.
wallaby pouch
Wallace technique
wall-echo shadow triad
wallet stomach
Walsh radical retropubic prostatectomy
Walter
W. Reed classification
W. Reed classification for HIV infection
W. Reed operation
Walther
W. canal
W. duct
W. fracture
W. ganglion
W. plexus
waltzed flap
wandering
w. abscess
w. kidney
w. liver
w. organ
w. spleen
Wangensteen drainage
Wanger reduction technique
Wang pleural stoma
ward
observation w.

Wardill
- W. four-flap method
- W. pharyngoplasty

Wardill-Kilner
- W.-K. advancement flap method
- W.-K. four-flap uranoplasty
- W.-K. procedure

Ward-Mayo vaginal hysterectomy
Wardrop method
warm
- w. condensation
- w. ischemia
- w. ischemic time

warmer
- fluid w.
- high-capacity fluid w.

warming
- forced-air w.
- preanesthetic skin-surface w.
- preoperative skin-surface w.

Warner-Farber ankle fixation technique
Warren
- W. flap
- W. incision

Warren-Marshall classification
Wartenberg syndrome
Warthin-Starry staining method
wart-like excrescence
Warwick and Ashken technique
washed
- w. clot
- w. intrauterine insemination

washed-field technique
washing
- cytologic w.
- endometrial jet w.
- peritoneal w.

washout
- peritoneal w.
- seminal tract w.
- w. test

wash technique
Wasmann gland
Wassel
- W. thumb duplication
- W. thumb duplication classification

wasting
- muscle w.

Watanabe
- W. classification of discoid meniscus
- W. discoid meniscus classification

water
- degasified distilled w.
- w. density line
- w. displacement
- w. dissection
- distilled w.
- extravascular lung w.
- hydration layer w.
- lung w.
- total body w.
- w. vapor monitoring

Waterhouse transpubic procedure
Waterman osteotomy
Waters
- W. operation
- W. projection

watershed
- vascular w.

water-soluble
- w.-s. contrast enema
- w.-s. contrast esophagogram

Waterston
- W. extrapericardial anastomosis
- W. method
- W. operation

Waterston-Cooley procedure
water-suppression technique
Waters-Waldron position
watertight closure
water-trap stomach
Watkins fusion technique
Watson
- W. capsule biopsy
- W. method
- W. operation
- W. scaphotrapeziotrapezoidal fusion
- W. technique

Watson-Cheyne-Burghard procedure
Watson-Cheyne technique
Watson-Crick method
Watson-Jones
- W.-J. anterior approach
- W.-J. fracture repair
- W.-J. incision
- W.-J. lateral approach
- W.-J. procedure
- W.-J. reconstruction
- W.-J. tibial fracture classification
- W.-J. tibial tubercle avulsion fracture classification

Watzke operation
Waugh-Clagett pancreaticoduodenostomy
Waugh operation
wave
- abdominal fluid w.
- contraction w.
- phasic pressure w.
- pressure w.

waveform
- aortic root velocity w.
- electrical stimulator w.
- epidural pressure w. (EPWF)
- pressure w.

wavelength frequency

wavy respiration
wax
w. expansion
w. pattern thermal expansion technique
wax-matrix technique
waxy
w. exudate
w. kidney
w. liver
Wayne County reduction
Way operation
weakened bowel
weakness
contralateral w.
muscle w.
weaning
ventilator w.
weapon
stand-off w.
wear
three-body w.
Weaver-Dunn
W.-D. acromioclavicular technique
W.-D. procedure
W.-D. resection
weaving
head w.
web
antral w.
cell w.
w. corn
duodenal w.
esophageal w.
w. eye
finger w.
w. formation
hepatic w.
intestinal w.
laryngeal w.
mucosal w.
postcricoid w.
pulmonary arterial w.
w. space
w. space flap
w. space incision
w. space infection
terminal w.
thumb w.
tracheal w.
venous w.
webbed penis
Weber
W. humeral osteotomy
W. organ
W. physical injury classification
W. point
W. procedure
W. subcapital osteotomy
W. triangle
Weber-Brunner-Freuler-Boitzy technique
Weber-Brunner-Freuler open reduction
Weber-Danis ankle injury classification
Weber-Fergusson
W.-F. incision
W.-F. procedure
Weber-Vasey traction-absorption wiring technique
Webril immobilization
Webster operation
Weck-cel vitrectomy
Weckesser technique
weddellite calculus
Wedensky facilitation
wedge
arterial w.
ball w.
bone w.
w. bone
closing base w.
compensatory w.
w. compression fracture
dental w.
disconnect w.
w. excision
w. graft
w. hepatectomy
w. hepatic biopsy
w. hepatic venography
w. incision
light-reflecting w.
w. liver biopsy
Livingston peribulbar w.
mediastinal w.
open w.
w. osteotomy
w. pressure
pulmonary artery w.
w. resection
temporal w.
wedge-and-groove
w.-a.-g. joint

NOTES

wedged
w. hepatic vein pressure (WHVP)
w. hepatic venous pressure
wedge-shaped
w.-s. erosion
w.-s. fasciculus
w.-s. osteotomy
w.-s. tubercle
w.-s. uncomminuted fragment
w.-s. uncomminuted tibial plateau fracture
w.-s. vertebra
Weeker operation
Weeks operation
weeping lesion
Wegner line
weight
body w.
w. estimation and assessment
graft w.
gut mucosal w.
ideal body w.
lean body w.
mucosal w.
w. reduction
w. reduction surgery
total body w. (TBW)
weight-based peritoneal exchange volume
Weiland
W. classification
W. iliac crest bone graft
Weinberg modification of pyloroplasty
Weinstein-Ponseti technique
Weinstock desyndactylization
Weir
W. incision
W. operation
Weisinger operation
Weiss logarithmic method
Weissman classification
Weitbrecht
W. cartilage
W. cord
weitbrechti
Welch technique
Welcker method
weld
laser tissue w.
welding
fusion w.
laser tissue w.
pressure w.
tissue w.
well-circumscribed lesion
well-defined mass
well-localized adenoma
Wells posterior rectopexy
Wendell Hughes operation
Wepfer gland
Werb operation
Wernekinck decussation
Wernicke radiation
Wertheim
W. operation
tunnel of W.
Wertheim-Bohlman technique
Wertheim-Schauta operation
Wesenberg-Hamazaki body
Westberg space
Westcott Pyramid Program
Westergren sedimentation rate method
western
W. blot infection
w. boot in open fracture
Westin-Hall incision
West operation
West-Soto-Hall
W.-S.-H. patellar technique
W.-S.-H. patellectomy
wet
w. colostomy
w. field cautery
w. gangrene
w. lung
w. technique with liposuction breast reduction
wetting solution
Weve operation
Weyers-Thier syndrome
Wharton duct
Wharton-Jones operation
Wheeler
W. halving repair
W. method
W. operation
W. procedure
Wheeler-Reese operation
Wheelhouse operation
wheel rotation
wheezing
expiratory w.
whewellite calculus
whiplash injury
whipping condensation
Whipple
W. incision
W. operation
W. pancreatectomy
W. pancreaticoduodenectomy
W. pancreaticoduodenostomy
W. pancreatoduodenectomy
W. procedure
W. resection
whipstitch
w. suture technique

whipworm infection
whistle-tip
whistling deformity
Whitaker pressure-perfusion test
white
w. cell
W. classification
w. fixation
w. gangrene
w. graft
w. lesion
w. line response
w. line of Toldt
w. matter
w. muscle
w. patch
w. point
W. posterior ankle fusion
w. pulp
w. ring
W. slide procedure
w. without pressure
white-centered hemorrhage
Whitecloud-LaRocca fibular strut graft
whitegraft reaction
Whitehead
W. classification
W. deformity
W. operation
Whitesides-Kelly cervical technique
Whitesides technique
white-spot lesion
whitlow
melanotic w.
Whitman
W. femoral neck reconstruction
W. osteotomy
W. talectomy procedure
Whitman-Thompson procedure
Whitmore-Jewett (W-J)
W.-J. classification for staging of prostate cancer
Whitnall
W. ligament
W. orbital tubercle
W. sling operation
WHO
World Health Organization
WHO gastric carcinoma classification
whole
w. abdominal radiation
w. abdominopelvic irradiation
w. blood lysis technique
w. body radiation
w. lobar graft
whole-abdomen irradiation
whole-arm fusion
whole-body
w.-b. cooling
w.-b. extract
w.-b. hyperthermia
w.-b. irradiation
w.-b. scanning
w.-b. titration curve
whole-brain radiation therapy
whole-cell patch clamp recording
whole-gut
w.-g. irrigation
w.-g. lavage activating solution
whole-pelvis irradiation
whorl
coccygeal w.
whorled appearance
WHVP
wedged hepatic vein pressure
Wiberg patellar classification
Wicherkiewicz eyelid operation
Wick catheter technique
Wickham technique
wide
w. elliptical anastomosis
w. internal inguinal ring
w. local excision
w. mucosa-to-mucosa Roux-en-Y hepaticojejunostomy
w. plane
wide-field
w.-f. radiation therapy
w.-f. total laryngectomy
wide-mouth sac
widened retrogastric space
wide-open anastomosis
wide-range radiation therapy
widespread
w. portal system thrombosis
w. vasculitis
Widman flap
width
line w.
pulse w.
Wiener
W. operation
tract of Münzer and W.

NOTES

W

Wies
W. operation
W. procedure
Wigand maneuver
Wigby-Taylor incision
Wilcoxon signed-rank test
Wilde incision
Wiley-Galey classification
Wilkie artery
Wilkinson synovectomy
Wilkins radial fracture classification
Willett-Stampfer method
William
W. Dixon Cratex point
W. microlumbar disk excision
Williams
W. copulating pouch operation
W. diskectomy
W. procedure
W. vulvovaginoplasty
Williams-Haddad technique
Willi glass crown technique
Willis
W. antrum
artery of W.
circle of W.
W. cord
W. pancreas
W. pouch
willisii
willow fracture
will therapy
Willy Meyer mastectomy incision
Wilmer operation
Wilms
W. amputation
W. renal tumor
W. thoracoplasty
Wilson
W. ankle fusion
W. bone graft
W. bunionectomy
W. fracture
W. muscle
W. oblique displacement osteotomy
W. procedure
W. technique
Wilson-Jacobs
W.-J. patellar graft
W.-J. tibial fracture fixation technique
Wilson-McKeever
W.-M. arthroplasty
W.-M. shoulder technique
Wilson-White method
Wiltberger
W. anterior cervical approach
W. fusion
Wiltse
W. ankle osteotomy
W. bilateral lateral fusion
W. varus supramalleolar osteotomy
Wiltse-Spencer paraspinal approach
Winberger line
windblown deformity
window
aortic-pulmonic w.
aortopulmonary w.
dilating w.
oval w.
pericardial w.
peritoneal w.
soft-tissue w.
w. technique
uterine w.
vestibular w.
windpipe
windsock deformity
Windson-Insall-Vince
W.-I.-V. bone graft
W.-I.-V. grafting technique
windswept deformity
wind-up
second pain w.-u.
wing
winged V double flap
Winiwarter-Buerger disease
Winiwarter operation
Winkelmann rotationplasty
Winkler body
Winkler-Waldeyer
closing ring of W.-W.
Winnie landmark
Winograd
W. nail plate removal
W. partial matrixectomy
W. procedure
W. technique
Winquist femoral shaft fracture classification
Winquist-Hansen femoral fracture classification
Winslow pancreas
Winston-Lutz method
Winter
W. classification
W. convex fusion
W. procedure
W. spondylolisthesis technique
Wintrobe
W. and Landsberg method
W. sedimentation rate method
wire
w. arch
w. contour preparation
w. extrusion

w. insertion
w. knot
w. localization
w. loop fixation
w. loop test
w. osteosynthesis
w. passage
w. removal technique
w. stabilization

wire-guided
w.-g. balloon-assisted endoscopic biliary stent exchange
w.-g. biopsy sample
w.-g. breast biopsy
w.-g. placement

wire-loop lesion

wiring
compression w.
continuous loop w.
craniofacial suspension w.
facet fracture stabilization w.
facet subluxation stabilization w.
interspinous w.
Ivy loop w.

Wirsung
W. canal
W. dilation
W. duct

Wirth-Jager tendon technique

Wise
W. mastopexy
W. operation
W. pattern mammaplasty

with correction

within-list recognition (WLR)

without correction

Witzel
W. duodenostomy
W. gastrostomy
W. jejunostomy
W. operation

W-J
Whitmore-Jewett
W-J classification for staging of prostate cancer

WLR
within-list recognition

WOB
work of breathing

Wolfe
W. breast carcinoma classification
W. method
W. ptosis operation

Wolfe-Kawamoto bone graft

Wolfe-Krause graft

wolffian
w. body
w. cyst
w. duct
w. duct carcinoma

Wolff-Parkinson-White bypass tract

Wolf full-thickness free graft

Wölfler
W. gastroenterostomy
W. gland
W. suture technique

Womack procedure

womb

wood
W. light examination
w. point
w. wool

Woods screw maneuver

Woodward
W. esophagogastroscopy
W. esophagogastrostomy
W. operation wound
W. procedure
W. technique

Woofry-Chandler classification of Osgood-Schlatter lesion

Wookey reconstruction

wool
wood w.

Wooler-type annuloplasty

Woolf method

work
w. of breathing (WOB)
w. hardening program

working bite relation

workup
diagnostic w.
hematologic w.

World
W. Health Organization (WHO)
W. Health Organization classification

wormian bone

Worst operation

Worth ptosis operation

wound
abdominal gunshot w.
abraded w.

NOTES

W

wound *(continued)*
w. abscess
acute w.
anterior w.
w. approximation
avulsed w.
back gunshot w.
w. biopsy
bullet w.
w. cavity
central hepatic gunshot w.
w. closure
w. complication
crease w.
w. dehiscence
w. disruption
w. drainage
exit w.
w. failure
flank gunshot w.
w. fluid
fresh w.
glancing w.
gunshot w. (GSW)
gutter w.
w. healing
w. hematoma
hepatic gunshot w.
w. hernia
incised w.
w. infection
w. irrigation
laparoscopic trocar w.
lateral w.
nonpenetrating w.
open w.
penetrating w.
perforating w.
precordial w.
w. problem
puncture w.
w. recurrence
remodeling of w.
w. retraction
seton w.
shotgun w.
w. site
skin w.
skin deficit w.
stab w.
sucking w.
superficial w.
surgical w.
tangential w.
thoracoabdominal gunshot w.
w. tract
transpelvic gunshot w.
trocar w.
Woodward operation w.
wound-breaking strength
W-plasty
W-pouch
ileal W-p.
wrap
cardiac muscle w.
gastric w. (GW)
gastric fundus w.
w. hematoma
Nissen fundoplication w.
rectus fascial w.
smooth w.
total gastric w.
wraparound
w. neurovascular composite free tissue transfer
w. neurovascular free flap
w. periapical lesion
wrapping
omental pedicle w.
pedicle w.
valve w.
vein valve w.
Wright
W. maneuver
W. operation
Wright-Giemsa evaluation
wrinkler muscle
wrinkling membrane
Wrisberg
W. cartilage
W. lesion
W. nerve
W. tubercle
wrist
w. block
w. deformity
w. disarticulation
w. dislocation
w. extensor
w. extensor tendon
Wroblewski method
wryneck
W-shaped
W-s. ileal pouch-anal anastomosis
W-s. incision
W-sitting position

xanthoastrocytoma
xanthogranuloma
xanthogranulomatous
x. cholecystitis
x. pyelonephritis (XCP)
xanthomatosis
cerebrotendinous x.
xanthosarcoma
Xase complex
X body
XCP
xanthogranulomatous pyelonephritis
X-dimension
^{133}Xe intravenous injection technique
xenogeneic
x. graft
x. tissue
xenogenic
x. cell therapy
x. infection
xenograft
x. graft
x. transplantation
xenografting
xenon
x. arc photocoagulation
x. gas
x. lung ventilation imaging
x. method
xenon-washout technique
xenotransplantation
cellular x.
x. thymus
xenozoonosis
xeroma
xeroradiogram
xerosis
xerostomia
xiphisternal
x. joint
x. junction chondritis
xiphisternum
xiphocostal
xiphodynia
xiphoid
x. cartilage
x. process
xiphoidalgia
xiphoideus
xiphoid-to-pubis midline abdominal incision
xiphoid-to-umbilicus incision
xiphosternalis
synchondrosis x.
x-line method
X-pattern exotropia
x-radiation
x-ray
abdominal x-r. (AXR)
anteroposterior chest x-r.
barium contrast x-r.
chest x-r.
x-r. control
frontal x-r.
lateral chest x-r.
x-r. therapy

Y

Y body
Y cartilage
Y fracture
Y graft
Y incision

y

y angle
y mesh hernia repair

Yacoub and Radley-Smith classification

YAG

yttrium-aluminum-garnet

Yale Optimal Observation Score

Yancey osteotomy

Yasargil craniotomy

Yates correction

Y configuration

Y-dimension

yeast infection

Yee posterior shoulder approach

yellow

y. body
y. hepatization
y. lesion
y. ligament
y. nail
y. nail syndrome
y. point

yellow-ochre hemorrhage

yield

nodal y.

ympathectomy

yoke

alveolar y.
y. block
y. bone
cricoid y.
y. hanger
y. transposition procedure

yolk

y. membrane
y. sac
y. sac carcinoma
y. space

Yorke-Mason incision

York-Mason

Y.-M. procedure
Y.-M. repair

Y-osteotomy

Pauwels Y-o.

young

y. cyst
y. onset cancer
Y. operation
Y. pelvic fracture classification
Y. procedure
Y. technique
Y. type epispadias repair

Young-Dees

Y.-D. bladder neck reconstruction
Y.-D. operation
Y.-D. procedure
Y.-D. technique

Young-Dees-Leadbetter

Y.-D.-L. bladder neck reconstruction
Y.-D.-L. operation

Youngwhich modification

Yount

Y. fasciotomy
Y. procedure

yo-yo weight fluctuation phenomenon

Y-piece

Y-plasty

ypsiliform

Y-shaped incision

Y-suture technique

Y-T fracture

yttrium-90

yttrium-aluminum-garnet (YAG)

Yu

Y. osteotomy
Y. pyloroplasty

Y-V

Y-V anoplasty
Y-V plasty

Y-V-plasty incision

Z
- Z direction
- Z fashion
- Z incision
- Z line
- Z marginal tenotomy
- Z myotomy
- Z point
- Z procedure
- Z technique

Zadik total matrixectomy
Zaglas ligament
Zahn
- anomaly of Z.
- Z. line
- striae of Z.

Zaias nail biopsy
Zancolli
- Z. capsuloplasty
- Z. clawhand deformity repair
- Z. procedure for clawhand deformity
- Z. reconstruction
- Z. rerouting technique
- Z. static lock procedure

Zancolli-Lasso procedure
Zanelli position
Zang space
Zariczny technique
Zarins-Rowe
- Z.-R. ligament technique
- Z.-R. procedure

Zavala technique
Zavanelli maneuver
Zazepen-Gamidov technique
Z-dimension
ZEEP
zero end-expiratory pressure
Zeier transfer technique
Zeis gland
Zemuron
Zenker
- Z. diverticulum
- Z. pouch

zero
- z. end-expiratory pressure (ZEEP)
- z. end-inspiratory pressure
- z. line

zeta sedimentation ratio method
zeugmatography
- rotating-frame z.

Z-flap incision
Zickel
- Z. classification
- Z. subtrochanteric fracture operation

Ziegler
- Z. operation
- Z. puncture

Zielke technique
zig-zag
- z.-z. approach
- z.-z. compensatory deformity
- z.-z. finger incision

Zimany bilobed flap
Zimmerman-Brittin exchange model
Zimmerman operation
zinc
- z. sulfate

zinc-sulfate flotation method
Zinn
- Z. ligament
- Z. membrane
- tendon of Z.
- Z. zonule

zipped canal
zipper sphincterotomy
Zlotsky-Ballard acromioclavicular injury classification
Zoellner-Clancy procedure
Zollinger classification
Zöllner line
zona, pl. **zonae**
zonal anatomy
zone
- abdominal z.
- adherent z.
- anal transitional z. (ATZ)
- arcuate z.
- barrier z.
- basement membrane z.
- calcification z.
- cervical transformation z.
- ciliary z.
- dorsal root entry z. (DREZ)
- echo z.
- entry z.
- exudative z.
- gingival z.
- Head z.
- hemorrhoidal z.
- high pressure z. (HPZ)
- normal transformation z.
- orbicular z.
- pectinate z.
- proliferation z.
- pupillary z.
- transformation z.
- vascular z.

zonoskeleton
zonula, pl. **zonulae**

Z

zonular
- z. band
- z. fiber
- z. space

zonulares
zonule
- ciliary z.
- Zinn z.

zonulolysis
- Barraquer z.
- enzymatic z.

zonulotomy
zoodermic
zoograft
zoografting
zoonotic infection
zooplastic graft
zooplasty
zoospermia
Z-osteotomy
- scarf Z-o.

Z-osteotomy-bunionectomy
- scarf Z-o.-b.

Z-plasty
- Z-p. approach
- Broadbent-Woolf four-limb Z-p.
- Cozen-Brockway Z-p.
- four-flap Z-p.
- four-limb Z-p.
- Gudas scarf Z-p.
- Z-p. incision
- Z-p. local flap graft
- Peet Z-p.
- Z-p. procedure
- scarf Z-p.
- Spencer-Watson Z-p.
- Z-p. tenotomy
- Z-p. transposition

z-point pressure
Z-shaped
- Z-s. anastomosis
- Z-s. incision
- Z-s. suture line

Z-suture technique
Z-track intramuscular injection method
Z-type deformity
Zuckerkandl
- Z. diverticulum
- Z. fascia
- Z. perforating canal
- Z. tubercle
- Z. tuberculum

Zuker and Manktelow technique
Zung Depression Scale
zygapophyseales
zygapophyseal joint
zygapophysial
zygapophysis
zygion
zygoma
zygomatic
- z. arch
- z. arch fracture
- z. bone
- z. branch
- z. fossa
- z. maxillary complex fracture
- z. nerve
- z. region

zygomatica
zygomatici
zygomaticoauricular index
zygomaticoauricularis
zygomaticofacial
- z. artery
- z. branch
- z. canal
- z. foramen

zygomaticofaciale
zygomaticofrontalis
zygomaticofrontal suture
zygomaticomaxillaris
zygomaticomaxillary
- z. fracture
- z. suture

zygomaticoorbital
- z. artery
- z. foramen

zygomaticoorbitale
zygomatico-orbitalis
zygomaticosphenoid
zygomaticotemporal
- z. branch
- z. canal
- z. foramen
- z. space
- z. suture

zygomaticotemporale
zygomaticotemporalis
zygomaticum
zygomaticus
- z. major muscle
- z. minor muscle

zygomaxillare
zygomaxillary point
zygopodium
Zylik operation

Appendix 1

Anatomical Illustrations

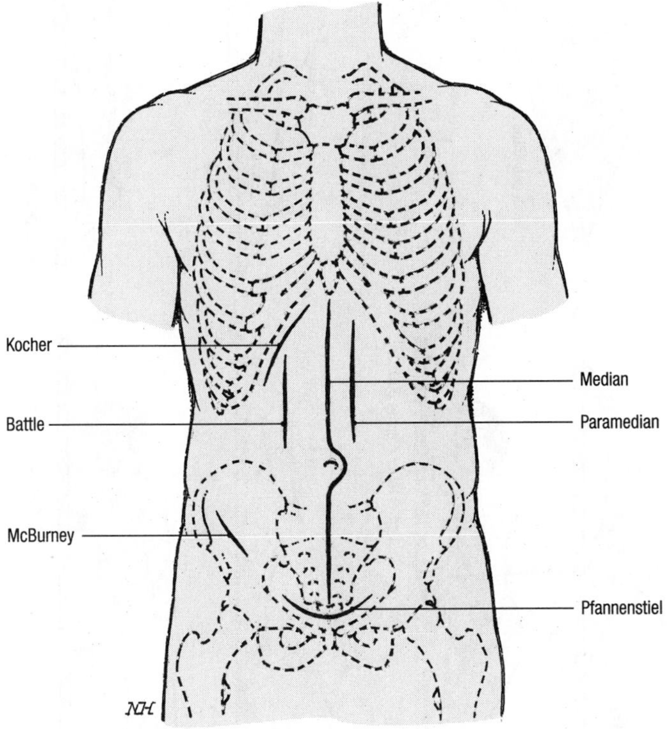

Figure 1. Surgical incisions.

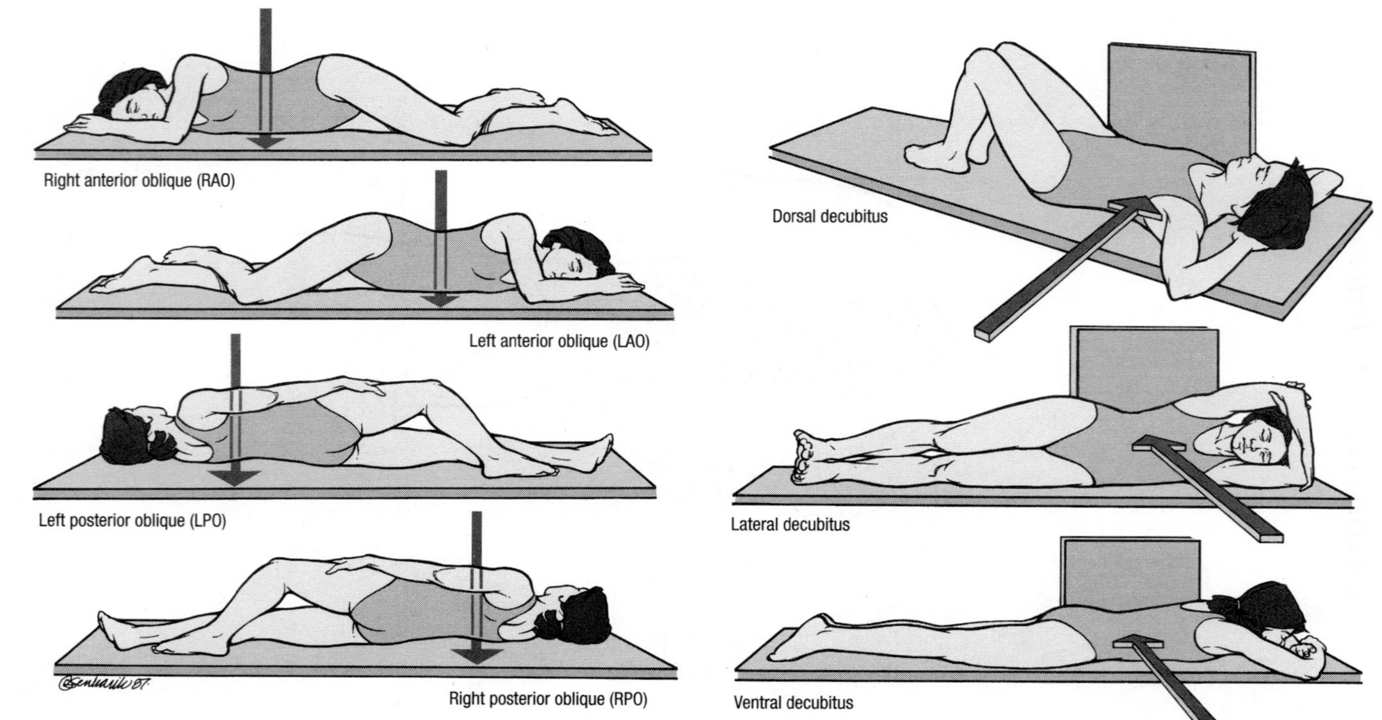

Figure 2. Patient positions.

Figure 3. Patient positions.

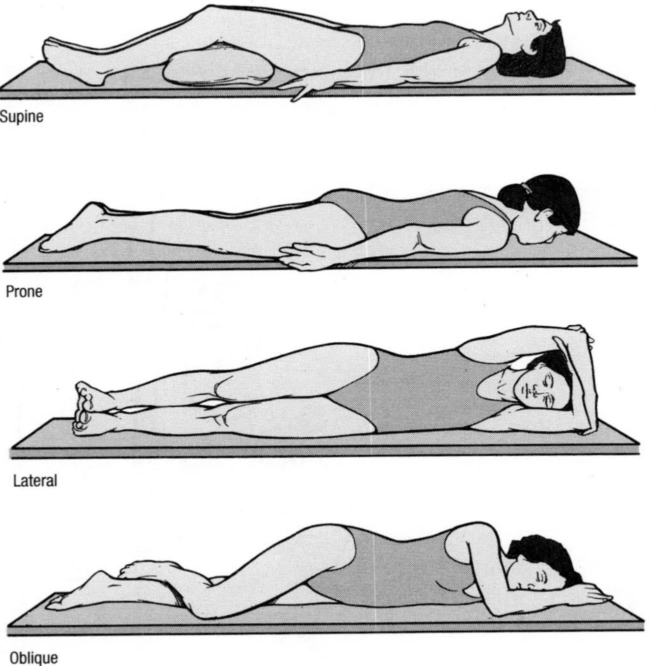

Figure 4. Patient positions.

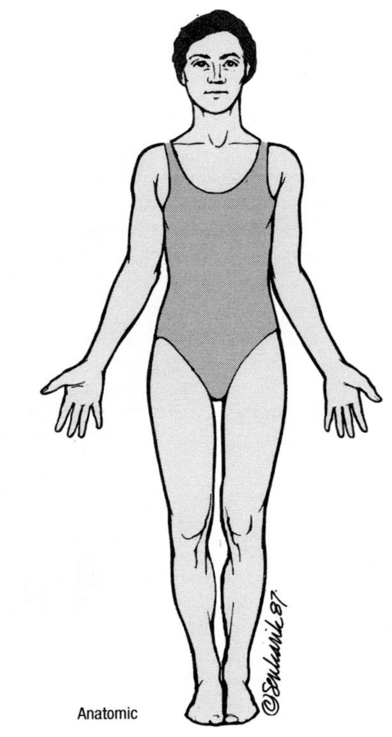

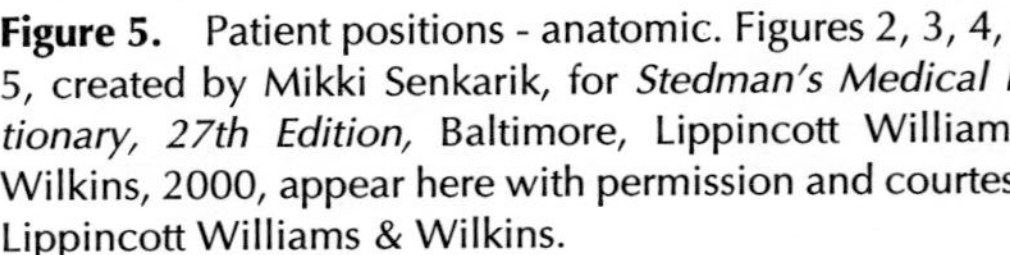

Figure 5. Patient positions - anatomic. Figures 2, 3, 4, and 5, created by Mikki Senkarik, for *Stedman's Medical Dictionary, 27th Edition,* Baltimore, Lippincott Williams & Wilkins, 2000, appear here with permission and courtesy of Lippincott Williams & Wilkins.

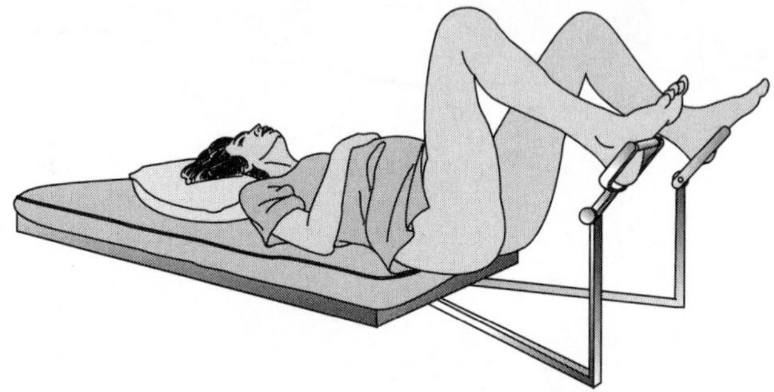

Figure 6. Lithomy position, inferolateral view.

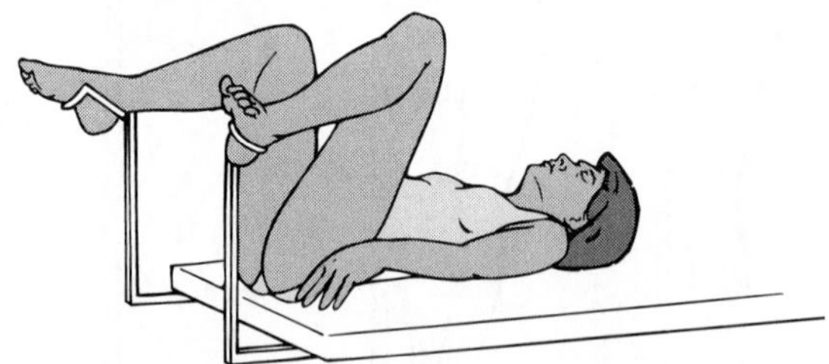

Figure 7. Dorsal lithomy position.

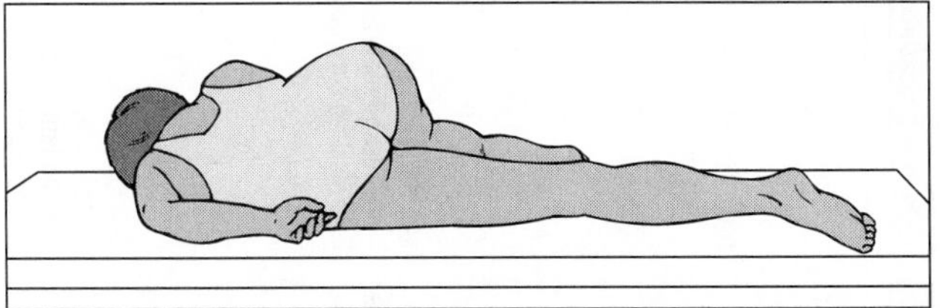

Figure 8. Sims position.

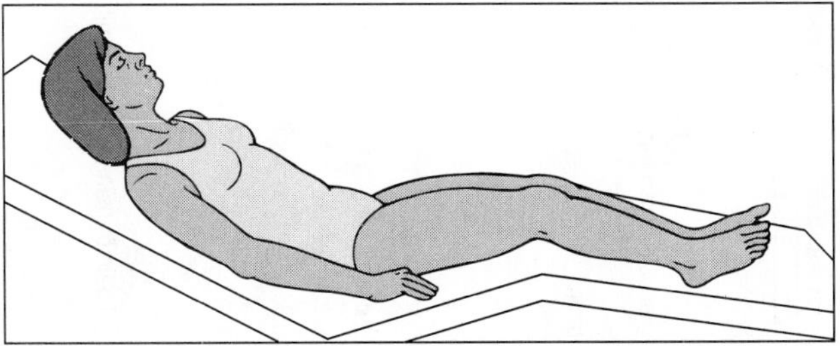

Figure 9. Fowler position.

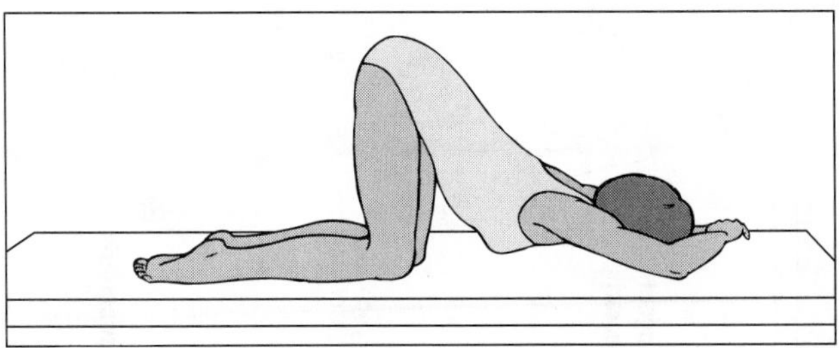

Figure 10. Knee-chest position.

Assessment of chest pain

Ailment	Character, location, and radiation	Duration	Precipitating conditions	Relieving measures
Angina pectoris	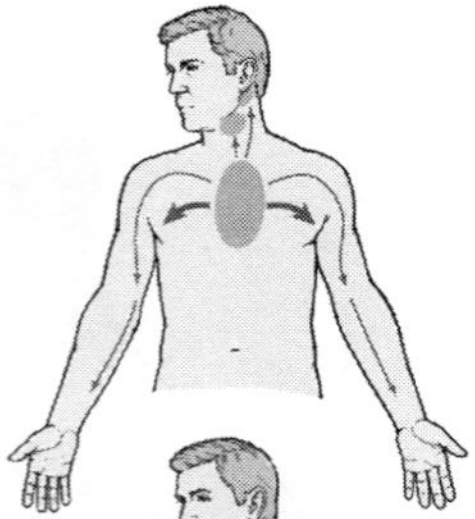 Substernal or retrosternal pain spreading across chest May radiate to inside of arm, neck, or jaws	5–15 min	Usually related to exertion, emotion, eating, cold	Rest, nitroglycerin, oxygen
Myocardial infarction	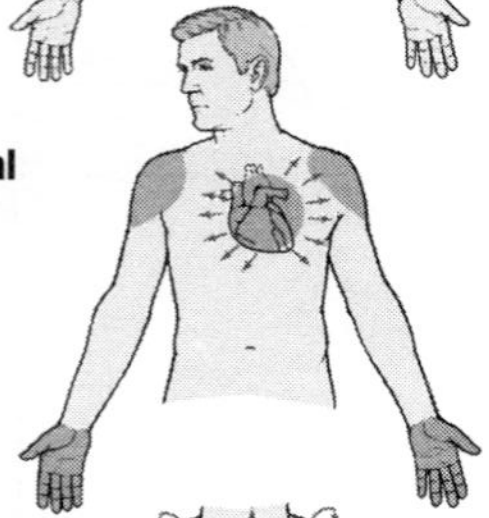 Substernal pain or pain over precordium May spread widely throughout chest Painful disability of shoulders and hands may be present	>15 min	Occurs spontaneously but may be sequela to unstable angina	Morphine sulfate, successful reperfusion of blocked coronary artery
Pericarditis	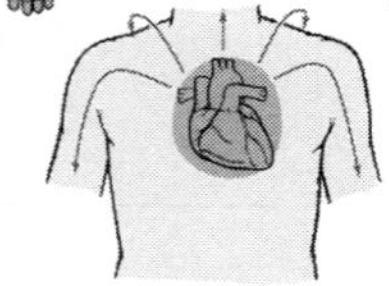 Sharp, severe substernal pain or pain to the left of sternum May be felt in epigastrium and may be referred to neck, arms, and back	Intermittent	Sudden onset Pain increases with inspiration, swallowing, coughing, and rotation of trunk	Sitting upright, analgesia, antiinflammatory medications

Assessment of chest pain (cont.)

Ailment	Character, location, and radiation	Duration	Precipitating conditions	Relieving measures
Pulmonary pain	Pain arises from inferior portion of pleura May be referred to costal margins or upper abdomen Patient may be able to localize the pain	30+ min	Often occurs spontaneously Pain occurs or increases with inspiration	Rest, time Treatment of underlying cause, bronchodilation
Esophageal pain (Hiatus hernia, reflux esophagitis, or spasm)	Substernal pain May be projected around chest to shoulders	5–60 min	Recumbency, cold liquids, exercise May occur spontaneously	Food, antacid Nitroglycerin relieves spasm
Anxiety	Pain over left chest May be variable Does not radiate Patient may complain of numbness and tingling of hands and mouth	2–3 min	Stress, emotional tachypnea	Removal of stimulus, relaxation

Figure 11. Assessment of chest pain. This table adapted from Smeltzer SC & Bare BG, *Brunner & Suddarth's Textbook of Medical Surgical-Nursing, 8th Edition,* Philadelphia, J.B. Lippincott Company, 1996, table 26.1, and created by Susan Caldwell, appears here with permission and courtesy of Lippincott Williams & Wilkins.

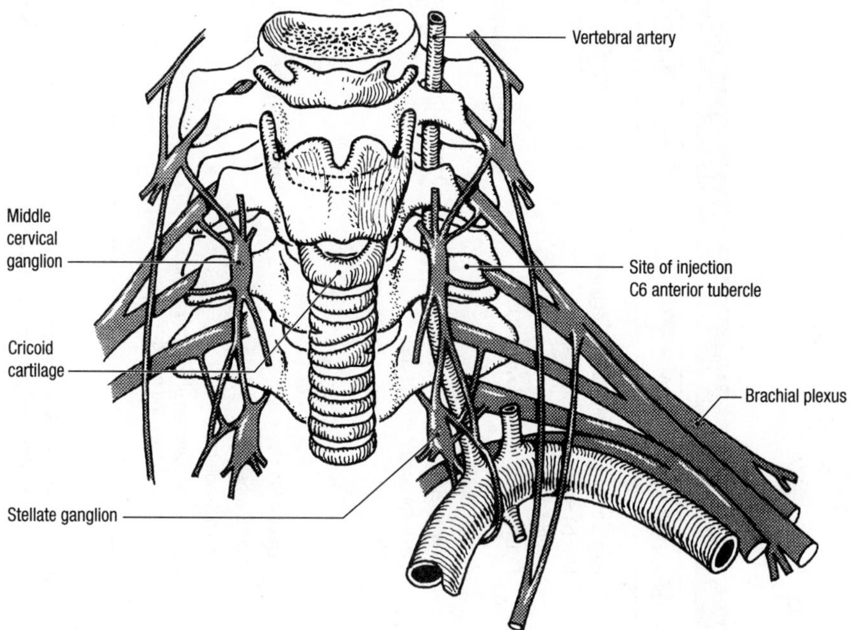

Figure 12. Site of injection for the C6 paratracheal approach to the stellate ganglion block. This image, from Benumof JL, *Clinical Procedures in Anesthesia and Intensive Care,* Philadelphia, J.B. Lippincott Company, 1992, appears here with permission and courtesy of Lippincott Williams & Wilkins.

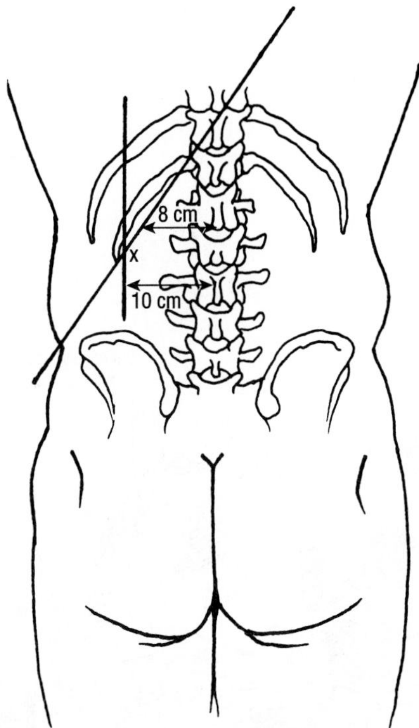

Figure 13. Landmarks for the lumbar sympathetic block (L2 paravertebral approach).

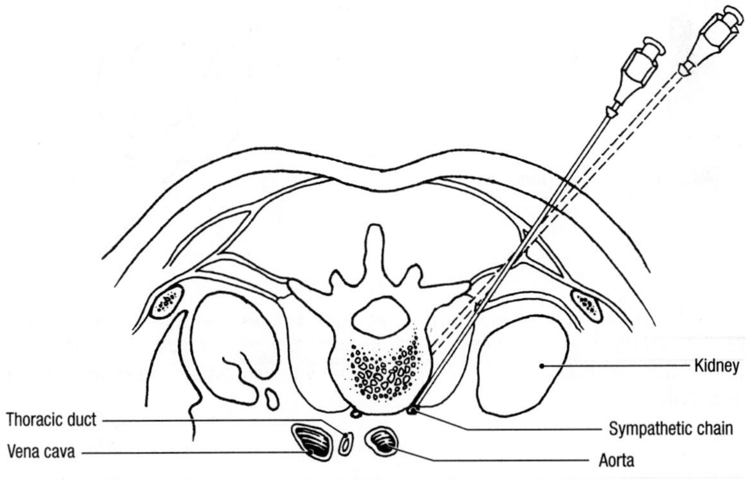

Figure 14. Initial and final needle position for the lumbar sympathetic block. The images on this page, from Abram SE & Haddox JD, *The Pain Clinic Manual, 2nd Edition,* Philadelphia, Lippincott Williams & Wilkins, 2000, figures 38-3, 38-4, appear here with permission and courtesy of Lippincott Williams & Wilkins.

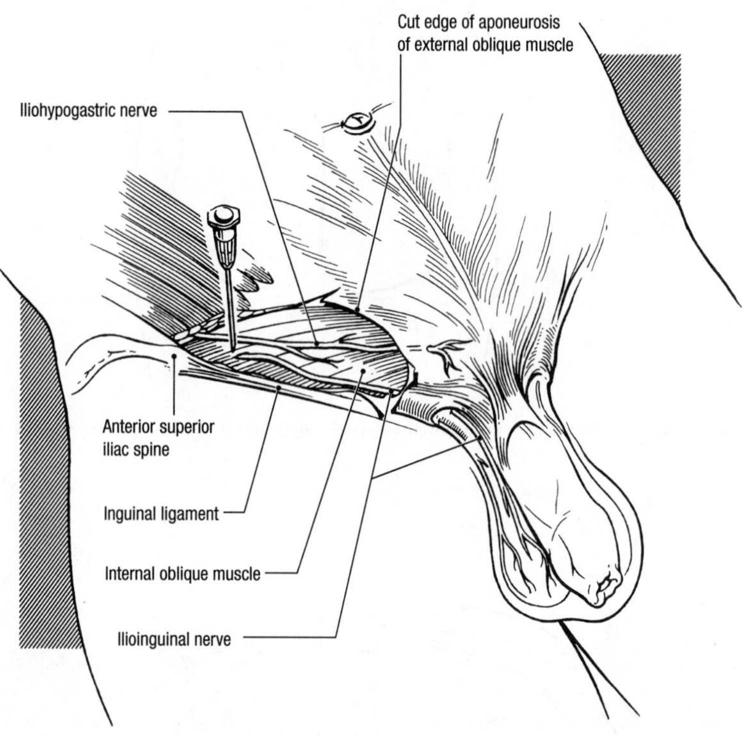

Figure 15. Ilioinguinal and iliohypogastric nerve block. Figures 15–18, from Cousins MJ & Bridenbaugh PO, *Neural Blockade in Clinical Anesthesia and Management of Pain, 3rd Edition,* Philadelphia, Lippincott-Raven Publishers, 1997, appear here with permission and courtesy of Lippincott Williams & Wilkins.

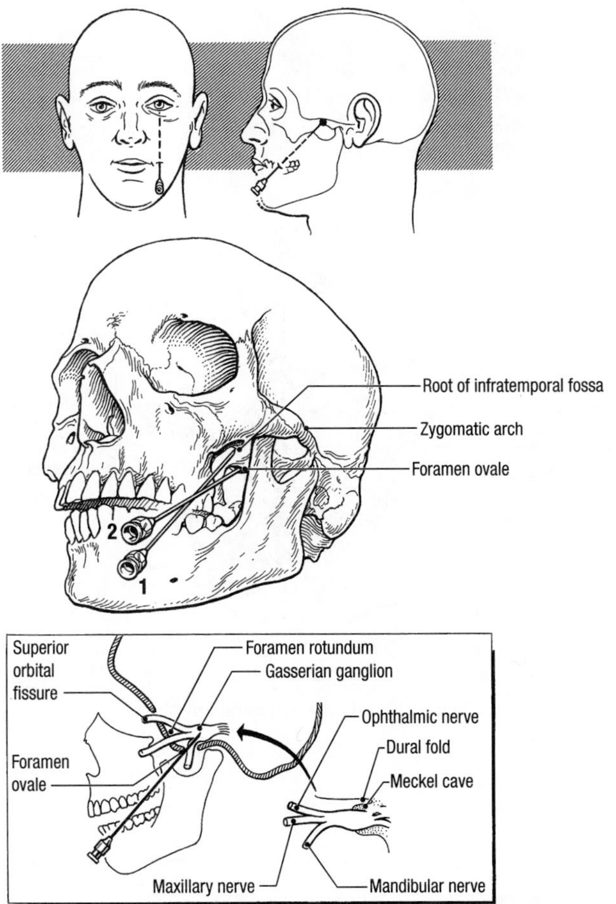

Figure 16. Gasserian ganglion block. Top panel: Note that the needle is inserted in the cheek about 1 cm posterior to the angle of the mouth as shown and directed toward the pupil in the anterior view and the midpoint of the zygoma in the lateral view. In patients with teeth, needle insertion in the cheek is superficial to the teeth of the upper jaw. In edentulous patients this may lie a variable distance between the angle of the mouth and the line midway between upper lip and nose. A palpating finger in the mouth helps to prevent needle penetration into the mouth. Middle panel: As the needle is advanced into the infratemporal fossa, it will usually strike the roof of the infratemporal fossa initially (1); this is the correct depth to seek the foramen ovale. The needle is then directed slightly posteriorly (2) to obtain a mandibular nerve (V3) paresthesia. Lower panel: The needle can then be advanced through the foramen ovale into the middle cranial fossa, where it will be adjacent to the gasserian ganglion, as shown. Note the relationships of the dural fold and Meckel cave, containing cerebrospinal fluid. A needle advanced too far through the foramen ovale can enter the Meckel cave, and subsequent injections could enter the cranial CSF and produce total spine anesthesia.

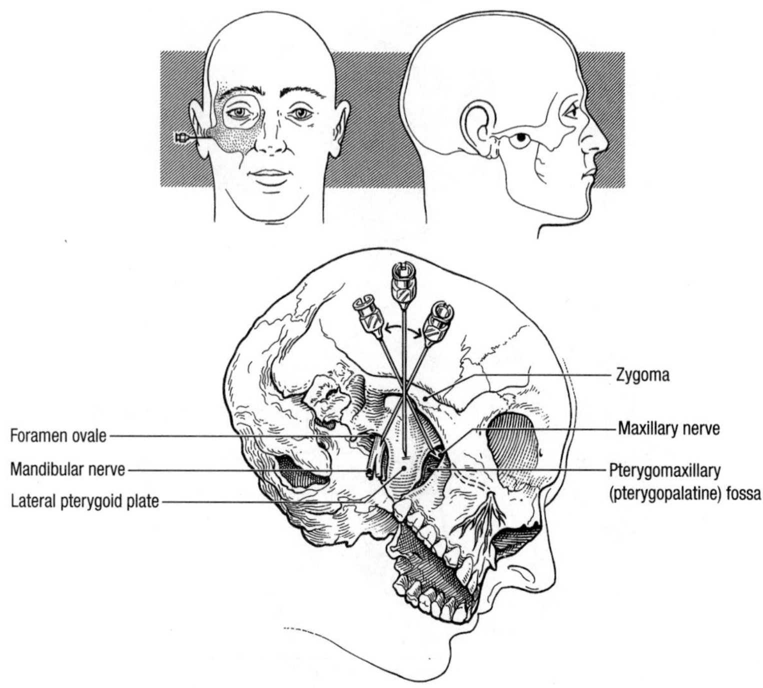

Figure 17. Gasserian ganglion block.

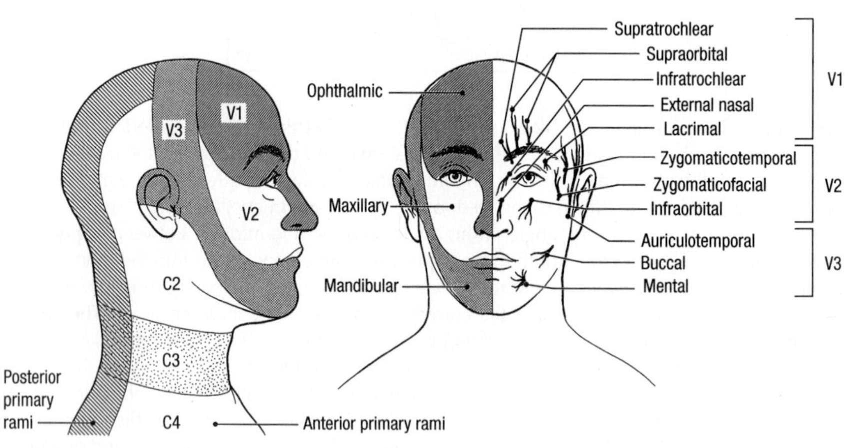

Figure 18. Dermatomes and cutaneous nerves of head, neck, and face.

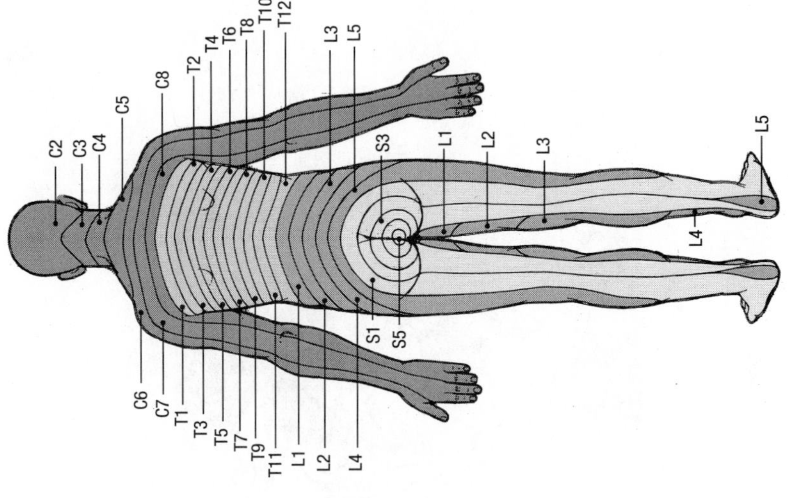

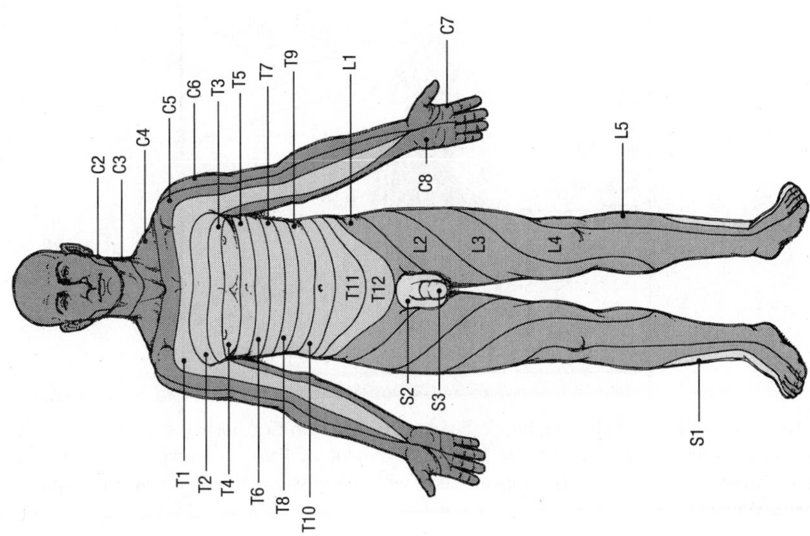

Figure 19. Dermatomes. Areas of the skin supplied by cutaneous branches of spinal nerves.

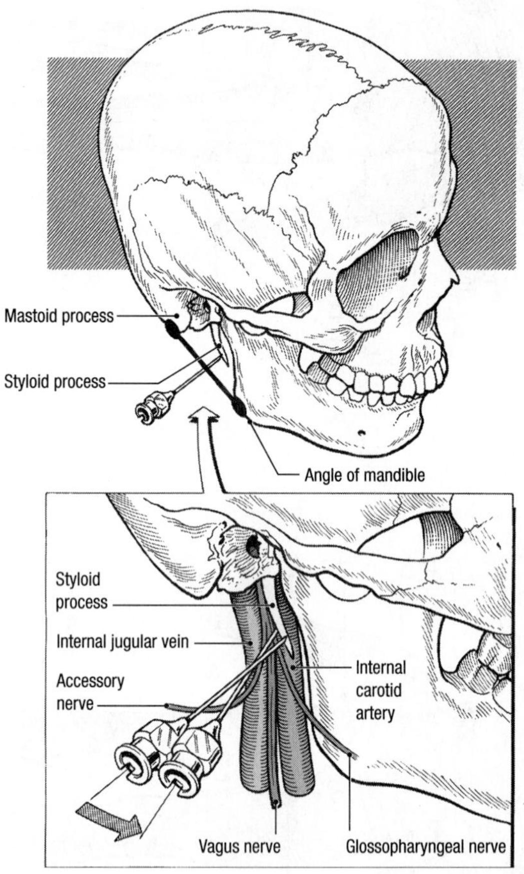

Figure 20. Glossopharyngeal nerve block. Figures 20–23, from Cousins MJ & Bridenbaugh PO, *Neural Blockade in Clinical Anesthesia and Management of Pain, 3rd Edition*, Philadelphia, Lippincott-Raven Publishers, 1997, appear here with permission and courtesy of Lippincott Williams & Wilkins.

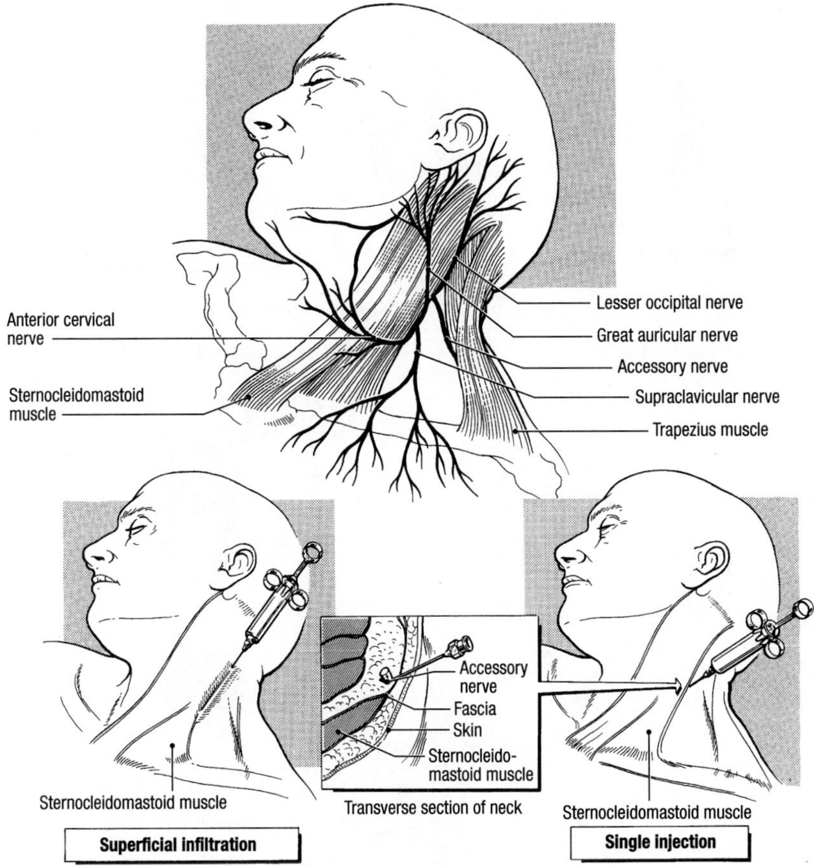

Figure 21. The superficial cervical plexus, which is blocked in the posterior triangle of the neck as it emerges adjacent to the midpoint of the posterior border of the sternocleidomastoid muscle.

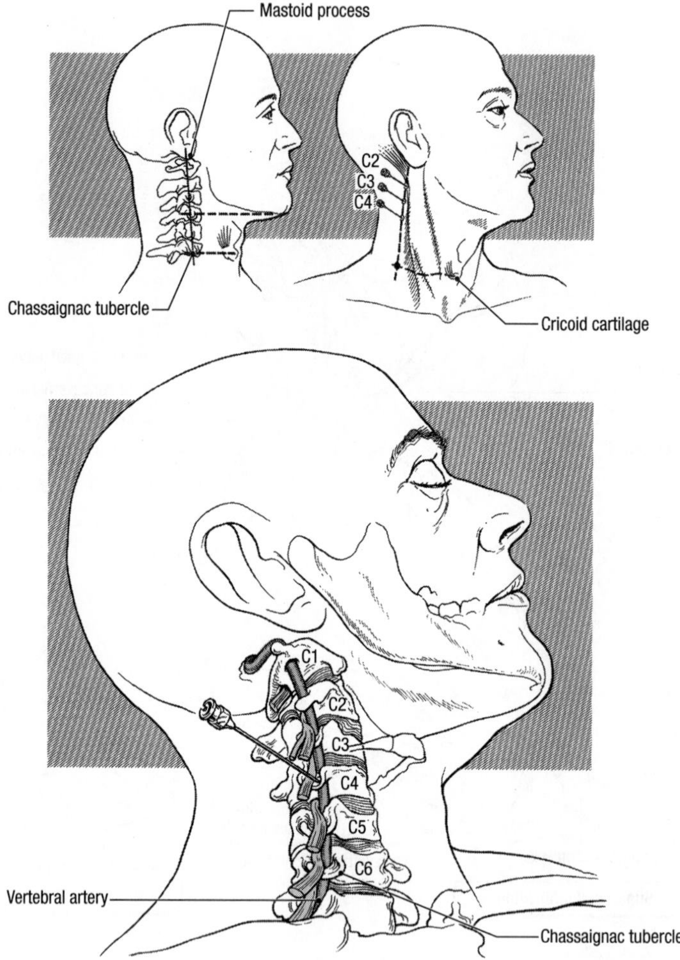

Figure 22. Deep cervical plexus block.

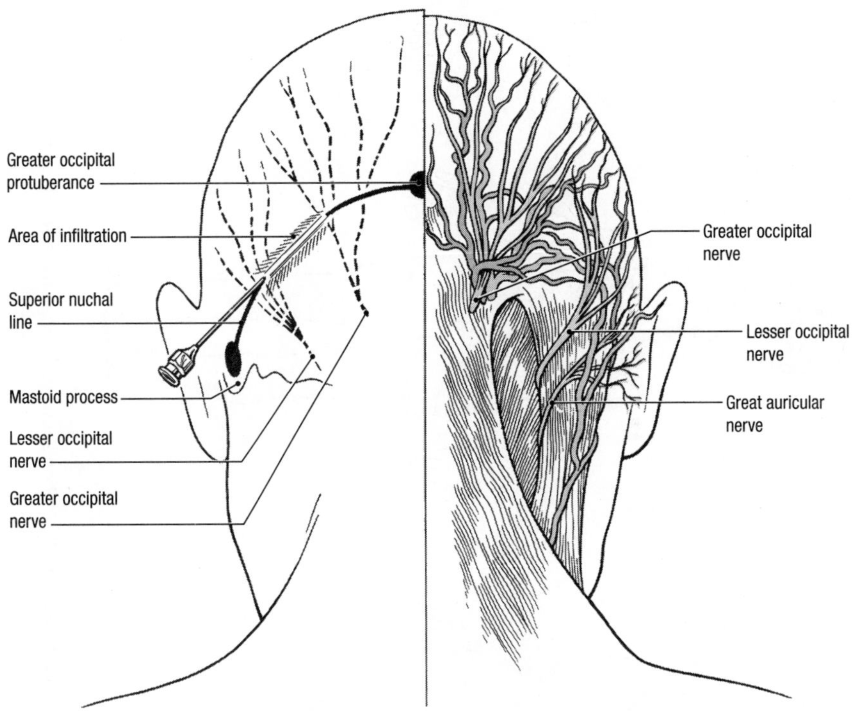

Figure 23. Greater and lesser occipital nerve block.

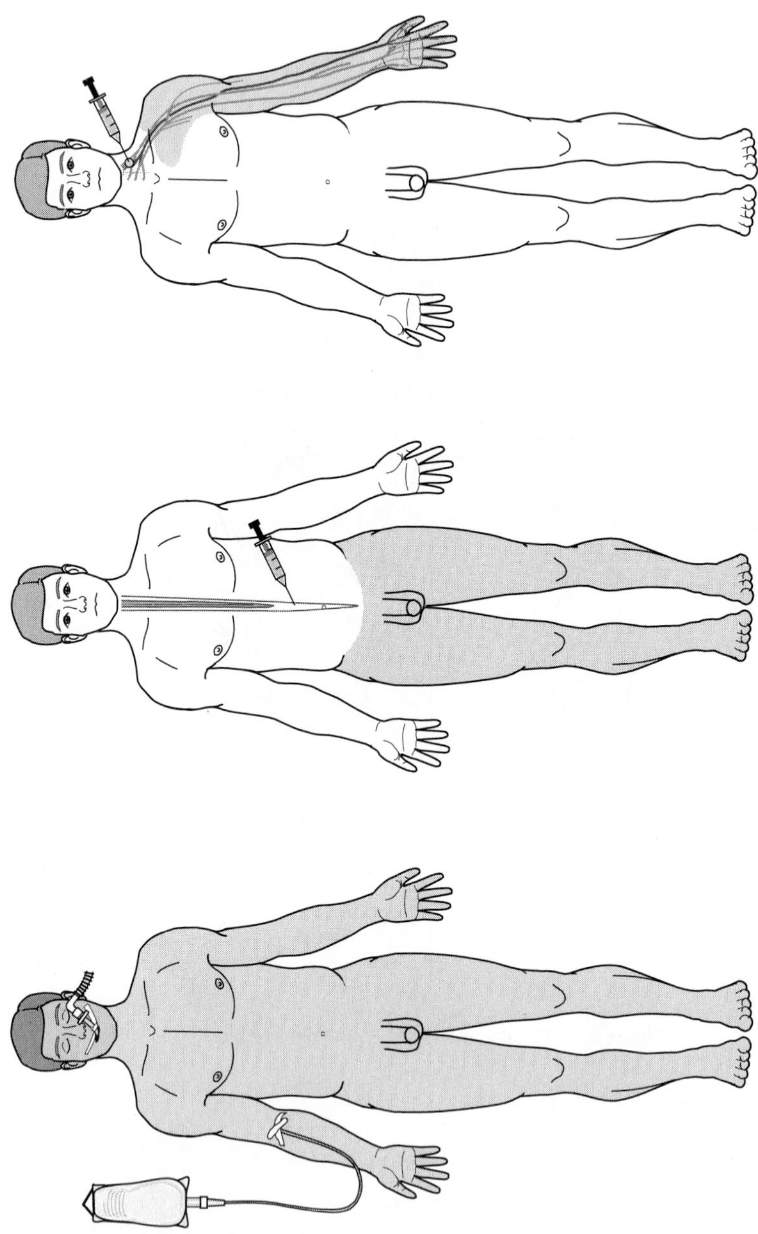

Figure 24. Types of anesthesia. Three-part illustration showing the regions affected by three types of anesthesia: general (left), regional (middle), and peripheral (right).

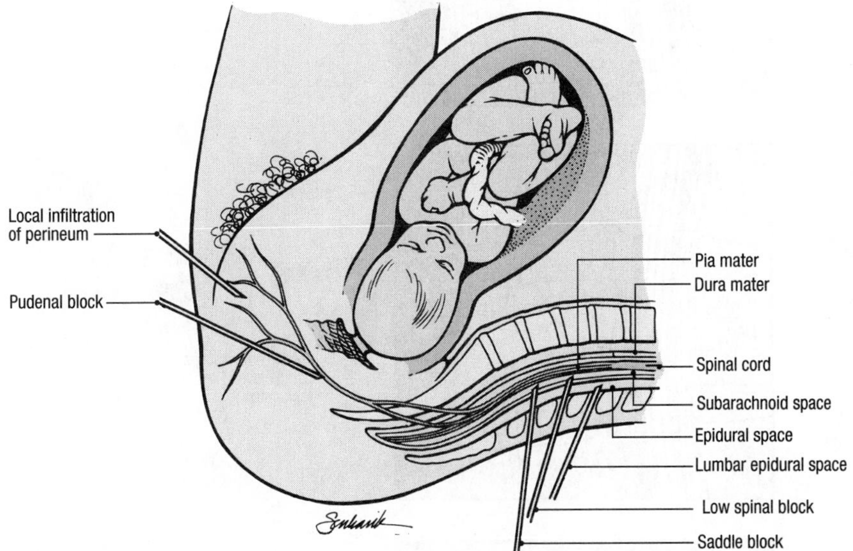

Figure 25. Regional anesthesia for childbirth. Sites of injections. This image, created by Mikki Senkarik, for Pillitteri A, PhD, RN, PNP, *Maternal & Child Health Nursing: Care of the Childbearing & Childrearing Family, 3rd Edition,* Philadelphia, Lippincott Williams & Wilkins, 1998, appears here with permission and courtesy of Lippincott Williams & Wilkins.

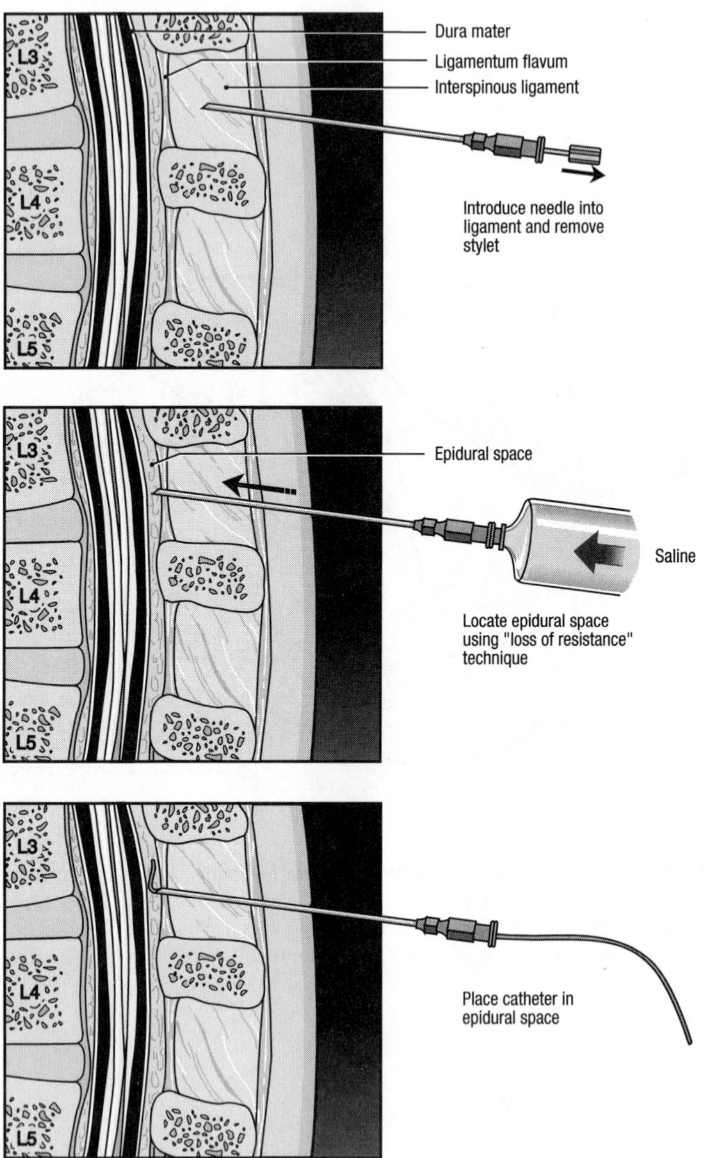

Figure 26. Epidural procedure. Three-step illustration showing the procedure used in giving an epidural.

Appendix 2

Pain Glossary

pain	an unpleasant sensory and emotional experience associated with actual or potential pain damage, or described in terms of such damage
allodynia	pain arising from stimulus that does not usually provoke pain
analgesia	absence of pain in response to stimulation that would usually be painful
anesthesia dolorosa	pain occurring in an anesthetic area
causalgia	a syndrome of sustained burning pain, allodynia, and hyperpathia after a traumatic nerve lesion, often combined with vasomotor and sudomotor dysfunction and later trophic changes
central pain	pain associated with a lesion of the central nervous system
dysesthesia	an unpleasant abnormal sensation, whether spontaneous or evoked
hyperalgesia	an increased response to a painful stimulus
hyperanesthesia	increased sensitivity to stimulation, excluding the special senses
hyperpathia	a painful syndrome characterized by increased reaction to a stimulus
hypoalgesia	diminished pain in response to normally painful stimulus
hypoesthesia	decreased sensitivity to stimulation, excluding the special senses
neuralgia	pain in the distribution of a nerve or nerves
neuritis	inflammation of a nerve or nerves

neuropathy	a disturbance of function or pathologic change in a nerve; in one nerve, mononeuropathy; in several nerves, mononeuropathy multiplex; if diffuse and bilateral, polyneuropathy
nociceptor	a receptor preferentially sensitive to a noxious stimulus or to a stimulus that would become noxious, if prolonged
noxious stimulus	stimulus that is damaging to normal tissue
pain threshold	the least experience of pain that a patient can recognize
pain tolerance level	the greatest level of pain that a patient is prepared to tolerate
paraesthesia	an abnormal sensation, whether spontaneous or evoked

Appendix 3

Pain Management Techniques

I. Pharmacologic Therapy

A. Nonsteroidal Antiinflammatory Drugs (NSAIDs)
B. Opioids
C. Adjuvant treatments
   1. Anticonvulsants
   2. Local anesthetics
   3. Corticosteroids
   4. Antispasmodics
   5. Clonidine
   6. Topical agents
D. Psychopharmacology
E. Antidepressants
F. Antipsychotics
G. Mood stabilizers
H. Anxiolytics
I. Psychostimulants

II. Nonpharmacologic Therapy

A. Blocks
   1. Epidural steroid injections
   2. Central nerve blocks
   3. Sympathetic nerve blocks
   4. Visceral nerve blocks
   5. Peripheral nerve blocks
   6. Facet joint blocks
   7. Sacroiliac joint blocks
   8. Trigger point injections
B. Intravenous lidocaine injection
C. Intravenous phentolamine infusion
D. Intravenous regional sympathetic blocks (Bier blocks)

III. Interventional Therapy

A. Spinal cord stimulation
B. Intrathecal therapy
C. Discography
D. Intradiscal electrothermal therapy
E. Vertebroplasty

IV. Neurosurgical Therapy

A. Ablative procedures
B. Augmentation procedures

V. Physical Therapy

A. Stretching exercises
B. Strengthening exercises
C. Endurance exercises
D. Electrical stimulation
E. Ultrasound
F. Local heat
G. Local cooling
H. Joint mobilization
I. Soft-tissue mobilization

VI. Acupuncture

VII. Radiotherapy and Radiopharmaceuticals for Cancer Pain

A. Palliative treatment
B. Radiation therapy for bone metastases
C. Hemibody irradiation
D. Systemic radioisotopes

Appendix 4

Sample Reports and Dictation

PAIN CLINIC CONSULTATION FOR MEDICATION MANAGEMENT

DIAGNOSES

1. Chronic axial low back pain with bilateral lower extremity radiculopathy.
2. Status post decompressive lumbar laminectomy with postlaminectomy pain syndrome.
3. Bilateral foraminal stenosis, L4–5 and L5-S1.

PROCEDURE PERFORMED: Follow-up outpatient consultation and medication management; recommendation for intrathecal narcotic trial.

INDICATIONS AND BACKGROUND INFORMATION: The patient was seen in our practice last year. Current regimen has included OxyContin 10 mg q.a.m., 10 mg q.p.m., 20 mg q.h.s., with Percocet one q.6h. p.r.n. The patient has had persistent symptoms of breakthrough pain. She has been able to work full time; however, increased dosages of medications have affected cognitive functioning and caused slight sedation.

The patient is requesting additional information concerning an intrathecal pump, given persistence of breakthrough pain and associated side effects with her current regimen. We have again discussed this procedure in great detail with the patient. We have provided an additional two months' worth of medication and asked the patient to contact our office in the interim if she wishes to discuss further the possibility of an intrathecal narcotic trial. Currently, to provide better management during the daytime hours, we have asked the patient to take OxyContin 20 mg t.i.d. in an attempt to reduce her current Percocet usage to one tablet t.i.d. p.r.n. The patient will contact our office in the interim with questions and concerns or to discuss further the possibility of an intrathecal narcotic trial.

PAIN MANAGEMENT PSYCHOMETRIC EVALUATION

REASON FOR EVALUATION: As part of the initial evaluation from a behavioral medicine standpoint for this patient, an MMPI was ordered for general personality evaluation.

TEST RESULTS AND OBSERVATIONS: This appears to be a valid and interpretable profile. The patient, however, did not answer 16 of the items. This is generally higher than would be expected for most patients. The Welsh code is 326941′07-8/5: F-LK:. The mean profile elevation is 69.9, indicating a moderate degree of emotional intensity at the time of testing.

Patients with similar profiles are often described as acting distressed and avoiding responsibility through development of physical symptoms. Such persons may report headaches, numbness, discomfort, chest pains, weakness, and other vague physical symptoms. These symptoms may appear and disappear suddenly. Such persons often lack insight concerning the causes of their symptoms and lack insight about their own motives and feelings. They are often described as psychologically immature. They may use indirect means to get attention and affection from others. They often have a difficult time expressing resentment or hostility openly. Such persons are often interested in what other people can do for them. These persons are often initially enthusiastic about treatment and view themselves as having medical problems and wanting medical attention. They are often resistant to psychological interpretations of their issues. Persons with similar profiles also often display depressive symptoms and are pessimistic about the future. They may have feelings of guilt or self-deprecation and often are given some form of depressive diagnosis. These persons lack self-confidence and often feel unable to function. They act helpless and give up easily on tasks. Such persons often have lifestyles characterized by withdrawal and lack of involvement with other people. Such persons have difficulty making decisions and feel overwhelmed when faced with major life decisions. Such persons often may exhibit disturbed thinking; feel mistreated; feel angry and resentful but have no way of expressing this directly, harbor grudges; and utilize projection as a defense mechanism. These persons also show high degrees of energy and they present themselves as agitated.

Overall, this profile indicates somebody who presents with multiple vague physical symptoms. These symptoms appear to be long-standing in nature and will not likely be alleviated by purely symptomatic and/or medical interventions. These persons have often adjusted to a lifestyle characterized by a focus on medical symptoms, lower levels of efficiency, depression, and social isolation. Such persons may resist psychological interpretations of their issues and prefer to see themselves as medically ill.

Caudal Epidural Steroid Injection

Diagnosis: Chronic sacral pain and back pain.

Procedure Performed: Initial outpatient consultation and caudal epidural steroid injection #1 with fluoroscopic guidance.

Indications and Background: The patient is referred to our service for evaluation and treatment of chronic low back pain. The pain is described as being located in the base of her sacrum. The patient states she has had back pain for the last 20 years and has undergone surgical intervention for lumbar disk disease as well as degenerative hip disease. The patient is now complaining of back pain located at the base of her sacrum, described as an aching-type pain, at worse 10/10. The patient states that resting on her back or spine causes the pain, lying on her side tends to somewhat relieve the pain. She denies any numbness or tingling in her lower extremities. She says the pain is affecting her sleep, appetite, and physical activity.

PAST TREATMENT MODALITIES: The patient has had three back surgeries, the last one three years ago, and uses heat for temporary relief. She has been taking Percocet, approximately four tablets per day. I note she has taken OxyContin in the past. She states that she is trying the Duragesic patch; however, this does not work for her.

PAST MEDICAL HISTORY: The patient's past medical history is significant for arthritis of both the spine and the hip.

PREVIOUS HOSPITALIZATIONS: The patient had surgery three times for her back, the last approximately three years ago. She also underwent hemiarthroplasty for her hip, approximately three years ago.

MEDICATIONS: She has been taking Percocet and OxyContin 20-mg tablets.

ALLERGIES: The patient has no known drug allergies.

SOCIAL HISTORY: The patient is married, lives with her family, and is retired. She has no known psychiatric history.

SUBSTANCE USE: She denies use of tobacco, alcohol, or recreational drugs.

PHYSICAL EXAMINATION: The patient's vital signs were taken, with her blood pressure 187/93, her pulse 61. Examination of her back revealed a well-healed midline scar, extending from the upper lumbar level to the top of the sacrum. There is tenderness over the scar area, but more significant tenderness is noted over the lower sacral area at approximately the level of the sacral hiatus. No significant sacroiliac joint pain was noted. No areas of localized infection were noted. There is an area of redness over the lower buttocks, but this did not extend to the area of discomfort.

DESCRIPTION OF PROCEDURE: Caudal epidural steroid injection with fluoroscopic guidance. The risks and benefits of the procedure were discussed with the patient. Written consent was obtained and placed in the chart. The patient was transported to the fluoroscopy suite and placed prone on the x-ray table with a roll under her abdomen. Her back was prepped with Betadine and draped in the usual aseptic fashion. The area over the sacral hiatus where it should be located was found to have bony prominence. The subcutaneous tissues above it were anesthetized with 1% lidocaine using a 27-gauge needle. Fluoroscopic view from a lateral projection showed what appeared to be a sharp angulation of the lower sacral element at approximately the sacral hiatus. A 20-gauge Tuohy needle was then advanced through the sacral hiatus, into the sacral epidural space. Entry into the epidural space was confirmed by injection of 3 cc of Isovue contrast material under continuous lateral fluoroscopic view. Typical sacral epidural spread was noted in both the lateral and the AP views. Then 80 mg of Depo-Medrol in 0.5% lidocaine was injected incrementally with frequent negative aspiration. The patient reported moderate to intense pressure paresthesias, which dissipated quickly and had no sequelae.

She was returned to our area, where she was observed for approximately one hour with periodic blood pressure monitoring.

ASSESSMENT AND PLAN: The patient presents with relatively localized back pain, located over the bottom of the sacrum. It was unclear whether an actual sacral fracture exists or whether her anatomy is somewhat aberrant. However, the locality of her pain corresponds to a rather strong angulation at the base of her sacrum. We hope that the epidural steroid injections will provide her with some relief.

The patient appears to have had some problems with using medication in the past; she was provided with a prescription of 25 Percocet tablets for pain relief, status post procedure. She is to return in approximately one week for the second in a planned series of three caudal epidural steroid injections.

CERVICAL EPIDURAL STEROID INJECTION

DIAGNOSES

1. Chronic right hand pain.
2. Cervical disk disease.
3. Chronic bilateral arm pain.

PROCEDURE: Cervical epidural steroid injection #3 with fluoroscopic guidance.

INDICATIONS AND BACKGROUND: The patient returns to our service today for the third in a planned series of three cervical epidural steroid injections. She reports that the injection provided on her last visit did provide some relief to her arm pain bilaterally. She states the right hand pain, particularly around the thenar eminence, is still present and has not been affected by either of the two injections. She does wish to proceed with the third injection at this time.

INTERIM PHYSICAL EXAMINATION: The patient's neck has good range of motion. The patient's shoulder area at her neck was palpated, and no significant areas of tenderness were noted.

DESCRIPTION OF PROCEDURE: The risks and benefits of the procedure were discussed with the patient. Written consent was obtained and placed on the chart. The patient was transported to the fluoroscopy suite, placed prone on the x-ray table with a roll under her chest. Her neck was prepped with Betadine and draped in the usual aseptic fashion. The C6-C7 interspace was identified using fluoroscopy, and the subcutaneous tissues above it were anesthetized with 1% lidocaine using a 27-gauge needle. A 20-gauge Tuohy needle was then advanced into the epidural space at the C6-C7 level from a midline approach, using loss-of-resistance-to-saline technique and fluoroscopic guidance. No heme, CSF, or paresthesias were encountered with needle placement. Injection of 2 cc of Isovue contrast material showed good epidural spread, more on the right than the left. Then 80 mg of Depo-Medrol in 6 cc of preservative-free normal saline was injected incrementally with frequent negative aspiration. The patient reported mild pressure paresthesias, which dissipated quickly with no sequelae. She was returned to our area, observed for approximately 15 minutes, and then discharged to home.

ASSESSMENT AND PLAN: The patient presents with residual arm pain post cervical diskectomy. The patient's pain apparently stems from cervical disk disease not addressed by her previous surgery. We hope that the injections provided will give her some relief. She is to follow up as needed.

L4–5 TRANSFORAMINAL EPIDURAL STEROID INJECTION

DIAGNOSES

1. Left lower extremity radiculopathy, recurrent.
2. Status post decompressive lumbar laminectomy.
3. Neuroforaminal stenosis, left L4–5 and L5-S1.

PROCEDURES PERFORMED

1. Follow-up outpatient consultation.
2. Left L4–5 transforaminal epidural steroid injection with fluoroscopic guidance and contrast confirmation, #3.

INDICATIONS AND BACKGROUND INFORMATION: The patient is returning to our practice for a third, and final, transforaminal epidural injection in this series. The patient has had no adverse side effects or sequelae. He is continuing to report approximately 50 to 60% overall benefit. We have again discussed the risks and benefits associated with the procedure to be performed today, and informed, written consent has been obtained and placed in the permanent medical record.

INTERIM PHYSICAL EVALUATION: Unchanged.

DESCRIPTION OF PROCEDURE: The patient was taken to our fluoroscopy suite, where he was positioned prone with the roll underneath the abdomen. The lumbosacral spine was aseptically prepared and draped. Utilizing oblique fluoroscopic image, the L4–5 foramen was visualized. The local anesthetic skin wheal was raised over this region, and a 22-gauge spinal needle inserted through this local anesthetic skin wheal, where it was guided with both oblique and AP fluoroscopic imaging to lie in the transforaminal aspect of L4–5. Confirmation of appropriate placement was performed with the injection of 3 cc of Isovue 200 contrast. This was followed by the injection of 80 mg of Depo-Medrol, diluted to a volume of 7 cc with preservative-free normal saline. This was injected slowly and incrementally, without adverse event. The patient was then monitored after the procedure, provided with our routine postprocedural instructions, and discharged to home.

FOLLOW-UP PLAN: The patient will follow up on an as-needed basis in the future for recurrent symptoms. We have encouraged him to contact our office in the interim with any questions or concerns regarding the procedure performed today. We have also asked him to follow up with his private physician for reevaluation. At the patient's request, we have provided a prescription of 5-mg Percocet, #60, to be used one q.12h. p.r.n.

L4–5 TRANSLAMINAR EPIDURAL STEROID INJECTION

DIAGNOSES

1. Multilevel symptomatic spinal stenosis.
2. Low back pain with bilateral lower extremity radiculopathy and neurogenic claudication.

PROCEDURES PERFORMED

1. Initial outpatient consultation.
2. L4–5 translaminar epidural steroid injection with fluoroscopic guidance and contrast confirmation, #1.

INDICATIONS AND BACKGROUND INFORMATION: The patient is a very pleasant female, who was referred to our practice on a semi-urgent basis for consideration of a series of lumbar epidural steroid injections for the symptomatic management of low back pain and lower extremity radiculopathy symptoms, which have been present for at least seven weeks. The patient has had progressive pain, which has restricted activity, and currently she is primarily restricted to a wheelchair. She has been using Darvocet one tab up to four times daily, has tried Celebrex, as well as Ultram, and physical therapy. There is no bowel or bladder dysfunction and no focal motor weakness. An MRI of the lumbosacral spine was obtained. Impression was degenerative disk disease, lumbosacral spine, resulting in severe central canal stenosis at L2–3 and L4–5, and moderate bilateral neuroforaminal narrowing at L4–5.

ALLERGIES: Penicillin.

MEDICATIONS: Caltrate, Fosamax.

PAST MEDICAL HISTORY: Osteoporosis.

PAST SURGICAL HISTORY: Appendectomy, hemorrhoidectomy.

PHYSICAL EVALUATION: The patient appears younger than her stated age. She appears to be in no acute distress at this time. Vital signs are stable. Peripheral neurological evaluation is nonfocal, and there is no evidence of peripheral cyanosis, clubbing, or edema. Examination of the lumbar spine reveals no signs of cutaneous infection or irritation and no palpable tenderness overlying the paraspinous musculature or the sacroiliac joints. There is mild kyphosis of the thoracic spine and flattening of the lumbar lordosis present.

DESCRIPTION OF PROCEDURE: After a discussion with the patient and her family concerning the risks and benefits of an empirical trial of lumbar epidural steroid injections for the symptomatic management of spinal stenosis, and specifically after the risks of infection, bleeding, postdural puncture headache, and neurologic sequelae had been fully disclosed, the patient was transported to our fluoroscopy suite, where she was positioned prone. The area overlying the lumbosacral spine was aseptically prepared and draped. The L4–5 interspace was identified, a local anesthetic skin wheal raised centrally, and a 20-gauge 3-1/2-inch Tuohy needle was inserted through this local anesthetic skin wheal, where it was advanced into appropriate epidural placement on the first attempt. No heme, CSF, or paresthesias were elicited. Then 3 cc of Isovue 200 contrast documented appropriate epidural layering. This was followed by the injection of 80 mg of Depo-Medrol, diluted to a volume of 7 cc with preservative-free normal saline. This was injected slowly and incrementally. The patient was monitored after the procedure, provided with postprocedural instructions, and discharged to home.

FOLLOW-UP PLAN: This patient will follow up in one week for reevaluation, a second epidural injection to be performed at that time. Based upon her overall level of improvement, we will determine the number of injections to be performed in this series.

L5-S1 TRANSFORAMINAL EPIDURAL STEROID INJECTION

DIAGNOSES

1. Recurrent left lower back pain and left lower extremity radiculopathy.
2. Status post diskectomy, L4–5, left.

PROCEDURES PERFORMED

1. Follow-up outpatient consultation.
2. L5-S1, left, transforaminal epidural steroid injection with fluoroscopic guidance and contrast confirmation.

INDICATIONS AND BACKGROUND INFORMATION: The patient is returning to our practice for routine follow-up care. Despite two translaminar epidural steroid injections on the left at L3–4, the patient has had no significant overall improvement in her pain symptoms. An MRI of the lumbosacral spine was obtained, revealing degenerative disk change with enhancing anular fissures, L4–5 and L5-S1. No focal disk herniations, neural impingement, or scar tissue is noted. The patient has had persistent radicular symptoms, continues to be a nonsurgical candidate, and therefore we will proceed with a transforaminal injection at this time. Based upon improvement, we will determine whether a fourth injection with a transforaminal approach is indicated. We have also provided educational information on spinal cord stimulation, in the event we do not obtain adequate relief of symptoms with interventional nerve blocks.

INTERIM PHYSICAL EVALUATION: Unchanged.

DESCRIPTION OF PROCEDURE: The patient was taken to our fluoroscopy suite and positioned. The area overlying the lumbar spine was aseptically prepared and draped. Utilizing oblique fluoroscopic imaging, the L5-S1 foramen was visualized. A local anesthetic skin wheal was raised, and a 22-gauge, 3-1/2-inch spinal needle entered through this local anesthetic skin wheal, where it was advanced into transforaminal placement with both oblique and AP fluoroscopic imaging. Confirmation of appropriate placement was performed with the injection of 3 cc of Isovue 200 contrast, in addition to provocative pressure paresthesias, which were transient in nature. The patient then received 80 mg of Depo-Medrol, diluted to a volume of 7 cc with preservative-free normal saline. This was injected slowly and incrementally, without adverse sequelae. The patient was then monitored after the procedure, provided with routine postprocedure instructions, and discharged to home.

FOLLOW-UP PLAN: The patient will follow up in two weeks for reevaluation, with consideration of an additional transforaminal injection at that time. If there is no significant improvement from this treatment series, we will ask the patient to consider a trial of spinal cord stimulation for chronic and intractable refractory pain.

TRIGGER POINT INJECTION

DIAGNOSES

1. Chronic chest wall pain.
2. Chronic abdominal pain.

PROCEDURE: Initial outpatient consultation and trigger point injections times three.

INDICATIONS AND BACKGROUND: The patient is a 31-year-old gentleman referred to our service for evaluation and treatment of pain and discomfort in the right upper quadrant of his abdomen and along the lower costal border. The patient stated that the pain began approximately one year ago and is located from the midline to approximately 5 cm lateral to the right. He states the pain is predictable in occurring when he eats. The pain occurs or intensifies shortly after eating and resolves after two to three hours.

PAST TREATMENT MODALITIES: The patient has tried Prilosec and Prevacid. He underwent an EGD, which showed some Candida esophagitis, but no peptic ulcer disease. He had a trial of Diflucan. The Candida was thought related to the Azmacort medication. The patient has also had a sonogram, a CT scan, and a HIDA scan, which have all been normal. He denies any generalized malaise, fevers, or weight loss. He denies any trauma to that area or any inciting event.

PAST MEDICAL HISTORY: The patient's past medical history is significant only for asthma. He was hospitalized several times in the past, however, not recently.

MEDICATIONS: The patient currently takes albuterol two to three puffs, six to eight times per day. He also uses Singulair and Tylenol for pain.

ALLERGIES: The patient has no known drug allergies.

SOCIAL HISTORY: The patient is married and works for a salvage corporation.

SUBSTANCE USE: The patient denies tobacco or recreational drug use. He occasionally uses alcohol.

PHYSICAL EXAMINATION: Vital signs reveal the patient has a blood pressure of 120/66 and pulse of 84. On physical exam, the patient is a well-developed male, looking his stated age. He arrives ambulatory, with no assistive devices. He is alert and oriented. Examination of his abdomen does not reveal any scars or signs of localized infection or inflammation. Palpation of his abdomen does not reveal any discomfort in the left upper or lower quadrants or in the right lower quadrant. There is tenderness over the lower costal border anteriorly and at the juncture of the lower rib at the sternum. Pressure on these structures causes tenderness but does not reproduce his pain. Pressure underneath the rib on the upper edge of the liver is not painful.

DESCRIPTION OF PROCEDURE: Trigger point injections times three. The risks and benefits of the procedure, including bleeding, infection, and possible pneumothorax were discussed with the patient. Written consent was obtained and placed in the chart. The patient was placed supine on the stretcher, and the area above his right lower costal border was prepped with Betadine. The area was palpated, and a total of three tender areas were identified, one at the sternal border and two more on the surface of the rib. Each area was injected with 3 cc of 0.5% bupivacaine containing 2 mg of Depo-Medrol per cc. The patient tolerated the procedure well.

ASSESSMENT AND PLAN: The patient presents with a complicated pain problem that has no apparent etiology. The patient's observation of temporal relationship to eating raises the question of gallbladder or pancreatic involvement. However, all studies thus far have been negative. The patient does display significant tenderness in the area of the lower costal border on the right. He has received local anesthetic injections in the area of his pain. He was instructed to immediately take food and to observe whether the expected discomfort was felt as usual or whether the injections provided did, indeed, cause him to be relieved. The patient is to follow up in approximately two weeks for reevaluation. If this procedure provides him with some relief, it will be repeated. If it does not, an intercostal block would be considered as a next step in eliminating musculoskeletal causes of his pain. Further investigation might include celiac plexus block. If the patient's pain appears to be visceral, the patient is to follow up in two weeks.

PARAVERTEBRAL FACET NERVE BLOCK

DIAGNOSES: Chronic low axial low back pain, lumbar disk disease, and lumbar facet arthritis with spondylolisthesis.

PROCEDURE: Initial outpatient consultation and medial branch blocks of the L3–4, L4–5, and L5-S1 levels bilaterally.

INDICATIONS AND BACKGROUND: The patient is referred to our service for evaluation and treatment of chronic axial low back pain. The patient first began experiencing pain in 1991, after being involved in a motor vehicle accident. The patient was involved in a second motor vehicle accident in 1996, which caused increase in his back pain. The pain currently is located in the low to mid lumbar area, in the mid back, radiates approximately 8 to 10 cm bilaterally. The patient has experienced some radicular pain in the past; however, this has not occurred for a number of years. He best describes the pain as an aching, burning-type pain with occasional stabbing component, at worst a 10/10, at best a 3/10. Sitting or standing tends to bring the pain on; lying down or using his inversion table tends to relieve the pain somewhat. He denies any numbness or tingling. He denies any weakness. The pain is affecting his sleep, appetite, physical activity, and concentration.

PAST TREATMENT MODALITIES: The patient has had physical therapy with no lasting results. He has undergone a course of acupuncture, without significant relief. The patient underwent a series of epidural steroid injections in 1996. These did provide relief of the radicular portion of his pain, however, did not affect the axial portion. He does use an inversion table, which he states does provide temporary relief on a consistent basis. He is using narcotic medications. The patient has been seen in the past by another doctor and had been placed on a Duragesic patch. The patient's last MRI shows degenerative arthritis and degenerative disk changes at L3-L4 and L4-L5 with mild disk bulging. These appear stable and unchanged compared to the prior exam. The lateral recesses and neural foramina are patent, and the patient is status post surgery at L5-S1 with minimal left epidural fibrosis, which appears to be slightly less prominent when compared to the prior exam. There is also mild spondylosis and mild to moderate concentric disk bulging at L5-S1, extending into the undersurface of both neural foramen, but slightly greater on the right than the left. This bulging is more pronounced compared to the prior exam. The exiting right L5 nerve root is not significantly affected. The lateral recesses at L5-S1 are patent, and no central stenosis is noted.

PAST MEDICAL HISTORY: The patient's past medical history is significant only for increased cholesterol and previous hospitalizations. The patient was hospitalized in 1996 for a motor vehicle accident. In 1991 the patient underwent L5-S1 laminectomy. In 1995 he had testicular cancer, which was treated by orchiectomy. He had an appendectomy in 1990.

MEDICATIONS: The patient currently taking Vioxx 25 mg q.d. He is using a Duragesic patch 75 mcg/h. He also uses Lipitor. He is taking Effexor and Zyban. It also states he is using Demerol 100 mg p.r.n. for breakthrough pain.

ALLERGIES: The patient has no known drug allergies.

SOCIAL HISTORY: The patient lives with his family and is on disability from his job as a plumber. He has a psychiatric history consisting of depression, for which he is currently being treated with antidepressants.

SUBSTANCE USE: The patient is a smoker, smoking approximately one-half pack per day, which he has done for approximately 20 years. He denies alcohol or recreational drug use.

PHYSICAL EXAMINATION: Vital signs reveal blood pressure 128/80, pulse 93. On physical exam, the patient is a well-developed male, in no apparent distress. He arrives ambulatory with a cane for assistance and is able to move about the examination area but does display some mild history of moderate pain behavior. Examination of his back reveals a well-healed scar over the lower lumbar area. No signs of infection are noted. The spinous processes are well aligned. Palpation reveals some mild tenderness over the lower lumbar spinous processes and paravertebral musculature. The patient has increased pain with flexion. However, range of motion in extension is normal.

DESCRIPTION OF PROCEDURE: Paravertebral facet nerve blocks bilaterally. The risks and benefits of the procedure were discussed in detail with the patient, and written consent was obtained. The patient was transported to the fluoroscopy suite and placed prone on the x-ray table with a roll under his abdomen. The patient's back was prepped with Betadine and draped in the usual aseptic manner. The patient's spine was visualized fluoroscopically, and the juncture of the L4 transverse process and the pedicle was located. A skin wheal was raised above it, and a 25-gauge spinal needle was advanced until contact was made with the superior edge of the transverse process at its juncture with the pedicle. Isovue contrast, 0.2 cc, was injected to visualize spread. Then 1 cc of 0.5% bupivacaine was injected incrementally with frequent negative aspiration. This process was repeated at the L5 transverse process and the juncture of the sacral ala, on both the right and the left-hand side, for a total of six injections. The patient tolerated the procedure well and was returned to our area, where he stayed for approximately 15 minutes, and was then discharged to home.

ASSESSMENT AND PLAN: The patient presents with a long history of chronic back pain. The patient has responded to epidural steroid injections in the past; however, it was noted that he had significant psychiatric reactions to the steroids, even though they helped with his sciatic pain. The patient's pain pattern is nonspecific but does suggest that either facet-joint disease or discogenic pain may be involved. We have provided the patient with a three-level bilateral medial branch block of his lumbar facets. If he receives significant pain relief, this would indicate that the facet joints are generating a substantial portion of his pain. The patient is to follow up in one week for reevaluation and possible repeat medial branch blocks. The patient is to continue on his Duragesic patch, 75 mcg/h. He was provided with a prescription for that medication at this time.

INTERROGATION AND REPROGRAMMING OF SPINAL CORD STIMULATOR

DIAGNOSES

1. Postlaminectomy pain syndrome.
2. Status post dual-lead spinal cord stimulator implantation.

PROCEDURES PERFORMED

1. Follow-up outpatient consultation.
2. Interrogation and reprogramming of spinal cord stimulator.

INDICATIONS AND BACKGROUND INFORMATION: The patient was seen in our practice last year for postoperative staple removal following spinal cord stimulator generator replacement. He has been taking one 20-mg OxyContin tablet per day, and Vicodin ES, approximately one twice daily for pain. We have been asked to reprogram the spinal cord stimulator for a change in his stimulation pattern due to inadequate coverage of his postlaminectomy pain symptoms. The patient is having no difficulty with this current medication regimen. Although we did not initially prescribe OxyContin at a dose of 20 mg once per day, the patient has found that this regimen offers him significant relief of pain symptoms, particularly late in the day and during the evening, and taking Vicodin early in the day offers less sedation; overall the patient is satisfied with this current regimen and, therefore, we will not change. The patient's spinal cord stimulator has been reprogrammed. Current settings have been placed into the current clinic chart. Channel one: 0 positive, 1 negative, 3 positive. Channel two: 6 positive, 7 negative. The patient's percent therapy time is 32%. An additional prescription for OxyContin 20 mg, #30, to be utilized one q.d., has been provided, dated today's date, and the patient is to follow up in one month for reevaluation and ongoing medical care.

INTERROGATION, REPROGRAMMING, AND REFILL OF INTRATHECAL PUMP

DIAGNOSES

1. Postlaminectomy pain syndrome.
2. Intractable low back pain and lower extremity radiculopathy.
3. Status post intrathecal pump implantation.

PROCEDURES PERFORMED

1. Follow-up outpatient consultation.
2. Interrogation and reprogramming of intrathecal pump.
3. Intrathecal pump refill, morphine 15 mg/mL mixed in 0.75% bupivacaine, daily rate increased to 2.4 mg per 24 hours.

DESCRIPTION OF PROCEDURE: The patient is returning for routine intrathecal pump maintenance and intrathecal pump refill. He is having no adverse side effects or sequelae, persistent of breakthrough pain, and is requesting an increase in his current intrathecal rate. The area overlying this gentleman's intrathecal pump was aseptically prepared and draped. The central port of the pump was localized, and a local anesthetic skin wheal raised. A 22-gauge Huber needle was inserted through this local anesthetic skin wheal, into the central port of the pump, to contact the posterior wall. The residual volume in the pump was aspirated, compared to calculated, and discarded. The intrathecal pump was then filled with the admixture above, a total of 18 mL. The tubing was opened to atmospheric pressure, to demonstrate no overpressurization, and the Huber needle was removed. The intrathecal pump was reprogrammed to reflect a current reservoir volume of 18 mL, an increased daily rate of 2.4 mg per 24, and a change in morphine concentration of 15 mg/mL, with a single-bolus bridge dose of 6.336 mg for 20 hours and 58 minutes. The patient has been given a follow-up appointment in two weeks for reevaluation and interrogation and reprogramming of the intrathecal pump at that time, if there is persistent breakthrough pain.

Percutaneous Insertion of Spinal Cord Stimulator Lead

Preoperative Diagnoses

1. Recurrent low back pain with left lower extremity radiculopathy.
2. Status post L5-S1 diskectomy.

Postoperative Diagnoses

1. Recurrent low back pain with left lower extremity radiculopathy.
2. Status post L5-S1 diskectomy.

Procedure Performed: Percutaneous insertion, T12-L1 Quad Plus 33-cm spinal cord stimulator lead, tip at T9-proximal.

Anesthesia: Monitored anesthesia care.

Estimated Blood Loss: Minimal.

IV Fluids: Lactated Ringer.

Preoperative Antibiotics: Ancef 1 g IV.

Complications: None.

Disposition: To ambulatory surgery department and then discharged home.

Followup: Five days for percutaneous lead removal.

Description of Operative Procedure: After failure of conservative management for residual back low back pain and left lower extremity radiculopathy, informed consent was obtained from the patient to proceed with a percutaneous spinal cord stimulation trial. The patient was taken to the operating room where she was positioned prone with the roll underneath the abdomen. The lumbosacral spine was aseptically prepared and draped.

Under fluoroscopic guidance, the T12-L1 interspace was visualized, and a local anesthetic skin wheal was raised in a left paramedian approach. A 15-gauge Medtronic Tuohy needle was inserted through this local anesthetic skin wheal, where it was advanced on the first attempt into epidural placement in the midline of T12-L1 with a loss-of-resistance technique. No heme, CSF, or paresthesias were elicited.

The Quad Plus spinal cord stimulator lead was easily threaded in a cephalad direction, initially central and then repositioned to a slightly left paramedian position, approximately 1 mm left lateral from midline, with the tip lying at the proximal aspect of the T9 vertebral body. Trial stimulation was performed and, with mild manipulation in a cephalocaudad direction, 90 to 100% coverage of the areas of this patient's pain were covered with spinal cord stimulation with several configurations and electrodes being used. The patient at this point was satisfied with this area of coverage and decision to trial the lead was made. The Tuohy needle was removed with continuous fluoroscopic evidence of no lead migration. The lead was secured at the level of the skin with one 2–0 silk suture and then aseptically dressed to the left lateral flank with 2 × 2 and Tegaderm.

The patient was then transported to the ambulatory surgery department in stable condition with an intact neurological evaluation, where postprocedural trial stimulation was performed and education on limitations for the percutaneous trial. The patient is to follow up in five days for percutaneous lead removal. An appointment has been provided. She has also been encouraged to contact our office in the interim if there is any change in stimulation pattern or any question that the trial would be unsuccessful so that we may reprogram her spinal cord stimulator lead before reaching the end of the trial period.

PERCUTANEOUS INSERTION, L2–3, OF QUAD PLUS SPINAL CORD STIMULATOR LEADS; SURGICAL IMPLANTATION OF SYNERGY SPINAL CORD STIMULATOR GENERATOR, LEFT POSTERIOR ILIAC FOSSA

PREOPERATIVE DIAGNOSES

1. Postlaminectomy pain syndrome with intractable low back pain and right lower extremity radiculopathy.
2. Status post sacroiliac joint fusion times three, right.
3. Status post successful outpatient spinal cord stimulation trial.

Postoperative Diagnoses

1. Postlaminectomy pain syndrome with intractable low back pain and right lower extremity radiculopathy.
2. Status post sacroiliac joint fusion times three, right.
3. Status post successful outpatient spinal cord stimulation trial.

Procedures Performed

1. Percutaneous insertion, L2–3, dual-lead Quad Plus spinal cord stimulator leads, with surgical implantation.
2. Surgical implantation Synergy spinal cord stimulator generator, left posterior iliac fossa.

Anesthesia: Monitored anesthesia care.

Estimated Blood Loss: Minimal.

IV Fluids: Lactated Ringer, 800 cc.

Preoperative Antibiotics: Ancef 1 g IV.

Complications: None.

Disposition: To home.

Followup: Nine days for percutaneous staple removal.

Description of Operative Procedure: Informed consent was obtained from the patient to proceed with permanent spinal cord stimulator implantation. After a successful spinal cord stimulation trial, we have elected to proceed with permanent implantation, with dual leads for improved coverage of the patient's lower back symptoms. She had at least 70% relief of her right lower extremity radiculopathy symptoms overall, with a single-lead trial.

The patient was taken to the operating room, where she was positioned prone with the roll underneath the abdomen. The area overlying the lumbosacral spine as well as the posterior iliac fossa on the left were all aseptically prepared and draped. Initially the L2–3 interspace was fluoroscopically imaged. Local anesthetic skin wheals were raised at both right and left paramedian approaches.

The Medtronic 15-gauge Tuohy needle was inserted through each of these local anesthetic skin wheals and directed to enter the epidural space in a midline position with a loss-of-resistance-to-saline technique bilaterally. No heme, CSF, or paresthesias were elicited.

At this point the Quad Plus leads were easily threaded cephalad, one lead in a slightly right paramedian position approximately 1 to 2 mm right lateral of midline, and a second lead in an essentially midline position anatomically. The leads were threaded up to approximately the T10 vertebral body height, and with minor manipulation in a cephalocaudad direction, excellent coverage of the right lower extremity and right sacroiliac joint area was able to be obtained with the right-sided lead, and excellent coverage of the patient's lower back and left buttock was able to be obtained with the physiologic midline lead.

The patient is documenting at least 90 to 100% coverage of her painful areas in a stimulation pattern, which was as good or better than her spinal cord stimulation trial.

A decision to implant the leads at this location was made, and with a local anesthesia, a skin incision was made in the midline at the needle insertion sites, and dissection to expose the supraspinous ligament at this level was performed. The leads were secured to the supraspinous ligament with two 2–0 silk sutures, and the spinal cord stimulator anchor. Documentation of no lead migration was performed. Trial stimulation was again performed to document no change in stimulation pattern.

This incision was then copiously irrigated with antibiotic irrigation, and strict hemostasis was obtained. Incision was made in the region of the posterior iliac fossa. Again, after local anesthetic infiltration and dissection to form a pocket, the spinal cord stimulator was implanted in the subcutaneous tissue. Again, copious antibiotic irrigation was utilized in this incision, and strict hemostasis was obtained.

The catheter passer was placed from the midline incision to the pocket, and the leads passed from midline lumbar incision to the pocket, connected to the extensions with the torque screwdriver, covered with the enclosed sheath, and secured with two 2–0 silk sutures each. The extensions were connected to the spinal cord stimulator generator with the midline lead in channel one and the right-sided lead in channel two. These leads were secured again with the torque screwdriver.

The generator was placed into the pocket with the lettering facing the skin, and excess extension and lead coiled underneath the generator. Both midline lumbar incision and pocket were closed with two layers of 2–0 Vicryl sutures, staples at the skin, and aseptically dressed with 4 × 4's and Tegaderm.

The patient was then transported to the ambulatory surgery department, with a stable neurological evaluation, and discharged to home. The Medtronic representative performed the postprocedure training, and adequate stimulation coverage was documented at the time of her discharge, and complete discharge instructions have been provided.

The patient is to contact our office in the interim with any questions or concerns or changes in spinal cord stimulation pattern.

Appendix 5

Common Terms by Procedure

Pain Clinic Consultation for Medication Management

axial low back pain
breakthrough pain
cognitive functioning
decompressive lumbar laminectomy
intrathecal narcotic trial
intrathecal pump
lower extremity radiculopathy
lumbar laminectomy
medication management
OxyContin
Percocet
postlaminectomy pain syndrome

Pain Management Psychometric Evaluation

behavioral medicine
depressive symptom
emotional intensity
interpretable profile
Minnesota Multiphasic Personal Inventory (MMPI)
psychological interpretation
psychologically immature
self-deprecation
Welsh code

Caudal Epidural Steroid Injection

aching-type pain
anesthetized
AP view (anteroposterior)
Betadine
bony prominence
caudal epidural steroid injection
degenerative hip disease
Depo-Medrol
Duragesic patch
epidural space
epidural spread
epidural steroid injection
fluoroscopic guidance
fluoroscopic view
fluoroscopy suite
frequent negative aspiration
hemiarthroplasty
injected incrementally
Isovue contrast material
lateral projection
lateral view
0.5% lidocaine
locality of pain
lumbar disk disease
negative aspiration
OxyContin
Percocet
pressure paresthesia
sacral element
sacral epidural space
sacral hiatus
sacral pain
sacroiliac joint pain
sequela
sharp angulation
strong angulation
subcutaneous tissue
surgical intervention
Tuohy needle
usual aseptic fashion
x-ray table

Cervical Epidural Steroid Injection

aseptic fashion
Betadine
C6-C7 level
cervical disk disease
cervical diskectomy
cervical epidural steroid injection

Depo-Medrol
dissipated quickly
epidural space
epidural spread
fluoroscopic guidance
fluoroscopy suite
frequent negative aspiration
injected incrementally
interspace
Isovue contrast material
1% lidocaine
loss-of-resistance-to-saline technique
midline approach
mild pressure paresthesia
needle placement
preservative-free normal saline
pressure paresthesia
sequela
subcutaneous tissue
thenar eminence
Tuohy needle
usual aseptic fashion
written consent
x-ray table

L4–5 Transforaminal Epidural Steroid Injection

adverse event
adverse side effect
AP fluoroscopic imaging
(anteroposterior)
appropriate placement
aseptically prepared and draped
as-needed basis
contrast confirmation
decompressive lumbar laminectomy
Depo-Medrol
fluoroscopic guidance
fluoroscopy suite
injected slowly and incrementally
Isovue 200 contrast
local anesthetic skin wheal
lower extremity radiculopathy
L4–5 foramen
lumbosacral spine
neuroforaminal stenosis
oblique fluoroscopic image
overall benefit
Percocet
positioned prone
preservative-free normal saline
recurrent symptom
risks and benefits
routine postprocedural instruction
sequela
skin wheal
slowly and incrementally
spinal needle
transforaminal aspect
transforaminal epidural steroid injection

L4–5 Translaminar Epidural Steroid Injection

appendectomy
appropriate epidural layering
aseptically prepared and draped
bilateral lower extremity radiculopathy
bilateral neuroforaminal narrowing
bowel or bladder dysfunction
Caltrate
Celebrex
central canal stenosis
contrast confirmation
cutaneous infection
cyanosis, clubbing or edema
Darvocet
degenerative disk disease
Depo-Medrol
empirical trial
epidural layering
epidural placement
first attempt
fluoroscopic guidance
fluoroscopy suite
focal motor weakness
Fosamax

heme, CSF, or paresthesia
hemorrhoidectomy
interspace
Isovue 200 contrast
kyphosis
local anesthetic skin wheal
lower extremity radiculopathy symptom
lumbar epidural steroid injection
lumbar lordosis
lumbosacral spine
multilevel symptomatic spinal stenosis
neurogenic claudication
neuroforaminal narrowing
neurologic sequela
no acute distress
nonfocal
osteoporosis
palpable tenderness
paraspinous musculature
penicillin
peripheral neurological evaluation
physical therapy
postdural puncture headache
postprocedural instruction
preservative-free normal saline
progressive pain
radiculopathy symptom
sacroiliac joint
semiurgent basis
skin wheal
spinal stenosis
symptomatic management
thoracic spine
translaminar epidural steroid injection
Tuohy needle
Ultram

L5-S1 Transforaminal Epidural Steroid Injection

adverse sequela
anular fissure
anteroposterior (AP) fluoroscopic imaging
aseptically prepared and draped
contrast confirmation
degenerative disk change
Depo-Medrol
diskectomy
epidural steroid injection
fluoroscopic guidance
fluoroscopy suite
focal disk herniation
interventional nerve block
intractable refractory pain
Isovue 200 contrast
L5-S1 foramen
local anesthetic skin wheal
lower extremity radiculopathy
lumbosacral spine
neural impingement
nonsurgical candidate
oblique fluoroscopic imaging
postprocedure instruction
preservative-free normal saline
provocative pressure paresthesia
radicular symptom
recurrent left lower back pain
refractory pain
scar tissue
skin wheal
slowly and incrementally
spinal cord stimulation
spinal needle
transforaminal approach
transforaminal epidural steroid injection
transforaminal placement
translaminar epidural steroid injection

Trigger Point Injection

Azmacort
Betadine
bupivacaine
Candida esophagitis
celiac plexus block

computerized tomography scan (CT)
costal border
Depo-Medrol
Diflucan
esophagogastroduodenoscopy (EGD)
gallbladder
generalized malaise
HIDA scan (dimethyl iminodiacetic acid)
intercostal block
local anesthetic injection
musculoskeletal cause
outpatient consultation
pancreatic involvement
peptic ulcer disease
pneumothorax
Prevacid
Prilosec
recreational drug use
Singulair
sternal border
temporal relationship
trigger point injection
Tylenol
visceral

Paravertebral Facet Nerve Block

acupuncture
antidepressant
appendectomy
axial low back pain
axial portion
Betadine
bupivacaine
burning-type pain
central stenosis
concentric disk bulging
degenerative arthritis
degenerative disk change
Demerol
discogenic pain
disk bulging
Duragesic patch
Effexor
epidural fibrosis
epidural steroid injection
facet joint
facet-joint disease
fluoroscopy suite
frequent negative aspiration
injected incrementally
inversion table
Isovue contrast
laminectomy
lateral recess
lumbar disk disease
lumbar facet arthritis
medial branch block
narcotic medication
negative aspiration
nerve root
neural foramina
numbness or tingling
orchiectomy
paravertebral facet nerve block
paravertebral musculature
pedicle
radicular pain
radicular portion
sacral ala
sciatic pain
series of epidural steroid injections
skin wheal
spinal needle
spinous process
spondylolisthesis
spondylosis
stabbing component
testicular cancer
transverse process
undersurface
usual aseptic manner
Vioxx
visualized fluoroscopically
well-healed scar

x-ray table
Zyban

Interrogation and Reprogramming of Spinal Cord Stimulator

dual-lead spinal cord stimulator implantation
inadequate coverage
interrogation and reprogramming
medication regimen
OxyContin
percent therapy time
postlaminectomy pain symptom
postlaminectomy pain syndrome
reprogram
spinal cord stimulator generator replacement
spinal cord stimulator implantation
stimulation pattern
Vicodin ES

Interrogation, Reprogramming, and Refill of Intrathecal Pump

adverse side effect
aseptically prepared and draped
aspirated
atmospheric pressure
breakthrough pain
bridge dose
bupivacaine
central port
compared to calculated
daily rate
Huber needle
interrogation and reprogramming
intractable low back pain
intrathecal pump implantation
intrathecal pump maintenance
intrathecal pump refill
local anesthetic skin wheal
lower extremity radiculopathy
morphine
overpressurization
posterior wall
postlaminectomy pain syndrome
reprogrammed
reservoir volume
residual volume
sequela
single-bolus bridge dose
skin wheal
tubing

Percutaneous Insertion of Spinal Cord Stimulator Lead

ambulatory surgery department
Ancef
aseptically dressed
aseptically prepared and draped
cephalad direction
cephalocaudad direction
configuration
conservative management
diskectomy
electrode
epidural placement
fluoroscopic evidence
fluoroscopic guidance
heme, CSF, or paresthesia
interspace
lactated Ringer
lead migration
lead removal
local anesthetic skin wheal
loss-of-resistance technique
lower extremity radiculopathy
lumbosacral spine
Medtronic Tuohy needle
neurological evaluation
paramedian approach
percutaneous insertion
percutaneous spinal cord stimulation trial
percutaneous trial

positioned prone
postprocedural trial stimulation
proximal aspect
Quad Plus spinal cord stimulator lead
recurrent low back pain
reprogram
residual low back pain
skin wheal
spinal cord stimulation trial
spinal cord stimulator lead
stimulation pattern
Tegaderm
trial stimulation
Tuohy needle
vertebral body

Percutaneous Insertion, L2–3, of Quad Plus Spinal Cord Stimulator Leads; Surgical Implantation of Synergy Spinal Cord Stimulator Generator, Left Posterior Iliac Fossa

ambulatory surgery department
Ancef
antibiotic irrigation
aseptically dressed
aseptically prepared and draped
catheter passer
cephalad
cephalocaudad direction
copiously irrigated
dual-lead Quad Plus spinal cord stimulator lead
epidural space
fluoroscopically imaged
heme, CSF, or paresthesia
informed consent
interspace
intractable low back pain
lactated Ringer
lead migration
local anesthetic infiltration
local anesthetic skin wheal
loss-of-resistance-to-saline technique
lower extremity radiculopathy
lumbosacral spine
Medtronic Tuohy needle
midline incision
midline position
monitored anesthesia care
needle insertion site
neurological evaluation
paramedian approach
paramedian position
percutaneous insertion
permanent implantation
permanent spinal cord stimulator implantation
physiologic midline lead
posterior iliac fossa
postlaminectomy pain syndrome
Quad Plus spinal cord stimulator lead
radiculopathy symptom
sacroiliac joint fusion
silk suture
single-lead trial
skin wheal
spinal cord stimulator anchor
spinal cord stimulator generator
spinal cord stimulator implantation
spinal cord stimulation trial
staple removal
stimulation coverage
stimulation pattern
strict hemostasis
subcutaneous tissue
supraspinous ligament
surgical implantation
Synergy spinal cord stimulator generator
Tegaderm
torque screwdriver
trial stimulation
Tuohy needle
Vicryl suture

Appendix 6

Dermatomal Explanation

Dermatome	Area Innervated and Reflex Elicited	Nerve Affected
C2	occiput, top part of neck	
C3	lower part of neck to clavicle	
C4	area just below the clavicle, deltoids	
C5	lateral arm, at and above the elbow, brachioradialis, infraspinatus, supraspinatus, deltoid, biceps	axillary
C6	forearm, radial side of hand wrist extensors	radial, thumb median, index finger
C7	pronator teres, flexor carpi ulnaris, latissimus dorsi, triceps, long finger	median, long finger
C8	lateral aspect of hand, wrist extensors and flexors, finger flexors	ulnar, small finger
T1	medial forearm, little finger adductor	medial brachial cutaneous
T2	sternal notch	intercostal
T3-T12	chest and back to hip girdle	
T4	nipples	intercostal
T6	xiphoid process	intercostal
T10	umbilicus	intercostal
L1	inguinal ligament	ilioinguinal, iliohypogastric

Dermatome	Area Innervated and Reflex Elicited	Nerve Affected
L2	iliopsoas, hip flexors	anterior femoral, lateral femoral
L3	adductor longus, hip adductors, quadriceps, patellar reflex	obturator
L4	vastus lateralis, knee extensors, vastus medialis, ankle dorsiflexors, anterior tibialis, patellar reflex	saphenous
L5	hip abductors, ankle dorsiflexion, eversion and inversion, long toe extensors, hallucis longus	deep peroneal
S1	hip extensors, ankle plantar flexors, gastrocnemius, heel, middle of back of leg, Achilles reflex	sural
S2	back of thigh	
S3	medial side of buttocks	
S4/5	perineal region, anal sphincter	
S5	skin at and adjacent to anus	

Appendix 7

American Academy of Pain Management (AAPM) Accredited Pain Programs

This list includes facilities that have passed the American Academy of Pain Management's rigorous Pain Program Accreditation testing and on-site inspection, and that participate in additional AAPM services and status. For additional information, please visit www.aapainmanage.org.

ALABAMA

A Center for Conservative Foot Care—Bessemer
519 4th Avenue SW
Bessemer, AL 35023

SRJR Health Care Inc.
2315 Lurleen Wallace Boulevard
Northport, AL 35476

CALIFORNIA

Pacific Center
2155 Webster Street
San Francisco, CA 94115

Pain and Rehabilitation Medical Group
3445 Pacific Coast Highway, #300
Torrance, CA 90505

Pasadena Rehabilitation Institute
1017 South Fairoaks
Pasadena, CA 91105

Robb Pain Managment Group
12840 Riverside Drive, #208
North Hollywood, CA 91607

COLORADO

Craniofacial Diagnostic Center
1660 South Albion, Suite 1008
Denver, CO 80222

FLORIDA

Springer Group
9120 NW 36th Place
Gainesville, FL 32606

Wuesthoff Pain Management Center
110 Longwood Avenue
Rockledge, FL 32955

GEORGIA

Pain Control & Rehabilitation Institute of Georgia, Inc.
2786 North Decatur Road, #220
Decatur, GA 30033

Southern Pain Control Center
P.O. Box 962677
Riverdale, GA 30296-6926

ILLINOIS

Interventional Pain Management
455 South Roselle Road, Suite 127
Schaumburg, IL 60193

Kishwaukee Healthcare Systems
c/o Kishwaukee Community Hospital
626 Bethany Road
DeKalb, IL 60115

INDIANA

Oliver Headache and Pain Clinic
2828 Mount Vernon Avenue
Evansville, IN 47712

KENTUCKY

Ephraim McDowell Regional Medical Center
Pain Management Center
217 South Third Street
Danville, KY 40422

Spine & Brain Neurosurgical Center
1721 Nicholasville Road
Lexington, KY 40503

MARYLAND

The Pain Center
Greater Baltimore Medical Center
6701 North Charles Street
Baltimore, MD 21204

MASSACHUSETTS

Catholic Memorial Home Pain Management Program
2446 Highland Avenue
Fall River, MA 02720

Madonna Manor Pain Program
85 North Washington Street
North Attleboro, MA 02760

Marian Manor
33 Summer Street
Taunton, MA 02780-3491

Our Lady's Haven Pain Management Program
71 Center Street
Fairhaven, MA 02719

Sacred Heart Home Pain Management Program
359 Summer Street
New Bedford, MA 02740

MICHIGAN

North Oakland Pain Management Service
1305 North Oakland Boulevard
Waterford, MI 48327

Patrick T. Kelly, DDS
1320 West Ridge Street
Marquette, MI 49855

MISSISSIPPI

Pain Treatment Center
Rush Foundation Hospital
1314 19th Avenue
Meridian, MS 39301

MISSOURI

Headache Care Center
1230 East Kingsley
Springfield, MO 65804

NEW HAMPSHIRE

Cottage Hospital Pain Clinic
P.O. Box 2001
90 Swiftwater Road
Woodsville, NH 03785

NEW JERSEY

North Jersey Center for Surgery
39 Newton Sparta Road
Newton, NJ 07860

Pain Control Center of New Jersey
561 Cranbury Road
East Brunswick, NJ 08816

The Back Rehab Institute (Hamilton)
1245 Whitehorse-Mercerville Road
Hamilton Township, NJ 08619

The Back Rehab Institute (Margate)
9401 Ventnor Avenue
Margate, NJ 08402

NEW YORK

Healthworks of Staten Island
585 North Gannon Avenue
Staten Island, NY 10314

The Kingston Hospital Pain Management Service
396 Broadway
Kingston, NY 12401

OHIO

Grandview Hospital & Medical Center
405 Grand Avenue
Dayton, OH 45405-4796

Hal Blatman, MD
10653 Techwoods Cr, #101
Cincinnati, OH 45242

The St. Joseph Pain Management Center
662 Eastland Avenue
Eastland Medical II Building, #201
Warren, OH 44484

Whiteamire Clinic P.A., Inc.
2031 Park Avenue West
Mansfield, OH 44906

PENNSYLVANIA

Gettysburg Rehabilitation Services
124 Carlisle Street
Gettysburg, PA 17325

Jefferson Pain & Rehabilitation Center
4735 Clairton Boulevard
Pittsburgh, PA 15236

John J. Bowden, Jr., DO
P.O. Box 14299
Philadelphia, PA 19138-0299

Joseph L. Kaczor
2606 Broad Avenue
Altoona, PA 16601

Latrobe Anesthesia Associates, Inc.
121 West Second Avenue
Latrobe, PA 15650

Michael S. Melnick, D.M.D., M.A.G.D.
The Park Plaza, #207
128 North Craig Street
Pittsburgh, PA 15213

Sarah and Benjamin Lincow Pain Foundation
7622 Ogontz Avenue
Philadelphia, PA 19150

The Montgomery Surgical Center
One Adington Plaza, #202
Jenkintown, PA 19046

TEXAS

Acute & Chronic Pain & Spine Center
5211-B West 9th Avenue
Amarillo, TX 79106

Center for Rehabilitative Medicine
1307 8th Avenue, #610
Ft. Worth, TX 76104

Central Imaging of Arlington
1015 West Randol Mill Road
Arlington, TX 76012

Healthsouth
3340 Plaza 10 Boulevard
Beaumont, TX 77707

Lake Arlington Center for Pain Management
6702 West Poly Webb Road
Arlington, TX 76016

Rio Grande Health Center
7230 Gateway East, Suite E
El Paso, TX 79915

Tri-County Pain Management Centre
200 North Arch Street
P.O. Box 758
Royse City, TX 75189

Warm Springs Rehab Center NW
7616 Culebra Road, Suite 115
San Antonio, TX 78251-1476

UTAH

Alpine Pain Clinic
1960 Sidewinder Drive, #106
Park City, UT 84060

VIRGINIA

Myofascial Pain Treatment Center
6417 Loisdale Road, #308
Springfield, VA 22150

WASHINGTON

The Mustard Clinic
North 1414 Vercler, #3
Spokane, WA 99216

Appendix 8

Drugs Commonly Used in Pain Practice

acetaminophen
acetylsalicylic acid
amitriptyline
amoxapine
Anafranil®
Anaprox®
Ansaid® Oral
Aristocort®
Asendin® (Can)
aspirin
Atarax®
Ativan®
baclofen
Benadryl® Injection
Benadryl® Oral [OTC]
Benylin® Codeine (Can)
butalbital-caffeine-Tylenol/ASA
capsaicin
carbamazepine
Catapres® Oral
Catapres-TTS® Transdermal
Celebrex™
celecoxib
chlorpromazine
choline magnesium trisalicylate
Clinoril®
clomipramine
clonazepam
clonidine
codeine
Compazine®
cyclobenzaprine
Demerol®
Depakene®
desipramine
dexamphetamine
dextromethorphan
D.H.E. 45
diazepam
diclofenac
diflunisal
dihydroergotamine
Dilantin®
Dilaudid-HP® Injection
Dilaudid® Injection
Dilaudid® Oral
Dilaudid® Suppository
diphenhydramine
Disalcid®
Dolobid®
Dolophine®
doxepin
droperidol
Elavil®
Ergomar®
etodolic acid
Feldene®
fenoprofen
Fioricet®
Fiorinal®
Flexeril®
fluoxetine
flurbiprofen
gabapentin
Haldol®
Haldol® Decanoate
haloperidol
hydrocodone
hydromorphone
hydroxyzine
ibuprofen
imipramine
Imitrex®
Inapsine®
Indocin® Oral
Indocin® SR Oral
indomethacin
Kenalog® Topical
ketoprofen
ketorolac

Klonopin™
lamotrigine
Levo-Dromoran®
levorphanol
Lioresal®
Lodine®
Lodine® XL
lorazepam
Lorcet® 10/650
Lorcet®-HD
Lorcet® Plus
meclofenamate
meperidine
methadone
methylphenidate
methylprednisolone
metoclopramide
mexiletine
morphine
Motrin®
Motrin® IB [OTC]
MS Contin® Oral
Nalfon®
naloxone
naproxen
naproxen sodium
Norpramin®
nortriptyline
ondansetron
Orudis®
Orudis® KT [OTC]
oxycodone
OxyContin®
Pamelor®
Percocet® 2.5/325
Percocet® 5/325
Percocet® 7.5/500
Percocet® 10/650
Percocet®-Demi (Can)
Percodan®
Percodan®-Demi
perphenazine
phenoxybenzamine
phentolamine
phenylbutazone
phenytoin
piroxicam
prednisolone
prilocaine
prochlorperazine
promethazine
protriptyline
Prozac®
rofecoxib
salsalate
senna
sertraline
Sinequan® Oral
sodium valproate
sulindac
sumatriptan
Tegretol®
Tegretol®-XR
Thorazine®
tizanidine
Tofranil®
Tofranil-PM®
Tolectin®
Tolectin® DS
tolmetin
topiramate
Toradol®
tramadol
triamcinolone
Trilisate®
Tylenol® [OTC]
Ultram®
Valium® Oral
valproic acid
Vicodin®
Vicodin® ES
Vioxx®
Vistaril®
Vivactil®
Voltaren® Oral
Voltaren Rapide® (Can)

Voltaren®-XR Oral
Zanaflex®
Zoloft®
Zostrix® [OTC]
Zostrix High Potency®
Zostrix®-HP [OTC]

Appendix 9

Drugs Used for Anesthesia

Actiq® Oral Transmucosal
AK-Taine®
Alcaine®
Alfenta®
alfentanil
Ametop™ (Can)
Amidate®
Anestacon® Topical Solution
Apo®-Diazepam (Can)
Arduan®
atracurium
Atropair®
atropine
Atropine-Care®
Atropisol®
Brevital® Sodium
Brietal Sodium® (Can)
bupivacaine
Buscopan® (Can)
Buprenex®
buprenorphine
carbetocin (Can)
Carbocaine®
Chirocaine®
chloroprocaine
cisatracurium
Citanest® Forte
Citanest® Plain
cocaine
Demerol®
desflurane
Diastat® Rectal Delivery System
diazepam
Diazepam Intensol®
Dilocaine® Injection
Diocaine® (Can)
Diprivan®
Dizac® Injectable Emulsion
doxacurium
doxapram
droperidol
droperidol and fentanyl
Duo-Trach® Injection
Duragesic® Transdermal
Duranest®
Duratocin™ (Can)
enflurane
Ethrane®
etidocaine
etomidate
fentanyl
Fentanyl Oralet®
Fluoracaine® Ophthalmic
Forane®
gallamine triethiodide
halothane
Inapsine®
Innovar®
Isocaine® HCl
isoflurane
Isopto® Atropine
Isopto® Hyoscine
I-Tropine®
Ketalar®
ketamine
levobupivacaine
Levo-Dromoran®
levorphanol
lidocaine
lidocaine and epinephrine
Lidodan™ (Can)
Marcaine®
meperidine
mepivacaine
methohexital
methoxyflurane
metocurine iodide
Mivacron®
mivacurium
Naropin™

Nervocaine® Injection
Nesacaine®
Nesacaine®-MPF
Nimbex®
Norcuron®
Novocain®
Numorphan®
Nuromax®
Ophthetic®
oxymorphone
pancuronium
pentazocine
pentazocine compound
Pentothal® Sodium
Penthrane®
pipecuronium
Polocaine®
Pontocaine®
prilocaine
procaine
proparacaine
proparacaine and fluorescein
propofol
rapacuronium
Raplon™
remifentanil
rocuronium
ropivacaine
Scopace® Tablet
scopolamine
Sensorcaine®
Sensorcaine®-MPF
sevoflurane
Sevorane™ (Can)
Sublimaze® Injection
Sufenta®
sufentanil
Suprane®
Talacen®
Talwin®
Talwin® Compound
Talwin® NX
tetracaine
tetracaine and dextrose
thiopental
Tracrium®
Transderm Scop®
Transderm-V® (Can)
tubocurarine
Ultane®
Ultiva™
vecuronium
Vivol® (Can)
Xylocaine® HCl I.V. Injection for Cardiac Arrhythmias
Xylocaine® Oral
Xylocaine® Topical Ointment
Xylocaine® Topical Solution
Xylocaine® Topical Spray
Xylocard® (Can)
Zemuron™

Appendix 10
Drugs by Indication

ANESTHESIA (GENERAL)

Barbiturate
- Brevital® Sodium
- Brietal Sodium® (Can)
- methohexital

General Anesthetic
- Amidate®
- desflurane
- Diprivan®
- enflurane
- Ethrane®
- etomidate
- Forane®
- halothane
- isoflurane
- Ketalar®
- ketamine
- methoxyflurane
- Penthrane®
- propofol
- sevoflurane
- Sevorane™ (Can)
- Suprane®
- Ultane®

ANESTHESIA (LOCAL)

Local Anesthetic
- AK-Taine®
- Alcaine®
- Americaine® [OTC]
- Ametop™ (Can)
- Anbesol® [OTC]
- Anbesol® Baby (Can)
- Anbesol® Maximum Strength [OTC]
- Anestacon® Topical Solution
- Anusol® Ointment [OTC]
- Babee® Teething® [OTC]
- benzocaine
- benzocaine, butyl aminobenzoate, tetracaine, and benzalkonium chloride
- benzocaine, gelatin, pectin, and sodium carboxymethylcellulose
- Benzocol® [OTC]
- Benzodent® [OTC]
- bupivacaine
- Caladryl® Lotion
- Carbocaine®
- Ceepryn® [OTC]
- Cēpacol® Anesthetic Troches [OTC]
- Cēpacol® Troches [OTC]
- Cetacaine®
- cetylpyridinium
- cetylpyridinium and benzocaine
- Chiggertox® [OTC]
- Chirocaine®
- chloroprocaine
- Citanest® Forte
- Citanest® Plain
- cocaine
- Cylex® [OTC]
- Dermoplast® [OTC]
- dibucaine
- Dilocaine® Injection
- Diocaine® (Can)
- Duo-Trach® Injection
- Duranest®
- Dyclone®
- dyclonine
- ethyl chloride
- ethyl chloride and dichlorotetrafluoroethane
- etidocaine
- Fleet® Pain Relief [OTC]
- Fluoracaine® Ophthalmic
- Fluro-Ethyl® Aerosol
- Foille® [OTC]
- Foille® Medicated First Aid [OTC]
- hexylresorcinol
- Hurricaine®
- Isocaine® HCl
- Itch-X® [OTC]

Lanacane® [OTC]
levobupivacaine
lidocaine
lidocaine and epinephrine
Lidodan™ (Can)
LidoPen® I.M. Injection Auto-Injector
Marcaine®
Maximum Strength Anbesol® [OTC]
Maximum Strength Orajel® [OTC]
mepivacaine
Mycinettes® [OTC]
Naropin™
Nervocaine® Injection
Nesacaine®
Nesacaine®-MPF
Novocain®
Numzitdent® [OTC]
Numzit Teething® [OTC]
Nupercainal® [OTC]
Ocu-Caine®
Ophthetic®
Orabase®-B [OTC]
Orabase®-O [OTC]
Orabase® With Benzocaine [OTC]
Orajel® Brace-Aid Oral Anesthetic [OTC]
Orajel® Maximum Strength [OTC]
Orajel® Mouth-Aid [OTC]
Orasept® [OTC]
Orasol® [OTC]
Parcaine®
Phicon® [OTC]
Polocaine®A10
Pontocaine®
Pontocaine® With Dextrose
PrameGel® [OTC]
pramoxine
Prax® [OTC]
prilocaine
procaine
ProctoFoam® NS [OTC]
proparacaine
proparacaine and fluorescein
Rhulicaine® [OTC]
Rid-A-Pain® Dental [OTC]
ropivacaine
Sensorcaine®
Sensorcaine®-MPF
Slim-Mint® [OTC]
Solarcaine® [OTC]
Spec-T® [OTC]
Sucrets® [OTC]
Sucrets® Sore Throat [OTC]
Tanac® [OTC]
tetracaine
tetracaine and dextrose
Trocaine® [OTC]
Tronolane® [OTC]
Unguentine® [OTC]
Vicks® Children's Chloraseptic® [OTC]
Vicks® Chloraseptic® Sore Throat [OTC]
Xylocaine® HCl I.V. Injection for Cardiac Arrhythmias
Xylocaine® Oral
Xylocaine® Topical Ointment
Xylocaine® Topical Solution
Xylocaine® Topical Spray
Xylocaine® With Epinephrine
Xylocard® (Can)
Zilactin®-B Medicated [OTC]

Local Anesthetic, Injectable
Chirocaine®
Levobupivacaine

ANESTHESIA (OPHTHALMIC)

Local Anesthetic
Fluoracaine® Ophthalmic
proparacaine and fluorescein

BACK PAIN (LOW)

Analgesic, Narcotic
codeine
Codeine Contin® (Can)

Analgesic, Non-narcotic

Anacin® [OTC]
Arthritis Foundation® Pain Reliever [OTC]
Arthropan® [OTC]
Ascriptin® [OTC]
aspirin
Asprimox® [OTC]
Bayer® Aspirin [OTC]
Bayer® Buffered Aspirin [OTC]
Bayer® Low Adult Strength [OTC]
Bufferin® [OTC]
Buffex® [OTC]
Cama® Arthritis Pain Reliever [OTC]
choline salicylate
Easprin®
Ecotrin® [OTC]
Ecotrin® Low Adult Strength [OTC]
Empirin® [OTC]
Extra Strength Adprin-B® [OTC]
Extra Strength Bayer® Enteric 500 Aspirin [OTC]
Extra Strength Bayer® Plus [OTC]
Halfprin® 81® [OTC]
Heartline® [OTC]
Regular Strength Bayer® Enteric 500 Aspirin [OTC]
St. Joseph® Adult Chewable Aspirin [OTC]
Teejel® (Can)
ZORprin®

Benzodiazepine
Apo®-Diazepam (Can)
diazepam
Valium® Injection
Valium® Oral
Vivol® (Can)

Nonsteroidal Anti-inflammatory Drug (NSAID)
Back-Ese M (Can)
Doan's Backache Pills (Can)
Doan's®, Original [OTC]
Extra Strength Doan's® [OTC]
Herbogesic (Can)
Magan®
magnesium salicylate
Magsal®
Mobidin®

Skeletal Muscle Relaxant
Aspirin® Backache (Can)
methocarbamol
methocarbamol and aspirin
Methoxisal (Can)
Robaxin®
Robaxisal®

NERVE BLOCK

Local Anesthetic
Ametop™ (Can)
Anestacon® Topical Solution
bupivacaine
Carbocaine®
chloroprocaine
Citanest® Forte
Citanest® Plain
Dilocaine® Injection
Duo-Trach® Injection
Duranest®
etidocaine
Isocaine® HCl
lidocaine
lidocaine and epinephrine
Lidodan™ (Can)
LidoPen® I.M. Injection Auto-Injector
Marcaine®
mepivacaine
Nervocaine® Injection
Nesacaine®
Nesacaine®-MPF
Novocain®
Polocaine®
Pontocaine®
Pontocaine® With Dextrose
prilocaine

procaine
Sensorcaine®
Sensorcaine®-MPF
tetracaine
tetracaine and dextrose
Xylocaine® HCl I.V. Injection for Cardiac Arrhythmias
Xylocaine® Oral
Xylocaine® Topical Ointment
Xylocaine® Topical Solution
Xylocaine® Topical Spray
Xylocaine® With Epinephrine
Xylocard® (Can)

NEURALGIA

Analgesic, Non-narcotic
Arthropan® [OTC]
choline salicylate
Teejel® (Can)
Analgesic, Topical
Antiphlogistine Rub A-535 No Odour (Can)
Arth Dr®
Arthricare Hand & Body®
Born Again Super Pain Relieving®
Caprex®
Caprex Plus®
Capsagel®
Capsagel Extra Strength®
Capsagel Maximum Strength®
Capsagesic-HP Arthritis Relief®
capsaicin
Capsin® [OTC]
Capzasin-P® [OTC]
D-Care Circulation Stimulator®
Dolorex®
Double Cap®
Icy Hot Arthritis Therapy®
Myoflex® [OTC]
Pain Enz®
Pharmacist's Capsaicin®
Rid-A-Pain®
Rid-A-Pain-HP®
Sloan's Liniment®
Sportscreme® [OTC]
Sportsmed®
Theragen®
Theragen HP®
Therapatch Warm®
triethanolamine salicylate
Trixaicin®
Trixaicin HP®
Zostrix® [OTC]
Zostrix High Potency®
Zostrix®-HP [OTC]
Zostrix Sports®
Nonsteroidal Anti-inflammatory Drug (NSAID)
Anacin® [OTC]
Arthritis Foundation® Pain Reliever [OTC]
Ascriptin® [OTC]
Aspergum® [OTC]
aspirin
Asprimox® [OTC]
Bayer® Aspirin [OTC]
Bayer® Buffered Aspirin [OTC]
Bayer® Low Adult Strength [OTC]
Bufferin® [OTC]
Buffex® [OTC]
Cama® Arthritis Pain Reliever [OTC]
Easprin®
Ecotrin® [OTC]
Ecotrin® Low Adult Strength [OTC]
Empirin® [OTC]
Extra Strength Adprin-B® [OTC]
Extra Strength Bayer® Enteric 500 Aspirin [OTC]
Extra Strength Bayer® Plus [OTC]
Halfprin® 81® [OTC]
Heartline® [OTC]
Regular Strength Bayer® Enteric 500 Aspirin [OTC]
St Joseph® Adult Chewable Aspirin [OTC]
ZORprin®

OPHTHALMIC SURGERY

Nonsteroidal Anti-inflammatory Drug (NSAID)
- diclofenac
- Voltaren® Ophthalmic

OPHTHALMIC SURGICAL AID

Ophthalmic Agent, Miscellaneous
- GenTeal™ [OTC]
- Gonak™ [OTC]
- Goniosol® [OTC]
- hydroxypropyl methylcellulose

PAIN

Analgesic, Narcotic
- acetaminophen and codeine
- Actiq® Oral Transmucosal
- Alfenta®
- alfentanil
- Anexsia®
- Anodynos-DHC®
- aspirin and codeine
- Bancap HC®
- belladonna and opium
- B&O Supprettes®
- Buprenex®
- buprenorphine
- butalbital compound and codeine
- butorphanol
- Capital® and Codeine
- codeine
- Codeine Contin® (Can)
- Co-Gesic®
- Coryphen® Codeine (Can)
- Damason-P®
- Darvocet-N®
- Darvocet-N® 100
- Darvon®
- Darvon® Compound-65 Pulvules®
- Darvon-N®
- Demerol®
- DHC Plus®
- dihydrocodeine compound
- Dilaudid® Cough Syrup
- Dilaudid-HP® Injection
- Dilaudid® Injection
- Dilaudid® Oral
- Dilaudid® Suppository
- Dolacet®
- Dolophine®
- droperidol and fentanyl
- DuoCet™
- Duradyne DHC®
- Duragesic® Transdermal
- Duramorph® Injection
- Empirin® With Codeine
- Endocet®
- Endocodone®
- Endodan®
- fentanyl
- Fentanyl Oralet®
- Fiorinal®-C (Can)
- Fiorinal® With Codeine
- Hydrocet®
- hydrocodone and acetaminophen
- hydrocodone and aspirin
- hydrocodone and ibuprofen
- Hydrogesic®
- Hydromorph Contin® (Can)
- hydromorphone
- Hy-Phen®
- Infumorph™
- Innovar®
- Kadian™ Oral
- Lenoltec No 1, 2, 3, 4 (Can)
- Levo-Dromoran®
- levorphanol
- Lorcet® 10/650
- Lorcet®-HD
- Lorcet® Plus
- Lortab®
- Lortab® ASA
- Margesic® H
- Mepergan®
- meperidine

meperidine and promethazine
M-Eslon® (Can)
Metadol™ (Can)
methadone
Methadose® (Can)
morphine sulfate
MS Contin® Oral
MSIR® Oral
nalbuphine
Norcet®
Norco®
Nubain®
Numorphan®
opium tincture
Oramorph SR™ Oral
Oxycocet® (Can)
Oxycodan® (Can)
oxycodone
oxycodone and acetaminophen
oxycodone and aspirin
OxyContin®
OxyIR™
oxymorphone
paregoric
pentazocine
pentazocine compound
Percocet® 2.5/325
Percocet® 5/325
Percocet® 7.5/500
Percocet® 10/650
Percocet®-Demi (Can)
Percodan®
Percodan®-Demi
Percolone®
Phenaphen® With Codeine #3
PMS-Hydromorphone (Can)
Pronap-100®
Propoxacet-N®
propoxyphene
propoxyphene and acetaminophen
propoxyphene and aspirin
Pyregesic-C®
remifentanil
RMS® Rectal
Roxanol™ Oral
Roxanol SR™ Oral
Roxanol-T™
Roxicet® 5/500
Roxicodone™
Roxilox™
Stadol®
Stadol® NS
Stagesic®
Statex® (Can)
Sublimaze® Injection
Sufenta®
sufentanil
Supeudol® (Can)
Synalgos®-DC
222® Tablets (Can)
282® Tablets (Can)
292® Tablets (Can)
624® Tablets (Can)
Talacen®
Talwin®
Talwin® Compound
Talwin® NX
Tecnal C (Can)
T-Gesic®
Triatec-8® (Can)
Triatec-8® Strong (Can)
Triatec-30® (Can)
Tylenol® With Codeine
Tylox®
Ultiva™
Vicodin®
Vicodin® ES
Vicoprofen®
Wygesic®
Zydone®

Analgesic, Non-narcotic
Abenol® (Can)
Acephen® [OTC]
Aceta® [OTC]
Aceta® Children's [OTC]
Acetagesic® [OTC]

acetaminophen
acetaminophen and diphenhydramine
acetaminophen and phenyltoloxamine
acetaminophen, aspirin, and caffeine
Aches-N-Pain® [OTC]
Actamin® [OTC]
Actron® [OTC]
Acular® Ophthalmic
Advil® [OTC]
Aleve® [OTC]
Altenol® [OTC]
Alti-Flurbiprofen (Can)
Alti-Piroxicam (Can)
Amdol 500® [OTC]
Amdol 650® [OTC]
Amdoplus® [OTC]
Amigesic®
Aminofen® [OTC]
Aminofen Plus® [OTC]
Anacin® [OTC]
Anacin® P.M. Aspirin Free [OTC]
Anagesic® [OTC]
Anaprox®
Ansaid® Oral
Apapedyn® Children's [OTC]
Apapedyn® Extra Strength [OTC]
Apaphen® [OTC]
Apo®-Diclo (Can)
Apo®-Diflunisal (Can)
Apo®-Etodolac (Can)
Apo®-Flurbiprofen (Can)
Apo®-Ibuprofen (Can)
Apo®-Indomethacin (Can)
Apo®-Keto (Can)
Apo®-Keto-E (Can)
Apo®-Ketorolac (Can)
Apo®-Mefenamic (Can)
Apo®-Nabumetone (Can)
Apo®-Napro-Na (Can)
Apo®-Naproxen (Can)
Apo®-Piroxicam (Can)
Apo®-Sulin (Can)
Argesic®-SA
Arthritis Foundation® Pain Reliever [OTC]
Arthropan® [OTC]
Ascriptin® [OTC]
Aspergum® [OTC]
aspirin
Asprimox® [OTC]
Bayer® Aspirin [OTC]
Bayer® Buffered Aspirin [OTC]
Bayer® Low Adult Strength [OTC]
Bufferin® [OTC]
Buffex® [OTC]
Cama® Arthritis Pain Reliever [OTC]
Cataflam® Oral
Cetafen® [OTC]
Cetafen® Extra [OTC]
Children's Advil® Suspension
Children's Motrin® Suspension [OTC]
choline magnesium trisalicylate
choline salicylate
Clinoril®
Daypro™
diclofenac
diflunisal
Disalcid®
Dolobid®
Dolono® [OTC]
Dolono® Infants [OTC]
Double-Action Pain Relief® [OTC]
Easprin®
Eckogesic® [OTC]
Ecotrin® [OTC]
Ecotrin® Low Adult Strength [OTC]
Empirin® [OTC]
etodolac
Excedrin®, Extra Strength [OTC]
Excedrin® IB [OTC]
Excedrin® P.M. [OTC]
Extraprin® [OTC]
Extra Strength Adprin-B® [OTC]

Extra Strength Bayer® Enteric 500 Aspirin [OTC]
Extra Strength Bayer® Plus [OTC]
Febrol® [OTC]
Feldene®
Fem-Prin® [OTC]
fenoprofen
Feverall™ [OTC]
Fexicam (Can)
Flextra-DS® [OTC]
flurbiprofen
Froben® (Can)
Gelpirin® [OTC]
Genapap® [OTC]
Genapap® Children [OTC]
Genapap® Extra Strength [OTC]
Genapap® Infant [OTC]
Genasec® [OTC]
Genebs® [OTC]
Genebs® Extra Strength [OTC]
Gen-Etodolac (Can)
Gen-Naproxen EC (Can)
Gen-Piroxicam (Can)
Genpril® [OTC]
Goody's® Fast Pain Relief® [OTC]
Goody's® Headache Powders [OTC]
Halenol® [OTC]
Halfprin® 81® [OTC]
Haltran® [OTC]
Headache Formula PM® [OTC]
Headache Relief PM® [OTC]
Headrin® Plus Pain Relief [OTC]
Heartline® [OTC]
Ibuprin® [OTC]
ibuprofen
Ibuprohm® [OTC]
Ibu-Tab®
Indocid® (Can)
Indocin® Oral
Indocin® SR Oral
indomethacin
Indotec® (Can)
Infantaire® [OTC]
Junior Strength Motrin® [OTC]
ketoprofen
ketorolac tromethamine
Legatrin® PM Advanced Formula [OTC]
Leg Cramp Relief PM® [OTC]
Lodine®
Lodine® XL
Major-Gesic® [OTC]
Mapap® [OTC]
Mapap® Children's [OTC]
Mapap® Extra Strength [OTC]
Mapap® Infants' [OTC]
Mapap-PM® [OTC]
Mardol® [OTC]
meclofenamate
Meda-Cap® [OTC]
Medipren® [OTC]
mefenamic acid
Menadol® [OTC]
Midol® IB [OTC]
Midol® PM [OTC]
Mono-Gesic®
Motrin®
Motrin® IB [OTC]
nabumetone
Nalfon®
Naprelan®
Naprosyn®
naproxen
Naxen® (Can)
Night-Time Cramp Relief® [OTC]
Night-Time Pain Reliever/Sleep [OTC]
Norgesic™
Norgesic™ Forte
Novagesic® [OTC]
Novo-Difenac-K (Can)
Novo-Difenac®-SR (Can)
Novo-Diflunisal (Can)
Novo-Flurprofen (Can)
Novo-Keto (Can)
Novo-Keto-EC (Can)

Novo-Ketorolac (Can)
Novo-Methacin (Can)
Novo-Naprox (Can)
Novo-Pirocam (Can)
Novo-Piroxicam (Can)
Novo-Profen® (Can)
Novo-Sundac (Can)
Novo-Tolmetin (Can)
Nu-Diclo (Can)
Nu-Diflunisal (Can)
Nu-Flurprofen (Can)
Nu-Ibuprofen (Can)
Nu-Indo (Can)
Nu-Ketoprofen (Can)
Nu-Ketoprofen-E (Can)
Nu-Mefenamic (Can)
Nu-Naprox (Can)
Nu-Pirox (Can)
Nuprin® [OTC]
Nu-Sulindac (Can)
Ocufen® Ophthalmic
Ohmni-Gesic® [OTC]
Orafen (Can)
Oraphen PD® [OTC]
orphenadrine, aspirin, and caffeine
Orphengesic®
Orudis®
Orudis® KT [OTC]
Oruvail®
oxaprozin
Pain-Eze® [OTC]
Pain-Gesic® [OTC]
Pain-Off® [OTC]
Pamprin IB® [OTC]
Pedia-Profen™
Pediatrix (Can)
Percogesic® [OTC]
Phenylgesic® [OTC]
piroxicam
piroxicam and cyclodextrin (Canada only)
PMS-Diclofenac (Can)
PMS-Mefenamic Acid (Can)
Ponstan® (Can)
Ponstel®
Pyrecot® [OTC]
Pyregesic® [OTC]
Q-Gesic® [OTC]
Q-Pap® [OTC]
Q-Pap® Children's [OTC]
Redutemp® [OTC]
Regular Strength Bayer® Enteric 500 Aspirin [OTC]
Relafen®
Relagesic® [OTC]
Rhodacine® (Can)
Rhodis™ (Can)
Rhodis-EC™ (Can)
Rhovail® (Can)
Riva-Naproxen (Can)
Saleto-200® [OTC]
Saleto-400®
Salflex®
salsalate
Silapap® Children's [OTC]
Silapap® Infant's [OTC]
sodium salicylate
Sominex® Pain Relief Formula [OTC]
Staflex® [OTC]
St Joseph® Adult Chewable Aspirin [OTC]
sulindac
Supac® [OTC]
Synflex® (Can)
Synflex® DS (Can)
Tactinal® [OTC]
Tactinal® Children's [OTC]
Tactinal® Extra Strength [OTC]
Teejel® (Can)
Tempra® 1 [OTC]
Tempra® 2 [OTC]
Tension® [OTC]
Tolectin®
Tolectin® DS
tolmetin
Toradol®

T-Painol® [OTC]
T-Painol® Extra Strength [OTC]
tramadol
Trendar® [OTC]
Tricosal®
Trilisate®
Tycolene® [OTC]
Tylenol® [OTC]
Tylenol® Arthritis [OTC]
Tylenol® Children's [OTC]
Tylenol® Extra Strength [OTC]
Tylenol® Infants [OTC]
Tylenol® Infants Original [OTC]
Tylenol® Junior Strength [OTC]
Tylenol® PM Strength [OTC]
Tylenol® Severe Allergy [OTC]
Tylenol® Sore Throat [OTC]
Tylex® [OTC]
Tylex® Extra Strength [OTC]
Tylophen® [OTC]
Tyltabs® [OTC]
Tyltabs® Children's [OTC]
Tyltabs® Extra Strength [OTC]
Tyltabs® PM [OTC]
Ultradol™ (Can)
Ultram®
UniPerr® [OTC]
Uni-Pro® [OTC]
Unison® w/Pain Relief [OTC]
Valorin® [OTC]
Valorin® Extra [OTC]
Vanquish® [OTC]
Vitoxapap® [OTC]
Vofenal™ (Can)
Voltaren® Ophthalmic
Voltaren® Oral
Voltaren Rapide® (Can)
Voltaren®-XR Oral
ZORprin®

Decongestant/Analgesic
Advil® Cold & Sinus Caplets [OTC]
Dimetapp® Sinus Caplets [OTC]
Dristan® Sinus Caplets [OTC]
Motrin® IB Sinus [OTC]
pseudoephedrine and ibuprofen
Sine-Aid® IB [OTC]

Local Anesthetic
AK-Taine®
Alcaine®
Diocaine® (Can)
ethyl chloride
ethyl chloride and dichlorotetrafluoroethane
Fluro-Ethyl® Aerosol
Ocu-Caine®
Ophthetic®
Parcaine®
proparacaine

Neuroleptic Agent
Apo®-Methoprazine (Can)
methotrimeprazine (Canada only)
Novo-Meprazine (Can)
Nozinan® (Can)

Nonsteroidal Anti-inflammatory Drug (NSAID)
Back-Ese M (Can)
Doan's Backache Pills (Can)
Doan's®, Original [OTC]
Extra Strength Doan's® [OTC]
Herbogesic (Can)
Magan®
magnesium salicylate
Magsal®
Mobidin®

Nonsteroidal Anti-inflammatory Drug (NSAID), COX-2 Selective
rofecoxib
Vioxx®

Nonsteroidal Anti-inflammatory Drug (NSAID), Oral
floctafenine (Canada only)
Idarac® (Can)

PAIN (LUMBAR PUNCTURE)

Analgesic, Topical

EMLA®
lidocaine and prilocaine

PAIN (MUSCLE)

Analgesic, Topical
dichlorodifluoromethane and trichloromonofluoromethane
Fluori-Methane® Topical Spray

PAIN (SKIN GRAFT HARVESTING)

Analgesic, Topical
EMLA®
lidocaine and prilocaine

PAIN (VENIPUNCTURE)

Analgesic, Topical
EMLA®
lidocaine and prilocaine

PREOPERATIVE SEDATION

Analgesic, Narcotic
Demerol®
Levo-Dromoran®
levorphanol
meperidine
Antihistamine
Apo®-Hydroxyzine (Can)
Atarax®
hydroxyzine
Hyzine® Injection
Novo-Hydroxyzin (Can)
PMS-Hydroxyzine (Can)
Restall® Injection
Vistacot® Injection
Vistaril®
Barbiturate
Luminal®
Nembutal®
pentobarbital
phenobarbital
Benzodiazepine
midazolam
Versed®
General Anesthetic
Actiq® Oral Transmucosal
Duragesic® Transdermal
fentanyl
Fentanyl Oralet®
Sublimaze® Injection

TOPICAL ANESTHESIA

Local Anesthetic
Americaine® [OTC]
Ametop™ (Can)
Anbesol® [OTC]
Anbesol® Baby (Can)
Anbesol® Maximum Strength [OTC]
Anestacon® Topical Solution
Anusol® Ointment [OTC]
Babee® Teething® [OTC]
benzocaine
Benzocol® [OTC]
Benzodent® [OTC]
Caladryl® Lotion
Chiggertox® [OTC]
Citanest® Forte
Citanest® Plain
cocaine
Cylex® [OTC]
Dermoplast® [OTC]
Dilocaine® Injection
Duo-Trach® Injection
ethyl chloride
ethyl chloride and dichlorotetrafluoroethane
Fleet® Pain Relief [OTC]
Fluro-Ethyl® Aerosol
Foille® [OTC]
Foille® Medicated First Aid [OTC]
Hurricaine®
Itch-X® [OTC]
Lanacane® [OTC]
lidocaine
Lidodan™ (Can)
LidoPen® I.M. Injection Auto-Injector

Maximum Strength Anbesol® [OTC]
Maximum Strength Orajel® [OTC]
Mycinettes® [OTC]
Nervocaine® Injection
Numzitdent® [OTC]
Numzit Teething® [OTC]
Orabase®-B [OTC]
Orabase®-O [OTC]
Orajel® Brace-Aid Oral Anesthetic [OTC]
Orajel® Maximum Strength [OTC]
Orajel® Mouth-Aid [OTC]
Orasept® [OTC]
Orasol® [OTC]
Phicon® [OTC]
Pontocaine®
PrameGel® [OTC]
pramoxine
Prax® [OTC]
prilocaine
ProctoFoam® NS [OTC]
Rhulicaine® [OTC]
Rid-A-Pain® Dental [OTC]
Slim-Mint® [OTC]
Solarcaine® [OTC]
Spec-T® [OTC]
Tanac® [OTC]
tetracaine
Trocaine® [OTC]
Tronolane® [OTC]
Unguentine® [OTC]
Vicks® Children's Chloraseptic® [OTC]
Vicks® Chloraseptic® Sore Throat [OTC]
Xylocaine® HCl I.V. Injection for
Cardiac Arrhythmias
Xylocaine® Oral
Xylocaine® Topical Ointment
Xylocaine® Topical Solution
Xylocaine® Topical Spray
Xylocard® (Can)
Zilactin®-B Medicated [OTC]

TRANSURETHRAL SURGERY

Genitourinary Irrigant
Arlex®
sorbitol